PRACTICAL
GYNECOLOGY

For a catalogue of publications available from ACP–ASIM, contact:

Customer Service Center
American College of Physicians–American Society of Internal Medicine
190 N. Independence Mall West
Philadelphia, PA 19106-1572
215-351-2600
800-523-1546, ext. 2600

Visit our Web site at www. acponline.org

PRACTICAL GYNECOLOGY

A GUIDE FOR THE PRIMARY CARE PHYSICIAN

EDITORS

JANICE RYDEN, MD, FACP

PAUL D. BLUMENTHAL, MD, MPH

JOHNS HOPKINS UNIVERSITY SCHOOL OF MEDICINE

WOMEN'S HEALTH SERIES EDITOR

PAMELA CHARNEY, MD, FACP

AMERICAN COLLEGE OF PHYSICIANS
PHILADELPHIA

Clinical Consultant: David R. Goldmann, MD
Acquisitions Editor: Mary K. Ruff
Manager, Book Publishing: David Myers
Developmental Editor: Vicki Hoenigke
Production Supervisor: Allan S. Kleinberg
Editorial Coordinator: Alicia Dillihay
Interior and Cover Design: Patrick Whelan
Index: Nelle Garrecht

Printed in the United States of America
Composition by Fulcrum Data Services, Inc.
Printing/binding by McNaughton & Gunn

American College of Physicians (ACP) became an imprint of the American College of Physicians—American Society of Internal Medicine in July 1998.

Library of Congress Cataloging-in-Publication Data

Practical gynecology: a guide for the primary care physician / [edited by] Janice Ryden, Paul D. Blumenthal
    p. cm. – (Women's health series)
    Includes bibliographical references and index.
    ISBN 0-943126-94-0
    1. Gynecology. 2. Primary care (Medicine). I. Ryden, Janice, 1962–.
II. Blumenthal, Paul D, 1952–. III. American College of Physicians–American Society of Internal Medicine (Philadelphia, Pa.). II. Women's health series
    [DNLM: 1. Genital Diseases, Female. WP 140 P895 2000]
RG101.P8855 2000
618.1–dc21

                                                    00-049599

02 03 04 05 06/9 8 7 6 5 4 3 2 1

To my parents,
for a lifetime of encouragement,
and to my husband, Don,
for his constant love and support.
J.R.

To Lynne and Joshua,
For their understanding and patience as we created a
work to help clinicians better understand their patients.
P.D.B.

Editors

Janice Ryden, MD, FACP
Assistant Professor of Medicine
Johns Hopkins University School of Medicine
Johns Hopkins Community Physicians
Baltimore, MD

Paul D. Blumenthal, MD, MPH
Associate Professor
Department of Gynecology and Obstetrics
Johns Hopkins University School of Medicine
Johns Hopkins Bayview Medical Center
Baltimore, MD

Women's Health Series Editor

Pamela Charney, MD, FACP
Clinical Professor of Medicine
Clinical Associate Professor of Obstetrics & Gynecology and Women's Health
Albert Einstein College of Medicine
Bronx, NY;
Program Director
Internal Medicine Residency
Norwalk Hospital
Norwalk, Connecticut

Contributors

Richard H. Baker, MD
Associate Program Director
Clinical Assistant Professor of Medicine
College of Medicine of the State University
York Hospital
York, Pennsylvania

David H. Barad, MD
Associate Professor of Obstetrics and
  Gynecology
Albert Einstein College of Medicine
Department of Obstetrics and Gynecology
Bronx, New York

Tamara G. Bavendam, MD
Associate Professor of Urology
MCP-Hahnemann University
Center for Pelvic Floor Disorders
Centers for Women's Health
Philadelphia, Pennsylvania

Paul D. Blumenthal, MD, MPH
Associate Professor
Department of Gynecology and Obstetrics
Johns Hopkins University School of
  Medicine
Johns Hopkins Bayview Medical Center
Baltimore, Maryland

Ursula Boynton, MD
UCSF School of Medicine
San Francisco, California

Laura D. Castleman, MD, MPH
Instructor
Department of Gynecology and Obstetrics
Johns Hopkins University School of
  Medicine
Johns Hopkins Bayview Medical Center
Baltimore, Maryland

Pamela Charney, MD, FACP
Clinical Professor of Medicine
Clinical Associate Professor of Obstetrics &
  Gynecology and Women's Health
Albert Einstein College of Medicine
Bronx, New York
Program Director
Internal Medicine Residency
Norwalk Hospital
Norwalk, Connecticut

Vanessa E. Cullins, MD, MPH
Vice President, Medical Affairs
Planned Parenthood Federation of America
New York, New York

Michele G. Cyr, MD, FACP
Associate Professor of Medicine
Brown University School of Medicine
Director
Division of General Internal Medicine
Rhode Island Hospital
Providence, Rhode Island

Alan H. DeCherney, MD
Professor and Chairman
Department of Obstetrics and Gynecology
UCLA School of Medicine
Los Angeles, California

Dee E. Fenner, MD
Vice-Chairman for Academic Affairs
Associate Professor
Department of Obstetrics and Gynecology
University of Washington
Seattle, Washington

Jodi L. Friedman, MD
Associate Clinical Professor of Medicine
Department of Internal Medicine
UCLA Medical School
Los Angeles, California

Francisco A. R. Garcia, MD, MPH
Assistant Professor
Department of Obstetrics and Gynecology
University of Arizona
Tucson, Arizona

Mark Gibson, MD
Professor and Chairman
Obstetrics and Gynecology Department
Robert C. Byrd Health Sciences Center of
  West Virginia University
Morgantown, West Virginia

Meera C. Kataria, MD
Department of Obstetrics and Gynecology
University of Illinois School of Medicine
Chicago, Illinois

Audrey S. Koh, MD
Clinical Instructor
San Francisco, California

Delbert J. Kwan, MD
Fellow
Department of Urology
University of Washington
Seattle, Washington

Carol Landau, PhD
Clinical Professor of Psychiatry and
    Human Behavior
Brown University Medical School
Division of General Internal Medicine
Rhode Island Hospital
Providence, Rhode Island

Jeanne McCauley, MD, MPH, FACP
Assistant Professor of Medicine
Johns Hopkins University School of
    Medicine
Medical Director for Clinical Research and
    Outcomes
Johns Hopkins Community Physicians
Baltimore, Maryland

James A. McGregor, MD, CM
Professor of Obstetrics and Gynecology
Department of Obstetrics and Gynecology
University of Arizona
Tucson, Arizona

Anne W. Moulton, MD
Associate Professor of Medicine
Brown University Medical School
Division of General Internal Medicine
Rhode Island Hospital
Providence, Rhode Island

Ann Butler Nattinger, MD, MPH, FACP
Professor of Medicine
Chief of General Internal Medicine
Division of Internal Medicine
Medical College of Wisconsin
Milwaukee, Wisconsin

Anita L. Nelson, MD
Associate Professor
Department of Obstetrics and Gynecology
Medical Director
Women's Health Care Clinic
Harbor-UCLA Medical Center
Torrance, California

Sharon J. Parish, MD
Assistant Professor of Medicine
Department of Medicine
Albert Einstein College of Medicine
Montefiore Medical Center
Bronx, New York

John C. Petrozza, MD
Assistant Professor of Obstetrics and
    Gynecology
Harvard University School of Medicine
Massachusetts General Hospital
Boston, Massachusetts

Samantha M. Pfeifer, MD
Assistant Professor of Obstetrics and
    Gynecology
Division of Human Reproduction
University of Pennsylvania Medical Center
Philadelphia, Pennsylvania

Nicole Pilevsky, MD
Department of Obstetrics and Gynecology
University of Pennsylvania
Philadelphia, Pennsylvania

Andrea J. Rapkin, MD, FACOG
Professor
Department of Obstetrics and Gynecology
UCLA School of Medicine
Los Angeles, California

Janice Ryden, MD, FACP
Assistant Professor of Medicine
Johns Hopkins University School of
    Medicine
Johns Hopkins Community Physicians
Baltimore, Maryland

William H. Salazar, MD, FACP
Associate Professor of Medicine and
  Psychiatry
Co-Director
Section of General Internal Medicine
Medical College of Georgia
Augusta, Georgia

Bert Scoccia, MD
Associate Professor and Clinical Director
Division of Reproductive Endocrinology
  and Infertility
University of Illinois College of Medicine
Chicago, Illinois

Robert M. Sinow, MD
Associate Professor
Department of Radiological Sciences
UCLA School of Medicine
Harbor-UCLA Medical Center
Torrance, California

Barbara L. Smith, MD, PhD
Comprehensive Breast Cancer Center
Boston, Massachusetts

Steven J. Sondheimer, MD
Professor of Obstetrics and Gynecology
University of Pennsylvania Medical Center
Department of Obstetrics and Gynecology
Philadelphia, Pennsylvania

Gerda Ellen Tapelband, MD
Chief of Medical Services
St. Charles Medical Center
Bend Memorial Clinic LLP
Bend, Oregon

L. Chesney Thompson, MD
Assistant Professor
Department of Obstetrics and Gynecology
University of Colorado Health Sciences
  Center
Denver, Colorado

Catherine Todd, MD
Instructor
Department of Gynecology and Obstetrics
Johns Hopkins University School of
  Medicine
Johns Hopkins Bayview Medical Center
Baltimore, Maryland

Maria L. Chanco Turner, MD
Clinical Professor of Dermatology
Dermatology Branch
National Institutes of Health
Bethesda, Maryland

Rebekah Wang-Cheng, MD, FACP
Professor of Medicine
Department of Medicine
Division of General Internal Medicine
Medical College of Wisconsin
Milwaukee, Wisconsin

Jocelyn C. White, MD, FACP, FAAPP
Assistant Professor
Department of Medicine
Oregon Health Sciences University
Legacy Portland Hospital
Portland, Oregon

Preface

Over the years many have recognized the benefits of patients receiving routine gynecologic care from their primary care physician. After a period of time during which health care was fractionated among specialists, a more unified structure of health care delivery has become standard again. However, while patients commonly present to primary care offices with gynecologic issues, the field of gynecology lies outside the confines of what is classically considered internal medicine. Consequently, clinical experience in gynecology during internal medicine residency training has often been insufficient to prepare physicians for careers in primary care.

At our institution, a formal survey in 1993 found that the internal medicine residents described their basic gynecology experience to be inadequate. In response to this, a team of five gynecologists and general internists (led by Dr. Jeanne McCauley and including Drs. Richard "Hal" Baker, Jessica Bienstock, Vanessa Cullins, and Janice Ryden) was assembled. Under the direction of Drs. David Kern, Randy Barker, Eric Bass, Pat Thomas and Donna Howard, and as part of the Johns Hopkins Faculty Development Program, the team created a formal gynecology curriculum. The curriculum consisted of a written syllabus, a series of lectures, and a well-defined clinical experience. It was first implemented in the primary care residency track in 1994, and today it continues to be a highly valued component of residency training.

The essence of *Practical Gynecology: A Guide for the Primary Care Physician* originated from this curriculum at Johns Hopkins Bayview Medical Center, although the book version quickly evolved and expanded to include a much wider range of topics. Contributions were solicited from authors from across the United States, all of whom are leading authorities in their field, and to whom we are greatly indebted. The resulting volume is the latest in the ACP Women's Health series, a collection that highlights the College's ability to recognize and respond to the needs of its members and that attests to its commitment to the field of women's health.

The intended audience for *Practical Gynecology* is the primary care physician already established in practice. The editors recognize that some readers will use this text in order to fill perceived gaps in their training in basic gynecology, while others will read it to further their knowledge in areas of particular interest. Consequently, the book has been tailored to meet the needs of physicians with different levels of gynecologic knowledge and clinical experience. The fundamentals are reviewed, yet current and detailed evidence-based information on a wide variety of topics is also offered. The clinical care of the patient is central to the book, and we have made this information easily accessible to the busy clinician through the liberal use of tables and by highlighting important points.

Our intent and hope is that *Practical Gynecology* will provide the reader with valuable information, and that it will kindle enthusiasm for the practice of basic gynecology.

Janice Ryden
Paul D. Blumenthal

Acknowledgments

First and foremost, special thanks must go to Dr. Pamela Charney, editor of the ACP Women's Health series, whose vision was instrumental in the conception of this text. Her ideas and suggestions were crucial to the development of *Practical Gynecology* and her assistance in the creation of the editorial team was most helpful.

We would also like to express our appreciation to Mary K. Ruff for her guidance and invaluable knowledge regarding practical aspects of academic publishing and for her troubleshooting abilities. We wish to thank our outstanding developmental editor Vicki Hoenigke, particularly for her gentle way of trying to keep the book on schedule. We extend our sincere appreciation also to editorial assistant Alicia Dillihay, production supervisor Allan Kleinberg, and publishing manager David Myers, for their expertise and hard work.

Closer to home, we are indebted to our colleagues and residents. In particular, we acknowledge the expert input of Drs. Lisa Beck, Jeff Bender, Robert Bristow, Joel Fradin, and David Smith, as well as Suzanne J. Smith. In addition, the librarians of the Harrison Library at the Johns Hopkins Bayview Medical Center deserve much thanks and praise for their prompt, cheerful, and most able research assistance.

Lastly, we extend our heartfelt thanks to the authors, whose contributions have little tangible reward, but without whom *Practical Gynecology* would not have been possible.

Contents

CHAPTER 1

The Gynecologic Examination

PAMELA CHARNEY, MD
URSULA BOYNTON, MD
DAVID H. BARAD, MD

The complete gynecologic examination can provide information about several organ systems: reproductive, gastrointestinal, musculoskeletal, urologic, and neurologic. The information obtained during the gynecologic examination is determined in part by the provider's skill and by the degree of attention devoted to each element of the examination. This description of the gynecologic examination will emphasize how to maximize opportunities to obtain valuable information during the patient encounter.

The pelvic examination may be performed to screen an asymptomatic woman or to assess a specific symptom. Symptoms commonly evaluated by the gynecologic examination include changes in menstrual bleeding patterns, vaginal discharge, lower abdominal pain, dyspareunia, and urinary incontinence. Screening for infectious diseases is another important reason for the pelvic examination. Pelvic examinations are also necessary to screen for cervical cancer or dysplasia. A complete gynecologic examination will also screen for breast, colon, uterine, and ovarian cancer, although the detection rates are substantially lower than for cervical cancer.

Today most primary care physicians receive training in the gynecologic examination as residents. Unfortunately, many physicians already in practice have had minimal training in these skills, so self-education after residency has been essential. Recently physicians in practice have had the opportunity to learn or to improve their pelvic examination skills in continuing medical education courses under the guidance of genital teaching associates. Genital teaching associates are women trained to teach breast and pelvic examina-

1

tions using themselves as models, aiding in the development and improvement of examination skills for both medical students (1) and residents. This type of instruction has been shown to improve individual skills substantially, especially in examination of the adnexae.

A complete gynecologic evaluation includes several components: a careful history, preparation, and the breast and pelvic examinations. In the following sections, we discuss each component, with particular emphasis on the pelvic examination.

Gynecologic History

The complete gynecologic history addresses many issues that the patient may consider deeply personal (Box 1-1). Discussion of sensitive issues can trigger emotional reactions that may cause the patient to withhold information (1). Therefore the physician must take measures to gain the patient's trust. The gynecologic history should be obtained in a private consultation room with the patient fully clothed. Preparing for the pelvic examination by discussing it before the patient disrobes may foster communication. Most patients have a reason for seeking a gynecologic examination, and the examiner should be sure to adequately address the patient's concern.

The initial reproductive history includes the patient's developmental history, menstrual pattern, and history of all previous pregnancies. Developmental landmarks that sometimes can be recalled include the patient's age at initial breast development, axillary and pubic hair growth, menarche, growth spurt, and the age at which the patient achieved her adult height.

The result of any recent Pap smear and the initial day of the most recent menses should be recorded. A review of the patient's usual menstrual pattern should include the interval between menses, duration of menses, and any menstrual problems such as midcycle pain, intermenstrual bleeding, or dysmenorrhea. The physician should inquire about past gynecologic problems

---

Box 1-1 Elements of the Gynecologic History

- Presenting problems
- Medical and surgical history
- Medications
- Developmental history
- Menstrual history

- Sexual history
- Reproductive history
- Urinary symptoms
- Rectal symptoms

such as abnormal Pap smear, fibroids, endometriosis, sexually transmitted diseases, pelvic infections, or *in utero* exposure to DES.

An understanding of the patient's current and past sexual activity is important in assessing her risk of sexually transmitted disease and contraceptive needs. The physician should strive to avoid assumptions about a patient's sexuality. One way to explore sexual activity is to ask, "Are you sexually active with women, men, or both?" Similarly, inquiring whether the patient is interested in birth control rather than assuming a patient is only choosing between birth control methods will lead to a more productive interaction. Obviously, current and prior expression of sexual identity may vary. A more detailed sexual history would include discussion of the frequency of sexual activity and an estimate of the number of lifetime and recent partners. Women with more than one sexual partner are at greater risk for sexually transmitted diseases as are women with an earlier age of first intercourse. A complete sexual history would include discussion of potential sexual difficulties such as recent changes in libido, difficulties with arousal or lubrication, painful intercourse, postcoital bleeding, and vaginal burning or itching following intercourse.

The examiner should next obtain the obstetrical history including any abortions, miscarriages, or live births. A standard shorthand is used for tallying the patient's obstetrical history. Gravidity represents the total number of pregnancies. Parity is recorded as four sequential numbers representing the number of full-term infants, premature infants, abortions (gestational age less than 20 weeks), and living children. The physician can elicit information about previous deliveries including name, health, birth date, mode of delivery, gestational age, and birth weights of each infant, as well as pregnancy complications.

A general medical history will provide important information about non-gynecologic symptoms, previous diagnoses, and previous surgeries. The physician should perform a complete review of symptoms with emphasis on the genitourinary and gastrointestinal systems. A review of urinary symptoms should include previous urinary tract infections, dysuria, hematuria, renal calculi, and urinary incontinence. Urinary tract infections (UTIs) are sometimes triggered by sexual activity and are one of the most common reasons to seek medical care. Urinary incontinence is an increasingly recognized health problem that patients are eager to address (see Chapter 10), and both urinary and rectal incontinence may be a consequence of childbirth. Other rectal symptoms include changes in the stool pattern such as a change in frequency, diameter, or color (black or bloody). The details of onset, duration, and pattern of development of all these symptoms often help to establish the diagnosis and determine the optimal management, which sometimes includes referral.

Finally, screening for current or previous physical, emotional, or sexual abuse is an essential part of the patient history. The prevalence of this problem has been substantiated by a survey of physicians from California, which found that most of the providers had encountered a victim of intimate partner violence (2). Women who have experienced domestic violence report a preference for direct questioning by the examining physician (3). Potential exploratory questions include "Have you ever experienced physical, emotional, or sexual violence?" and "When couples disagree, some use words. Other couples shout or use fists, knives, or guns. What happens in your relationship?" Possible interventions are discussed in Chapter 21.

Gynecologic Examination

A complete gynecologic examination includes a breast examination and a pelvic examination. Most physicians perform the breast examination first. Note that examination of the abdomen and inguinal areas usually preceedes the pelvic examination.

Breast Examination

The breast examination has both visual and tactile components. Ideally, the physician performs the visual examination of the anterior chest wall and axilla while the patient is sitting with arms lifted overhead first and then while the patient places her hands on her waist and leans forward. These positions allow for best assessment of pigmentation changes and surface irregularities suggesting a mass or adenopathy. However, for reasons of modesty, inspection is commonly performed in the recumbent position.

The tactile examination of the breast and axilla is best performed with the patient recumbent with her arm raised above her head. Sometimes the placement of a small pillow under her upper back helps to further distribute the breast tissue over the chest wall. The tactile examination is performed using the base of the fingertips in small circular motions that vary in depth. Different methods to cover all the potential breast tissue include moving in vertical stripes, following imaginary lines in and out like the spokes of a wheel, and making concentric circles of increasing size. In a study of the effectiveness of different methods among young women, the vertical stripe method resulted in the most complete breast self-examination (4). However, no study of physician behaviors has focused on this issue. It is critical to completely assess all breast tissue, noting that breast tissue extends beyond the region usually defined by a bra.

The physician should next palpate all sides of the axilla. This pyramidal-shaped space can be examined with the patient's arm remaining above her head, but sometimes more effectively if she moves her arm to her side, where the examiner supports it at the elbow. The supraclavicular nodes should also be palpated. Lastly, each nipple is gently squeezed to assess for the presence of nipple discharge.

The accurate identification of breast abnormalities has been correlated with a longer breast examination time. Thus, if the physician chooses to make efficient use of the time required for a thorough breast examination, the tactile portion of the breast exam provides an ideal opportunity for patient education. The use of a set verbal message also allows the physician to monitor the duration of the examination. Chapter 18 provides a more detailed discussion of the breast examination and reviews the evaluation of any abnormalities that are detected.

In many states, another member of the medical team is legally required to be present during a pelvic examination or a breast examination. The rationale is to prevent sexual misconduct by the examiner or charges of the same. These additional staff may also provide assistance in preparing the patient and attending to her comfort. However, the logistics of having adequate staffing to provide this support is problematic at many clinical sites, and lack of available staff may create a barrier to examination. In several surveys of patients and providers, wide variation of the use of a chaperone was reported (5,6).

Pelvic Examination

Anatomy Review

Familiarity with the superficial and deep pelvic anatomy aids in performing the pelvic examination.

The vulva consists of the labia majora, the labia minora, the clitoris, the hymen, and the vulvar vestibule. The superficial anatomy of the female external genitalia (Fig. 1-1) is subject to normal variations including the size and shape of the labia. Before puberty, the labia majora hide the folds of the labia minora and the clitoral hood. After puberty, these midline structures enlarge enough to be visible without manipulation. The openings of the urethra, vagina, Skene's glands, Bartholin's glands, and minor vestibular glands are located within the vestibule. Bartholin's glands are located in the posterior third of the labia majora, but with the glandular meatus in the vagina. The hymeneal ring is located superior to the posterior fourchette. The hymen may or may not be intact, irrespective of the patient's previous sexual activity. An imperforate hymen is rare but can impede menstrual flow and be a cause of cyclic pain and primary amenorrhea. In women of reproductive age, the vaginal mucosa is thick and folded into rugae. A small-to-moderate amount of vaginal discharge may be normal. The vaginal mucosa and its secretions are influenced by estrogen levels and therefore vary throughout the lifespan and during each menstrual cycle.

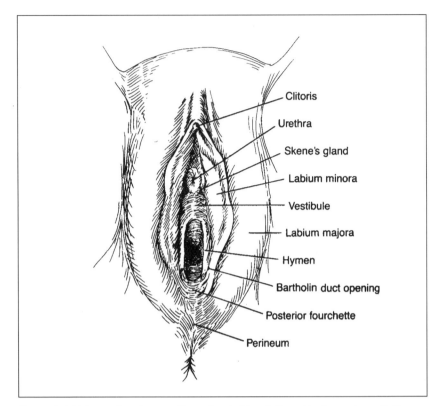

Clitoris

Urethra

Skene's gland

Labium minora

Vestibule

Labium majora

Hymen

Bartholin duct opening

Posterior fourchette

Perineum

Figure 1-1 Vulva and perineum. (From Berek SJ, ed. Norvak's Gynecology. Baltimore: Williams & Wilkins; 1988:110; with permission.)

The cervix is the inferior external surface of the uterus that extends into the vaginal vault (Fig. 1-2). The endocervix is that portion of the cervix contained within the cervical canal, while the ectocervix is the surface of the cervix visible in the vagina. The transformation zone is the area surrounding the junction where the squamous and columnar epithelia meet; it most often lies just inside the cervical os (the opening of the cervix) but varies in its location. Exposure to increased estrogen is thought to be associated with columnar epithelium extending externally from the os onto the ectocervix.

A woman who has borne children may have a larger uterus that one who has not because uterine size increases with each pregnancy and does not fully return to its pregravid size.

The uterus is attached to the lateral pelvis walls by the broad, cardinal, and infundibulopelvic ligaments (Fig. 1-3). Uterine size varies throughout the life cycle. Pregnancy is the most common etiology of an enlarged uterus. A woman who

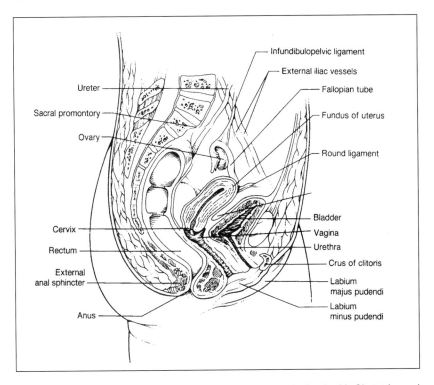

Figure 1-2 Lateral view of the pelvic viscera. (From Danforth D. Danforth's Obstetrics and Gynecology. Philadelphia: Lippincott Williams & Wilkins; 1999; with permission.)

has borne children may have a larger uterus than one who has not because uterine size increases with each pregnancy and does not fully return to its pregravid size. Uterine fibroids, adenomyosis, and uterine cancer are pathologic causes of uterine enlargement. After menopause uterine size begins to gradually decrease.

The pelvic adnexae include the fallopian tubes and ovaries. The fallopian tubes lie within the upper margin of the broad ligament extending from the lateral superior aspect of the uterus. The proximal end of each fallopian tube opens into the uterine cavity while the distal end curves over the surface of an ovary, placing the open fimbriated end in close proximity to the ovary.

The ovaries are a pair of peach pit–shaped organs located close to the lateral walls of the uterus. The infundibulopelvic ligament of the ovary connects the superior end of the ovary to the lateral wall of the pelvis and contains the ovarian artery. The ovarian ligament connects the infe-

The appendix, which can vary in location, may be close to the right ovary and fallopian tube.

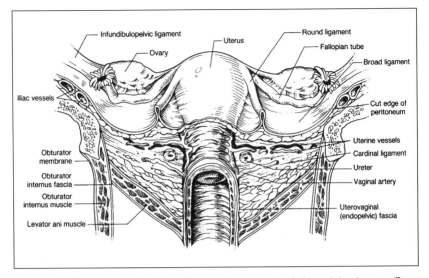

Figure 1-3 Ligamentous, fascial, and muscular support of the pelvic viscera. (From Danforth D. Danforth's Obstetrics and Gynecology. Philadelphia: Lippincott Williams & Wilkins; 1999; with permission.)

rior border of the ovary to the uterus. The appendix, which can vary in location, may be close to the right ovary and fallopian tube, and is rightly considered a pelvic structure.

Ovarian size varies through the life cycle. In general, ovaries increase in size throughout childhood, plateau in adulthood, then decrease in size beginning in the postmenopausal period (5). The size of the postmenopausal ovary is affected by the number of years since menopause and the number of prior pregnancies (7). Ovaries may also vary in size over the course of the menstrual cycle, ranging from the size of a small almond to that of a golf ball.

Because small variations in ovarian size are very difficult to assess on routine pelvic examination, pelvic ultrasound has contributed greatly to our understanding of functional ovarian anatomy and physiology. An ovary with a volume more than twice that of its companion ovary should be regarded with concern (8). However, a follicular or corpus luteum cyst is a common cause of adnexal enlargement or fullness on pelvic examination. On the other hand, symmetric enlargement of the ovaries is often palpable in women with polycystic ovary syndrome (PCOS). Ultrasound studies confirm that most (but not all) women with this condition have multiple (1 to 3 mm) cysts just below the surface of their ovaries, as well as increased ovarian stroma, both of which contribute to ovarian enlargement.

Preparation for the Examination

DISCUSSION WITH PATIENT

Before performing the examination, the physician should discuss with the patient what to expect. Ideally, this discussion should occur before the patient undresses, especially with a patient who is not well known to the physician. Asking whether the patient has any questions or concerns about the pelvic examination may help identify women who require additional reassurance or alternative approaches to the examination. A frank discussion before the examination also provides the patient opportunity to reveal previous life experiences and discuss any sexual symptoms or concerns without another person present.

Common reasons for fearing or avoiding pelvic examinations include embarrassment, lack of information, cultural or language barriers, pain with previous examinations, or posttraumatic stress related to sexual abuse. Each of these circumstances requires additional sensitivity by the physician and efforts to minimize emotional or physical discomfort. Often, given an opportunity, the patient can articulate ways to decrease her personal discomfort. The use of an additional professional female staff member as a chaperone, special draping, or a variation in position may also help to decrease patient anxiety. If the patient is concerned about pain, it may help to perform the examination using a small, well-lubricated speculum, and with only one digit during the bimanual exam.

Women about to have their first pelvic examination especially benefit from a full description of the process, including seeing the speculum and having the testing procedures explained. It may be helpful to have the patient make a fist to approximate the size of her uterus and to define the cervix as the entry site within the curvature of the second digit. This also allows illustration of speculum entry and specimen collection. This visual model also facilitates the reminder that the vagina can stretch to accept examination without discomfort. Some physicians provide the patient with a handheld mirror, so anatomy can be visualized by the patient as it is described during the examination (1, 9).

CHAPERONES

As discussed earlier, chaperones may be legally required to be present during the pelvic examination. In addition to protecting the patient from the possibility of sexual misconduct and the examiner from such charges, the presence of a chaperone may lessen patient anxiety during the examination. The chaperone also typically assists in specimen procurement and processing.

GOWNING

Before the patient undresses and sits on the examination table, she should be asked to empty her bladder in order to both decrease possible discomfort during the examination and make the pelvic organs more easily palpable. Patient privacy is best maintained when the gown is closed posteriorly. If there are no covers on the examination table stirrups, the patient may prefer to wear her shoes during the examination. A sheet placed over the gown can provide additional draping if desired.

SUPPLIES

All supplies required should be gathered before beginning the pelvic examination (Box 1-2).

• *Specula*—Specula are made of either metal or plastic and available in many different sizes (Fig. 1-4). In general, the smallest speculum that will allow adequate visualization of the cervix will cause the least discomfort. A small pediatric speculum is appropriate for virgins and women who are post-menopausal for years without multiple births. The Pedersen speculum is narrow and is most often used for nulliparous women. A large speculum is often necessary to examine multiparous women, especially those who are obese. Involution of the vaginal folds into lateral spaces around the large speculum can prevent visualization of the cervix. In such cases, a condom with its tip cut off and then placed over the speculum may provide visualization of the cervix by holding back the vaginal walls.

Both metal and plastic specula are in common use. Metal specula can be reused after proper processing but need to be warmed before insertion because the metal feels cold. Plastic specula are intended for single use. Because the plastic is transparent, there may be greater visualization of the vaginal walls. However, plastic specula may be difficult to adjust once they are in an open locked position, and may lack the necessary strength to open wide enough to allow for adequate inspection of the cervix and upper vagina in some women.

• *Other Equipment*—Equipment for specimen collection of vaginal secretions, cervical cultures, Pap smear, and possibly for endometrial biopsy

---

Box 1-2 Supplies for the Pelvic Examination

- Gloves
- Water-based lubrication
- Light source
- Speculum
- Pap collection supplies (including spatula, cytobrush, slides, and fixative)
- Glass slides and cover slips
- Saline for wet mount, KOH solution
- Narrow-range pH paper
- Culture or immunofixative for chlamydia and gonorrhea
- Cotton balls on a stick

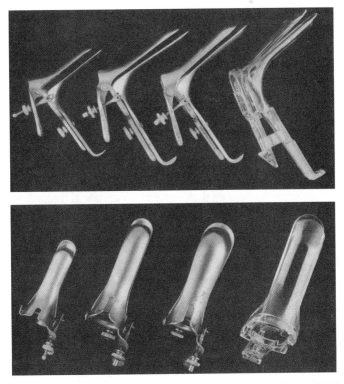

Figure 1-4 Specula. *From left to right:* Small metal Pedersen, medium metal Pedersen, medium metal Graves, and large plastic Pedersen. (From Bates B. A Guide to Physical Examination and History Taking. Philadelphia: JB Lippincott; 1995:383; with permission.)

should be easily accessible. It is poor practice to begin searching for this equipment after the speculum is already in place in the patient's vagina.

• *Alternatives to the Exam Table*—If the patient is in a bed and an examination table is not available, then the patient can most easily be examined with something firm placed under the buttocks. For example, in the inpatient setting, an upside-down bedpan can provide such a firm surface.

Performing the Examination

A pelvic examination that minimizes pain triggers less muscular guarding and therefore can more effectively define anatomy. The physician's initial attitude and touch as well as the level of attention to the patient's comfort can affect the patient's ability to cooperate. It is helpful to tell the patient what is being done to her and why. The physician should avoid technical terms and instead use language that is easily understandable to the patient. Regardless of whether there has been earlier explanation, consistently keeping the patient apprised of each upcoming action helps to demystify the examination. The pelvic examination is divided into three components: the external examination, the speculum examination, and the bimanual examination.

EXTERNAL EXAMINATION

The pelvic examination begins with a visual inspection of the external genitalia from the mons to the peri-rectal area using the assistance of a good light source. The labia majora and minora should be completely visualized. Any skin lesions or color changes should be noted. Although skin cancer is rare in this region, it is often diagnosed late because women cannot easily inspect this area themselves. Hyperpigmented, erthymatous, and hypopigmented areas are all of concern and may require further evaluation. Lichen sclerosus is a relatively common condition in which the vulvar skin may appear like parchment. It occurs more commonly in postmenopausal women, but may occur in all age groups, and can be associated with cancer. Other problems to be alert for include folliculitis, cellulitis, pubic lice, and scabies.

In addition to the assessment of the labia majora and minora, the visual survey should include the clitoris, urethra, introitus, and anus. Significant enlargement of the clitoris may signify excess androgens and a likely adrenal or ovarian tumor. After childbirth, prolapse or scarring from an episiotomy may be present. Bartholin's glands may swell from a retention cyst, infection, or trauma. In elderly patients, however, a swollen Bartholin's gland should raise the possibility of an underlying cancer. After menopause, atrophic changes may be evident, such as a urethral caruncle, which appears as a cherry red polypoid mass extending from the urethral opening and represents prolapse of the urethral mucosa.

When prolapse (pelvic relaxation) is severe, it is sometimes evident on examination of the external genitalia. Bladder, uterine, and rectal prolapse are not uncommon sequelae of childbirth. At times, bulging is obvious on initial inspection, but at other times severe prolapse is evident only when the patient is asked to bear down as if she were attempting to void and then defecate. While the patient bears down, the perineum should be observed for evidence of bladder, uterine, or rectal prolapse. Some women with stress urinary incontinence will lose urine with this maneuver; the examiner should be appropriately positioned before undertaking this evaluation. For most women with prolapse, however, the speculum examination is necessary to make the diagnosis (see below).

SPECULUM EXAMINATION

The speculum examination includes entry, positioning, opening, use, and removal. The metal speculum should be warmed, and both metal and plastic speculums should be examined before use to ensure normal functioning. Lubrication should be used to decrease friction. Most examiners use water for lubrication, so that if cultures, a Pap smear, or wet mount is required, results are not altered.

Before inserting the speculum, an initial light touch on the inner thigh, rather than the genitalia, helps to decrease patient guarding. After apprising the patient in advance what is to follow, the speculum is inserted. One technique for inserting the speculum is to first insert a gloved index finger slowly into the introitus and then apply gentle pressure posteriorly. By doing so the examiner can sense when the patient has relaxed, at which time the speculum is inserted directly over the finger.

When inserting, positioning, and removing the speculum, minimal pressure should be exerted on the urethra. This is achieved with slight downward pressure on the speculum, by positioning the speculum so that the blades are at a 30-degree angle from the vertical axis, and by pointing the speculum directly toward the sacrum. Once the speculum is placed deep in the vagina, the blades are rotated to the horizontal position. Next, the speculum is withdrawn slightly as the blades are slowly opened, allowing the cervix to fall between the two blades. If the cervix is not easily observed, the speculum should be partially withdrawn and redirected. Most commonly, the cervix is more posterior than anticipated, and appropriate adjustment is usually successful.

If a patient's uterus is retroflexed, the cervix will often be located more anteriorly.

If, however, the examiner experiences great difficulty finding the cervix, then the speculum is removed so that the location of the cervix can be identified with a single gloved finger lubricated with water. If a patient's uterus is retroflexed, the cervix will often be located more anteriorly. Some clinicians routinely locate the cervix using a gloved examining finger before initial speculum insertion.

If a patient has previously undergone a hysterectomy, the cervix is usually no longer present and only a vaginal cuff remains. Available evidence indicates that such women no longer require Pap smears (10). However, if the hysterectomy was performed for cervical cancer or dysplasia, one should continue Pap smear screening on the vaginal cuff. This is because remnants of cervical tissue may be present, and also because women with such a history are at higher risk for vaginal intraepithelial neoplasia (VAIN) and vaginal cancer. If the hysterectomy was not performed for cancer, yet the patient has had documented human papillomavirus (HPV) infection or multiple sexual partners, she is at slightly higher risk for vaginal cancer, and some physicians would still screen with periodic Pap smears (11). After a supracervical hysterectomy, the cervix remains *in situ*, and such women require continued routine screening for cervical cancer.

Once the cervix is visualized, the shape of the os, the surface of the cervix, and any adherent secretions can be assessed. The nulliparous os is small and round (Fig. 1-5/Plate 1). Following vaginal delivery, the cervical os normally increases in size and becomes more horizontal and irregular in contour. Nabothian cysts are a common finding in normal reproductive age women. The cysts often appear in clusters over the surface of the cervix with only a section of the cyst visible above the cervical surface (Fig. 1-6/Plate 2). Previous cryosurgery for cellular abnormalities can lead to scarring and a stenotic appearance of the os. Cervical or endometrial polyps may extrude from the cervix and can cause bleeding or dysmenorrhea (Fig. 1-7/Plate 3).

The ectocervix is typically covered by squamous epithelium, whereas the endocervix is lined with columnar epithelium. The transition zone between the pale pink of the squamous epithelium and the red color of the columnar epithelium is most commonly located just inside the cervical os (see Fig. 1-5/Plate 1). In some young women the columnar epithelium may extend from the cervical canal well onto the ectocervix (an "ectropion" or a "cervical ectopy") and appear as a red and beefy area (Fig. 1-8/Plate 4). This normal variant is sometimes difficult to distinguish from chronic cervicitis because both appear dark red and can be associated with an adherent discharge. In the case of ectopy, however, close inspection easily reveals the demarcation where the squamous epithelium begins. After menopause the transition zone recedes from the surface of the cervix and deeper into the endocervical canal (11). Cervical warts (Fig. 1-9/Plate 5) are another possible finding; they may result from infection of the cervix by the human papilloma virus.

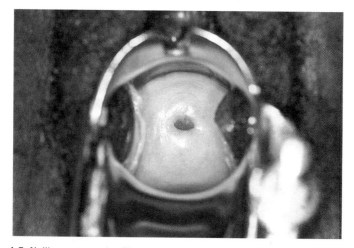

Figure 1-5 Nulliparous cervix. The nulliparous os is smooth and round. Childbirth or abortion results in a more irregular, "worn" cervix. With close inspection the squamo-columnar junction can be seen just inside the os. (From Atlas of Visual Inspection of the Cervix with Acetic Acid. Baltimore: JHPIEGO Corporation; 1999; with permission.) (For color reproduction, see Plate 1 at back of book.)

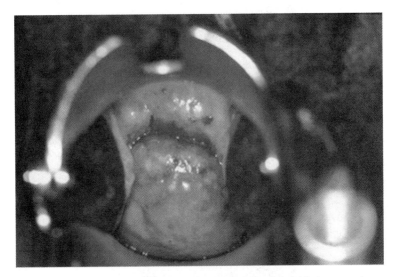

Figure 1-6 Nabothian cysts are formed when glandular tissue is folded over and covered by squamous epithelium. Nabothian cysts are common, may become quite large, and should not be confused with pathologic lesions. (From Atlas of Visual Inspection of the Cervix with Acetic Acid. Baltimore: JHPIEGO Corporation; 1999; with permission.) (For color reproduction, see Plate 2 at back of book.)

The cervix should be examined for gross abnormalities of the epithelium (Fig 1-10/Plate 6). If these are present, the patient should be referred for further assessment by a gynecologist, regardless of Pap smear results.

The secretions present on the cervix and in the vaginal vault should be noted. The amount and character of secretions may vary both individually and physiologically throughout the menstrual cycle. Clear and white secretions are expected. If the amount is profuse, possibilities include a vaginal infection or hormonal exposure. A yellow or green discharge may indicate chlamydia or gonorrhea infection, while a foamy gray or green discharge is typical of trichomonas infection. Bacterial vaginosis is associated with a profuse, white, homogeneous discharge. Yeast vaginitis is most classically associated with a discharge that resembles cottage cheese curds. In the setting of a yeast infection, the vaginal mucosa usually has a most pronounced beefy-red and inflamed appearance. A similar presentation can sometimes result from irritant or allergic vaginitis.

> *If gross abnormalities are visible on the cervix, the patient should be referred for further assessment by a gynecologist, regardless of Pap smear results.*

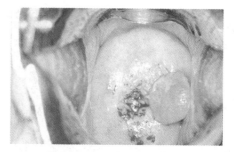

Figure 1-7 A cervical polyp appears as a finger-like projection in the cervical os and may emanate from cervical or endometrial tissue. Polyps may cause menorrhagia and post-coital bleeding. Although almost always benign, they are usually removed and sent for pathologic evaluation. In postmenopausal women polyps occasionally signal underlying endometrial hyperplasia. (From Atlas of Visual Inspection of the Cervix with Acetic Acid. Baltimore: JHPIEGO Corporation; 1999; with permission.) (For color reproduction, see Plate 3 at back of book.)

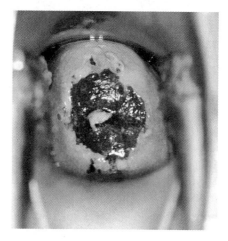

Figure 1-8 Cervical ectopy (or "ectropion"), defined as the presence of columnar epithelium on the ectocervix, is a normal variant. Here the squamocolumnar junction is obvious at first inspection, at the color change. (From Atlas of Visual Inspection of the Cervix with Acetic Acid. Baltimore: JHPIEGO Corporation; 1999; with permission.) (For color reproduction, see Plate 4 at back of book.)

Notwithstanding these generalizations, there is significant variation and overlap in the appearance of all of these entities and therefore objective testing should always be undertaken. Any symptomatic, colored, or foul-smelling discharge should be sampled from the lateral vaginal wall for microscopic examination. Such specimens are usually obtained before the Pap test is performed to decrease the presence of red blood cells. Secretions are mixed with a small amount of normal saline either in a test tube or on a slide with a pro-

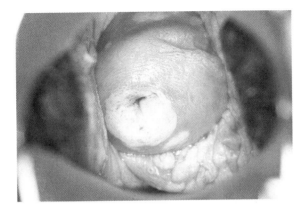

Figure 1-9 Cervical warts. Warts are more readily seen following the application of dilute acetic acid (vinegar solution). Genital warts are caused by HPV, which is responsible for cervical dysplasia and squamous cell cancers of the cervix. (From Atlas of Visual Inspection of the Cervix with Acetic Acid. Baltimore: JHPIEGO Corporation; 1999; with permission.) (For color reproduction, see Plate 5 at back of book.)

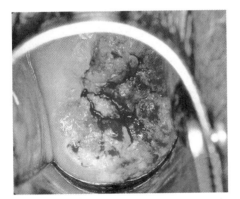

Figure 1-10 Invasive cancer of the cervix can assume a variety of appearances. Here a dark mass appears on the ectocervix, but at other times a mass may protrude from the cervical os or the cervix may appear densely white. Bimanual examination reveals an enlarged, hard cervix that may or may not be mobile. (From Atlas of Visual Inspection of the Cervix with Acetic Acid. Baltimore: JHPIEGO Corporation; 1999; with permission.) (For color reproduction, see Plate 6 at back of book.)

tective cover slip to prevent air-drying. The saline wet mount is examined under the microscope for trichomonas, excess leukocytes, and "clue cells." A similar specimen is prepared using KOH 10% solution, which aids in diagnosis of bacterial vaginosis and candida. If bacterial vaginosis is present, an amine (fishy) odor is released. The KOH also disrupts surrounding cellular material but not the yeast, allowing for easier identification upon microscopic examination. If narrow-range pH paper is available, the vaginal secretions can be placed on the paper to assess the pH of the vaginal discharge. Whenever an abnormal vaginal discharge is present, cervical testing for chlamydia and gonorrhea is often warranted.

If testing is done for the presence of chlamydia and gonorrhea infection, cervical specimens are usually collected immediately before or after the Pap smear. Because the presence of blood interferes somewhat with the interpretation of both the Pap smear and nonculture testing for infection, whichever test is more important for the given clinical setting should be performed first.

Rates of both gonorrhea and chlamydia infection have been noted to be inversely related to age, with the highest risk below age 17 (12). Although both infections may sometimes be completely asymptomatic, substantial sequelae may nonetheless ensue. Some have advocated universal screening in all women until age 24, and then only in women at higher risk. However, because screening and treatment decreases the rate of ectopic pregnancy and infertility, others have recommended screening all women interested in maintaining fertility (13).

The proper technique for collection of the Pap smear is reviewed in Box 1-3. For a more detailed discussion, see Chapter 7.

Before the metal speculum is removed, the screw should be loosened so the speculum blades can close. As the speculum is withdrawn, the vaginal vault mucosa should be carefully inspected. It is normally pink but may be erythematous if the vaginal mucosa is inflamed, as occurs in the setting of a yeast infection. Atrophic mucosa usually appears pale, unless there is associated inflammation. The speculum should gradually partially close upon withdrawal. If using a plastic speculum, the patient should be warned that there is a loud clicking noise as the speculum is released from the open locked position.

When one wishes to better assess for mild pelvic relaxation the two blades of the speculum are separated and only one is inserted at a time. The posterior blade is introduced alone and pressed against the posterior vaginal wall so that the resting location of the bladder is seen. Normally, the anterior vaginal wall of the nulliparous patient is barely visible. Therefore impression of the bladder base on the upper half of the vagina constitutes a mild cytocoele. Moderate relaxation is diagnosed when the bladder impression is located in the lower half of the vagina; severe relaxation is diagnosed when the bladder is through the introitus. The patient is next asked to cough or "bear down" to assess whether the bladder or urethra are hypermobile (move a distance greater than 2 cm). The speculum blade is then removed and the other blade is lifted against the anterior wall in order to assess for the presence of a rectocoele.

BIMANUAL EXAMINATION

The head of the examining table should be raised so that the patient is partially upright and her internal organs move nearer the perineum. This is es-

---

Box 1-3 Obtaining the Pap Smear

---

1. The speculum should be carefully positioned so that the entire cervix is seen. If excess mucus or other secretions obscure the cervix, they should be gently removed with a proctoswab. Any abnormalities of the epithelium on gross inspection necessitate colposcopy and/or second opinion and possible biopsy. This is true even when the Pap smear is ultimately interpreted as normal, because cytology may be unreliable. Normal variants such as Nabothian cysts and cervical ectopy (or "ectropion") are common and should be recognized (see Figs. 1-5 to 1-9).

2. The Ayres spatula is placed in the cervical os and rotated 360 deg to sample the entire ectocervix. This specimen is then smeared on the glass slide. When cervical ectopy is present, the red endocervical lining extends to the ectocervix, and an additional circumferential scraping at the outside edge of this tissue is necessary to ensure that the squamocolumnar junction is sampled.

3. The cytobrush is next inserted into the cervical os and rotated 360 deg. The brush is then rolled onto the slide, ensuring that the entire circumference of the brush makes contact with the slide. A cotton applicator moistened with saline is an alternative to the cytobrush but is less effective in retrieving cells.

4. The slide must be immediately sprayed with fixative to prevent desiccation of the cells, which begins to occur in as quickly as 15 seconds.

5. The patient should be instructed to anticipate vaginal spotting following use of the cytobrush and told that this does not indicate a problem.

---

pecially important when examining a very obese woman. Positioning the patient so she can abduct her flexed knees away from her perineum increases the examiner's access. The examiner may sometimes benefit from placing one foot on the examining table step to bring the body nearer to the patient.

Adequate lubrication during the bimanual examination serves to improve tactile sensitivity for the examiner as well as to minimize patient discomfort. Water-based lubricants are more effective than water alone; however, the use of lubricants should be deferred until the Pap smear and cultures are obtained. Water-based lubricants feel cold, and, if they are not warmed before use, the patient should be warned of the cool sensation before initial contact.

If throughout the bimanual examination the examiner describes to the patient what to expect and how she may cooperate, the examiner's accuracy and patient's comfort will both be maximized. Again, an initial light touch on the thigh, rather than the genitalia, helps to decrease patient guarding. Then, after verbal cuing, one or two fingers are placed at the perineum followed by slow entrance into the introitus. After evaluation of the uterus, the adnexae and ovaries are palpated. The fornices are next assessed followed by a recto-vaginal examination. Each step is described in detail below.

The examiner begins by assessing the cervix. The surface of the nonpregnant cervix is usually nontender and firm and feels like the tip of a nose. The cervix is next moved from side to side between the examiner's fingers. Movement of the cervix is usually possible without discomfort, although some patients normally experience a mild pressure sensation. Cervical motion tenderness is defined as discomfort that occurs with lateral movement. This finding signifies a localized peritonitis and may occur with tubo-ovarian infections, ectopic pregnancy, and other causes of adnexal or uterine pathology.

The examiner next defines the location, shape, and size of the uterus. One or two fingers are inserted posterior to the cervix and gently pushed upward while the fingers of the abdominal hand are placed on the lower abdominal wall to feel the upward movement of the uterus. When necessary, physicians may choose to brace their elbow against their hip in order to create greater leverage for the vaginal examination. The uterus is usually located in the midline but may be deviated to either side. The uterine contours may be irregular if fibroids are present. The uterine fundus will be most accessible when the uterus is anteverted (fundus tipped anteriorly). If the uterus is retroverted (fundus tipped posteriorly), the fundus may be more difficult to assess, even with the rectovaginal examination. Normally, the uterus is fairly mobile; limited mobility can result from scarring related to surgery or endometriosis. Palpation of the uterus may feel odd to the patient but should not elicit tenderness. Infection, degenerating or bleeding fibroids, and adnexal masses may be sources of discomfort with palpation.

Sizing of the uterus is more accurate if the patient has voided within 30 min (14, 15). For the nulliparous woman without abnormalities, the uterus is approximately the size of a closed fist. Increases in uterine size are recorded using descriptors associated with pregnancy (Table 1-1). After menopause the uterus progressively involutes and becomes smaller.

Sizing of the uterus is more accurate if the patient has voided within 30 minutes.

The ovaries are usually situated immediately lateral to the uterine fundus. Many physicians have been inadequately trained to assess for ovarian size and consistency. However, with the aid of the patient being examined, normal ovaries as well as ovarian masses can often be appreciated. The first step for the physician is to explain to the patient that ovaries are small organs that produce eggs. These organs have innervation similar to a man's testicles, meaning that the ovaries are delicate and sensitive to pressure. If a woman pays close attention, she can often tell when the ovaries are being palpated,

Table 1-1 Uterine Sizing

Measurement	Weeks Since Last Menstrual Period			
	6	8	10	12
Length (cm)	7.3	8.8	10.2	11.7
Fruit model (diameter in cm)	Small orange (7.8)	Large orange (9.0)	Grapefruit (10.2)	Cantaloupe (13.7)
Balls (diameter in cm)	Hardball (7.6)	Softball (9.8)	. . .	. . .

Adapted from Fox GN. Teaching first trimester uterine sizing. J Fam Pract. 1985;21:400–1.

and she is instructed to inform the physician when she feels a slight tenderness. The examiner needs to remember that tenderness will also be elicited when the ureter is tugged. However, when this occurs the patient will have the sensation of needing to void.

A patient can aid in the examination of her ovaries by informing the physician when she feels a slight tenderness.

To palpate the ovaries, the physician uses the abdominal hand to apply downward pressure and concentrate on tactile sensation. The internal hand sweeps from the highest level by the fundus inferiorly, causing the adnexae to slip between the two examining hands. Often the observant examiner and patient will concur when the ovary was felt. Focusing on the activity together decreases the patient's guarding and improves the physician's ability to appreciate the ovary.

Careful examination of the fornices, the clefts of the vagina created by the cervix, can provide information regarding many other structures in the pelvic cavity. Gentle palpation of the anterior fornix allows for assessment of the bladder wall; the patient will feel the pressure as a desire to void. In the patient with acute lower abdominal pain, significant bladder tenderness may suggest a urinary tract infection. The lateral fornices provide access to the intestines as well as to the adnexal structures. Asymmetry between the lateral fornices, especially when bulging is associated with tenderness, may indicate an intra-abdominal process such as appendicitis or diverticulitis. The posterior fornix, below the uterus, is adjacent to the rectum. Palpation of this region can assess for the presence of stool and can aid in the diagnosis of constipation, for instance.

The rectovaginal examination is particularly helpful in the assessment of lower abdominal pain, in the setting of a retroverted uterus, and in the evaluation of rectal symptoms or endometriosis. Although not a necessary component of all routine pelvic exams in women younger than age 40, patients undergoing evaluation for lower abdominal or pelvic pain should always have a rectovaginal examination. For any patient in whom the presence of a sexually transmitted disease is suspected, it is important for the examiner to change gloves between the bimanual and rectovaginal exams to avoid inoculating the rectum. Following completion of the rectovaginal exam and in the absence of vaginal bleeding, any secretions or stool found on the glove should be tested for occult blood.

When the presence of a sexually transmitted disease is suspected, it is important for the examiner to change gloves between the bimanual and rectovaginal exams to avoid inoculating the rectum.

In suspected appendicitis, right-sided discomfort and possibly fullness on rectovaginal examination help to confirm the diagnosis. In the setting of a retroverted uterus, sizing often can be performed more effectively using the rectovaginal examination. In patients with endometriosis, pelvic nodules can occasionally be appreciated on deep examination along the uretosacral ligament or rectovaginal septum, and are best detected during menstruation (16).

At the conclusion of the pelvic examination the physician should inform the patient that "everything appears healthy" or "normal" when appropriate.

Special Considerations

The commonest situations warranting special consideration are the patient undergoing her first pelvic examination and the women with previous negative experiences. These have been reviewed in the Preparation for the Examination section along with discussion of performing a pelvic exam when an examination table is unavailable. The care of the lesbian patient is facilitated mostly by avoiding assumptions (see Chapter 22). In this section special considerations regarding the adolescent, geriatric, and handicapped patient are reviewed.

The most common situations warranting special consideration are the patient undergoing her first pelvic examination and the woman with previous negative experiences.

ADOLESCENT PATIENT In some states information between physicians and adolescents remains confidential, whereas in others parental consent is required for access to medical care. The pelvic examination is usually performed in adolescent patients because of gynecologic symptoms, STD screening, or care during pregnancy. Note that a pelvic examination is not necessary before provision of hormonal contraception.

It is common for adolescents to have limited knowledge regarding the examination and to have concerns that the examination will be painful or about what may be found. Discussion before the examination and a step-by-step description may be helpful. The adolescent patient may have strong preferences about who is present during her pelvic examination. Choices include a staff chaperone, a family member, or a friend. Providing a handheld mirror for the patient to observe the examination provides an opportunity for education (17).

Before attempting to insert a speculum, placement of a gloved index finger in the introitus with pressure directed posteriorly can aid the patient in observing what muscles to relax and allow assessment of whether a speculum can be tolerated. If a speculum cannot be tolerated, then the importance of the information to be gained must be weighed against the potential discomfort of the examination. Referral to a gynecologist can be considered. If the purpose of the examination is primarily to assess for the presence of possible vaginitis, vaginal secretions can be sampled without a speculum.

In about one-third of adolescents (18), columnar epithelium is visible on the cervix; this is termed "cervical ectopy" or "ectropion" (see Fig. 1-8/Plate 4). The columnar epithelium is beefy appearing and has a mucous covering.

At the conclusion of the pelvic examination, it is most important to remember to inform the adolescent that all appears "normal" (when appropriate) and to advise her to expect spotting when this is anticipated.

GERIATRIC PATIENT

The older patient should be assessed without assumptions. Sexual issues may be important to discuss, especially low libido or atrophic changes (19). Urinary or rectal incontinence or prolapse issues are more likely to be revealed if the possibility is first raised by the physician. A focused history will identify women who have not had cervical cancer screening for years because these women are at increased risk for unidentified cervical cancer (20).

An examination table that can be lowered to stool height is an advantage for the patient with limited mobility. Some women are unable to use the stirrups but can extend their legs laterally. Other women find the lithotomy position impossible, yet can tolerate a pelvic examination in the left lateral decubitus position.

For a patient who is many years postmenopause and not sexually active, atrophic changes may limit the pelvic examination. The smallest speculum available should be used, and the bimanual examination first be attempted with a single lubricated digit. Other atrophic changes include a shift in the vaginal flora from a predominance of lactobacillus to fecal bacteria (21), which is sometimes associated with inflammation. Ovaries are typically not palpable after menopause, and any adnexal enlargement requires further evaluation with ultrasound.

PATIENTS WITH PHYSICAL DISABILITIES

Recent literature reveals that women patients with conditions that limit mobility or the ability to follow instructions are less likely to have regular health maintenance examinations such as cervical cancer screening (22). Inability to climb onto a traditional examination table may pose a substantial barrier. As was discussed for the geriatric patient, performing the pelvic examination with the patient in the left lateral decubitus position and the use of a motorized exam table both may facilitate provision of care for many physically challenged patients.

Conclusion

There are many elements to the complete gynecologic examination. When performed skillfully, it may provide an abundance of information about several organ systems. Proper attention to preparation of the patient and to her individual needs helps ensure that the exam is neither unpleasant nor painful.

REFERENCES

1. **Frye CA, Weisberg RB.** Increasing the incidence of routine pelvic examinations: behavioral medicine's contribution. Womens Health. 1994;21:33-55.

2. **Rodriquez MA, Bauer HM, McLoughlin E, et al.** Screening and interventions for intimate partner abuse: practices and attitudes of primary care physicians. JAMA. 1999; 282:468-74.

3. **Warshaw C, Alpert E.** Integrating routine inquiry about domestic violence into daily practice. Ann Intern Med. 1999;131:610-2.

4. **Saunders KJ, Pilgrim CA, Pennypacker HS.** Increased proficiency in breast self-examination. Cancer. 1986;58:2531-7.

5. **Ehrenthal DB, Farber NJ, Collier VU, Aboff BM.** Chaperone use by residents during pelvic, breast, testicular and rectal exams. J Gen Intern Med. 2000;15:573-6.

6. **Broadmore J, Carr-Gregg M, Hutton JD.** Vaginal examinations: women's experiences and preferences. N Z Med J. 1986;99:8-10.

7. **Goswany RK, Campbell S, Royston JP, et al.** Ovarian size in postmenopausal women. Br J Obstet Gynaecol. 1988:95:795-801.

8. **Goswamy RK, Campbell S, Whitehead MI.** Screening for ovarian cancer. Clin Obstet Gynecol. 1983;10:621.

9. **Feldman RJ, Driscoll CE.** Evaluation of the patient-centered pelvic examination. J Fam Pract. 1982;15:990-3.

10. **Pearce KF, Haefner HK, Sarwar SF, Nolan TE.** Cytopathological findings on vaginal Papanicolaou smears after hysterectomy for benign gynecologic disease. N Engl J Med. 1996;335:1559-62.

11. **American Geriatrics Society.** Screening for cervical carcinoma in older women. J Am Ger Soc. 2001;49:655-7.

12. **Gaydos, CA, Howell MR, Pare B, et al.** Ligase chain reaction screening for chlamydia yielded a high prevalence of chlamydial infection in female military recruits. N Engl J Med. 1998;229:739-44.

13. **Charney P, Walsh J, Nattinger AB.** Update in women's health. Ann Intern Med. 1999: 131:952-8.

14. **Engstrum JL, Ostrenga KG, Plass RV, Work BA.** The effect of maternal bladder volume on fundal height measurements. Br J Obstet Gynaecol. 1989;96:987-91.

15. **Worthen N, Bustillo M.** Effect of urinary bladder fullness on fundal height measurements. Am J Obstet Gynecol. 1980;138:759-62.

16. **Koninckx PR, Meuleman C, Oosterlynck D, Cornillie FJ.** Diagnosis of deep endometriosis by clinical examination during menstruation and plasma CA-125 concentration. Fertil Steril. 1996;65:280-7.

17. **Koadlow E.** The pelvic examination: the first vaginal examination for a healthy young woman. Aust Fam Physician. 1990;19:665-9.

18. **Rimsza ME.** An illustrated guide to adolescent gynecology. Pediatr Clin North Am. 1989;36:639-63.

19. **Walsh JM, Dolan NC, Charney P, et al.** Update in women's health. Ann Intern Med. 2000;133:808-14.

20. **Mandeblatt J, Gopaul I, Wistreich M.** Gynecological care of elderly women: another look at Papanicolaou smear testing. JAMA. 1986;256:367-93.

21. **Milsom I, Arvidsson L, Ekelund P, et al.** Factors influencing vaginal cytology, pH and bacterial flora in elderly women. Acta Obstet Gynecol Scand. 1993;72:286-91.

22. **Wee CC, McCartney EP, Davis RB, Phillips RS.** Screening for cervical and breast cancer: is obesity an unrecognized barrier to preventive care? Ann Intern Med. 2000: 132:697-704.

CHAPTER 2

Sexuality

SHARON J. PARISH, MD
WILLIAM H. SALAZAR, MD

Sexuality is an entity that involves the integration of an individual's intellectual aspects, personal development, social mores, and biologic function (1). It influences happiness and affects interpersonal relationships. Given the complexity of the human sexual response, it is not surprising that it is vulnerable to dysfunction. Female sexual problems are typically multifactorial in origin and best understood through a biopsychosocial approach.

Sexual problems are common in women. The prevalence of sexual dysfunction ranges from 20% to 63% in sexually active women of all ages (2). Frank and colleagues (3) surveyed couples with a high degree of marital satisfaction and found that 63% of the women reported arousal or orgasmic dysfunction and even a higher percentage (77%) reported sexual "difficulties." A recent analysis of a survey of adult sexual behavior revealed that 43% of women experience sexual problems that negatively affect their quality of life (4).

Although sexual disorders are prevalent, only 10% to 20% of affected women spontaneously volunteer these concerns to medical practitioners. Because clinicians rarely ask about sexual problems, detection rates are consequently low. In one study (5) in which clinical physicians were trained to take a screening sexual history, 53% of patients reported a sexual problem. When polled, 91% of the patients said they considered questions about sexuality an appropriate part of the interview. These data demonstrate the high prevalence of sexual problems, improved detection with focused training in history-taking skills, and patient acceptance of such discussions.

Although our understanding of the etiology and treatment for women's sexual disorders is limited, new data are rapidly emerging from recent and ongoing research. Available information will be presented as it applies to the primary care setting.

Sexual Response Cycle

The human sexual response is best characterized by a sexual cycle consisting of four phases:

1. *Desire* consists of fantasies about and interest in sexual activity.
2. *Excitement* is a phase of a subjective sexual pleasure and the physiologic changes of pelvic vasocongestion, vaginal lubrication, and expansion and swelling of the external genitalia.
3. *Orgasm* consists of a peaking of sexual pleasure and rhythmic contractions of the perineal muscles, reproductive organs, anal sphincter, and the outer third of the vagina. Although women do not have an emission phase, they may have an analogous sense of orgasmic inevitability (6).
4. *Resolution* consists of a sense of muscular relaxation and well-being. In contrast to males, females may respond to additional stimulation almost immediately.

Sexual disorders can occur within one or more of these phases except during resolution.

Normal Physiology, Sexual Normalcy, and Sexual Concerns

Female sexual response is governed by neurologic, vascular, and hormonal mechanisms. Among hormonal factors the androgens are of paramount importance because they maintain sexual desire when present in normal levels. Estrogens preserve local genital blood flow and mucosal lubrication. Neurologic function is important for arousal, which is achieved via a local reflex pathway in which pudendal sensory nerve fibers stimulate parasympathetic fibers from S2-S4 ganglia, resulting in arterial dilatation, labial and clitoral vasocongestion, and vaginal wall relaxation. The vascular supply to the genitals is derived from the internal iliac arteries via the pudendal arteries. Increased blood flow, combined with the effect of the neurotransmitter vasoactive intestinal polypeptide (VIP), results in the lubrication-swelling response characteristic of arousal. Vaginal smooth muscle relaxation and clitoral engorgement, both arousal events, are considered separate entities. It is important to note that although clitoral engorgement is similar to penile erection, there are no sinusoidal lacunae and no process of veno-occlusion, which has implications for biological treatments of female arousal disorders. Orgasm is achieved by skeletal muscle contractions via the pudendal motor nerve; however, autonomic (sympathetic) components probably also play a role. The subjective pleasurable sensation is an intrapsychic and purely cortical phenomenon.

Although sexuality is a subjective phenomenon and sexual behavior varies widely, definitions of what is "normal" have been proposed. The World Health Organization defines "normalcy" for biological, psychological, social, and temporal components (7). Biological dimensions include the usual sequence of sexual development and the ability to experience the physical events of the sexual response cycle. Psychological aspects involve psychosexual maturation and the capacity for intimacy. Social elements relate to societal norms of sexual behavior as they compare with an individual's sexual expression.

The sexual response cycle has been the standard framework for understanding normal sexual functioning, but this approach has been challenged. Tiefer (8) and others have argued that the sexual response model assumes that the sexual experience of men and women is equivalent, when in fact female sexual response does not always proceed in accordance with the prescribed sequence. For example, many women only experience desire after sexual stimulation has led to arousal (9). Furthermore, the sexual response cycle may be too "genitally focused" and limited, defining heterosexual intercourse as the normative sexual experience (8). This model therefore fails to adequately account for the wide spectrum of sexual expression, and it does not promote attention to the communication and intimacy that is central to female sexual satisfaction.

Despite the prevalence of classic sexual dysfunction, patients in the primary care setting often present instead with questions regarding the "normalcy" of their sexual practices.

Moreover, despite the prevalence of the classic sexual dysfunctions, what is commonly seen in the primary care setting are what may be termed "sexual concerns". Namely, individuals may have questions about the "normalcy" of their sexual practices with regard to frequency, technique, masturbation, and fantasy. Women may have concerns about communication, disparate attitudes or value systems, and about the role of sexuality in their overall relationship. These "sexual concerns" may evolve into sexual dysfunctions if they result in intrapsychic distress or conflict between partners.

Etiology of Sexual Dysfunction

The causes of female sexual dysfunction encompass a continuum from organic to psychogenic etiologies and often include a combination of factors.

Biological Causes

Organic factors influence all phases of the sexual response cycle. The biological causes include impairment in neurologic, vascular, and hormonal systems; local structural abnormalities; drug/medication effects; and chronic, debilitating systemic medical illnesses (Box 2-1). Therefore the medical history of a patient with a sexual disorder should include an evaluation of behaviors or conditions that might affect these biological categories (e.g., cigarette smoking, the course of a medical illness, the timing of the administration of a medication relative to the sexual symptom).

Psychological Causes

Many sexual problems are purely psychogenic. Even when an organic cause is identified, psychological and social factors often also contribute to or influence the problem. Psychological reactions, such as anger, can impair sexual responsiveness. In addition, psychological responses to a specific organic problem may interfere with sexual functioning. For example, atrophic vaginitis and decreased lubrication can lead to a fear of pain, which then impairs sexual arousal. The symbolic implications of medical conditions, such as infertility or a mastectomy, may influence a woman's body image and sexual self-esteem. Remote psychological issues, such as sexual trauma, often have a long-term detrimental impact on sexuality (4).

Patients with psychiatric illnesses may present with sexual symptoms. For example, major depression and anorexia nervosa commonly manifest with a loss of sexual desire and arousal, whereas manic or bulimic women may present with hypersexuality. Schizophrenic women may have lowered sexual desire and may experience arousal and orgasm difficulties that appear to be independent of the neuroleptic medication (7). Personality problems may interfere with attachment, communication, and intimacy.

Social Causes

Social factors can have a significant impact on sexual expression. Examples include child-rearing responsibilities, professional demands, and relationship conflicts regarding concerns such as money, schedules, and relatives. Unequal power, intimidation, or abuse in a relationship may result in severe dis-

---

Box 2-1   Organic Factors That May Affect Sexual Function

Angina pectoris, recent myocardial infarction
Chronic obstructive pulmonary disease
Chronic systemic disease (anemia, uremia, cirrhosis)
Degenerative arthritis
Diabetes mellitus
Disc disease of lumbosacral spine
Endocrine disorders
  Adrenal insufficiency (Addison's disease, adrenalectomy, oophorectomy)
  Cushing's disease
  Estrogen deficiency
  Hyperprolactinemia
  Hypopituitarism
  Hypothyroidism and hyperthyroidism
Hyperlipidemia
Hypertension
Neurologic disorders
  Cord lesions (low and high)
  Multiple sclerosis
  Neurogenic bladder
  Neuromuscular disease
  Peripheral neuropathy (alcoholic, diabetic)
  Temporal or cortical lobe lesions
Pelvic fracture
Pelvic radiation
Radical pelvic or urologic surgery
Sickle cell disease
Vascular disease
  Large artery vessel
  Small artery vessel (pelvic vascular insufficiency)
  Venous insufficiency

Adapted from Schmidt CW. Sexual disorders. In: Barker LR, Burton JR, Zieve PD, eds. Ambulatory Medicine, 4th ed. Baltimore: Williams and Wilkins; 1995:188–203.

---

tress and sexual alienation. Declining economic status, low educational attainment, and stress-related problems correlate with increased sexual difficulties, whereas, overall, married women have lower rates of sexual complaints (4). Lesbians may suffer from internalized homophobia or the impact of societal stigmatization.

Culture, Ethnicity, and Race

Women's social and cultural environments may influence or prevent the expression of biological sexual capacities. In some societies the sexual desires and satisfaction of women are given less relevance (especially when fertility is the primary concern) than for males. Cultural norms, which often originate from family, educational, or religious values, may convey conflicting messages about sex. For example, young women are encouraged to appear sexually attractive but then admonished for sexual behavior. This contradiction may generate guilt about sex, which can then lead to future sexual dysfunction. Women in "machismo" cultures are expected to maintain their virginity until marriage, whereas premarital sexual experiences are seen as a sign of virility in men. In Asian and Hispanic cultures, premarital sex may be labeled as an act of prostitution. Hispanic women, however, report overall lower rates of sexual disorders than black and white women, who have more desire and sexual pain disorders, respectively (4).

Organic versus Psychogenic Problems

In some patients a problem with sexual function may be clearcut and amenable to an organic or psychosocial approach. Psychogenic problems usually begin abruptly, are situational or episodic, and are related to specific events or stressors, whereas organic problems start gradually and are often persistent and progressive (Table 2-1) (10). Most commonly, sexual problems are multifactorial, especially in older patients with complex medical illnesses. In these cases the optimal approach is to identify and address contributing factors that are amenable to intervention.

Table 2-1 Distinguishing Psychogenic and Organic Dysfunction

	Psychogenic Dysfunction	Organic Dysfunction
Onset	Usually abrupt	Usually gradual
Course	Selective, intermittent, episodic, or transient	Usually persistent, often progressive
Degree of impairment	Partial: may respond to strong erotic stimulation or change of partner or situation	Partial in earlier stages; absolute later
Associated features	Onset temporally related to specific psychosocial stress	Onset temporally related to organic disease

Adapted from Williams S. The sexual history. In: Lipkin M Jr, Putnam SM, Lazare A, eds. The Medical Interview: Clinical Care, Education, and Research. New York: Springer-Verlag; 1995:235–50.

Explanatory Model for Sexual Problems

The etiology of sexual dysfunction can be conceptualized as having "predisposing", "precipitating", and "maintaining" factors (11). Predisposing factors such as prior life experiences (e.g. sexual trauma) and medical conditions (e.g. diabetes) render an individual vulnerable to the development of a sexual problem. Precipitating factors are those emotional reactions, cognitions, and biological determinants that immediately impinge on sexual responsiveness. Examples include arguments, fear of pain, medication side effects, performance anxiety, and spectatoring (obsessive self-observation during sex). Precipitating factors transform predisposing factors into sexual problems. Maintaining factors are ongoing psychosocial issues or medical conditions that contribute to the persistence of a sexual problem. Furthermore, sexual function and dysfunction is understood to be a learned phenomenon, subject to behavioral conditioning and learned inhibition.

The Sexual History

As stated earlier, physicians do not regularly screen for sexual problems, and only 10% of women with chronic illness will initiate requests for assistance with sexual problems (7). Practitioners are sometimes reluctant to discuss sexual issues because of lack of knowledge, discomfort with sexual language, and concern over the effect of such a discussion (12). Patients fear their doctor will dismiss their sexual concerns or that the topic might embarrass their physician. Consequently, they are often grateful when their practitioner initi-

---

Box 2-2   Goals of Sexual History Taking in Primary Care

1. Identify sexual dysfunction and assess possible organic or psychological etiologies.
2. Identify high-risk sexual behavior requiring education or counseling.
3. Assess effects of illness, disability, surgery, or medication on sexual function.
4. Assess effects of other psychosocial problems on sexual function.
5. Identify sexual problems that are symptoms of psychosocial problems.
6. Identify sexual problems that may be clues to an organic illness.
7. Identify any other questions or concerns related to sexuality.

From Williams S. The sexual history. In: Lipkin M Jr, Putnam SM, Lazare A, eds. The Medical Interview: Clinical Care, Education, and Research. New York: Springer-Verlag; 1995: 235–50; with permission.

ates discussions. Furthermore, because sexual concerns often manifest as physical or psychosomatic symptoms, such as headaches, pelvic pain, or fatigue, detecting sexual problems is particularly important in the primary care setting. To detect sexual problems the clinician must actively screen for them.

Information Gathering

The goals of sexual history taking are highlighted in Box 2-2. The screening sexual history is aimed at detecting sexual disorders that are of concern to the patient. It should begin with determining whether a patient is in a sexual relationship and understanding the nature of that relationship. Examples include *Are you having a meaningful relationship at this time? How is it? Are you sexually involved in this relationship?* Screening questions for sexual problems might include *Are you satisfied with your sexual functioning? How has your illness affected your sexual functioning?*

Once a problem is detected, the clinician can further define it using standard techniques such as the narrative thread and facilitating comments. Contrary to what is recommended for the general medical interview, for sexual history gathering it may be useful to start with a close-ended question instead of open-ended questions. Examples include *Do you experience any difficulty with lubrication? Have you ever reached orgasm with your partner?* Thereafter one can proceed with open-ended questions such as *Would you tell me more about that?* This approach helps overcome barriers to discussing difficult topics and models the desired level of explicitness.

To clarify the nature of a sexual problem, the interviewer can lead a patient through a description of a typical sexual experience, using the sexual response cycle as a guide. It is important to remember that a dysfunction in one phase may actually be the result of a dysfunction in another phase (e.g., decreased lubrication may cause pain and lead to decreased sexual desire), so a problem should be characterized from its onset and as it evolves over time. The interviewer should determine whether the problem occurs in specific situations or is generalized, as well as explore the nature of the nonsexual aspects of the relationship, the biopsychosocial context, and sexual difficulties in the partner.

The sexual history can be inserted into the medical interview where the clinician finds it appropriate and when the questions arise naturally. Good opportunities for the introduction of the topic are during the urogenital or gynecologic review of systems, when asking about social habits such as smoking and alcohol intake, or when discussing relationship issues. It is important not to make assumptions about the patient's sexuality or to assume that the relationship under discussion is the only one that the patient is having. A married patient may be having an affair, and an apparently happily married woman may be having homosexual contacts. Therefore the interviewer may conclude with "safety net" questions such as *Do you have any other questions or concerns about sex? Are there other sexual relationships that I should know about?*

Responding to Emotions

When taking a history of sexual problems, responding to emotions requires the practitioner to attend and respond to his or her own feelings, the patient's feelings, and to the emotional aspects of the physician-provider relationship. Effective empathy promotes the therapeutic alliance, comforts and supports the patient, encourages the discussion of difficult or embarrassing issues, and facilitates information gathering. The clinician may initially feel uncomfortable, but this discomfort tends to dissipate as the skills of sexual history taking are mastered. In addition, the interviewer may discover issues the patient has never discussed with a practitioner or her partner and which may require specific interventions. For example, a woman may disclose a history of sexual trauma in a very emotional manner, and thus it is important that the clinician be familiar with a qualified resource person who could provide timely and appropriate therapeutic follow-up.

Language

Providers and patients are both unaccustomed to talking frankly about sexual issues. However, it is necessary to use language that is clear, explicit, and mutually understood. It may be useful to begin by following the patient's lead, although Williams' guidelines suggest avoiding euphemisms (e.g., "losing one's nature") and clarifying any that the patient uses (13). One should avoid language that is excessively technical on the one hand or too informal on the other and instead use language that the patient understands and that is also comfortable for the provider.

Physical Examination

When evaluating a patient with sexual disorders, the clinician should conduct a general physical examination. Most importantly, one should look for changes in body habitus or evidence of chronic systemic illness, disfiguring problems, signs of endocrine dysfunction (e.g. diabetes mellitus, thyroid disease, hyperprolactinemia, adrenal disease), and indications of pregnancy. In addition, signs of peripheral vascular disease (diminished peripheral pulses and skin changes) and neurologic impairment (especially peripheral nerve, sacral sensation, and motor function) should be identified. The pelvic examination should include a thorough examination of the vulva (to rule out warts, ulcers, or other lesions), speculum exam (to assess estrogenization of the vaginal mucosa and to identify abnormalities of the cervix), and bimanual exam (to rule out fibroids, endometriosis, and cysts). The pelvic examination should include an assessment of perineal muscle tone, and evaluation for pelvic relaxation, as indicated. During the examination it may be helpful to encourage a woman to point out genital concerns herself, having her use a mirror if needed.

Laboratory Evaluation

The laboratory examination is most useful when evaluating sexual desire disorders and sexual pain disorders. For problems of apparently psychogenic origin, no laboratory testing is necessary. When clinical suspicion warrants, however, the clinician may obtain tests for organic causes of sexual disorders. Depending on the history and physical findings, this might include tests such as fasting glucose, complete blood count, urinalysis, and profiles to evaluate thyroid, liver, and renal functions. Further evaluation may sometimes include cervical cultures, pelvic ultrasound, and syphilis testing. Prolactin and androgen (testosterone and dihydroepiandrosterone sulfate [DHEA-S]) levels are sometimes ordered in the evaluation of disorders of sexual desire. Low estradiol levels have also been associated with low frequency of sexual activity. However, there is no definitive evidence indicating that knowing the level of estrogen, androgens, and progesterone is helpful in understanding the cause of a woman's sexual problem (7); thus such testing should only be used in select clinical situations.

Nocturnal vaginal blood flow monitoring has shown that vaginal engorgement cycles in women take place during rapid eye movement (REM) sleep with the same frequency that erectile cycles occur in men. This technique has also shown that postmenopausal women presenting with vaginal atrophy lack basal levels of vaginal capillary blood flow and that during arousal these women have less engorgement than do control women (14). Estrogen replacement therapy reverses this physiological abnormality. However, among reproductive-age women who have impaired vaginal blood flow and arousal during erotic stimulation in the laboratory, it is unclear whether the cause is physiologic, psychogenic, or both. Direct measurements of sensory, motor, or autonomic nerve function have provided inconclusive results. Similarly, indirect measure of peripheral sensory or autonomic neuropathy in diabetic women does not correlate well with sexual functioning. Newer technology, which measures both large fiber vibratory and small fiber thermal sensation, may prove more promising in understanding the cause of arousal phase problems.

Classification of Sexual Dysfunction

Sexual dysfunction, as defined in the *Diagnostic and Statistical Manual of Mental Disorders* (DSM IV), is characterized by a disruption in the sexual response cycle or by pain associated with sexual intercourse (15). The categories of dysfunction therefore include sexual desire disorders, sexual arousal disorder, orgasm disorder, and sexual pain disorders (Box 2-3). Also, by definition, a sexual disorder must cause intrapsychic distress or interpersonal conflict. The DSM IV classification distinguishes disorders exclusively related to general medical conditions or to substances and medications as separate entities from those of psychogenic origin. The International Consensus Development Conference on Female Sexual Dysfunction modified these definitions by combining psychogenic and physiological etiologies in sexual dysfunction categories, adding a category of noncoital sexual pain disorders, and emphasizing

> *By definition, a sexual disorder must cause intrapsychic distress or interpersonal conflict.*

Box 2-3   Classification of Sexual Dysfunctions in Women

Desire disorders
  Hypoactive sexual desire disorder
  Sexual aversion disorder
Arousal disorder
  Sexual arousal disorder
Orgasm disorder
  Inhibited orgasm
Pain disorders
  Dyspareunia
  Vaginismus
  Noncoital sexual pain
Disorder due to a general medical condition
Disorder due to substance abuse or medication

satisfaction and personal distress criteria (16). The following discussion will incorporate both schemata.

The dysfunctions are further classified as lifelong (no prior history of normal functioning) or acquired (previous normal function), as generalized (all partners, activities, situations, forms of sexual expression) or situational (certain partners, situations, practices). Dysfunctions may have mixed, psychogenic, organic, or unknown etiologies and often present as co-morbid conditions. Management of these disorders requires an understanding of their causes and pathogenesis. This typically requires a thorough evaluation using history, physical examination, and sometimes laboratory testing; initiation of treatment strategies; and, if necessary, referral to other appropriate professionals.

Sexual Desire Disorders

Hypoactive Sexual Desire

Hypoactive sexual desire affects at least 22% of women and is the most common female sexual disorder seen in primary care. It is defined as the persistent or recurrent deficiency (or absence) of sexual fantasies and/or desire for or receptivity to sexual activity, which causes personal distress (16). The woman with this disorder usually does not initiate sexual activity and participates only reluctantly when her partner initiates sex. Sexual activity is often infrequent. When the disorder is situational the woman may continue to masturbate or have partners outside the primary relationship but have decreased interest in her primary partner. Standards for frequency and degree of sexual desire do not exist; therefore the diagnosis of this disorder is mainly based on clinical judgment, evaluating the individual's characteristics, her interpersonal situation, the life stage and circumstances, and socio-cultural factors. It is important to remember that it is normal for the female sex drive to be receptive and governed more by the need for intimacy than for sexual release. When discrepancies in a couple's sexual desire are present, it is important to evaluate the woman's partner as well, because an apparently low sexual desire in one partner may in fact reflect an excessive need for sexual expression by the other. Also, partners may have similar sexual desire but at different times.

The most common relationship difficulty that underlies hypoactive sexual desire disorder is an unresolved conflict that leads to covert anger, buried resentment, and unconscious alienation. A past history of sexual trauma is also associated with chronic and intermittent desire disorders that are strongly influenced by the individual's comfort with safety and intimacy in a relationship. Psychological factors are usually implicated in the development and persistence of primary, chronic hypoactive sexual desire disorder, which is complicated in origin and difficult to treat (17).

Hormonal abnormalities can influence sexual desire. These include thyroid dysfunction and androgen deficiency caused by panhypopitituitarism, oophorectomy, or adrenalectomy. Following bilateral oophorectomy, testosterone levels decrease by approximately 50%, and many women report impaired sexual functioning (18). A more gradual decline in androgens occurs after menopause (19). Oral contraceptives may decrease sex drive by increasing sex hormone binding globulin (SHBG), thereby decreasing free testosterone. Progesterone treatment and hyperprolactinemia (by suppressing CNS dopamine) can depress libido, as can excess endogenous beta-endorphins (as seen in athletes or in the setting of starvation) or exogenous opioids (from prescription and recreational drugs). Pregnancy and premenstrual syndrome may alter desire, in the latter setting most likely due to cyclic changes in mood. In addition to the decline in androgens, falling estrogen levels at the time of menopause result in decreased lubrication and impaired arousal, and may secondarily affect desire.

Although controversial, evidence suggests that some postmenopausal women who do not respond to hormone replacement therapy (HRT) alone may experience improvement in their sexual function with the addition of androgens (19–21). Studies show that oral testosterone included in an HRT regimen may improve desire, pleasure, and psychological well-being (20). Combined estrogen/testosterone formulations are available in the form of Estratest (conjugated estrogens 1.25 mg/methyltestosterone 2.5 mg) and Estratest H.S. (half-strength) (conjugated estrogens 0.625 mg/methyltestosterone 1.25 mg). Although initial data regarding testosterone therapy have not shown harm, subjective improvement must be weighed against the potential detrimental effects (e.g., lipid abnormalities, virilization [hirsutism, male pattern baldness, deepening of the voice, acne], changes in body composition, unknown long-term cardiovascular effects). More long-term data are needed. (For further discussion see Chapter 16.) Even less well studied is the precursor to testosterone, DHEA.

Sexual Aversion

Sexual aversion disorder, which is rare, is characterized by the aversion to, and active avoidance of, genital sexual contact. A sexual opportunity with a partner may produces marked anxiety and even extreme emotional distress. The aversion may be focused on a specific aspect of the sexual experience (e.g., penile erection, vaginal penetration). Severe cases of sexual aversion disorder are often rooted in early sexual trauma, conflicts with family of origin, or serious psychopathology.

Sexual Arousal Disorder

The patient with female sexual arousal disorder presents with a persistent or recurrent inability to attain or maintain sufficient sexual excitement, manifest either as a lack of subjective arousal, an inadequate lubrication-swelling response or other somatic response, and which causes personal distress (16). Of note, the diagnosis of female arousal disorder cannot be made if sexual stimulation is inadequate in focus, intensity, and duration. The prevalence of this disorder is 14% in women aged 14 to 59 (4) and may be higher in older women in whom it may be under-reported.

The reduction in estrogens in menopausal and postmenopausal women may lead to vaginal dryness and atrophic vaginitis. Reduced lubrication can also occur in the setting of lactation. Drugs may contribute to this disorder and those that have been implicated include antihypertensive, antihistaminic, and anticholinergic medications, as well as tricyclic antidepressants. Depression may lead to a lack of emotional involvement and subsequently a diminished sexual response. Women who have diminished lubrication may develop performance anxiety or have concerns about pain during intercourse; these psychological reactions may maintain or worsen an existing arousal disorder. Lifelong arousal problems are usually psychogenic in origin.

Organic causes of female excitement disorder have not been studied as extensively as in men and further research is needed. However, it is clear that physiological arousal relies on vascular and neurological systems and that impairment in either domain may lead to difficulties. Neurological impairment resulting from spinal cord injury, local damage (blunt perineal trauma, compression of a neurovascular bundle, laceration), and diseases of the peripheral nerves (diabetes mellitus, multiple sclerosis) can impair arousal. Decreased lubrication may also result from pelvic vascular disease affecting either large or small arteries, with common underlying etiologies being diabetes mellitus, hypertension, hyperlipidemia, and smoking. Vascular mechanisms are probably more important than neurological ones for diabetic women with impaired arousal. Although data are less clear than for diabetic men, studies suggest that women with diabetes types 1 and 2 are significantly affected. Other contributors to excitement disorders include pelvic relaxation, clitoral phimosis, and distension of the urethral meatus.

Presently, medical treatment is limited. Surgical repair of uterine prolapse and pelvic relaxation may be helpful when indicated. Preliminary data suggest that a new vacuum therapy device that enhances clitoral engorgement may help sexual arousal problems (22). A recent study using sildenafil (Viagra) in postmenopausal women with sexual dysfunction demonstrated increases in vaginal lubrication and clitoral sensitivity, although overall self-reported global sexual function did not improve significantly (23). Subsequent studies are underway, and the role of this medication in the treatment of arousal disorder in females remains to be determined.

Orgasm Disorder

Orgasm disorder is characterized by the persistent or recurrent difficulty, delay in, or absence of orgasm following a normal sexual excitement phase, and which causes subjective distress. Orgasm dysfunction is more common in younger women, and the problem can affect the patient's well-being, self-esteem and relationship satisfaction. In assessing whether a woman has this disorder, the clinician should consider the wide variation in the type or intensity of stimulation that triggers orgasm. Many women require clitoral stimulation to reach orgasm, others require vaginal penetration, and some respond to both forms of stimulation. The clinician should appraise a woman's orgasm capacity in the context of her age and sexual experience.

The prevalence of primary lifelong orgasm disorders, defined as a woman having never reached orgasm by any means, is approximately 10%. In the lifelong situational disorder the woman can reach orgasm in some circumstances (e.g., masturbation or manual clitoral stimulation) but not in others (e.g., in the presence of her partner or with intercourse). With situational disorders the clinician should assess the female's satisfaction and concern for the problem.

Once a female learns how to reach orgasm, she will usually not lose that capacity unless problems intervene, such as ineffective sexual communication, a relationship issue, a traumatic experience, a mood disorder, or an organic factor. Medications and severe neurological conditions may also contribute to secondary orgasm disorders. Approximately 50% of spinal cord injured women maintain their orgasmic capacity; preservation depends on the level, completeness, and type of lesion. Studies show that those who do develop an orgasm disorder following injury may respond to sildenafil (Viagra) (24).

Of women taking serotonin reuptake inhibitors (SSRIs) at least 50% complain of delayed or absent orgasm, which appears most pronounced with paroxetine (Paxil) and sertraline (Zoloft). SSRI-induced sexual dysfunction may respond to a weekend drug holiday. However, it is sometimes necessary to discontinue SSRI and substitute a sexual-sparing antidepressant such as nefazodone (Serzone), bupropion (Wellbutrin), or mirtazapine (Remeron).

Another strategy is to continue the daily SSRI and add a second agent. For example, although not FDA approved for this indication, limited data suggest that sildenafil (Viagra) may be helpful for this group of women, and this is becoming an increasingly common strategy (25). Sildenafil is contraindicated in patients taking nitrate medications. Alternatively, bupropion 75 to 150 mg

1 to 2 hr before sexual activity or taken on a daily basis (at a total dose range of 75 to 225 mg/day) has documented efficacy (25a,25b). This drug should be avoided in patients with seizure or eating disorders and used with caution in patients with anxiety, obsessive-compulsive symptoms, or uncontrolled hypertension. Reports suggest cyproheptadine (Periactin) is another effective antidote; in similar fashion it can be dosed either daily or episodically at 4 to 6 mg (25c). An open trial demonstrated that SSRI-induced sexual dysfunction may also respond to ginkgo biloba extract, dosed in a range of 60 mg/day to 120 mg bid (25d). Of note, anecdotal reports suggest possible benefit from ginseng, however, there are concerns regarding the safety of this herb.

Aside from neurologic pharmacologic agents, other organic causes of primary inhibited orgasm have not been identified and, therefore, psychological causes are implicated. Common etiologies include spectatoring, unresolved marital conflict, religious guilt, and fear of pregnancy. Anorgasmia in the female may also be related to a sexual disorder, such as premature ejaculation, in the partner. Patients with disorders of sexual desire and arousal usually also have orgasm disorder. Lastly, sexual pain disorders may lead to orgasm difficulties.

Sexual Pain Disorders

Dyspareunia

Dyspareunia is genital pain that occurs before, during, or after intercourse. In women the prevalence ranges from 7% to 20%. The pain is classified as superficial (on initial penetration), vaginal (from the introitus to the cervix), or deep (from the cervix into the pelvic or abdominal cavities, during penile thrusting). By definition, the problem cannot be caused by vaginismus or lack of lubrication. Women with this disorder usually seek care from medical providers rather than mental health practitioners. The pain during intercourse may result in the avoidance of sexual intimacy, which may disrupt existing sexual relationships or limit the development of new sexual ones.

Dyspareunia is associated with an array of organic (Box 2-4) and psychological factors. Certain medical conditions have clear associations. For example, women with urinary tract symptoms are eight times as likely to complain of dyspareunia (4). However, an organic cause is identified in only 30% to 40% of patients (26). In fact, treatment, such as vulvectomy for severe vulvodynia, does not reliably cure the pain. Psychological components, fear of pain, and anxiety may inhibit arousal and lead to a vicious cycle, thus sustaining the sexual disturbance. Women with organically based dyspareunia may develop vaginismus as a result of anticipatory pain.

Psychological factors that may contribute to dyspareunia include anxiety or guilt about intercourse, memories of distressing early sexual experiences, fear of penetration, unresolved anger, feelings of shame and guilt, and inadequate precoital stimulation or technique.

Noncoital Sexual Pain Disorder

Noncoital sexual pain disorder is defined as recurrent or persistent genital pain during noncoital sexual stimulation. This new category recognizes that sexual activity for women does not always include vaginal penile penetration and may include nonheterosexual women who have alternative sexual practices (16).

Vaginismus

Vaginismus is characterized by the recurrent or persistent involuntary contraction of the perineal muscles of the outer third of the vagina during attempts or with anticipation of vaginal penetration with a penis, finger, object, tampon, or speculum. The contraction may range from mild (inducing some tightness and discomfort) to extreme (preventing penetration). Vaginismus is a psychological disorder with varied clinical presentations. The clinician may diagnose this disorder when contraction of the vaginal outlet occurs during routine pelvic examination. However, some women may exhibit vaginismus during sexual activity but not during a gynecological examination and vice versa. Vaginismus is more common in females who are younger or who have a history of being sexually traumatized.

Substance-Induced Sexual Dysfunction

The effects of substances on the sexual function in women vary according to the particular drug, and include decreased sex drive, decreased vaginal lubrication, inhibited or delayed orgasm, and decreased vaginal contractions (Box 2-5). Less commonly substances may enhance the sexual response and increase the sex drive (26).

Medications may affect sexual function by interfering with adrenergic function, by causing central nervous system depression or sedation, and by causing anticholinergic or antihistaminic effects. As discussed above, common agents that impair sexual function include all classes of antidepressants and antihypertensives, antipsychotics, and benzodiazepines. Tricyclic antidepressants may decrease vaginal lubrication due to their anticholinergic effects, and selective serotonin re-uptake inhibitors may impair sex drive and cause delayed or absent orgasm (see Orgasm Disorder section). However, many patients on antidepressant medication report progressive improvement in sexual function as their depression resolves with treatment. Benzodiazepines may improve sexual function in those inhibited by anxiety. The effect of antihypertensive medications on women is less well studied than for men,

Box 2-4   Dyspareunia in Women: Organic Factors

Minor
  Atrophic vaginitis
  Bartholin's gland inflammation
  Clitoral phimosis
  Episiotomy scar
  Glomus tumor
  Human papilloma virus infection
  Hymenal fibrosis
  Imperforate/tender/rigid hymen
  Infections (bacterial vaginosis, chlamydia, *Candida albicans*, herpes,
    trichomoniasis)
  Irritants (contraceptives, douches)
  Painful hymenal tag
  S/P radiation
  Sjögren's syndrome
  Vaginal adhesions, scar tissues, stenosis
  Vulvar vestibulitis, vulvodynia
Major
  Adhesions (surgical)
  Cervical cancer
  Cervicitis
  Ectopic pregnancy
  Endometriosis
  Fibroid uterus
  Hemorrhoids
  Intrauterine device complications
  Ovarian cysts, tumors
  Pelvic inflammatory disease
  Pelvic tumors
  Posthysterectomy scarring
  Retroverted uterus
  Uterine prolapse
Miscellaneous
  Bulimia
  Constipation
  Cystitis
  Cystocele
  Female circumcision
  Hemorrhoids
  Irritable bowel syndrome
  Lactation
  Oophorectomy
  Proctitis
  Rectocele
  Urethritis

Box 2-5   Drugs That May Affect Sexual Response

Alcohol (high dose)	Digoxin
Androgens	Disopyramide
Antidepressants	Disulfiram
Serotonin re-uptake inhibitors	Diuretics
Tricyclic antidepressants	L-Dopa
Antihistamines	Estrogens
Antihypertensives	Lithium
Central acting	Marijuana (high dose)
β-blockers	Narcotics
Clonidine	Neurotoxic chemotherapy agents
Methyldopa	(particularly vincristine)
Reserpine	Phenytoin
Peripherally acting	Progesterone
ACE inhibitors	Sedatives (high dose)
Calcium channel blockers	Spironolactone
Hydrochlothiazide	Stimulants (high dose)
Antipsychotics	Amphetamines
Benzodiazepines	Cocaine
Bromocriptine	Tobacco
Cimetidine	

---

but high dose medication and combined therapy are associated with a increased rate of sexual dysfunction and noncompliance (27).

Recreational substances such as marijuana and small doses of alcohol may enhance performance by decreasing inhibition and anxiety, but increasing amounts can impair arousal and orgasmic capacities. Sedatives, barbiturates, and opiates depress desire. Substance abusers may have difficulty with intimacy and with the social skills necessary for a successful sexual relationship.

Female alcoholics may develop low desire, orgasmic dysfunction, and vaginismus. Newly sober alcoholics may worry about life's problems, have concern for their relationship, and consequently may experience performance anxiety that interferes with sexual responsiveness (11).

Medical Illness and Sexual Dysfunction

Chronic illness can produce negative emotional responses, physical discomfort, altered body image, and a stigma of fragility, all of which may have a detrimental effect on sexuality. Examples include chronic obstructive pulmonary disease, musculoskeletal deformities, cancer, and uremia. Disabled individuals may have issues that impair sexual function, such as poor self-image and neurological problems, as well as social concerns, such as lack of privacy.

Chronic pain disorders may be complicated by sexual problems. In one study of arthritic women, 54% had sexual difficulties; patients in their mid-30's and 40's had the highest incidence (7). Narcotics may impair neurological regulation of all phases of the sexual response cycle. Medical illnesses with a predominant psychophysiological component (e.g., irritable bowel syndrome, low back pain) are associated with disrupted sexual function, as are psychiatric illnesses that present with pain such as somatization disorder.

Patients who have undergone female circumcision may experience impaired desire or anorgasmia from a complex interaction of predominantly psychosocial issues and a poorly understand biological component. Egyptian psychologists have suggested that the sexual impairment correlates with both the extent of surgery and the internalization of the social messages. However, the relationship between anatomical damage and the ability to reach orgasm is not substantiated by research (28).

Hysterectomy for benign conditions will generally not impair sexual functioning and, in fact, some women note enhanced desire, comfort, and responsiveness (29). However, if the surgery involves oophorectomy or abdominal or pelvic nerve damage, sexual problems may ensue.

Cancer has both direct and indirect effects on sexual function. For example, mastectomy results in the loss of erotic sensation from the breast. However, breast surgery may also affect sexual function indirectly via effects such as arm pain and swelling and sometimes from a resulting negative body image. However, the most important causes of subsequent sexual difficulties in women with breast cancer are 1) premature menopause resulting from the chemotherapy and 2) dyspareunia (30). For women with early stage ovarian and uterine cancer who receive surgery, radiation, or combination therapy, 50% develop a new sexual dysfunction in the subsequent year (31).

Sexuality Throughout the Lifecycle

During each of the three phases of the adult lifecycle (adolescence through early adulthood, middle adulthood, and late middle age through old age), women experience specific concerns regarding their sexuality (Box 2-6).

As women age, they normally experience changes in their physiologic sexual response. Women may note decreased vaginal muscle tension and expansion, delay in reaction time in the clitoris, and lack of breast size increase during stimulation. Estrogen levels decline with menopause, and women may experience atrophic changes and dyspareunia. Appropriate treatment of this

---

Box 2-6 Lifecycle and Sexuality

Adolescence and Early Adulthood
Developing a sexual identity, including sexual preference
Romantic and intimate relationships
Decisions about beginning sexual activity
Concerns about attractiveness, body normality, sexual adequacy, and
    performance
Need for information about sexuality, safe sex, and birth control
Anorgasmy

Middle Adulthood
Relationship issues (fears of commitment, boredom and stasis, long-term or
    recent incompatibilities or conflicts)
Decisions about starting a family; fertility issues
Extrarelationship affairs
Parenthood (lack of time and energy for sex, changes in role, re-emergence
    of developmental issues affecting sexuality)
If single, evaluation of this choice and of desirable and safe sexual activity in
    the age of AIDS
Work and career pressures or disappointments
Secondary anorgasmia or problems with sexual desire

Late Middle Age and Old Age
Departure of children and/or retirement, prompting changes in identity
    and roles
Concerns about loss of youthful attractiveness and function
Illness in self or partner affecting sexual function
Death of partner; return to singlehood
Menopause and related biological changes and psychological reactions to
    the loss of reproductive potential
Prejudices of family and health care providers against sexual activity in the
    elderly
Difficulty finding partners

From Williams S. The sexual history. In: Lipkin M Jr, Putnam SM, Lazare A, eds. The Medical Interview: Clinical Care, Education, and Research. New York: Springer-Verlag; 1995: 235–50; with permission.

---

condition can often restore sexual function. Although orgasmic capacity is retained with age, there is a decrease in the number and intensity of vaginal contractions. Despite these changes, sexual dysfunction rates in older women are lower overall. The most important factors for maintaining sexual activity are partner availability and the partner's physical health (32).

Many physicians assume that older women are not interested in sexuality or discussing sexual issues. This myth creates a physician barrier in caring for older adults.

Lesbian Issues

Lesbians constitute approximately 3% to 8% of the female population. Their choices regarding sexual activity include celibacy and sex exclusively with women or men, or with both (33). It is important to become familiar with their sexual practices (see Chapter 22). Whenever taking a woman's sexual history the clinician should avoid assumptions about heterosexual orientation and need for birth control. Lesbians may, however, have questions related to reproductive or parenting issues, including artificial or alternative insemination.

Sexual dysfunction occurs in some lesbians and bisexual women, although lesbians do not have significant rates of orgasmic dysfunction, dyspareunia, or vaginismus, probably due to technique and less emphasis on genital stimulation and orgasm. Compared with heterosexual women, lesbians have lower sexual frequency in long-term relationships and may complain more often of low sexual desire. Discrepancies in libido between partners may lead to affairs and dissolution of relationships (33).

Therapy

A sensible approach to the management of sexual problems is to identify and examine the interplay of biological, psychological, and social contributions and simultaneously address those factors that are amenable to intervention. Specific biological treatments have been discussed in the context of the individual sexual disorders. The following section will focus on educational, behavioral, and psychological approaches.

When initiating a treatment plan, the clinician may suggest the patient include her partner. This intervention helps to gain the partner's perspective and initiates the therapeutic process of reframing the problem. It communicates to the couple that sexual problems are manageable, orients them toward problem solving, and offers relief.

The P-LI-SS-IT Model

The P-LI-SS-IT model (11, 34) is a widely used and highly accepted approach to managing sexual problems. Some of the elements may be implemented in the primary care setting. The following interventions are applied in a sequential manner:

P - Permission

Patients are given permission to discuss their questions and emotions, as well as to explore new solutions to their sexual concerns. Effective empathic listening can serve as communication skills training for the patient to employ with her partner. The clinician may normalize, universalize, and reframe sexual issues.

LI - Limited Information

The practitioner may provide education about sexual functioning, such as anatomic descriptions and physiologic changes with age. Diagrams and the recommendation of lay press materials may be employed. The clinician may offer technical information about the use of lubricants, sexual positions, and stimulation devices such as vibrators.

SS - Specific Suggestions

Sex therapy approaches that are designed to improve sexual and emotional communication may be applied to the primary care setting. The sensate focus exercises involve initially replacing intercourse with gradual, nondemanding pleasuring techniques. Intercourse is reintroduced when the couple improves their trust and sexual communication. Other modalities of treatment include cognitive-behavioral therapy, relaxation training, hypnosis, and guided imagery. Specific techniques, such as direct self-stimulation (masturbation training), systematic desensitization, and Kegel exercises (contraction of pubococcygeus muscles) may be added.

Hypoactive desire is treated with sensate focus exercises, use of erotic material, and masturbation training with fantasy. *Sexual aversion disorder* treatment involves systematic desensitization with sensate focus exercises and the addition of anti-anxiety medications if phobic symptoms are present.

Vaginismus often responds to the progressive use of dilators or fingers, vaginal lubricants, Kegel exercises, and sometimes anxiolytics. By performing a digital pelvic exam and demonstrating vaginal muscle spasm, the clinician can demonstrate to the woman that, although vaginismus is involuntary and not her fault, she may gain conscious control over the problem, particularly by practicing Kegel exercises. Eventually intercourse is attempted in the female superior position, whereby the woman can gradually insert her partner's erect penis into her vagina with the assistance of relaxation techniques and lubricants.

In *primary arousal dysfunction* the best approach is directed self-stimulation and lubricants combined with sex therapy. *Total anorgasmia* is treated with fantasy material, masturbation training, and Kegel exercises. The practitioner may also recommend that the patient and partner use the sensate focus exercises and the back protected (male in seated position with female between his legs with back against his chest) or female superior positions, both of which allow the woman control of stimulation and pelvic thrusting. When a woman experiences anorgasmia during intercourse, the clinician may recommend the "bridge technique," during which the clitoris is stimulated manually or with a vibrator after penile insertion (35).

IT - Intensive Therapy

Intensive therapy may involve individual therapy to deal with intrapsychic issues, couples therapy to improve communication and resolve conflict, or group therapy. Other indications for referral include psychiatric disorders requiring diagnosis and treatment and past sexual or other trauma requiring specific treatment.

Prognosis

Long-term prognosis varies with the type of disorder and its causes. Generally good results (80% to 95% satisfaction) are obtained when treating vaginismus and primary female orgasmic disorders. The outcome in secondary anorgasmia depends on the factors involved. The prognosis for dyspareunia depends on the ability to successfully treat identified organic factors. Long-term success is poorest when treating sexual desire disorders.

Conclusion

Because of the complex mosaic of biopsychosocial factors and the impact of sexual disorders on patients, sexual dysfunctions are very much part of the primary care provider practice domain. With appropriate interest and practice, the clinician can better understand, identify, and manage these problems, either independently or through referral.

REFERENCES

1. **Klingman EW.** Office evaluation of sexual function and complaints. Clin Geriatr Med. 1991;7:15–36.
2. **Spector IP, Carey MP.** Incidence and prevalence of the sexual dysfunctions: a critical review of the empirical literature. Arch Sex Behav. 1990; 19:389–407.
3. **Frank E, Anderson C, Rubenstein D.** Frequency of sexual dysfunction in "normal" couples. N Engl J Med. 1978; 299:111–5.

4. **Laumann E, Paik A, Rosen RC.** Sexual dysfunction in United States: prevalence and predictors. JAMA. 1999:281;537–44.

5. **Ende J, Rockwell S, Glasgow M.** The sexual history in general medicine practice. Arch Intern Med. 1984;144:558–61.

6. **Bohlen JG, Held JP, Sanderson MO, Alhgren A.** The female orgasm: pelvic contractions. Arch Sex Behav. 1982;11:367–86.

7. **Schover LR, Jensen SB.** Sexuality and Chronic Illness: A Comprehensive Approach. New York: Guilford Press; 1988.

8. **Tiefer L.** Sex is Not a Natural Act and Other Essays. Boulder, CO: Westview Press, 1995.

9. **Basson R.** The female sexual response revisited. J Soc Obstet Gynecol Can. 2000;22: 383–7.

10. **Schmidt CW.** In: Barker LR, Burton JR, Zieve PD, eds. Sexual Disorders: Ambulatory Medicine. Baltimore: Williams & Wilkins; 1995:188–203.

11. **Wincze JP, Carey MP.** Sexual Dysfunction: A Guide for Assessment and Treatment. New York: Guilford Press; 1991.

12. **Risen CD.** A guide to taking a sexual history. Psychiatr Clin North Am. 1995;18:39–53.

13. **Williams S.** The sexual history. In: Lipkin M, Putnam SM, Lazare A, eds. The Medical Interview: Clinical Care, Education, and Research. New York: Springer-Verlag; 1995: 235–50.

14. **Semmens JP, Wagner G.** Estrogen deprivation and vaginal function in postmenopausal women. JAMA. 1982; 248:445–8.

15. Diagnostic and Statistical Manual of Mental Disorders, 4th ed. Washington, DC: American Psychiatric Association; 1994.

16. **Basson R, Bergman J, Burnett A, et al.** Report of the International Consensus Development Conference on Female Sexual Dysfunction: Definitions and Classification. J Urol. 2000;163:888–93.

17. Leiblum SR, Rosen RC, eds. Sexual Desire Disorder. New York: Guilford Press, 1988.

18. **Shifren JL, Braunstein GD, Simon JA, et al.** Transdermal testosterone treatment in women with impaired sexual function after oopherectomy. N Engl J Med. 2000;343: 682–8.

19. **Davis SR, McCloud P, Strauss BJG, Burger H.** Testosterone enhances estadiol's effects on postmenopausal bone density and sexuality. Maturitas. 1995;21:227–36.

20. **Sarrel PM.** Psychosexual effects of menopause: role of androgens. Am J Obstet Gynecol. 1999;180:S319–24.

21. **Sarrel PM, Dobay B, Wiita B.** Estrogen and estrogen-androgen replacement in postmenopausal women dissatisfied with estrogen-only therapy: sexual behavior and neuroendocrine responses. J Reprod Med. 1998;43:847–56.

22. **Billups KL, Berman L, Berman J, et al.** A new non-pharmaological vacuum therapy for female sexual dysfunction. J Sex Marital Ther. 2001;27:435-41.

23. **Kaplan SA, Kohn IJ, et al.** Safety and efficacy of sildenafil in postmenopausal women with sexual dysfunction. Urology. 1999;53:481–6.

24. Female Sexual Function Forum 2000. J Sex Marital Ther (in press).

25. **Nunberg HG, Hensley PL, Lauriello J, et al.** Sildenafil for women with antidepressant-induced sexual dysfunction. Psychiatr Serv. 1999;50:1076–8.

25a. **Masand PS, Ashton AK, Gupta S, et al.** Sustained-release bupropion for selective serotonin reuptake inhibitor-induced sexual dysfunction: a randomized, double-blind, placebo-controlled, parallel-group study. Am J Psychiatry. 2001;158:805–7.

25b. **Ashton AK, Rosen RC.** Bupropion as an antidote for serotonin re-uptake inhibitor-induced sexual dysfunction. J Clin Psychiatry. 1998;59:112–5.

25c. **Cohen AJ.** Fluoxetine-induced yawning and anorgasmy reversed by cyproheptadine treatment. J Clin Psychiatry. 1992;53:174.

25d. **Cohen AJ, Bartlik B.** Ginkgo biloba for antidepressant-induced sexual dysfunction. J Sex Marital Ther. 1998;24:139–43.

26. **Sadock V.** Normal human sexuality and sexual and gender identity disorders. In: Saddock BJ, Kaplan HI, eds. Comprehensive Textbook of Psychiatry. Baltimore: Williams & Wilkins; 1995; 21:1295–1333.

27. **Prisant LM, Carr AA, Bottini PB, et al.** Sexual dysfunction with antihypertensive drugs. Arch Intern Med. 1994;154:730–6.

28. **Toubia N.** Female circumcision as a public health issue. N Engl J Med. 1994;331: 712–6.

29. **Rhodes JC, Kjerulff KH, Langenberg PW, Guzinski GM.** Hysterectomy and sexual functioning. JAMA. 1999;282:1934–41.

30. **Ganz PA, Rowland JH, Desmond K, et al.** Life after breast cancer: understanding women's quality of life and sexual functioning. J Clin Oncol. 1998;16:501–13.

31. **Anderson BL, Anderson B, deProsse C.** Controlled prospective longitudinal study of women with cancer: II. Sexual functioning outcomes. J Consult Clin Psychol. 1989;57: 692–7.

32. **Greendale GA, Hogan P, Shumaker S.** Sexual functioning in postmenopausal women. The Postmenopausal Estrogen/Progestin Intervention (PEPI) Trial. J Womens Health. 1996;5:445–58.

33. **White J, Levinson W.** Primary care of lesbian patients. J Gen Intern Med. 1993;8:41–7.

34. **Annon JS.** Behavioral Treatment of Sexual Problems: Brief Therapy. Hagerstown, MD: Harper & Row; 1976.

35. **Shafer L.** Sexual dysfunction. In: Carlson KJ, Eisenstat SA, eds. Primary Care of Women. St. Louis: Mosby; 1995;40:270–4.

CHAPTER 3

Menstrual Disorders and Dysfunctional Uterine Bleeding

MARK GIBSON, MD

CATHERINE TODD, MD

Normal menstruation in a woman of reproductive age is an indicator of health, whereas menstrual abnormalities may signify pathology in a wide variety of systems. The menstrual history can therefore often provide a window to the state of not only the reproductive system but the general health of the patient. This chapter first reviews the physiology of the normal cycle to provide a context for interpreting complaints of abnormal bleeding. Next, categories of abnormal bleeding patterns are defined. The salient aspects of the history and physical exam are reviewed, and the appropriate use of diagnostic modalities and referrals is described. Finally, the evaluation and management of common menstrual disorders are organized by age group to guide the clinical care of the patient.

Physiology of the Normal Menstrual Cycle

Ovary, Pituitary, and Hypothalamus

Although the pattern of reproductive hormones in the normal menstrual cycle appears complex, there is an underlying simplicity to the key endocrine events. The behavior of the dominant ovarian follicle and its post-ovulatory remnant, the corpus luteum, determines the sequence and timing of events of the cycle through secretion of steroid and peptide signals (Fig. 3-1) (1). These hormones elicit facilitating gonadotropin secretory responses, which are in

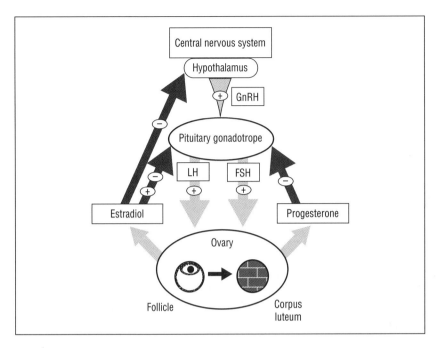

Figure 3-1 Contemporary understanding of the menstrual cycle recognizes the central role of the ovarian follicle and its remnant, the corpus luteum. The complex processes of steroid synthesis, oocyte maturation, and luteal transformation are all determined by the cellular mechanisms of the follicle itself. Although the hypothalamus and pituitary do mediate key steps, their function is in turn influenced by the estrogen and progesterone produced by the ovary. (From Harman SM, Blackman MR. Common problems in reproductive endocrinology. In: Barker LR, Burton JR, Zieve PD, eds. Principles of Ambulatory Medicine, 5th ed. Baltimore: Williams & Wilkins, 1999; with permission.)

turn supported by the pulsatile release of gonadotropin releasing hormone from the medial basal hypothalamus.

The emergence of candidate ovarian follicles from the fixed pool of primordial follicles is continuous from prenatal life until ultimate exhaustion at the menopause and is marked functionally by the appearance of FSH receptors in the granulosa cells. Given sufficient FSH, follicular maturation continues. This process includes granulosa cell mitosis, estrogen synthesis, elaboration of follicular fluid, and the appearance of LH receptors. The emergence of a single follicle that will dominate hormone production and release its oocyte occurs in the middle of the follicular phase (about day seven). Selection occurs as a result of increasingly negative feedback (which results in gradually falling FSH levels) combined with an increasing FSH receptiveness in this lead ("dominant") follicle. Less "receptive" secondary follicles are not sustained by the declining FSH levels and undergo atresia.

In the several days preceding ovulation, estrogen synthesis by the dominant follicle rapidly increases as a result of intrafollicular positive feedback, and final maturation (completion of meiosis) of the oocyte occurs. Rising estrogen levels alter pituitary gonadotropin secretion such that a rapid increase in LH secretion (the midcycle LH surge) is timed to coincide with oocyte maturation to effect follicular rupture and ovulation. The LH surge triggers not only follicular rupture but steroidogenesis by the corpus luteum, resulting in sustained progesterone secretion. The corpus luteum has a programmed lifespan of 12 to 14 days, unless there is support in the form of hCG from an implanted pregnancy. As progesterone secretion falls with demise of the corpus luteum, FSH levels rise and stimulate a new cohort of follicles, and the ovulatory process is repeated.

The most important principle to emerge from this model of the cycle is that the complex processes of steroid synthesis, oocyte maturation, and luteal transformation are all determined by the cellular mechanisms of the follicle itself. Gonadotropic signals from the pituitary that mediate key steps in the cycle are directed by estrogen and progesterone produced by the ovary. Although pituitary function is also enabled by pulsatile release of GnRH from the hypothalamus (2), even GnRH release is in turn influenced by ovarian signals. However, this latter modulation appears not to be critical, as illustrated by the success of unvarying, pulsatile administration of exogenous GnRH to induce ovulation in infertile women lacking hypothalamic function (3).

The Endometrium

The exquisitely coordinated sequencing of hormonal signals that accompany follicular growth and assure oocyte maturation not only enables timely release of a fertile oocyte but prepares the endometrium for implantation of the fertilized oocyte (Fig. 3-2). During follicular maturation and under the influence of circulating estrogen, endometrial proliferation of several millimeters occurs. After ovulation, circulating progesterone effects an orderly sequence of altered glandular secretion and stromal differentiation that leads to a receptive environment for blastocyst implantation. In cycles without conception, these same factors produce a tissue state that will undergo orderly desquamation and subsequent regeneration so that a new cycle can be repeated. Menses, the bleeding event that marks endometrial breakdown in the ovulatory nonconceptual cycle, is an orderly, physiologic, time-limited process characterized by a predictable pattern of bleeding (initially heavy, then decreasing) with a predictable duration (up to 7 days). It is typified by a predictable and familiar rhythm and pattern and is usually preceded by subjective awareness of impending menses (see the discussion of molimina below).

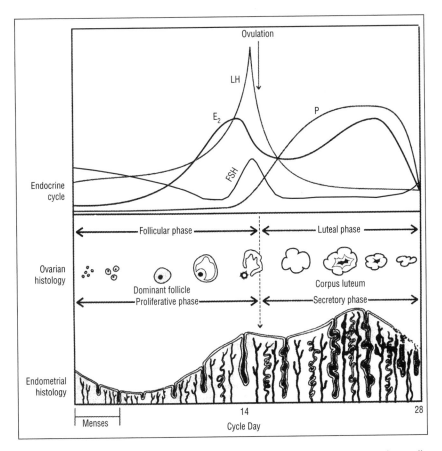

Figure 3-2 Physiology of the normal menstrual cycle. The top panel shows the cyclic changes of FSH, LH, estradiol (E_2), and progesterone (P) relative to the time of ovulation. The bottom panel correlates the ovarian cycle in the follicular and luteal phases and the endometrial cycle in the proliferative and secretory phases. (From Berek JS, ed. Novak's Gynecology, 12th ed. Baltimore: Williams & Wilkins; 1996:160; with permission.)

It should be noted that a minority of normal women experience periovulatory bleeding that usually amounts to brief spotting. The cause of periovulatory bleeding is unknown, but it may be related either to endometrial shedding resulting from the abrupt midcycle decline in estrogen levels or to bleeding from rupture of the follicle. The diagnosis is easy if the symptoms are coincident with Mittelschmerz, but confirmation can be accomplished with a basal body temperature record when necessary.

Abnormal Bleeding Patterns

The various causes of abnormal bleeding patterns are summarized in Box 3-1.

Distinguishing Dysfunctional Uterine Bleeding from Bleeding Due to "Local" Pathology

Dysfunctional uterine bleeding is a clinical term referring to abnormal bleeding in premenopausal women that is not due to identifiable gynecologic pathology. The causes of dysfunctional uterine bleeding are numerous. It is almost always related in part to anovulatory bleeding, although bleeding patterns resulting from an admixture of both ovulatory and anovulatory episodes will produce dysfunctional bleeding as well. The latter is often the case in perimenopausal women. Types of endometrial bleeding and their characteristics are summarized in Table 3-1.

Bleeding from "local" (gynecologic) pathology is generally superimposed on an underlying discernable menstrual pattern (in premenopausal women) and can present as erratic bleeding throughout the cycle, accentuated menstrual flow, or both.

Box 3-1   Etiologies of Abnormal Bleeding

- Pituitary neoplasm
  Space occupying (prolactinoma, other) and destructive (Sheehan's syndrome)
- Psychoneuroendocrine
  Anorexia nervosa, obesity
- Nutrition/metabolic
  Insulin resistance
- Gonadal dysgenesis
  Neoplastic change in the dysgenic gonad
- Ovarian failure
  Generalized autoimmune diathesis
- Uterine/endometrial
  Neoplasm, benign and malignant

- Cervical/vaginal
  Neoplasm, malignant
- Functional gonadal neoplasm
  Masculinizing and estrogen producing tumors
- Nongonadal endocrinopathy
  Thyroid, adrenal dysfunction
- Altered sex steroid metabolism
  Hepatic, renal disease
- Hemostatic
  Thrombocytopenia, platelet dysfunction

Table 3-1   Types of Endometrial Bleeding

Type	Rhythm	Pattern	Amount	Molimina
Ovulatory	Regular	Predictable	Moderate	Present
Estrogen withdrawal (anovulatory)	Erratic	Unpredictable	Variable	None
Atrophic	Erratic	Unpredictable	Light	None
Progestational atrophy	Erratic	Unpredictable	Light	None
Local pathology	◄— Abnormal pattern & amount superimposed on ovulatory pattern —►			
Bleeding dyscrasia	Regular	Predictable	Heavy	Present

Anovulatory Bleeding

Endometrial breakdown and vaginal bleeding may occur without ovulation. Anovulation is most common at both ends of the reproductive lifespan. Anovulation is caused by disturbances in the pituitary-hypothalamic axis but also occurs in conditions such as the polycystic ovary syndrome. Anovulation may present in a variety of ways, from amenorrhea to chronic spotting to intermittent heavy bleeding. Bleeding occurs because extended unopposed estrogen exposure may lead to a proliferative or hyperplastic endometrium that lacks the normal structural support and that subsequently may disintegrate as a result of transient fluctuations in the estrogen stimulation. Because the endometrial stimulation occurs without secretory transformation

Anovulation can manifest in various ways, ranging from amenorrhea to intermittent spotting to prolonged, heavy menses.

by progesterone, such bleeding can be prolonged, unduly heavy, or both. Bleeding may also occur from an endometrium rendered unstable by prolonged exposure to progestins. This occurrence is limited to circumstances where exogenous progestins, such as depot medroxyprogesterone acetate (Depo-Provera), are administered either for hormonal contraception or gynecologic disorders such as endometriosis.

Excessive Bleeding

Blood loss during a typical menstrual cycle is approximately 30 cc; blood loss in excess of 80 cc is defined as *menorrhagia*. With normal menses typically four to six super or regular sanitary pads or tampons are required per day, with perhaps one change during the night. Requiring a pad every 2 hr, needing to change pads frequently at night, or soiling of bed linens is indicative of heavy bleeding, as is reported clot passage or symptoms of anemia without another identified source.

The most common reason for heavy menstrual bleeding is an anatomic disruption of the endometrium, typically by leiomyomata (fibroids). This type of menorrhagia is not necessarily confined solely to the menses and may persist for the entire month, with occasional fluctuations in flow, defined as *menometrorrhagia.*

Bleeding dyscrasias from disorders of platelet function or number typically present as menorrhagia in otherwise normal cycles. Usually this is easily diagnosed by history because it is accompanied by evidence of bleeding diathesis at other mucosal surfaces, such as epistaxis or excessive bleeding following dental work. Anovulation may also cause menorrhagia due to the lack of normal hormonal sequencing required for orderly maturation and shedding of the endometrium. Lastly, infection of the endometrium (chronic endometritis) may present with heavy, prolonged periods.

Amenorrhea

Amenorrhea is divided into two categories: primary and secondary. Primary amenorrhea is diagnosed in women without onset of menses by age 16 when normal secondary sexual features are present, or by age 14 if they also lack development of secondary sexual characteristics. The evaluation of primary amenorrhea is complex and falls outside the scope of this text but includes a pelvic examination and endocrine evaluation (4). Secondary amenorrhea is diagnosed in women with previously normal cycles who have had no menses for 6 months or have missed three consecutive menstrual cycles. Any complaint of missed menses necessitates a pregnancy test, because pregnancy is the most common etiology.

For women of reproductive age, it is important to first exclude pregnancy as the cause of amenorrhea or abnormal uterine bleeding.

Postcoital/Intermenstrual Bleeding

Metrorrhagia, bleeding that occurs between menses, has a variety of possible etiologies. It is important to distinguish whether the bleeding occurs spontaneously or following coitus. Postcoital bleeding is typically related to mechanical trauma to the cervix or vagina and can be due to benign or malignant causes. The cervix in pregnancy and in women in whom the glandular surface of the cervix is everted can bleed easily as a result of exposure of the glandular cells. Such glandular eversion (termed *ectropion of the cervix* or *cervical ec-*

topy) is common and visible on exam. Cervical polyps or a cervical or vaginal malignancy may also have a fragile epithelium and cause postcoital bleeding.

Lesions higher in the genital tract, such as submucous myomata (fibroids), may disturb the endometrium independently of coitus and can cause intermenstrual bleeding in addition to menorrhagia. Recall also that brief and light periovulatory spotting following follicular rupture is observed in some menstruating women and is normal.

Aside from these local causes, however, hormonal causes may be responsible for metrorrhagia. For example, an erratic bleeding pattern may be seen in women using combination oral contraceptives for the first few months due to transient dyssynchrony of the endometrium.

Postmenopausal and Atrophic Bleeding

Postmenopausal bleeding (any bleeding occurring at least 12 months after the last menses) is abnormal and must be investigated. Postmenopausal bleeding following 6 months of amenorrhea is also suspicious and usually warrants assessment. Postmenopausal bleeding that occurs in women taking hormone replacement can be managed by following well-accepted guidelines (see Chapter 16).

One of the most common forms of postmenopausal bleeding is that occurring from an atrophic endometrium. Such bleeding may occur after coitus or other mechanical trauma due to the thinning and subsequent fragility of nonestrogenized endometrium. However, this diagnosis cannot be established without first ruling out endometrial carcinoma or premalignant conditions with endometrial sampling. Similarly, while atrophic vaginitis may predispose the postmenopausal women to postcoital bleeding (sometimes manifest as vaginal tears on speculum examination), it is wise to exclude an endometrial source.

Postmenopausal bleeding is only rarely a symptom of nonuterine pelvic malignancies. If, during the investigation of the bleeding, an abnormality is noted on pelvic exam, appropriate imaging studies should be undertaken to rule out ovarian or fallopian tube etiologies. A thorough history and physical should also be performed to rule out the gastrointestinal or urinary tract as the bleeding source.

Evaluation of Abnormal Bleeding

History

The patient history provides the crucial clues that will guide the rest of an evaluation. The history can help establish whether complaints are due to either pregnancy or a complication thereof, may be associated with an evolving systemic disorder, related to hormonal therapy, of recent onset and superimposed on normal menstrual cycles, or reflect a lifelong pattern of anovulatory bleeding.

The patient history can distinguish bleeding resulting from completion of a normal ovulatory cycle from other bleeding with remarkable accuracy. The normal cycle is marked by a duration that varies from 21 to 35 days (5,6). Bleeding generally lasts 4 to 7 days, peaks early, then subsides gradually. Most importantly, in ovulatory cycles, systemic symptoms before the onset of flow warn the subject of impending menses. These symptoms, collectively termed *molimina*, exhibit considerable variation between individuals, yet are consistent and familiar from month to month for each woman. The spectrum of moliminal symptoms includes fluid retention, pelvic and lower back discomfort, mastalgia, and, often, psychological changes that include increased lability and lowered mood (see Chapter 4). Therefore a menstrual history that includes a predictable cycle length and is accompanied by the regular occurrence of molimina familiar to the patient virtually guarantees the presence of normal ovulatory physiology, regardless of the nature or extent of the superimposed abnormal bleeding.

For example, extremely heavy menses are nevertheless likely to be ovulatory in origin when the cycles are regular and accompanied by molimina; therefore nonendocrine causes for the menorrhagia must be sought. Similarly, the patient who reports a chaotic pattern of bleeding but who can detect an underlying regular cyclic recurrence of molimina is likely to harbor nonendocrine pathology as a cause for her superimposed bleeding. On the other hand, a patient who fails to sense molimina is likely not ovulating, and bleeding episodes in such a patient are therefore probably anovulatory, or less likely due to local pathology. In addition to occurring without subjective warning, such bleeding is most often without a consistent pattern, varying from prolonged to brief, light to extremely heavy. Menstrual diaries can be extremely helpful in determining the cause of abnormal bleeding, and the patient can be asked to record daily moliminal symptoms as well as bleeding pattern and volume.

Physical Examination

Findings on the general physical examination can provide important clues to the diagnosis of abnormal bleeding. Abnormally high or low body mass index, galactorrhea, hirsutism, and stigmata of nonreproductive endocrine disorders such as Cushing's syndrome and thyroid dysfunction all suggest possible anovulation. The skin should be examined for evidence of petechiae, ecchymoses, or systemic illness, and the abdominal examination should include careful assessment for tumors or liver disease. The pelvic examination is of chief importance in identifying lesions that may be the source of abnormal bleeding. Benign or malignant tumors, infections, ulcerated lesions, cervical polyps, or foreign bodies such as misplaced tampons are sometimes identified. One should carefully inspect the external genitalia, vagina, and cervix, and palpate the adnexae and uterus for abnormally large size or irregular shape. It should be noted, however, that clinically important lesions of the uterus affecting the endometrial cavity are not reliably detected by physical examination.

Laboratory Tests

The Pap Smear

A Pap smear is commonly performed in the initial work-up of abnormal vaginal bleeding, although it should be pointed out that this test rarely identifies the cause. Although the Pap smear is an important screening tool for precancerous changes of the cervix, these abnormalities, unlike cervical cancer, do not generally cause abnormal bleeding. (For details on the interpretation and management of Pap smear abnormalities, please refer to Chapter 7.) Also, it should also be noted that the Pap smear is most often normal in patients with endometrial carcinoma (7).

Occasionally endometrial cells will be detected on the Pap smear; their presence during the luteal phase has often raised concern for a possible endometrial abnormality (8,9). However, a recent longitudinal study of 206 Pap smears reporting the presence of normal endometrial cells was unable to find an association between normal endometrial cells on the Pap smear and significant endometrial disease, with a review of the literature supporting this finding (10). Thus, in the absence of worrisome symptoms, such as abnormal bleeding, the finding of normal endometrial cells does not warrant further investigation, regardless of the patient's age or menopausal status. Patients with abnormal bleeding require further evaluation; however, this is dictated by their symptoms, not by their Pap smear findings. Thus the presence of normal endometrial cells on Pap smears should prompt the physician to clarify whether the patient has had any abnormal bleeding, but it otherwise has no clinical relevance.

The finding of atypical glandular cells (AGUS), especially in patients with abnormal bleeding, may indicate malignancy.

However, the finding of atypical glandular cells on Pap smear always requires further investigation. Unlike the more commonly seen atypical squamous cells of undetermined significance (ASCUS), the presence of atypical glandular cells of undetermined significance (AGUS) may signify a malignancy involving the cervical canal or a higher site in the reproductive tract up to 20% of the time (11). Atypical glandular cells, especially in the patient with abnormal bleeding, necessitate prompt, thorough gynecologic evaluation. This includes endometrial biopsy and, if negative, pelvic ultrasound to rule out fallopian tube or ovarian pathology.

Grossly visible lesions of the external genitalia, vagina, and cervix require biopsy, because superficial cytologic examination lacks sensitivity.

The Pap smear is not an appropriate tool for the evaluation of grossly evident lesions. Visible lesions of the external genitalia, vagina, and cervix require biopsy, because superficial cytologic evaluation lacks sensitivity secondary to inflammation and necrosis (12).

Endometrial Biopsy

The principal use of the endometrial biopsy is to exclude malignancy or premalignant states in the endometrium; thus it is indicated for evaluation of postmenopausal bleeding, abnormal bleeding in the perimenopausal woman, and, less often, abnormal bleeding in younger women at risk for neoplasia owing to anovulation (13). Sampling of endometrial tissue by blind transcervical biopsy accurately reflects the histologic state of the endometrium to a remarkable degree given the small portion of endometrial surface retrieved. Current sampling devices are small (3 mm), flexible, and retrieve tissue by aspiration. The procedure is briefly uncomfortable but easily performed in the office setting without local anesthesia or systemic analgesia.

Numerous studies have validated the accuracy of histologic results achieved by endometrial biopsy using dilatation and curettage as a reference standard. The sensitivity of endometrial biopsy in detecting endometrial carcinoma is as high as 90% in several series (14,15). Despite these reassuring statistics, further evaluation should be considered when the uterus is enlarged or irregular, when imaging suggests gross lesions in the endometrial cavity, or when suspicious unexplained symptoms persist in patients with benign results. Histologic samples demonstrating progestational atrophy (as may be seen with HRT regimens containing continuous progestin) or simple atrophy may be insufficient for pathologic interpretation. Such results require clinical correlation with the bleeding history, findings on pelvic examination, and ultrasound demonstration of a thin endometrial stripe before being passed as reassuring. When diagnostic confidence is lacking, further assessment with dilatation and curettage is warranted.

Classification of endometrial biopsy findings is based on the degree and normality of proliferation. Proliferative endometrium signifies a normal endometrial response to the presence of endogenous or exogenous estrogen, and is benign. Atrophy is seen in low estrogen states and is normal in the un-replaced postmenopausal woman (Table 3-2). Progestational atrophy is also seen in women using hormonal contraceptives and in women using HRT that includes continuous progestin. Simple hyperplasia, likewise benign, is de-fined as a variant of cystic hyperplasia and consists of dilated glands and abundant stroma. This can be seen with prolonged, unopposed estrogen expo-sure, and in most cases simply calls for use of progestational agents to inter-rupt the chronic proliferative stimulus.

Complex hyperplasia and complex hyperplasia with atypical features are more serious histologic findings. Complex hyperplasia, which describes pro-liferation of endometrial glands accompanied by irregularities in their shape, has a low premalignant potential (16). However, treatment with progestins and in many cases further investigation to rule out the presence of more se-vere lesions within the endometrium are indicated. Complex hyperplasia with atypical features is more clearly premalignant. The glands often appear se-verely crowded with architectural distortions and/or the glandular epithelial cells have increased nuclear-to-cytoplasmic ratio. Further evaluation by dila-tation and curettage is warranted, because areas containing carcinoma may be missed by office sampling. Even when more thorough sampling does not reveal cancer, progression of atypia to malignancy has been observed in ap-proximately one fourth of patients (16). (The management of these more seri-ous entities is discussed in detail in the Endometrial Neoplasia section.)

Finally, an endometrial biopsy may reveal evidence of endometrial polyps. It is important to emphasize that even though polyps are almost always benign, particularly in the premenopausal woman, they may

In postmenopausal women, endometrial polyps may signify co-existent malignancy.

Table 3-2   Endometrial Biopsy Results.

Type	Significance	Management
Atrophy	Low estrogen levels, usually postmenopause	Exclude coexistent pathology
Progestational atrophy	Contraceptive steroids, some HRT	Treat any bleeding complaints with NSAID or estrogen
Simple hyperplasia or adenomatous hyperplasia	Unopposed estrogen	Progestin therapy
Hyperplasia (complex)	Neoplasia	Exclude coexistent carcinoma
Polyp	Neoplasia	Exclude carcinoma if menopausal

signify coexistent malignancy in postmenopausal women (11,17). Postmenopausal women with biopsy results indicating the presence of polyps should undergo further investigation of endometrial architecture to exclude other polyps or other endometrial lesions possibly missed by endometrial biopsy.

Imaging of the Reproductive Tract

The chief value of imaging procedures in the patient with abnormal bleeding is to identify lesions in or near the endometrial cavity and to assess the appearance of the endometrium. Transvaginal sonography can provide high-resolution images that permit evaluation of endometrial thickness, endometrial contour, and presence of leiomyomata in the subjacent myometrium. It is a cost-effective complement to endometrial biopsy in the evaluation of abnormal bleeding (18). Simultaneous transcervical instillation of fluid (sonohysterography) can add sensitivity to detection of lesions affecting the endometrial cavity (19,20). Computed tomography and magnetic resonance imaging (MRI) are not superior to ultrasound and are considerably more costly.

In women of reproductive age the endometrium may achieve a thickness of 1 cm or more during the proliferative phase of a normal cycle. The endometrium can appear as distinct layers due to the stromal edema in the opposing anterior and posterior surfaces, then subsequently appears homogenous and more echogenic during the secretory phase. Excessive thickness, with or without irregularity, can be consistent with hyperplasia or may suggest the presence of endometrial polyps. Leiomyomata are easily distinguishable by ultrasound. Those that are subjacent to or that distort the uterine cavity are more likely to be associated with abnormal bleeding.

The significance of endometrial thickness in the evaluation of postmenopausal bleeding has received considerable study. Malignancy or other abnormal proliferation is unlikely when the endometrial thickness is less than 5 mm (20,21). Therefore if endometrial biopsy in such a patient yields insufficient tissue for histologic interpretation, as may commonly occur, malignancy has been adequately ruled out. Further investigation should be done when tissue sampling is insufficient for diagnosis and endometrial thickness is 5 mm or more, depending on the entire clinical picture, including age, symptoms, and risk factors.

Age-Specific Guidelines for Evaluation of Abnormal Bleeding

The Adolescent

The possibility of pregnancy should never be overlooked in the young woman with bleeding complaints, even in the absence of supporting history. The principal causes of menorrhagia in the young patient are anovulatory bleeding and bleeding diathesis (22). History will provide important clues to the evaluation. An erratic and unpredictable bleeding pattern suggests a disturbance of ovulation, whereas regular but heavy menses associated with bleeding problems at other mucosal sites suggest bleeding diathesis.

Careful examination is sufficient to exclude neoplasm, which is uncommon in this group.

Anovulatory Bleeding

Irregular and anovulatory cycles should be regarded as normal in the first year after menarche due to immaturity of the ovarian-hypothalamic axis. Transient ovulatory disturbances in young women are common and, if the history and examination are otherwise normal, a short course of symptomatic management and observation is indicated. When evidence of persistent ovulatory disturbance is present more than a year after menarche, endocrine evaluation should be undertaken. Endocrine assessment for persistent anovulation and anovulatory bleeding in the very young woman is sufficiently investigated with assessment for thyroid dysfunction (TSH), hyperprolactinemia (serum prolactin), and ovarian failure or dysfunction, including the polycystic ovary syndrome (LH and FSH), unless findings and history point to other, nonreproductive endocrine disorders. In the adolescent all values are most commonly normal, and a pattern consistent with chronic anovulation is revealed. When this is the case it is likely that normal cycles will be established with further maturation.

Although hypothalamic dysfunction is common in younger women, a history should investigate the possibility of substance abuse, excessive exercise, weight loss, or eating disorders (see discussions in the Athletic Amenorrhea and Weight Loss/Eating Disorders sections). Psychological stress can also affect GnRH release through excess corticotropin-releasing hormone and vasopressin (23), and attention should be given to the possibilities of adjustment problems or stress at home or in school.

Acute episodes of menorrhagia related to anovulation can usually be arrested with high doses of oral progestational agents in the form of either medroxyprogesterone or, because all combined oral contraceptives are progestin dominant, contraceptive pill packs (Box 3-2). Medroxyprogesterone 10 mg daily is prescribed for 1 to 2 weeks. The oral contraceptives are administered in various regimens but often as one pill twice daily for the first 4 days, then one pill daily for the remainder of the pack. Bleeding typically decreases by the second day and often ceases altogether by the fourth day. A normal withdrawal bleed will then occur within a few days of the last active pill. Typically the oral contraceptives are continued (henceforth in standard fashion as one pill daily) for two or more cycles, at which point a trial of discontinuing

---

Box 3-2   Arresting Menorrhagia Due to Anovulatory Bleeding*

- Medroxyprogesterone acetate (Provera) 10 mg q day × 1-2 wk
  or
- Combined oral contraceptive pills: 1 pill bid × 4 days, then 1 pill daily for the remainder of pill pack; continue oral contraceptives (as 1 pill daily in standard fashion) for 1-2 more cycles

If the above measures are unsuccessful, intravenous estrogen may be required.

*Pregnancy should be excluded before initiating treatment.

---

treatment can be attempted. When prescribing oral contraceptives for this purpose it is wise to carefully communicate to the patient and/or her parent that the medication is being prescribed not for contraception but rather for a convenient form of hormonal medication to treat the menorrhagia.

Extensively disrupted anovulatory endometrium may sometimes not respond to progestational treatment. When this occurs, unopposed intravenous estrogen (ethinyl estradiol 40 mcg/d or conjugated estrogens 5 mg/d) may be required and will generally halt bleeding within two days, sometimes within hours. A course of progestins is added in 1 to 2 weeks to induce a withdrawal bleed. Endometrial curettage is almost never necessary.

PRIMARY AMENORRHEA

Primary amenorrhea is defined as absence of menses by age 16 with development of secondary sexual characteristics or without development of secondary sexual characteristics/menstruation by age 14. After pregnancy has been ruled out, an examination should be undertaken to rule out absence/ malformation of pelvic organs. Absence of pelvic organs on examination necessitates referral to a gynecologist and MRI or ultrasound to assess the extent of any malformation. Genetic work-up is necessary in the presence of the physical stigmata associated with Turner's syndrome. Patients with congenital absence of GnRH function, anosmia, and infantile sexual development (Kallman's syndrome) have a mutation in the X chromosome that disrupts olfactory axonal and GnRH neuronal migration (see section on Kallman's Syndrome). In addition to Kallman's syndrome, endocrine evaluation must exclude other neurologic lesions or masses and late-onset congenital adrenal hyperplasia.

SECONDARY AMENORRHEA

Secondary amenorrhea is diagnosed in women with a previously normal cycle who have had no menses for 6 months or who have missed three consecutive menstrual cycles. There are several etiologies for this condition that occur during adolescence, though one of the most prevalent and easily diagnosed is pregnancy. This must be ruled out before proceeding with work-up. As a general rule, patients who do not respond to progesterone challenge (progesterone to induce withdrawal bleeding; see Box 3-3) should be assessed for cessation of estrogen production.

AMENORRHEA FOLLOWING DISCONTINUATION OF HORMONAL CONTRACEPTION

Amenorrhea following discontinuation of oral contraceptives or depot medroxyprogesterone acetate is not unusual. Typically menstrual function resumes within 3 months, before the criteria for secondary amenorrhea are met, but may take as long 22 months in the case of depot medroxyprogesterone acetate. Amenorrhea persists until re-establishment of ovarian signaling to the hypothalamus, which had been suppressed by the contraceptive. It is important to stress to the patient that it is still possible to become pregnant in the absence of menses. Pregnancy testing should therefore always first be performed and, if negative, barrier or other nonhormonal method should be recommended. If the amenorrhea persists for more than 3 months, however,

---

Box 3-3   Progesterone Challenge and Estrogen-Progesterone Challenge

Progesterone Challenge Test*

- Medroxyprogesterone actate (Provera) 10 mg PO × 7 days

  or

- Progesterone in oil 100 mg IM × 1 dose

If adequate estrogen levels are present, withdrawal bleeding will occur 2-5 days following the oral regimen or 7-10 days following IM progesterone.

If the progesterone challenge fails to induce a withdrawal bleed, the estrogen-progesterone challenge is next performed.

Estrogen-Progesterone Challenge Test

- Conjugated estrogen 1.25 mg PO q day × 21 days with medroxyprogesterone acetate (Provera) 5-10 mg PO q day added for the last 7 days

Lack of a withdrawal bleed usually signals absent or damaged endometrium (i.e., Asherman's syndrome).

*Pregnancy must first be excluded in all patients presenting with secondary amenorrhea.

a careful history should be obtained, including inquiry regarding the presence of premature menopausal symptoms (hot flashes, vaginal dryness), weight changes, and medication history. If there are no endocrine etiologies suggested in the history, a withdrawal bleed can be induced by a 10-day course of medroxyprogesterone actetate 10 mg daily, which may lead to normal cycling in the next month. Although discontinuing contraception for the purpose of conception is uncommon among adolescents, whenever this occurs one should recommend or prescribe prenatal vitamins (see Chapter 19).

ATHLETIC AMENORRHEA

Irregular menses, delayed onset of menarche, and secondary amenorrhea are not uncommon in female athletes and dancers. This results from decreased GnRH secretion by the hypothalamus. There are many theories as to the exact mechanism by which the hypothalamus is suppressed; however, a significant determinant is amount of body fat. As body fat decreases, there is a measurable decrease in LH pulsatile frequency and amplitude before onset of irregular menses. The minimum percentage of body fat associated with menarche is 17%, and secondary amenorrhea is associated with levels falling under 22% (4). In addition to body fat percentage the stress of extreme activity may also impact on the menses. This phenomenon has been observed in dancers performing without any changes in body fat content or weight (24).

The treatment for athletic amenorrhea focuses on preventing unwanted pregnancy and bone loss. It is still possible to ovulate with this condition and, in the presence of irregular or absent menses, much more difficult for the individual to detect a pregnancy. It must be stressed to these patients that contraception is necessary to ensure that an undesired pregnancy is avoided. Secondly, decreased estrogen levels can result in bone demineralization. Several studies have established a radiologically detectable decrease in bone mineral density in amenorrheic female athletes, despite a normal rate of bone turnover (25-27). One study noted a 25% to 44% decrease in circulating progesterone and estradiol levels in amenorrheic runners, with a concomitant 10% decrease in lumbar bone density (26). Fortunately, this can be reversed, as studies demonstrate that bone mineral density increases following a year's treatment

Many young patients with amenorrhea are unaware that they are at risk for pregnancy and bone loss.

with cyclic progesterone—significantly more than after treatment with calcium alone—regardless of calcium supplementation (27). Extrapolating from this evidence, both contraception and osteopenia concerns can be addressed with the use of hormonal contraception, preferably with combined oral contraceptives or, alternatively, with progestin-only contraceptives.

Those desiring conception should be advised to decrease the level of activity with the hope of establishing a regular menstrual cycle or at least enough GnRH secretion to result in ovulation.

AMENORRHEA SECONDARY TO WEIGHT LOSS AND EATING DISORDERS

Anorexia nervosa and bulimia nervosa are distinguished by disordered perceptions of appearance and abnormal eating behaviors. These eating disorders may be associated with depression, social isolation, secretive eating habits, an obsession with calorie content and exercise, other obsessive-compulsive behaviors, and an overwhelming fear of being perceived as fat. Despite having received increased attention in the last decade, eating disorders are underdiagnosed. This is particularly true for bulimia nervosa, as patients with this condition most often fall in the normal weight range.

Patients with anorexia nervosa develop amenorrhea as a result of hypothalamic suppression from loss of body fat, similar to that seen from athletic amenorrhea. Given that anorexia nervosa is associated with a 5% to 15 % mortality rate, menstrual disorders are a relatively benign symptom of the disease. In patients with bulimia, amenorrhea is possibly related to weight fluctuations, nutritional deficiencies, or emotional stress.

Individuals with amenorrhea and any of the aforementioned risk factors, including low body mass index, should be asked about their behaviors with food as well as their family relationships, because abrupt lifestyle changes may cause tendencies towards anorexia to become active disease. Patients diagnosed with eating disorders should be referred to psychiatry and hospitalized as needed. The amenorrhea will resolve in up to 70% of these women when normal body weight is attained (4).

Pregnancy must always be ruled out, because the severe self-imposed malnutrition of eating disorders confers significant risk to the fetus as well. Contraception should be offered to all patients who are sexually active. If hormonal contraceptives are not desired, then the amenorrheic or irregularly cycling patient should at least be given hormone replacement therapy, because she is at risk for bone loss due to lack of estrogen. A daily dose of conjugated estrogen 0.625 mg and progesterone 2.5 mg is adequate for bone protection, though it will not result in menstrual bleeding.

HYPOTHALAMIC AMENORRHEA/KALLMAN'S SYNDROME/HYPOGONADOTROPIC HYPOGONADISM

This group of disorders is characterized by deficient gonadotropin secretion and mimics the endocrine state of the prepubertal girl. Gonadotropin levels are inadequate only relative to the lack of ovarian estrogen production and therefore often fall within the normal range. Thus this condition is diagnosed by a lack of withdrawal bleed following challenge with a progestational agent.

When fully expressed, these disorders are markedly hypoestrogenic; vasomotor symptoms such as hot flashes and night sweats are sometimes present.

The differential diagnosis includes conditions associated with destruction of hypothalamic and pituitary tissue (e.g., ischemic necrosis [Sheehan's syndrome]), head trauma, and neoplasms (e.g., craniopharyngioma and pituitary adenoma). Evaluation should consider both destructive and functional origins of hypogonadotropism through careful history, physical examination, and, when a functional or nutritional cause is not evident, imaging of the pituitary and juxtapituitary structures. One of the more common intracranial lesions in women is a pituitary microadenoma or macroadenoma, which may often be treated with bromocriptine and followed with serial prolactin levels and imaging.

Because all of these patients are anovulatory and hypoestrogenic, bone loss must be prevented with estrogen replacement, which can be prescribed either in the form of combined oral contraceptives or hormone replacement therapy. The patient should be reassured that when pregnancy is desired ovulation induction is possible with GnRH analog injections.

Bleeding Diathesis

Heavy menses accompanying a history of easy bruising, epistaxis, or prolonged bleeding following dental work should prompt a work-up for underlying hematologic disease. Screening for bleeding diathesis should focus on platelet number and function, because coagulopathy is less commonly implicated without an obvious underlying source.

Adult of Reproductive Age (Between 18 and 45 Years)

The reproductive-age adult female (loosely, a woman between the ages of 18 and 45) falls into a category where many different conditions may surface, some of which are more typical for other age groups and which are discussed in those sections. However, there are conditions related to bleeding patterns that significantly affect fertility, typically more an issue of concern during this time period than at any other. Because anovulation can occur despite menstruation, all women who present with the complaint of infertility for more than 12 months (or 6 months if 35 years or older) should first have basic endocrine labs (prolactin, TSH, LH, and FSH) assessed to exclude these causes of anovulation (see Chapter 20).

Towards the end of the reproductive age interval there is an increased incidence of irregular bleeding, with dysfunctional bleeding patterns caused either by hormonal or mechanical etiologies. The most common of these etiologies are discussed here, along with the effects of certain chronic conditions or medications. However, many endocrine disorders begin during this time period and may have menstrual manifestations. Some of these etiologies (such as Sheehan's syndrome) have been discussed in the preceding Adolescent section. As before, pregnancy must always be considered as an etiology for absent or light menses.

Premature Ovarian Failure

Premature ovarian failure by definition occurs in women under age 40, although it can occur at very young ages and even before menarche. Ovarian failure in women of reproductive age may be due to antineoplastic therapy (radiation, alkylating agents), autoimmune endocrinopathy, or idiopathic and familial mechanisms. The menstrual presentation is classically that of amenorrhea, but antineoplastic effects may be partial or transient, and autoimmune and idiopathic mechanisms may fluctuate. Therefore patients may either present as though perimenopausal, with oligomenorrhea and anovulatory bleeding, or may have intermittent episodes of amenorrhea interspersed with normal menstrual function. Some but not all women will have hot flashes, and given the varying presentations the diagnosis is not always obvious. Elevated levels of FSH are confirmatory, however.

The history will often implicate possible underlying causes, including identification of women in whom early menopause is clearly familial. When premature ovarian failure is diagnosed in women less than 30 years of age, karyotype testing should be performed to exclude gonadal dysgenesis. Among the remainder, precise distinction between autoimmune and idiopathic causes is difficult, and all patients should be screened periodically for evidence of associated autoimmune endocrinopathy affecting the adrenal, parathyroid, and thyroid glands and the gastric parietal cells. Also, these patients are essentially menopausal and must be given HRT for bone protection. Although spontaneous resumption of ovarian function and even pregnancy have been known to (rarely) occur, in general future fertility is not possible from a native oocyte. However, if desired, the patient may be referred to a reproductive endocrinologist to explore the option of pregnancy with oocyte donation (see Chapter 20).

Polycystic Ovary Syndrome

Polycystic ovary syndrome (PCOS), also known as Stein-Leventhal syndrome, was originally described as a triad of obesity, hirsutism, and oligomenorrhea in the setting of morphologically polycystic ovaries. However, this disorder is now understood to be very heterogeneous, and about half of all women with PCOS are nonobese. Also, despite the name, women with PCOS sometimes lack the classic polycystic ovary morphology; conversely, polycystic-appearing ovaries are sometimes observed in women without an ovulatory disorder (28,29). Thus the contemporary understanding of PCOS is one of chronic anovulation and hyperandrogenism in the absence of other endocrine disorders.

PCOS affects approximately 4% to 7% of women of reproductive age (30). Patients usually present with the complaint of primary infertility or secondary amenorrhea, or infrequent heavy menses that became irregular soon after menarche. Women with this disorder classically have visceral obesity with increased waist-to-hip ratio, acne, male-pattern alopecia, and some degree of hirsutism, though this is often not apparent due to successful hair removal. However none of these findings is required. Pelvic examination sometimes reveals enlarged, bilaterally cystic ovaries. It should be emphasized that patients with evidence of rapid onset or significant virilization (such as clitoromegaly) may have an androgen-producing tumor rather than PCOS and should undergo further testing (see section on Other Endocrine Causes of Anovulatory Bleeding).

PCOS is commonly diagnosed by an abnormally high LH-to-FSH ratio (2 or greater). However, this finding lacks both sensitivity and specificity. A more contemporary approach is to suspect the diagnosis of PCOS on the basis of the history and physical, then to exclude the other relatively common causes of chronic anovulation-hyperprolactinemia, premature ovarian failure, and hypothalamic dysfunction—by serum prolactin level, FSH level, and progesterone challenge, respectively. It should be noted that while serum androgen levels are elevated in patients with PCOS, such testing is unnecessary if masculinization is not present.

The clinical concerns of PCOS are anovulation and the effects of chronic estrogen stimulation. Anovulation occurs due to impairment of the LH surge and can be diagnosed in a variety of ways, though irregular menses implies that ovulation is unlikely (28). A basal body temperature chart can be used to confirm anovulation if the menses are somewhat regular. If pregnancy is desired, referral to a reproductive endocrinologist for ovulation induction is indicated. However, even if fertility is not immediately desired, the danger of prolonged unopposed estrogen secretion on the endometrium must be addressed.

In women with an anovulatory bleeding pattern for more than 1 year (similar to that seen with PCOS), endometrial biopsy should be performed to rule out endometrial hyperplasia or cancer.

Women who have had this bleeding pattern for longer than 1 year should undergo endometrial biopsy to rule out endometrial hyperplasia or cancer. Patients diagnosed in adolescence or in the early 20's with this disorder or with 6 months or less of amenorrhea benefit from an immediate course of Provera 10 mg daily for 10 to 12 days to induce a withdrawal bleed and restore secretory endometrium. Following this, these women are best maintained on low-dose combined oral contraceptives in order to protect the endometrium, suppress new cyst formation and, via its suppression of androgen production, decrease the incidence of acne and new abnormal hair growth and improve lipid abnormalities. In addition, oral contraceptives are sometimes needed for contraception, because ovulatory cycles may occur following progesterone withdrawal.

Another treatment is weight loss. Studies have demonstrated that a 7% reduction in body weight can restore reproductive function, and in fact such weight control is probably the best treatment for preventing chronic disease. Insulin-sensitizing agents such as metformin or the thiazolidinediones are also sometimes effective in restoring ovulatory cycles (31,32).

In addition to unopposed estrogen stimulation, PCOS involves other metabolic derangements—in particular, elevated androgen levels and, frequently, hyperinsulinemia. The significance of insulin resistance in PCOS has been increasingly appreciated, with the most direct correlates being impaired glucose tolerance in almost one third of obese women with PCOS and a three-fold risk of type 2 diabetes mellitus (30). In addition, the hyperinsulinemia and hyperandrogenism together lead to lipid derangements of the male pattern, namely elevations of total cholesterol, triglyceride and low-density lipoprotein levels, and lowered high-density lipoprotein levels. Hypertension is another association and, though uncommon in the young patient with PCOS, the incidence increases to approximately 40% by perimenopause (33). Not surprisingly, atherosclerosis is prevalent, and in fact women with PCOS have an approximately seven-fold increased risk for myocardial infarction (34). Therefore it is important that women with PCOS seek regular care from a generalist, particularly after age 35 or 40.

Although the etiology of PCOS is not fully understood, one theory holds that insulin resistance may be the root cause. Hyperinsulinemia stimulates excess production of ovarian androgens and increases peripheral androgen action by decreasing the concentration of serum sex hormone-binding globulin. Local intraovarian androgen excess likely is responsible for the anovulation. Excess insulin and androgens likely both act on the pituitary to chronically alter the secretion of gonadotropins in favor of excess LH (31). PCOS appears to have an autosomal dominant mode of inheritance, with premature baldness being the male counterpart (35).

Hyperprolactinemia

Irregular bleeding patterns may also be seen with elevated prolactin levels, a relatively common cause of anovulation. Hyperprolactinemia suppresses GnRH secretion and may arise through autonomous secretion by pituitary adenomas or unrestrained secretion by normal pituitary tissue owing to disruption of portal hypophyseal vascular communication ("stalk section"). Elevations of prolactin also occur in primary hypothyroidism owing to the effect of excess thyrotropin releasing hormone on prolactin release. In addition, because dopamine normally inhibits prolactin release, antidopaminergic medications can often lead to anovulation. Agents typically implicated are the phenothiazines, isoniazid opiates, metoclopramide, tricyclic antidepressants, alpha-blockade antihypertensives, and even exogenous hormones such as danazocrine, oral contraceptives and medroxyprogesterone acetate.

The classic clinical presentation of hyperprolactinemia is amenorrhea with galactorrhea, although both symptoms are variable and the latter is frequently not present. More typically, patients with hyperprolactinemia complain of irregular, sparse menses and infertility from anovulation. Screening for prolactin elevation is therefore appropriate when the menstrual history suggests only minor degrees of disruption of regular ovulation such as oligomenorrhea or anovulatory bleeding. A prolactin level above 20 is abnormal, and a level above 100 is unlikely to be caused by exogenous medication and should prompt work-up for a pituitary tumor. If not explained by drugs or hypothyroidism, evaluation of hyperprolactinemia should include MRI imaging of the sellar and juxtasellar areas. With medical treatment, surgical correction, or removal of the offending medication, ovulation and regular menses are usually restored.

It should be noted that galactorrhea is often functional and unrelated to important degrees of hyperprolactinemia in reproductively normal women. Therefore screening for hyperprolactinemia when galactorrhea occurs in the presence of regular, ovulatory cycles is unnecessary.

Other Endocrine Causes of Anovulatory Bleeding

Recall that hypothyroidism, hyperprolactinemia, and premature ovarian failure sometimes lack other symptoms and signs aside from anovulation; therefore laboratory testing (TSH, prolactin level, FSH, and LH) should be routinely sought for these three conditions when evaluating anovulatory bleeding. In contrast, other endocrine causes, such as androgen secreting neoplasm, adult-onset adrenal hyperplasia, and Cushing's disease, can generally be excluded using history and physical examination alone. Laboratory evaluation for these less common endocrine conditions is required only when indicated by clinical presentation.

A patient with features of only mild virilization and irregular menses dating back to adolescence most likely has polycystic ovary syndrome. In contrast, women with onset of hirsutism after the age of 25, or evidence of significant virilization (such as clitoromegaly) or a very rapid progression of masculinization over several months, may likely have an androgen-producing tumor. Such patients should undergo further testing with serum testosterone and dehydroepiandrosterone sulfate (DHEA-S) levels as well as imaging. Similarly, screening anovulatory patients for adult-onset adrenal hyperplasia is of low yield (well under 5%) and should be limited to those presenting with hypernatremia or symptoms of androgen excess. In general, ovulation resumes with treatment of these underlying endocrine problems.

Dysfunctional Bleeding Secondary to Chronic Conditions
Irregular bleeding is frequently observed in patients with chronic renal or hepatic disease. This pattern is caused by impairment in clearance of estrogen or its breakdown products. Ovulation will sometimes but not always resume upon initiation of dialysis. Diabetes mellitus also sometimes leads to impairment in ovulatory function.

Leiomyomata (Fibroids)
Menorrhagia in the setting of otherwise normal cycles requires evaluation to exclude pathology affecting the endometrium. The commonest etiology is leiomyomata (fibroids), which are benign tumors of the smooth muscle that comprises the myometrium. These growths are stimulated by estrogen, and typically become symptomatic from the late 30's onward. Patients often present with a history of heavy, prolonged menses with possible clot passage and sometimes menometrorrhagia. An enlarged, irregularly shaped uterus on pelvic examination usually suggests leiomyomata. Evaluation by an experienced examiner and endometrial biopsy for those patients over the age of 40 are warranted. In addition, pelvic ultrasound is performed to exclude other neoplasm masquerading as a leiomyoma as well as possible asymptomatic complications such as hydronephrosis. Patients with a presumed leiomyoma should undergo regular pelvic examinations every 6 to 12 months to ensure stable size. Those with rapid uterine growth should be referred to a gynecologist for evaluation and possible hysterectomy, because, although rare, leiomyomata can undergo malignant degeneration (less than 1%). Leiomyomata may also undergo other types of degeneration (cystic, hemorrhagic), typically when they outgrow their blood supply, and this may result in a significant amount of abdominal and pelvic pain.

Abnormal bleeding due to leiomyomata may respond to hormonal management. Options include high-dose progestins (depot medroxyprogesterone acetate 150 mg or more IM as frequently as monthly to control symptoms), oral contraceptive pills, or GnRH agonists. GnRH agonists (leuprolide, goserelin, nafarelin) not only correct the anemia but decrease the size of the fibroids. However, because GnRH agonists effectively induce a temporary menopausal state, their adverse effects on bone metabolism and lipid profiles limit their use to only 6 months, and probably the optimal use of the GnRH agonists is to decrease the size of the uterus before surgery.

Surgical options include hysterectomy or myomectomy, depending on the patient's preferences for future fertility, but newer options are also available (see Chapter 14). Patients who are asymptomatic and decline any intervention may simply be followed with regular examinations, because these tumors generally decrease in size after the onset of menopause. Fibroids should not be considered a contraindication to hormone replacement therapy or hormonal contraceptive use.

Endometrial Polyps

The cause of menorrhagia accompanying otherwise normal cycles in the presence of a normal pelvic examination can be due to submucous leiomyomata or endometrial polyps that usually are revealed by ultrasound, especially if performed with fluid contrast in the endometrial cavity (sonohysterography) (13). These polyps rarely bleed enough to cause a clinically significant anemia but may cause 1) intermenstrual bleeding that is sometimes related to defecation or 2) postcoital bleeding if located in the endocervical canal. If examination and these studies fail to detect polyps, thorough endometrial sampling should be done to exclude endometrial hyperplasia or more severe lesions. The patient's bleeding may be observed after definitive benign histologic diagnosis is made with endometrial biopsy or dilatation and curettage.

Other Etiologies of Intermenstrual Bleeding

Abnormal bleeding episodes superimposed on normal menstrual cycles are approached in the same manner as menorrhagia: the focus of evaluation is on the possibility of neoplasm in the vagina, cervix, or uterus. Careful examination and Pap smear are indicated in all cases; ultrasound imaging and dilatation and curettage, with or without hysteroscopy, are indicated in many cases. Recall that brief, isolated periovulatory bleeding is normal in some women. Premenstrual spotting with an otherwise negative evaluation is also not uncommon and can be managed expectantly. This bleeding pattern has been associated with the presence of pelvic endometriosis, but this possibility should not be pursued (by laparoscopic evaluation, for example) unless dictated by other symptoms or findings.

The Perimenopausal Patient

The Perimenopause

Perimenopause usually commences in the fifth decade, heralded by alterations in menstrual rhythm. It is in this age group that the term *dysfunctional uterine bleeding* is most commonly applied to the menstrual history. Although the transition to the postmenopausal state for some is brief and uncomplicated, the normal perimenopause is characterized in many women by the unpredictable occurrence of both shortened and lengthened ovulatory cycles as well as by anovulatory episodes commencing well before menopause (36,37). The resulting menstrual chaos causes inconvenience, frustration, and anxiety. For the physician, distinguishing those patients whose symptoms are the result of the expected dysfunction of this transition from those who harbor gynecologic pathology can be particularly challenging.

The perimenopausal woman is at increased risk for endometrial hyperplasia, endometrial polyps, and leiomyomata. The age-specific incidence of cervical cancer also peaks at this time and that of endometrial cancer begins to increase. In addition to excluding pregnancy many patients with abnormal patterns and amounts of flow will require endometrial biopsy and ultrasound. If biopsy results indicate hyperplasia with atypical features, then dilatation and curettage, with or without hysteroscopy, should be performed to exclude more severe coexistent pathology. Dilatation and curettage is also indicated when the ultrasound detects discrete abnormalities or irregularity of the endometrial canal or endometrial lining, which suggests that endometrial biopsy may not be representative (19).

When combined with sonography of the endometrial stripe, endometrial biopsy has a high sensitivity in detecting endometrial carcinoma. However, further evaluation with D&C is sometimes needed, particularly when the uterus is enlarged or irregular, when imaging suggests gross lesions in the endometrial cavity, or when unexplained bleeding persists.

Dysfunctional Uterine Bleeding

Women approaching the end of the reproductive spectrum often exhibit menstrual changes up to a decade before the onset of menopausal symptoms. Because of declining ovarian function, many but not all women first develop a briefer luteal phase, manifest as a gradual shortening of the menstrual cycle from 28 to 30 days to approximately 3 weeks. With time, the number of remaining oocytes further decreases. The menstrual cycle then typically lengthens, and patients may often note bleeding patterns consistent with ovulatory cycles interspersed with anovulatory ones.

When intermenstrual spotting occurs in the perimenopausal patient, the possibility of underlying pathology is suggested. Also of concern are cycles that are unexpectedly short, shortened cycles that occur in the patient with risk factors for endometrial carcinoma (see Endometrial Neoplasia section), and menstrual changes that are particularly alarming to the patient. Such patients should all undergo evaluation to exclude other etiologies of disordered

Although menstrual irregularity is common in this age group, cycles shorter than 3 weeks and intermenstrual spotting in perimenopausal patients both suggest the possibility of underlying disease.

bleeding, in particular endometrial neoplasia, and usually require endometrial biopsy and pelvic ultrasound.

When the endometrial biopsy and ultrasound are normal or indicate uncomplicated hyperplasia, or for the patient at low risk for endometrial neoplasia diagnosed with dysfunctional uterine bleeding on the basis of history and physical alone, hormonal management can be prescribed. Low-dose combined oral contraceptives are often helpful. Women may safely take combined oral contraceptives after the age of 35 if they do not smoke cigarettes and have no other contraindication. Patients who are not candidates for oral contraceptives may be given cyclic progestins in the form of medroxyprogesterone acetate 10 mg orally daily for 10 consecutive days each month. This will induce regular withdrawal bleeding, although this approach lacks the advantage of providing contraception. Alternatively, an injectable progestin (e.g., Depo-Provera) can be used in an attempt to suppress bleeding altogether. Note that postmenopausal HRT generally provides inadequate doses of hormone to correct dysfunctional uterine bleeding.

If hormonal treatment fails to regulate bleeding within a few cycles, then the low-risk patients who did not first undergo endometrial evaluation must now do so. However, frequently no pathology is found, because ongoing superimposed, dyssynchronous ovulatory and anovulatory ovarian function can confound attempts at hormonal management. In such situations, when faced with the prospect of persistent unpredictable bleeding, the patient will sometimes opt for definitive surgical management. However, physician support and vigilance may avert hysterectomy, a common outcome for bleeding complaints in this age group (17). (For further discussion see Chapter 14.)

The Postmenopausal Patient

Bleeding after the Menopause

There are several different etiologies for bleeding after the menopause, though this symptom is the only symptom many women have of endometrial neoplasia and this must be ruled out first. When *unexpected* bleeding occurs in the setting of HRT, similar concern should be raised (see Chapter 16) (18). Fortunately, however, the most common form of postmenopausal bleeding is that occurring from a nonestrogenized, atrophic endometrium. Atrophic changes may also affect the vagina, causing thinning and fragility of the vaginal mucosa. This condition predisposes to bleeding after pelvic examination or coitus, and a vaginal tear is often evident. Aside from the expected bleeding in the setting of HRT, all vaginal bleeding in the postmenopausal woman should be regarded as resulting from a genital tract malignancy until proven otherwise. Careful clinical examination and endometrial biopsy are mandatory.

Endometrial Neoplasia

Endometrial carcinoma is the most common of the gynecologic malignancies and is also one of the most treatable due to the fact that it is usually diagnosed at an early stage. The heralding symptom is typically postmenopausal bleeding, which always requires immediate investigation.

The underlying cause of endometrial neoplasia is unopposed estrogen stimulation. This has been clearly documented in studies of women receiving unopposed estrogen HRT. Indeed, as little as 1 year of therapy with low dose (0.625 mg/d) unopposed conjugated estrogen carries a 20% incidence of endometrial hyperplasia and a more than doubled risk of endometrial carcinoma over the general population. Thus estrogen-only HRT is almost never acceptable in women who still have a uterus (see Chapter 16). Patients

> *Because endometrial neoplasia is caused by unopposed estrogen stimulation, patients at higher risk include those with diabetes mellitus, obesity, nulliparity, PCOS, early menarche, and late menopause.*

prescribed combination HRT must be counseled as to the importance of the progestin and be advised not to self-discontinue this component.

It logically follows that other patients at higher risk for endometrial neoplasia have conditions resulting in prolonged, excessive estrogen exposure, such as nulliparity, obesity, diabetes mellitus, early menarche, late menopause, and history of PCOS. Hypertension is also a risk factor for endometrial neoplasia, though the mechanism is unclear. Because it is progestin dominant, hormonal contraception confers a protective effect.

All patients must be counseled to inform their physician immediately if postmenopausal bleeding should occur, regardless of the quantity. The patient should be examined as soon as possible, and an endometrial biopsy should be performed in the office. If the biopsy cannot be performed or reveals tissue insufficient for histologic diagnosis, then formal dilation and curettage is indicated. A possible exception to this rule is the woman using combined continuous hormonal replacement in whom pelvic ultrasound is completely reassuring with the finding of a thin (5 mm or less) endometrial lining lacking irregularity, because the risk of hyperplasia is very low in this setting (20,21). Such a patient should be offered the option of either dilatation and curettage to obtain definitive histologic diagnosis or continued observation. Should she opt for observation, persistence of symptoms dictates the need for further evaluation.

Treatment strategies are determined by the degree of proliferation found on endometrial biopsy. Recall that atrophy and progestational atrophy are benign, as well as proliferative endometrium, which can be seen in the reproductive-age patient or some patients receiving exogenous estrogen. However, the finding of simple hyperplasia without atypia suggests prolonged, unopposed estrogen exposure, and should be treated with a 6-month course of progestins (e.g., medroxyprogesterone actetate daily for 10 consecutive days each month or Depo-Provera injection every 2 months). After 6 months of progestin therapy the endometrial biopsy is often repeated to confirm transformation back to a secretory pattern. The risk of simple hyperplasia progressing to endometrial carcinoma is low (1% to 3%) (1).

Although complex hyperplasia is also of low malignant potential (16), endometrial biopsy is only up to 90% accurate; therefore further evaluation with dilatation and curettage is usually performed to exclude more serious endometrial foci. The vast majority of patients with complex hyperplasia will demonstrate regression with progestin therapy and can be followed with serial endometrial biopsies. Hysterectomy is sometimes appropriate for postmenopausal women and for patients desiring definitive surgical therapy.

Complex hyperplasia with atypical features is clearly premalignant. Dilatation and curettage is warranted to exclude concomitant carcinoma that office sampling with endometrial biopsy may have missed. Even in the absence of cancer, this diagnosis is treated aggressively, because complex atypical hyperplasia will progress to adenocarcinoma in up to 28% of patients (1). Hysterectomy is considered the management of choice in the woman who has completed childbearing, unless her operative risks mandate a trial of medical therapy (17). For patients who strongly desire future fertility (relevant in the setting of polycystic ovary disease) or for those who decline surgery, aggressive high-dose progestin therapy may reverse atypia. After 6 months of treatment, the endometrial biopsy is repeated to confirm transformation back to a secretory pattern. When possible, all patients with this histologic diagnosis should be managed by a gynecologist.

Endometrial carcinoma is treated with hysterectomy and staging, although it should be noted that sometimes gynecologists manage well-differentiated carcinoma more conservatively in the young patient who desires future fertility.

Conclusion

Patients with abnormal bleeding complaints have widely variable presentations and a multitude of potential etiologies that may at first seem daunting to the generalist. However, knowledge of the normal menstrual cycle, careful history taking, and thorough physical examination can often quickly distinguish dysfunctional uterine bleeding from bleeding due to "local" gynecologic causes. Identification of the common etiologies in each age group can then help shorten the differential diagnosis. When necessary, laboratory testing, endometrial biopsy, imaging studies, and referral to specialists are appropriate. One can then assign an etiology to the abnormal bleeding and intervene with a safe and effective course of management.

REFERENCES

1. **Erickson GF.** An analysis of follicle development and ovum maturation. Semin Reprod Endocrinol. 1986;4:233.

2. **Filicori M, Santoro N, Merriam GR, Crowley WF.** Characterization of the physiological pattern of episodic gonadotropin secretion throughout the human menstrual cycle. J Clin Endocrinol Metab. 1986;62:1136.

3. **Carr JS, Reid RL.** Ovulation induction with gonadotropin-releasing hormone (GnRH). Semin Reprod Endocrinol. 1990;8:174.

4. "Amenorrhea" and "anovulation" and the polycystic ovary. In: Speroff L, Glass RH, Kase NG, eds.Clinical Gynecologic Endocrinology and Infertility, 5th ed. Baltimore: Williams & Wilkins; 1994:401-82.

5. **Vollman RF.** The menstrual cycle. In: Friedman E, ed. Major Problems in Obstetrics and Gynecology. Phildelphia: WB Saunders; 1977.

6. **Lenton EA, Landgren B, Sexton L, Harper R.** Normal variation in the length of the follicular phase of the menstrual cycle: effect of chronologic age. Br J Obstet Gynecol. 1984;91:681.

7. **Gusberg SB, Milano C.** Detection of endometrial carcinoma and its precursors. Cancer. 1981;47:1173.

8. **Ng ABP, Reagan JW, Hawliczek CT, Wentz BW.** Significance of endometrial cells in the detection of endometrial carcinoma and its precursors. Acta Cytol. 1974;18:356.

9. **Zucker PK, Kasdon EJ, Feldstein ML.** The validity of Pap smear parameters as predictors of endometrial pathology in menopausal women. Cancer. 1985;56:2256.

10. **Gomez-Fernandez CR, Ganjei-Azar P, Capote-Dishaw J.** Reporting normal endometrial cells in Pap smears: an outcome appraisal. Gynecol Onc. 1999;74:381-4.

11. **Zweizig S, Noller K, Reale F, et al.** Neoplasia associated with atypical glandular cells of undetermined significance on cervical cytology. Gynecol Oncol. 1997;65:314-8.

12. **Gay JD, Donaldson LD, Grellner JR.** False negative results on cervical cytologic studies. Acta Cytol. 1985;29:1043-6.

13. **Ash SJ, Farrell SA, Flowerdew G.** Endometrial biopsy in DUB. J Reprod Med. 1996;41:892-6.

14. **Langer RD, Pierce JJ, O'Hanlan KA, et al.** Transvaginal ultrasonography compared with endometrial biopsy for the detection of endometrial disease. Postmenopausal Estrogen/Progestin Interventions Trial. N Engl J Med. 1997;337:1792-8.

15. **Youssif SN. McMillan DL.** Outpatient endometrial biopsy: the pipelle. Hosp Med. 1995;54:198-201.

16. **Kurman RJ, Kaminski PF, Norris HJ.** The behavior of endometrial hyperplasia: a long-term study of "untreated" hyperplasia in 170 patients. Cancer. 1985;56:403.

17. **Ferenczy A, Gelfand MM.** Hyperplasia vs. neoplasia: two tracks for the endometrium? Contemp Obstet Gynecol. 1986;28:79.

18. **Meuwissen JH, Oddens BJ, Klinkhamer PJ.** Endometrial thickness assessed by transvaginal ultrasound insufficiently predicts occurrence of hyperplasia during unopposed oestrogen use. Maturitas. 1996;24:21-30.

19. **O'Connell LP, Fries MH, Zeringue E, Brehm W.** Triage of abnormal postmenopausal bleeding: a comparison of endometrial biopsy and transvaginal sonohysterography versus fractional curettage with hysteroscopy. Am J Obstet Gynecol. 1998;178:956-61.

20. **Goldstein SR, Zeltser I, Horan CK, et al.** Ultrasonography-based triage for perimenopausal patients with abnormal uterine bleeding. Am J Obstet Gynecol. 1997;177: 102-8.

21. **Weber AM, Belinson JL, Bradley LD., Piedmonte MR.** Vaginal ultrasonography versus endometrial biopsy in women with postmenopausal bleeding. Am J Obstet Gynecol. 1997;177:924-9.

22. **Kadir RA, Economides DL, Sabin CA, et al.** Frequency of inherited bleeding disorders in women with menorrhagia. Lancet. 1998;351:485-9.

23. **Xiao E, Ferin M.** Stress-related disturbances of the menstrual cycle. Ann Med. 1997;29:215-9.

24. **Rencken ML, Chesnut CH 3rd, Drinkwater BL.** Bone density at multiple skeletal sites in amenorrheic athletes. JAMA. 1996;276:1384-5.

25. **Warren MP.** Effect of exercise and physical training on menarche. Semin Reprod Endocrinol. 1985;3:17.

26. **Hetland ML, Harbo J, Christiansen C, Larsen T.** Running induces menstrual disturbances but bone mass is unaffected except in amenorrheic female athletes. Am J Med. 1993;95:53-60.

27. **Prior JC, Vigne YM, Barr SL, et al.** Cyclic medroxyprogesterone treatment increases bone density: a controlled trial in active women with menstrual cycle disturbances. Am J Med. 1994;96:521-30.

28. **Hull HGR.** Epidemiology of infertility and polycystic ovarian disease: endocrinological and demographic studies. Gynecol Endocrinol. 1987;1:235.

29. **Polson DW, Wadsworth J, Adams J, Franks S.** Polycystic ovaries: a common finding in normal women. Lancet. 1988;2:870.

30. **Lobo RA, Carmina E.** The importance of diagnosing the polycystic ovary syndrome. Ann Intern Med. 2000;132:989-93.

31. **Valaszquez E, Acosta A, Mendoza SG.** Menstrual cyclicity after metformin therapy in polycystic ovary syndrome. Obstet Gynecol. 1997;90;392-5.

32. **Ehrmann DA.** Insulin-lowering therapuetic modalities for polycystic ovary syndrome. Endocrinol Metab Clin North Am. 1999;28:423-8.

33. **Dahlgren E, Johansson S, Lindstedt G, et al.** Women with polycystic ovary syndrome wedge resected in 1956 to 1965: a long-term follow-up focusing on natural history and circulating hormones. Fertil Steril. 1992;57:505-13.

34. **Mather KJ, Kwan F, Corenblum B.** Hyperinsulinemia in polycystic ovary syndrome correlates with increased cardiovascular risk independent of obesity. Fertil Steril. 2000;73:150-6.

35. **Govind A, Obhrai MS, Clayton RN.** Polycystic ovaries are inherited as an autosomal dominant trait: analysis of 29 polycystic ovary syndrome and 10 control families. J Clin Endocrinol Metab. 1999;84:38-43.

36. **Santoro N, Brown JR, Adel T, Skurnick JH.** Characterization of reproductive hormonal dynamics in the perimenopause. J Clin Endocrinol Metab. 1996;81:1495-1501.

37. **Prior JC.** Perimenopause: the complex endocrinology of the menopausal transition. Endocr Rev. 1998;19:397-428.

CHAPTER 4

Premenstrual Syndrome

JANICE RYDEN, MD

On approach of a woman in this state, new wine becomes sour, grass withers away, and fruit falls from the tree beneath which she sits.

Pliny the Elder [23–79], NATURAL HISTORY

The above observation, nearly 2000 years old, attests to the long-standing recognition of what is now known as premenstrual syndrome (PMS). However, no scientific papers were published on the topic until 1931, when an American physician, R. T. Frank, vividly described a cyclical state that he termed *premenstrual tension* (1). Considerable research in the past few decades has shed light on the syndrome, but the etiology remains elusive. This is reflected in the vagueness of the current definition of PMS: a collection of physical, emotional, and behavioral symptoms that recur in a monthly pattern and begin approximately 1 week before menses and remit within 1 week following the onset of the menstrual period.

More than 100 symptoms of PMS have been described in the literature, many of which are listed in Table 4-1. The more commonly noted symptoms include depressed or labile mood, irritability, fatigue, concentration and memory difficulties, emotional "oversensitivity," social withdrawal, insomnia, abdominal bloating, edema, headache, acne, breast tenderness, gastrointestinal upset, appetite changes, and food cravings (2). Also frequently noted are anxiety, anger, increased interpersonal conflicts, hypersomnia, and a subjective sense of feeling overwhelmed or "out of control" (3). The clinical appearances of PMS can vary from person to person, although the syndrome is generally consistent across menstrual cycles in a given women.

Table 4-1 Common Premenstrual Symptoms*

Psychological Symptoms	Somatic Symptoms
• Depressed mood	• Fatigue
• Labile mood	• Insomnia
• Irritability	• Hypersomnia
• Difficulty concentrating	• Abdominal bloating
• Oversensitivity	• Edema
• Social withdrawal	• Headache
• Insomnia	• Breast tenderness
• Anxiety	• Acne
• Anger	• Gastrointestinal upset
• Memory difficulties	• Appetite changes
• Subjective sense of feeling overwhelmed or "out of control"	• Food cravings

*Patients with PMS often report both somatic and psychological symptoms. Note that dysmenorrhea ("painful menses") is not part of the premenstrual syndrome, because it is a menstrual complaint that results from prostaglandin activity.

To meet criteria for PMS the symptoms must affect predominantly the late luteal and early menstrual phases, with a significant decline in or absence of symptoms during the week immediately before and following ovulation. The symptoms must be documented by means of prospective self-reported diaries over a minimum of two or three menstrual cycles. All authors agree that by definition the syndrome must be diagnosed in the absence of any pharmacologic therapy, hormone administration (including oral contraceptives), or drug or alcohol abuse. Various authors have added their own specific restrictions to the diagnosis of PMS, whereas others have argued that such formal limitations are premature given our limited understanding of the syndrome. For example, some authors stipulate that the symptoms must be of great enough severity to affect the patient's social life or work performance. In this regard their definitions resemble the DSM-IV entity for premenstrual dysphoric disorder.

Premenstrual dysphoric disorder (PMDD) (Table 4-2), called "late luteal phase dysphoric disorder" (LLPDD) when introduced in the DSM III-R, focuses predominantly on psychological symptoms. As a consequence of this and its requirement for socioeconomic dysfunction, it is actually a more severe subset of PMS, although the terms PMDD and PMS are often used interchangeably in the literature. One should note that neither LLPDD nor PMDD has been placed in the main body of the DSM due to "insufficient information to warrant inclusion" but instead have been relegated to an appendix (3).

The timing of premenstrual symptoms coincides with falling levels of serum estrogen and progesterone in the latter half of the luteal phase and the

Table 4-2 DSM-IV Research Criteria for Premenstrual Dysphoric Disorder

A. In most menstrual cycles during the past year, five (or more) of the following symptoms were present for most of the time during the last week of the luteal phase, began to remit within a few days after the onset of the follicular phase, and were absent in the week post-menses, with at least one of the symptoms being either (1), (2), (3), or (4):*
  (1) markedly depressed mood, feelings of hopelessness, or self-deprecating thoughts
  (2) marked anxiety, tension, feelings of being "keyed up" or "on edge"
  (3) marked affective lability (e.g., feeling suddenly sad or tearful, increased sensitivity to rejection)
  (4) persistent and marked anger or irritability or increased interpersonal conflicts
  (5) decreased interest in usual activities (e.g., work, school, friends, hobbies)
  (6) subjective sense of difficulty in concentrating
  (7) lethargy, easy fatigability, or marked lack of energy
  (8) marked change in appetite, overeating, or specific food cravings
  (9) hypersomnia or insomnia
  (10) a subjective sense of being overwhelmed or out of control
  (11) other physical symptoms, such as breast tenderness or swelling, headaches, joint or muscle pain, a sensation of "bloating," weight gain
B. The disturbance markedly interferes with work or school or with usual social activities and relationships with others (e.g., avoidance of social activities, decreased productivity and efficacy at work or school).
C. The disturbance is not merely an exacerbation of the symptoms of another disorder, such as major depressive disorder, panic disorder, dysthymic disorder, or a personality disorder (although it may be superimposed on any of these disorders).
D. Criteria A, B, and C must be confirmed by prospective daily ratings during at least two consecutive symptomatic cycles. (The diagnosis may be made provisionally prior to this confirmation.)

*In menstruating females, the luteal phase corresponds to the period between ovulation and the onset of menses, and the follicular phase begins with menses. In nonmenstruating females (e.g., those who have had a hysterectomy), the timing of luteal and follicular phases may require measurement of circulating reproductive hormones. (From Diagnostic and Statistical Manual of Mental Disorders, 4th edition (DSM-IV). American Psychiatric Association; with permission.)

first week of the follicular phase (Fig. 4-1). A possible casual relationship is suggested but cannot be assumed, because not every menstruating woman suffers from PMS. The cyclical pattern of symptoms has been replicated in numerous studies of women with PMS but is not seen in controls. Women who suffer from PMS will generally be free of symptoms during pregnancy or the occasional anovulatory cycle (4). Ovariectomy will also lead to the disappearance of the clinical symptoms, but hysterectomy alone will not (5).

Epidemiology

Estimates of the prevalence of PMS vary widely, from 5% to 90%, with the most commonly cited figure being one third of all ovulating women. Clearly,

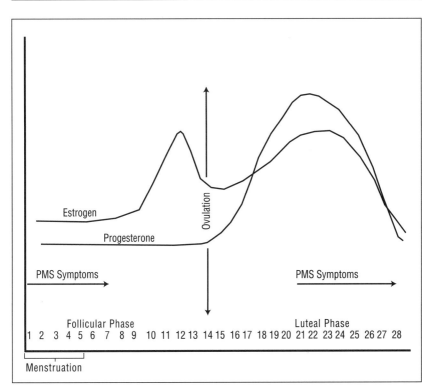

Figure 4-1 Schematic of the timing of PMS symptoms in relation to menstrual cycle events and hormone levels. Women with PMS suffer cyclic symptoms that begin at any time during the latter half of the luteal phase and continue into the first week of the next follicular phase (i.e., during menses). Some sufferers also report one day of PMS symptoms immediately following ovulation.

the prevalence estimates vary in part due to differences in the severity requirements of definitions being used. Researchers generally agree that the majority of women (approximately 75%) report minor or isolated, mostly somatic, premenstrual changes, and that 5% of ovulating women are severely affected, with this latter figure demonstrating consistency across different cultures.

The onset of PMS may be at any time but as early as menarche, with cessation of symptoms occurring reliably by or sometimes before menopause. Although some researchers have described the typical course as one of gradual worsening of symptoms over time until menopause, other studies have observed peak symptom severity to be in the late twenties to mid-thirties (6). Overall, however, epidemiologic studies of PMS have failed to demonstrate any age-specific association. Also, there does not appear to be a consistent correlation with personality traits, parity, menstrual cycle characteristics, socioeconomic status, diet, exercise habits, or stress (7). A study of twins suggests a possible genetic susceptibility to PMS, because the correlation coefficient of PMS symptom scores for monozygotic twins (0.55) was found to be nearly double that for dizygotic ones (0.28) (8).

PMS appears to be a universal phenomenon. It has been identified in every culture studied, from industrialized settings to less developed communities such as the Apache Indians (9). Two cross-cultural studies are worthy of mention. The first examined girls and women in the general population of a remote farming village in Italy (10). When questioned in a retrospective fashion the study subjects reported that the menstrual phase was the worst time of the month for them. However, their completed prospective symptom diaries exhibited classic premenstrual syndrome patterns, with symptoms starting in the late luteal phase and continuing into the menstrual phase. Moreover, when compared with data previously collected from American women, their PMS symptom scores were generally higher. This despite the fact that 78.7% of the Italian subjects reported never having heard of PMS.

The second study was a retrospective questionnaire presented to 400 Kenyan nursing students and nurses (11). Nearly 96% of the women reported at least one premenstrual complaint, but 98.4% considered it a normal part of their menstrual cycles and femininity, and only 6.5% reported having sought medical treatment. Unlike findings in the Italian study, the PMS symptoms in the Kenyans did not result in any sick role behavior such as absences from school or work. However, 26% of the surveyed women did admit to curbing voluntary activities such as going shopping or visiting relatives. Overall, the symptom complaints resembled those of Western women, with the exception of an absence of reported cravings for sweets, which was attributed to a lack of familiarity with such food.

Etiology

Until the latter half of the 20th century PMS was felt to be a psychological disorder stemming from an internal conflict surrounding the feminine role. This theory is no longer tenable, in part due to nonhuman primate studies in which animals have been observed displaying distinct changes in their feeding and social activities during the premenstrual and menstrual period. In a study of yellow baboons in the wild, for example, observers noted that during the five days before and after menstrual onset there was an abrupt increase in the time spent feeding and a decrease in the rate of participation in social interactions of all types (Fig. 4-2) (12).

A second primate study examined captive rhesus monkeys and revealed a similar sharp decline in copulation rates four to six days before the onset of menstruation (13). Another observation was a lack of cooperation for vitamin

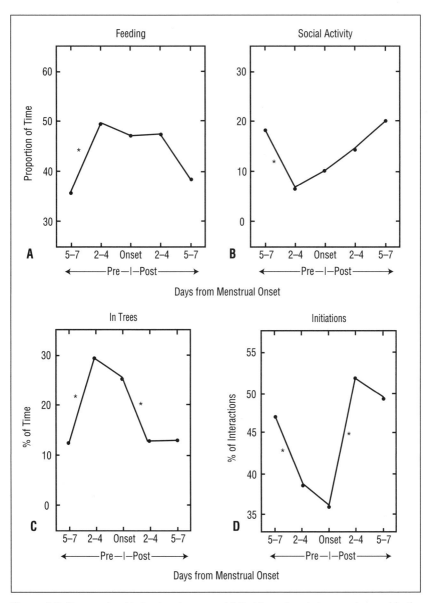

Figure 4-2 Premenstrual behavior changes exhibited by yellow baboons observed in the natural setting. The four graphs depict abrupt changes in the behavior of the yellow baboons beginning approximately 5 days before the onset of the menstrual period. The first plot (panel *A*) demonstrates a sudden increase in the time spent in feeding; the second plot (panel *B*) shows a simultaneous decrease in the time devoted to social acitvities. The lower pair of graphs (panels *C* and *D*) illustrates similar information using different data points. During the premenstrual period, the baboons spend more time in trees (where they feed) and initiate fewer social interactions. (From Hausfater G, Skoblick B. Premenstrual behavior changes among female yellow baboons: some similarities to premenstrual syndrome (PMS) in women. Am J Primatol. 1985;9:165-72; with permission.)

administration throughout both the premenstrual and menstrual phases. Also, in contrast to the solitary behavior of the baboons, this study observed a premenstrual rise in the incidence of aggression. As the female monkeys entered the premenstrual phase there was an abrupt and striking increase in their being frequently attacked and bitten. Shortly thereafter, during their menstrual period, the females themselves displayed an increase in initiating aggressive behavior towards others. It is unclear whether this observed cyclic increase in aggressive behavior by the rhesus monkeys represents an interspecies difference or the effect of captivity.

Hormonal and Neuroendocrine Studies

The obvious question as to whether women with PMS have altered levels of gonadal hormones has been raised and investigated. Most studies have failed to detect a difference in estrogen, progesterone, or androgen levels, despite initial data that misled practitioners for decades. Moreover and despite common practice, well-designed trials have shown that empiric administration of progesterone during the luteal phase does not ameliorate PMS symptoms (2). Similarly, treatment with oral contraceptives has not proven effective, and indeed these can exacerbate PMS symptoms in some but not all sufferers (14). Curiously, a clinical picture resembling PMS can also occur in some postmenopausal women when progesterone is added to their estrogen replacement therapy (15). Such findings lead one to wonder whether women with PMS have altered end-organ sensitivity to gonadal hormones, progesterone in particular.

One experimental study administered the potent progesterone antagonist mifepristone (Mifeprex, or "RU486") to PMS suffers immediately after ovulation in order to, in effect, bypass the luteal phase by inducing an early menses (16). Quite surprisingly, such manipulation of the menstrual cycle failed to prevent PMS symptoms, because they nevertheless occurred during the arti-

Symptoms resembling PMS can result from postmenopausal hormone replacement that contains progesterone.

ficially premature follicular phase. This unexpected result has been difficult to reconcile with previous implications of progesterone activity.

However, recent research may help crystallize available data with its finding of altered progesterone *metabolism* in women with PMS (17,18). Luteal phase levels of the progesterone metabolite allopregnanolone have recently been found to be lower in PMS sufferers compared with controls. Because allopregnanolone normally acts as an agonist on the gamma-aminobutyric acid (GABA-A) pathway in the central nervous system (CNS) (similar to the benzodiazepine class of drugs), a deficiency would be expected to lead to anxiety, tension, and depression—thereby explaining many of the PMS symptoms.

Such a direct connection between ovarian steroids and CNS activity may at first seem unexpected; however, earlier research has revealed other instances of sex hormone activity in the realm of neuroendocrinology. For example, it has long been established that progesterone metabolites protect against epileptic seizures. The increased incidence of seizure episodes (for most seizure types) during the late luteal and menstrual phases is attributable to the cyclic decline of levels of these hormones. The progesterone metabolites raise the seizure threshold through their agonistic action on the GABA-A receptors—similar to their effect on mood. Although other biochemical pathways are not as clearly elucidated, many experimental findings support the concept that cyclical changes in the CNS environment are responsible for the generation of PMS and PMDD symptoms. For example, studies reveal lower plasma levels of beta-endorphins around the time of ovulation in PMS sufferers compared with controls (19). Also, the plasma levels of beta-endorphins in normal women are equal in the follicular and luteal phases, whereas levels in PMS patients are lower during the luteal phase compared with their own levels during the follicular phase and with luteal phase levels of nonsufferers (20). Also, in normal women, plasma levels of GABA-A increase from the mid-follicular to the late luteal phase, whereas they remain low during both phases in women who suffer from PMS, as well as in women with a past history of major depressive disorder (21).

Evidence for serotonergic dysfunction is also quite striking and it may very well play the central role in the generation of PMS symptoms, in particular the classic disturbances in affect, carbohydrate cravings, impulsivity, and sleep disruption. For example, while in normal women whole-blood serotonin levels rise beginning one week before menstruation, serotonin levels decline during the luteal phase in women who suffer PMS (22). Also, women who suffer from PMS have decreased platelet uptake of serotonin in the late luteal phase (23).

Two studies that experimentally altered plasma levels of tryptophan, the precursor of serotonin, lend further support. The first employed the dietary technique of acute tryptophan depletion, which suppresses serotonin synthesis in the brain. PMS symptoms were acutely aggravated in half of the subjects tested (24), similar to what has previously been observed in remitted depressives, but not in control women. A second study examined the converse: the effect on PMS symptoms of a specially formulated, carbohydrate-rich beverage that increases the relative amount of tryptophan. Self-reported scores for anger, depression, carbohydrate craving, and cognitive function all improved significantly 90–180 min following ingestion (25). Experimental trials with dex-fenfluramine (a serotonergic agent) also significantly decreased premenstrual depression, anxiety scores, and cravings for carbohydrates. As will be discussed later (see Treatment section below), selective serotonin reuptake inhibitors (SSRIs) have also been shown to be highly effective for PMS symptoms, lending further support to the serotonin hypothesis.

An alternative theory holds that PMS is merely a variant of affective disorder, as there are obvious links between affective disorders and PMS. For example, the family history prevalence and personal lifetime occurrence of major depression is higher for those who suffer from PMS than for unaffected controls (26). Also, a single night of partial sleep deprivation early in the luteal phase can prevent PMS symptoms for that entire cycle (27). Such improvement resembles the temporary improvement in mood seen in persons suffering from major depression, but contrasts with the effect of sleep deprivation on normal subjects, in whom dysthymia results.

Explanations for these connections between PMS and major depression include the possibility that repetitive, monthly episodes of premenstrual depression lead to the development of a later major depression. Conversely, perhaps women with major depression that is incompletely resolved experience monthly periods of depression exclusively during the "biologically vulnerable time."

Perhaps the association of the two conditions simply points to a common underlying predisposing factor. It must be emphasized, however, that PMS is clearly distinguishable both clinically and biochemically from major depression. Women with major depression have continuous symptoms throughout the menstrual cycle, and sometimes have demonstrable endocrine abnormalities such as cortisol nonsuppression after dexamethasone administration, which is never seen in women with PMS (28).

Diagnosis

The typical woman with PMS goes to the physician with any of a variety of somatic or psychological symptom complaints that begin during the latter half of the luteal phase of the menstrual cycle and remit within one week after the onset of menstruation—sometimes within a few hours. A significant proportion of PMS sufferers experience a biphasic pattern, with symptoms also occurring briefly for one day immediately following ovulation. In taking the history, one should screen carefully for other disorders that are frequently diagnosed in women who present with a chief compliant of PMS (viz., major depression, anxiety disorders, eating disorders, substance abuse, hypothyroidism). When depression or anxiety disorders are suspected, suicidality and homicidality need to be assessed. No physical findings are evident in PMS, although an examination could potentially uncover signs of a medical problem such as hypothyroidism or stigmata of substance abuse or eating disorders. Similarly, no laboratory testing is currently available.

The diagnosis of PMS is therefore established solely on the basis of reported symptoms. Given that none of the symptoms of PMS is pathognomonic, the key to diagnosing the syndrome hinges on detecting its cyclical pattern. Authors agree that the diagnosis can be made only by means of a diary of self-rated daily symptoms recorded over a minimum period of two menstrual cycles (Fig. 4-3). The symptom diary is currently the only available diagnostic tool for research and clinical purposes.

The importance of the symptom diary cannot be overemphasized. In some clinics the recording of symptoms in this manner excluded the diagnosis of PMS in the majority of the women presenting with such a chief complaint. The reason for this is uncertain, but for many women with a substance abuse problem or other psychiatric illness, PMS may simply represent a more acceptable label than their actual diagnosis. Also, the symptoms of certain medical conditions (e.g., hypothyroidism, migraines, irritable bowel syndrome, allergies and asthma) (29) and psychiatric conditions (e.g., major depression, anxiety disorders) typically worsen during the late luteal phase. This "premenstrual magnification" of an underlying condition is actually more common than pure PMDD. Patients who sense this cyclic worsening of their symptoms may incorrectly self-diagnose their condition as PMS. In such situations the symptom diary would clarify the diagnosis, because it would demonstrate symptoms persisting throughout the month with a superimposed cyclic exacerbation during the late luteal phase. Thus, although patients are often eager to start treatment at their first visit to a physician, it is of utmost importance to first make the diagnosis properly through the use of the symptom diary.

Although patients are often eager to start treatment for PMS, it is of utmost importance to first make the diagnosis properly through the use of a symptom diary maintained over a minimum of two menstrual cycles.

It is often helpful to orient the patient to the symptom diary at the time of her office visit by helping her articulate and list the symptoms she wishes to track and instructing her in its use. Starting that night and each night upon retiring she should reflect upon the magnitude of her symptoms for that day and self-rate and record them, using a numbered scale (typically 0 for "none" to 5 for "severe"). She should also record the dates of her menstrual period on the calendar so that her luteal phase is apparent. She should be given three copies of the calendar and use it nightly until her next scheduled follow-up appointment in approximately 8 to 10 weeks.

1. Circle dates of menstrual period.   2. Rate symptoms on a scale of 1 to 5 (1 = mild, 5 = severe).   3. Leave blank if no symptoms.

MONTH: _August_

Symptom	1	2	3	4	5	6	7	8	9	10	11	12	13	(14)	(15)	(16)	(17)	(18)	(19)	20	21	22	23	24	25	26	27	28	29	30	31
fatigue	2	2	3	3	3	3	3	3	3	3	3	3	3	3	1												1	1	1	1	2
bloating	2	2	3	3	3	3	3	3	3	3	3	3	3	3		1											1	1	1	1	2
sleeplessness	2	2		3	2		3	3	2	3	3	2	3	3													1	2			2
irritable	2	2	2	3	3	2	3	3	3	3	3	3	3	3	2												2	2	2	2	2
craving chocolate	2	3	3	3	3	3	3	3	3	3	3	3	3	3														1	1	1	1
sadness	2	3	3	3	3	3	3	3	3	3	3	3	3	3	2												2	2	2	2	2
can't concentrate	2	3	3	3	3	3	3	3	3	3	3	3	3	3	2												2	2	2	2	2

Day

MONTH: _September_

Symptom	1	2	3	4	5	6	7	8	9	(10)	(11)	(12)	(13)	(14)	15	16	17	18	19	20	21	22	23	24	25	26	27	28	29	30	31
fatigue	2	2	2	2	3	3	3	3	3	3																2	2	2	2	2	2
bloating	2	2	2	2	3	3	3	3	3	3		1														1	2	2	2	2	2
sleeplessness	2	2	2	2	2	2	3	3	1	3																	1	2	2	1	
irritable	2	2	2	2	3	2	3	3	2	3	3															1	1	1	2	1	2
craving chocolate	2	2	2	3	3	3	3	3	3	3	3												1			1	1	1	2	2	2
sadness	2	2	3	3	3	3	3	3	3	3	3	3	3											1			1	2	2	2	2
can't concentrate	2	2	3	3	3	3	3	3	3	3	3	3	3											1			1	2	2	2	2

Day

Figure 4-3 Sample PMS symptom diary from a patient with severe documented PMS. Note the concentration of symptoms in the late luteal and early menstrual phases and the virtual absence of symptoms in the week surrounding ovulation. This pattern readily distinguishes the patient's PMS from a luteal phase exacerbation of another underlying disorder such as major depression. (Adapted from Figure 4 in Johnson SR. Clinician's approach to the diagnosis and management of PMS. Clin Obstet Gynecol. 1992;35:637-57.)

At the follow-up appointment the physician and patient should review the diary and discuss diagnosis and treatment options. To meet criteria established by the National Institute of Mental Health, the total symptom scores during the five days before menses must exceed those of the five days after completion of menses by at least 30% (30). Failure to meet the criterion of 30% exacerbation of symptom scores suggests either a premenstrual magnification of another disorder (detectable by persistence of symptoms across the cycle with a mild premenstrual exacerbation) or an altogether different diagnosis. Once the diagnosis of PMS is confirmed by the symptom diary, the severity of the patient's problem is assessed primarily on the basis of her history, particularly the impact of the PMS symptoms on her psychological, social, or economic functioning.

Even if an ovulating woman has undergone a hysterectomy, she can still use the symptom diary. She simply records her basal body temperature each morning so that the luteal phase is detectable by the expected rise in temperature. If a woman is on any form of hormonal contraception or therapy, the medication confounds the clinical picture and by definition she cannot be assigned the diagnosis of PMS. For her to use the symptom diary (and for the physician to make the diagnosis) she must first stop the hormones. Given that oral contraceptives have been shown to often exacerbate PMS symptoms, such an intervention may be at times therapeutic as well as diagnostic. Of course, the severity of the patient's symptoms and her need for a diagnosis and treatment should be weighed carefully against her desire for this reliable form of contraception. The effects of other forms of hormonal contraception on PMS symptoms have not yet been studied.

The diagnosis of PMS can be made only in the absence of hormonal medication, including contraceptives.

Oral contraceptives exacerbate PMS symptoms in some but not all sufferers.

Although PMS can begin at any time and occurs as early as menarche, the symptoms usually worsen with time; consequently the typical patient is in her thirties by the time she seeks medical attention. One can sometimes generalize that those women who present in their early twenties with the complaint of "PMS" are more likely to be suffering from dysmenorrhea, which is easily treatable with nonsteroidal anti-inflammatory drugs (NSAIDs) or oral contraceptives. Women who present for the first time in their mid to late forties are often experiencing symptoms of early menopause, which can be treated with hormone replacement therapy.

Treatment

General Issues

Given that the etiology of PMS is unknown, it should not be surprising that multiple and various treatment regimens have been proposed. In choosing to treat PMS with medications, however, there are several caveats. Few large controlled therapeutic trials have been conducted, the patients are often fertile, and long-term treatment is usually required. Also, potential side effects must be carefully weighed against the actual severity of PMS symptoms. Lastly, "proven" efficacy must be interpreted in light of the fact that most of the research trials have revealed a significant placebo response.

The decision to treat PMS with medication requires a careful risk-benefit analysis.

Fortunately, the symptom diary itself is often therapeutic in addition to being diagnostic. Recognition of the pattern of symptoms sometimes can be adequate therapy, because it validates the patient's symptoms, educates her, and offers her a sense of control over the problem. It also affords an opportunity for the physician to express empathy regarding the patient's symptoms.

Should the patient opt for a particular treatment, however, the symptom diary remains an integral part of the program. The patient should continue to chart her symptom severity for the first few months of therapy in order to document efficacy. A treatment is deemed efficacious when it yields a 30% or greater reduction in late luteal/menstrual phase symptom scores, although a more ambitious goal of 50% or greater reduction has recently become the research standard.

Nutritional Therapies

Mineral and vitamin supplements have long been promoted in the professional and lay literature as remedies for PMS, often without solid evidence. Some traditional and popular but unproven regimens have included magnesium, calcium, and vitamin B_6 supplementation, often given in combination. A recent meta-analysis of vitamin B_6 use concluded that the quality of the studies was poor and that there was insufficient evidence to recommend this treatment (31). Similarly, the studies that purport that magnesium supplementation is effective bear significant methodolologic flaws. Moreover, long-term use of this mineral may not risk-free, because excess magnesium may compete with calcium for absorption in the gastrointestinal tract and potentially lead to osteoporosis.

The evidence for possible benefit of calcium supplementation is more convincing. One randomized, double-blind study involving 466 patients showed that 600 mg of elemental calcium twice daily with meals throughout the mouth decreased PMS symptom scores by 48% compared with a 30% reduction with placebo (32). Further evidence for possible calcium dysregulation comes from a study that demonstrates an association between PMS and later osteoporosis (33). Also, the finding that perturbations in intracellular calcium in patients with primary hyperparathyroidism affect CSF levels of the serotonin precursor tryptophan suggests the possible mechanism by which calcium dysregulation may be linked with the mood and behavior changes seen in PMS.

Another nutritional intervention calls for decreasing sugar, salt, caffeine, and alcohol consumption despite the lack of any controlled trials to support this recommendation. Others have recommended increasing carbohydrate intake, for which there is suggestive evidence for efficacy. Carbohydrate intake can stimulate an insulin-mediated muscle uptake of large neutral amino acids that normally compete with tryptophan for transport across the blood-brain barrier. The resulting increase in CNS availability of tryptophan, the precursor to serotonin, can help elevate brain serotonin levels (25). Thus the carbohydrate craving typically seen in patients with PMS may represent not only a symptom but possibly either 1) a physiologic response or 2) a learned response and attempt at self-treatment.

Exercise

Two dissertation studies that examined the effect of exercise on PMS symptoms in a randomized fashion were reviewed. The results suggest that high-, moderate-, and low-intensity aerobic training all reduced symptom scores compared with baseline luteal-phase scores, with greater intensity exercise yielding greater improvement (34).

Sleep Deprivation

As mentioned earlier, experimental trials demonstrate that a single night of partial sleep deprivation early in the luteal phase can prevent PMS symptoms for that entire cycle (27). This form of treatment is infrequently prescribed in the clinical setting, however.

Psychotherapy

Cognitive-behavior therapy, relaxation training, and group therapy may have some benefit for the management of PMS; however, study results have been mixed and certainly not compelling (34).

Hormonal Agents

Gonadotropin-releasing hormone (GnRH) agonists, which with continuous use paradoxically inhibit ovulation, have been shown to be beneficial in relieving PMS symptoms (35). Similarly, danazol (36) and high-dose estradiol implants (37), both of which suppress ovarian function, are successful in abolishing cyclical mood changes. However, these three treatments are impracticable because of their attendant side effects and risks. Treatment of PMS with oral contraceptives has been disappointing; in fact, as stated before, most women report worsening of their PMS symptoms upon exposure to oral contraceptives (14). The reason for this is unclear and worthy of investigation, since other forms of ovarian suppression are beneficial. The effects of the newer forms of hormonal contraception (injectable medroxyprogesterone acetate [Depo-Provera], injectable medroxyprogesterone acetate/estradiol cypionate [Lunelle], and levonorgestrel implants [Norplant]) on PMS have not been studied.

Surgical Treatment

Surgical treatment that includes bilateral oophorectomy (but not hysterectomy alone) is an effective but radical treatment reserved for women who suffer severe debilitating PMS unresponsive to conventional measures (38). Concomitant hysterectomy is performed so that estrogen replacement therapy can be subsequently administered without progesterone, which, in some postmenopausal women, can induce a constellation of symptoms resembling PMS (15).

Psychotropic Agents

In general, women who suffer from severe PMS are most affected by the psychological symptoms (7). Moreover, of the women who refer themselves for PMS and whose diagnosis is confirmed by the symptom diary, the overwhelming majority also meet criteria for PMDD. Therefore one frequently must turn to psychotropic agents. Many classes of psychotropic agents have been studied in well-designed double-blind placebo-controlled trials and proven effective. Surprisingly, use of psychotropic agents yields improvement not only for psychological symptoms but for somatic PMS complaints (e.g., edema, headache, bloating) as well.

SSRIs appear to be the most effective pharmacologic agents for treating PMDD.

Of all the classes of psychotropic agents studied, the SSRIs appear the most effective. In a small well-designed trial (39) studying fluoxetine (Prozac) 20 mg daily, fully 90%

or more of PMS subjects enjoyed marked improvement of their symptoms and approximately half reported complete remission (Fig. 4-4). Other trials examining fluoxetine showed good benefit of less dramatic proportions, with response rates ranging from 41% to 77% (40–43). Long-term treatment with fluoxetine provides persistent benefit without loss of efficacy (44). Fluoxetine has received FDA approval for the treatment of PMDD and is also marketed in the form of blister cards of seven capsules under the trade name Sarafem. Other SSRIs, namely paroxetine (Paxil) (begun at 10 mg daily and gradually titrated to 20 to 30 mg daily) (45) and sertraline (Zoloft) (begun at 50 mg daily and titrated as needed to a dose of 100 mg daily) (46), have shown similar efficacy.

Recently three small studies examined intermittent dosing with sertraline 100 mg (Fig. 4-5), fluoxetine 20 mg (49), and paroxetine (50) administered exclusively in the luteal phase. The intermittent regimen was found to be as efficacious as treatment continued throughout the menstrual cycle. The predictable, cyclic nature of PMS lends itself to intermittent treatment, the advantages of which include limiting the patient's exposure to side effects and reducing cost.

Such a rapid onset of clinical response to the SSRI medications suggests that they exert beneficial effect through modes different from that for major depression, in which maximum benefit is typically not seen until one month of continuous use. A second but less fortunate distinction is that, unlike with major depression, sustained remission does not follow long-term treatment with SSRIs. PMS symptoms recur in the next luteal phase immediately following medication discontinuation.

Because studies reveal that not all PMS sufferers respond to SSRIs, treatment must be individually tailored. The tricyclic antidepressants nortriptyline (51), maprotriline (45), desipramine (46), and clomipramine (47) have all demonstrated some benefit for improving PMS symptoms. These drugs are usually begun at a dose of 10 mg nightly and gradually titrated to 25 to 75 mg qhs. While comparison trials confirm that SSRIs are more effective in reducing total PMS symptom scores (45,46), the noradrenergic agents are efficacious in relieving the depression and anxiety symptoms, and are a reasonable alternative for the minority of patients who do not respond to SSRIs. It should be noted that most studies report a high dropout rate for the subjects given tricylic antidepressants, the side effects of which appear to be less well tolerated by PMS sufferers than by women with major depression. In general, therefore, the superior efficacy and tolerability of SSRIs make tricyclic antidepressants a lesser choice for most women with PMS.

Benzodiazepines have long been prescribed for PMS symptoms. The benzodiazepine alprazolam (Xanax) has been studied and shown to be effective, with 70% of women responding, and most symptom scores reduced—some by as much as 50% (52). Patients usually begin the medication during the late

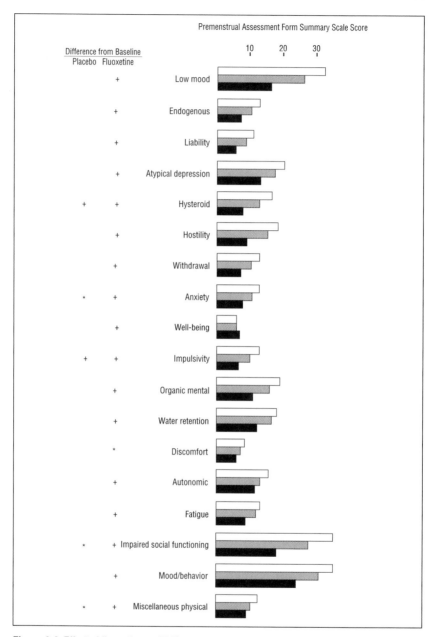

Figure 4-4 Effect of fluoxetine on PMS symptom scores. Fluoxetine (Prozac) use reduced PMS symptom scores (as measured by the Premenstrual Assessment Form) compared with baseline symptoms (*open bars*). As with most PMS trials, some placebo response was noted (*gray bars*); however, fluoxetine was by far more effective (*black bars*). As is often seen when using psychotropic medications, improvement was documented for both physical and psychological symptoms. (From Menkes DB, Taghavi E, Mason PA, Howard RC. Fluoxetine's spectrum of action in premenstrual syndrome. Intern Clin Psychopharm. 1993;8:95-102; with permission.)

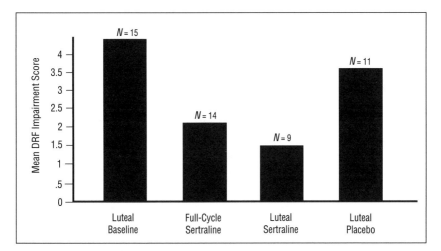

Figure 4-5 Continuous versus intermittent sertraline regimens. Data show effective reductions in PMS symptom scores using both continuous and intermittent (dosing confined to the luteal phase) regimens of sertraline (Zoloft). Studies using intermittent paroxetine (Paxil) and fluoxetine (Prozac) show similar benefits. The optimal timing for initiating and discontinuing treatment in each cycle has not yet been established. (From Halbreich U, Smoller JW. Intermittent luteal phase sertraline treatment of dysphoric premenstrual syndrome. J Clin Psychiatry. 1997;58:399-402; with permission.)

luteal phase of each cycle upon the first appearance of symptoms, gradually increase the dose as needed, then start tapering the dose upon the onset of menses. Gradual tapering is necessary to avoid withdrawal symptoms, which may include seizures. Other potential concerns are sedation, tolerance, and dependence. Certainly one would carefully select patients for this form of treatment, perhaps choose a different benzodiazepine with less addictive potential, and, given the current availability of safer medications, consider a trial of another class of psychotropic agent first.

Many other agents from various classes have been studied in clinical trials and shown to improve at least some PMS symptoms, including beta-blockers, naltrexone, and buspirone (BuSpar). However, on the whole, compared with SSRI therapy, they neither appear as successful in treating the wide range of PMS symptoms nor do they show the same degree of improvement.

Summary

Premenstrual syndrome is a universal phenomenon that has been identified in all cultures studied to date and that has been observed in other primate species as well. The etiology has not been fully delineated, but many of the symptoms appear to result from the action of sex steroids on the neuroendocrine systems. Recent research implicates abnormal progesterone metabolism, but confirmatory studies are needed.

At the present time the only accepted research and clinical tool for diagnosing PMS is a symptom diary maintained over at least two menstrual cycles. Making the diagnosis properly is essential, because a premenstrual exacerbation of another, underlying disorder is more common than pure PMDD, and some studies have found that the majority of the women who presented with a chief complaint of PMS were ultimately determined to have an altogether different diagnosis.

The decision to treat PMS with medication requires a careful risk-benefit analysis. For those patients with mild PMS symptoms or for those who hesitate to use medications, regular exercise, frequent carbohydrate ingestion, calcium supplementation, or a single night of partial sleep deprivation early in the luteal phase can be tried. For patients requiring aggressive treatment, certain means of ovarian suppression (excluding oral contraceptives and others) are efficacious but subject the patient to metabolic derangement and are now rarely used. Trials with various psychotropic agents demonstrate improvement in both psychological and somatic symptoms. Of all the agents studied, the SSRIs appear to be the most effective, and recent studies show equivalent efficacy with an intermittent regimen—daily dosing confined to the luteal phase—compared with daily administration throughout the menstrual cycle. For those who fail treatment with an SSRI, other psychotropic agents are often successful.

For most women PMS symptoms are merely a minor nuisance, but for approximately 5% of ovulating women the symptoms are severe enough to profoundly affect personal relationships and school or work performance. It is for these patients that proper diagnosis and appropriate treatment by the primary care physician can relieve significant suffering.

REFERENCES

1. **Frank RT.** The hormonal causes of premenstrual tension. Arch Neurol Psychiatry. 1931;26:1053-7.

2. ACOG committee opinion: premenstrual syndrome. No. 155, April 1995 (Replaces No. 66, January 1989). Int J Gynecol Obst. 1995;50:80-4.

3. **American Psychiatric Association.** Diagnostic and Statistical Manual of Mental Disorders, 4th ed. Washington, DC; 1994.

4. **Hammarback S, Elkholm UB, Backstrom T.** Spontaneous anovulation causing disappearance of cyclical symptoms in women with the premenstrual syndrome. Acta Endocrinol. 1991;124:132-7.

5. **Casson P, Hahn PM, VanVugt DA, Reid RL.** Lasting response to ovariectomy in severe intractable premenstrual syndrome. Am J Obstet Gynecol. 1990;162:99-105.

6. **Freeman EW, Rickels K, Schweizer E, Ting T.** Relationships between age and symptom severity among women seeking medical treatment for premenstrual symptoms. Psychol Med. 1995;25:309-15.

7. **Rubinow D.** The premenstrual syndrome: new views. JAMA. 1992;268:1908-12.

8. **Condon, JT.** The premenstrual syndrome: a twin study. Br J Psychiatry. 1993;162: 481-6.

9. **Janiger O, Riffenburgh R, Kersh R.** Cross-cultural study of premenstrual symptoms. Psychosomatics. 1972;13:226-35.

10. **Monagle L, Dan A, Krogh V, et al.** Perimenstrual symptom prevalence rates: an Italian-American comparison. Am J Epidemiol. 1993;138:1070-81.

11. **Rupani NP, Lema VM.** Premenstrual tension among nurses in Nairobi, Kenya. East Africa Med J. 1993;705:310-3.

12. **Hausfater G, Skoblick B.** Premenstrual behavior changes among female yellow baboons: some similarities to premenstrual syndrome (PMS) in women. Am J Primatol. 1985:9:165-72.

13. **Rowell TE.** Behavior and female reproductive cycles of rhesus macaques. J Reprod Fertil. 1963;6:193-203.

14. **Graham CA, Sherwin BB.** A prospective treatment study of premenstrual symptoms using a triphasic oral contraceptive. J Psychosomatic Res. 1992;36:257-66.

15. **Hammarback S, Backstrom T, Holst J, et al.** Cyclical mood changes in the premenstrual tension syndrome during sequential estrogen-progestagen post-menopause replacement therapy. Acta Obstet Gynecol Scand. 1985;64:393-7.

16. **Schmidt PJ, Nieman LK, Grover GN, et al.** Lack of effect of induced menses on symptoms in women with premenstrual syndrome. N Engl J Med. 1991;324:1174-9.

17. **Rapkin AJU, Morgan M, Goldman L, et al.** Progesterone metabolite allopregnanolone in women with premenstrual syndrome. Obstet Gynecol. 1997;90:709-14.

18. **Monteleone P, Luisi S, Tonetti A, et al.** Allopregnanolone concentrations and premenstrual syndrome. Eur J Endocrin. 2000;142:269-73.

19. **Chuong CJ, Bartholomew PH, Gibbons WE.** Periovulatory beta-endorphin levels in premenstrual syndrome. Obstet Gynecol. 1994;83:755-60.

20. **Chuong CJ, Coulam CB, Kao PC, et al.** Neuropeptide levels in premenstrual syndrome. Fertil Steril. 1985;44:760-5.

21. **Halbreich U, Petty F, Yonkers K, et al.** Low plasma gamma-aminobutyric acid levels during the late luteal phase of women with premenstrual dysphoric disorder. Am J Psychiatry. 1996;153:718-20.

22. **Rapkin AJ, Edelmuth E, Chang LC, et al.** Whole-blood serotonin in premenstrual syndrome. Obstet Gynecol. 1987;70:533-7.

23. **Ashby CR, Carr LA, Cook CL, et al.** Alteration of platelet serotonergic mechanisms and monoamine oxidase activity in premenstrual syndrome. Biol Psychiatry. 1988;24: 225-33.

24. **Menkes DB, Coates DC, Fawcett JP.** Acute tryptophan depletion aggravates premenstrual syndrome. J Affective Disord. 1994;32:37-44.

25. **Sayegh R, Schiff I, Wurtman J, et al.** The effect of a carbohydrate-rich beverage on mood, appetite, and cognitive function in women with premenstrual syndrome. Obstet Gynecol. 1995;86:520-8.

26. **Harrison W, Endicott J, Nee J, et al.** Characteristics of women seeking treatment for premenstrual syndrome. Psychosomatics. 1989;71:331-8.

27. **Parry BL, Cover C, Mostofi N, et al.** Early vs. late partial sleep deprivation in patients with premenstrual dysphoric disorder and normal comparison subjects. Am J Psychiatry. 1995;152:404-12.

28. **Rubinow DDR, Schmidt PJ.** Premenstrual syndrome: a review of endocrine studies. Endocrinology. 1992;2:47-54.

29. **Case AM, Reid RL.** Effects of the menstrual cycle on medical disorders. Arch Intern Med. 1998;158:1405-12.

30. National Institute of Mental Health. Premenstrual Syndrome Workshop Guidelines. Rockville, MD; 1983.

31. **Wyatt KM, Kimmock PW, Jones PW, O'Brien PM.** Efficacy of vitamin B-6 in the treatment of premenstrual syndrome: systemic review. BMJ. 1999;318:1375-81.

32. **Lee SJ, Kanis JA.** An association between osteoporosis and premenstrual and postmenstrual symptoms. Bone Miner. 1994;24:127-34.

33. **Thys-Jacobs S, Silverton M, Alvir J, et al.** Reduced bone mass in women with premenstrual syndrome. J Womens Health. 1995;4:161-8.

34. **Pearlstein T.** Nonpharmacologic treatment of premenstrual syndrome. Psychiatric Annal. 1996;26:9:590-4.

35. **Hammarback S, Backstrom T.** Induced anovulation as treatment of the premenstrual tension syndrome: a double-blind crossover study with GnRH-agonist versus placebo. Acta Obstet Gynecol Scand. 1988;67:159-66.

36. **Watts JFF, Butt WR, Edwards RL.** A clinical trial danazol for the treatment of premenstrual tension. Br J Obstet Gynaecol. 1987;94:30-4.

37. **Watson N, Studd J, Savvas M, Baber RJ.** The long-term effect of oestradiol implant therapy for the treatment of premenstrual syndrome. Gynecol Endocrinol. 1990;4:99-107.

38. **Casson P, Hahn PM, Van Vugt DA, Reid RL.** Lasting response to ovariectomy in severe intractable premenstrual syndrome. Am J Obstet Gynecol. 1990;162:99-105.

39. **Stone AB, Pearlstein TB, Brown WA.** Fluoxetine in the treatment of late luteal phase dysphoric disorder. J Clin Psychiatry. 1991;52:7:290-3.

40. **Menkes DB, Taghavi E, Mason PA, Howard RC.** Fluoxetine's spectrum of action in premenstrual syndrome. Int Clin Psychopharmacol. 1993;8:95-102.

41. **Steiner M, Steinberg S, Steward D, et al.** Fluoxetine in the treatment of premenstrual dysphoria. N Engl J Med. 1995;332:1529-34.

42. **Su T-P, Schmidt PJ, Danaceau MA, et al.** Fluoxetine in the treatment of premenstrual dysphoria. Neuropsychopharmacology. 1997;16:5:346-56.

43. **Wood SH, Mortola JF, Chan Y-F, et al.** Treatment of premenstrual syndrome with fluoxetine: a double-blind, placebo-controlled, crossover study. Obstet Gynecol. 1992;80:3:339-44.

44. **Pearlstein TB, Stone AB.** Long-term fluoxetine treatment in late luteal phase dysphoric disorder. J Clin Psychiatry. 1994;55:332-5.

45. **Eriksson E, Hedberg M, Andersch B, Sundblad C.** The serotonin reuptake inhibitor paroxetine is superior to the noradrenaline reuptake inhibitor maprotiline in the treatment of premenstrual syndrome. Neuropsychopharmacology. 1995;12:167-76.

46. **Freeman EW, Rickels K, Sondheimer SJ, Wittmaack FM.** Setraline versus desipramine in the treatment of premenstrual syndrome: an open-label trial. J Clin Psychiatry. 1996;57:7-11.

47. **Sundblad C, Hedberg M, Eriksson E.** Clomipramine administered during the luteal phase reduces the symptoms of premenstrual syndrome: a placebo-controlled trial. Neuropsychopharmacology. 1993;9:2:133-45.

48. **Halbreich U, Smoller JW.** Intermittent luteal phase sertraline treatment of dysphoric premenstrual syndrome. J Clin Psychiatry. 1997;58:399-402.

49. **Steiner M, Korzekwa M, Lamont J, Wilkins A.** Intermittent fluoxetine dosing in the treatment of women with premenstrual dysphoria. Psychopharm Bull. 1997;33: 771-4.

50. **Sundblad C, Wikander I, Andersch B, Eriksson E.** A naturalist study of paroxetine in premenstrual syndrome: efficacy and side-effects during ten cycles of treatment. Eur Neuropsychopharmacology. 1997;7:201-6.

51. **Harrison WM, Endicott J, Nee J.** Treatment of premenstrual depression with nortriptyline: a pilot study. J Clin Psychiatry. 1989;50:136-9.

52. **Smith S, Rinehart JS, Ruddock VE, Schiff I.** Treatment of premenstrual syndrome with alprazolam: results of a double-blind, placebo-controlled, randomized crossover clinical trial. Obstet Gynecol. 1987;70:37-43.

CHAPTER 5

Contraception

VANESSA E. CULLINS, MD, MPH
FRANCISCO A. R. GARCIA, MD, MPH

Almost half of all pregnancies in the United States are unintended (1). This extraordinarily high rate of unintended pregnancy is not seen in similarly developed countries. Although many explantations for this discrepancy have been invoked, data suggest that US women are more ambivalent (2), less effective (3,4) contraceptors. Because obstetrician/gynecologists often do not have contact with a woman until the unintended pregnancy has occurred, discussion of family planning issues should be an integral component of care provided by primary care physicians.

Facilitating the Choice of Contraceptive

Many factors influence a woman's contraceptive choices: cultural and religious beliefs; partner attitudes; previous contraceptive experiences; reproductive plans; medical risks associated with pregnancy; side effects and perceived risks associated with contraception; cost, convenience, and ease of method use; method effectiveness; and individual risk for sexually transmitted diseases. Because a provider cannot know the relative importance of each factor, his or her role in this discussion is clarification of misperceptions that may hamper the patient's informed decision making. Decision making can be facilitated through the use of a questionnaire but is usually best effected by doctor-patient conversation. The physician or other trained member of the health care team should initiate discussion of the patient's attitudes toward family planning, having children (e.g., desired family size, timing of pregnancy), sexual activities (e.g., number of sexual partners, need for protection against sexually transmitted diseases), and contraceptive experiences. Many of these questions may at first appear obtrusive, but they are generally well received in the context of assisting a patient in making an informed choice about contraception. Reproductive-aged women should have their contraceptive needs reassessed at least annually, because their plans for pregnancy, sexual practices, and risk profile may change.

When providing contraception it is important to apprise the patient of the typical failure rate with the chosen method (see Fig. 5-1 for comparison of the

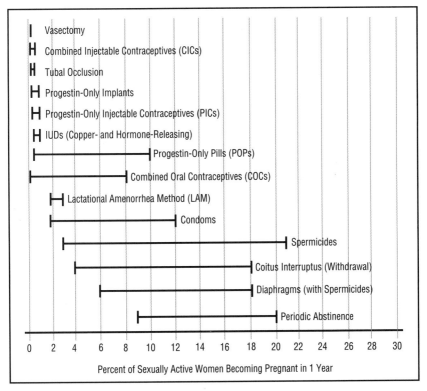

Figure 5-1 Range of theoretical and typical use pregnancy rates per 100 women during first year of use. Note that methods independent of the act of coitus and those more independent of the user are associated with lower failure rates. (From Blumenthal PD, McIntosh N. Pocket Guide for Family Planning Service Providers, 2nd ed. Baltimore: JHPIEGO Corp., 1996. Adapted from Labbok, Cooney and Coly 1994; Population Action International 1991; Trussel 1990; WHO 1993.)

failure rates of different contraceptive methods) and that, with the exception of some barrier methods, it likely lacks protection against sexually transmitted diseases. It is also helpful to point out the safety and noncontraceptive benefits of the method. Unfortunately, continuation rates with many contraceptive methods are low, often less than 50% at 1 year. The low continuation rates likely result from side effects associated with the method or from the fact that all forms of contraception represent some sort of compromise. Thus the physician's role in assisting a patient with contraception does not end with method selection.

Once the patient has chosen a contraceptive, scheduling a follow-up a few months later is important in helping to ensure that the patient will continue with the method. At this visit one can reassure the patient that the side effects she is experiencing are expected and not cause for alarm and in some instances, that these side effects are transient. Not uncommonly, however, the physician may need to work with the patient to select a different form of contraception with more tolerable side effects. The follow-up visit is also an opportunity to confirm that the patient is using the method properly. In the United States, 47% of unintended pregnancies are the result of contraceptive failure (5), mostly stemming from incorrect or inconsistent use. This statistic underscores the need for careful and thorough patient education and follow-up.

In part because no form of contraception has perfect efficacy, virtually all primary care physicians will encounter a patient with an unintended pregnancy. When this occurs the physician should thoroughly discuss the patient's options regarding the pregnancy so that timely referral can be made for prenatal care or pregnancy termination.

Hormonal Contraception

Hormonal contraception methods all contain a progestin, which is responsible for most of the contraceptive action. Some forms also contain an estrogen, which contributes to inhibiting ovulation but primarily serves to regulate bleeding so that it occurs only at expected intervals, simulating normal menses. Thus combined (i.e., a "combination" of an estrogen and a progestin) oral contraceptives and injectable contraception (Lunelle) usually allow for reliable, predictable withdrawal bleeding. In contrast, progestin-only methods, such as the progestin-only pill ("mini-pill"), injectable medroxyprogesterone acetate (Depo-Provera), and implanted progestins such as Norplant are all associated with a variety of possible bleeding patterns ranging from amenorrhea to episodic, unpredictable spotting to menorrhagia. The bleeding pattern can often be predicted according to the particular form of progestin-only method and the duration of its use. Aside from the rare occurence of anemia resulting from menorrhagia, these "abnormal" bleeding patterns are generally of no health consequence. However, irregular bleeding is likely a nuisance to the patient and a frequently cited reason for discontinuation of progestin-only methods.

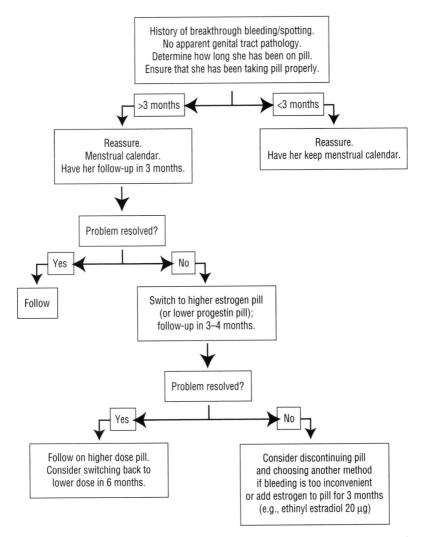

Figure 5-2 Management of bleeding/spotting occurring with combined oral contraceptive use. (Adapted from Pocket Guide for Family Planning Service Providers. Baltimore: JHPIEGO;1995.)

Progestins in moderate doses, such as in most combined oral contraceptives (COCs), the combined injectable (Lunelle), and medroxyprogesterone acetate (Depo-Provera), suppress ovulation. However, not all forms of hormonal contraception inhibit ovulation. Progestins have other important contraceptive actions, specifically, increasing the cervical mucous viscosity to inhibit sperm penetration and the ability to render the endometrium inhospitable for implantation. Methods such as the progestin-only pill and Norplant prevent pregnancy primarily via these latter two effects, because the doses of hormone in these agents are too low to reliably prevent ovulation.

Side effects of hormonal contraception can result from either the progestin or estrogen; sometimes the cause can be distinguished by the specific symptom (Table 5-1). Progestins have some weak androgen activity, and many of the side effects (e.g., acne, hirsutism) and adverse metabolic consequences (e.g., mild cholesterol elevation) can be attributed to this quality. The newer, third-generation progestins (gestodene [not available in the United States], desogestrel, or norgestimate) were developed to have fewer androgenic effects. Estrogens, in turn, are associated with side effects such as nausea and breast tenderness. However, the most serious effect associated with estrogen is the increased risk of thromboembolic events. Estrogen stimulates hepatic production of clotting factors, decreases antithrombin III levels, and increases platelet aggregation, all in a dose-dependent manner. This prothrombotic effect becomes particularly relevant for patients already at higher risk for heart disease and stroke, such as smokers 35 years of age or older. Lack of this estrogen-associated risk of thrombosis is a distinct advantage of progestin-only contraceptive methods.

Importantly, a pelvic examination is not necessary before the provision of hormonal contraception (5a). Although a pelvic examination and screening tests for sexually transmitted diseases and cervical cancer are desirable health behaviors, these have no relation to the safe use of hormonal methods and, in the interest of optimizing access to contraception, should not be considered

Table 5-1 Common Progestin and Estrogen Side Effects

Progestin-Related Side Effects	Estrogen-Related Side Effects
• Headaches	• Nausea
• Breast tenderness	• Breast tenderness
• Increased appetite	• Breast growth
• Decreased libido	• Fluid retention/bloating
• Acne/oily skin*	• Headaches
• Hirsutism*	• Thromboembolic events

*These androgenic side effects may be minimized by prescribing a pill containing desogestrel, or norgestimate, but note that most COCs improve acne.

mandatory before providing or continuing these methods. Before prescribing combined hormonal contraception the patient's medical history should be obtained to confirm that she lacks coronary artery disease, complex migraines, diabetes with vascular complications, hepatic disease, or previous history of stroke, breast cancer, or thromboembolic disease. Tobacco use should also be assessed and her blood pressure measured to exclude uncontrolled hypertension.

Combined Hormonal Contraception

Combined hormonal contraception methods include combined oral contraceptives and the combined monthly injectable, Lunelle.

Combined Oral Contraceptives

Combined oral contraceptives (COCs), which contain ethinyl estradiol or mestranol plus one of many possible progestins, are the most popular prescription-requiring, reversible contraceptives in the United States (6,7). In addition, COCs are one of the more effective forms of reversible contraception, with a perfect-use failure rate of 0.1% (8-11). The typical use failure rate ranges from 3% to 8% (11,12), meaning that of 100 women using the method, 3 to 8 will have an unintended pregnancy in a 12-month period.

In the 1960s, COCs contained 150 μg estradiol. Over time, this high estrogen content (as well as the progestin dose) was gradually reduced, and in 1974 "low-dose" oral contraceptives containing 35 μg ethinyl estradiol were introduced. Today low-dose COCs are standard, and COCs containing more than 35 μg estrogen are prescribed only in select circumstances. More recent developments include formulations using even lower doses (20 μg) of estrogen and the introduction of "third-generation" progestins (desogestrel, gestoden, and norgestimate), which have fewer androgenic effects than traditional progestins. The older COCs that contained higher doses of estrogen and progesterone worked by reliably inhibiting ovulation. Very low-dose COCs suppress ovulation to varying degrees; therefore important contraceptive effects are increased cervical mucus viscosity and poor receptivity of the endometrium (8,9,13,14).

Absolute contraindications and cautions to combined hormonal contraceptive use are given in Table 5-2 and 5-3, respectively.

Selection and Implementation
Many COCs are available in the United States (Table 5-4). If contraceptive efficacy is a woman's only concern, any low dose (≤35 μg ethinyl estradiol) COC

Table 5-2 Absolute Contraindications to Combined Hormonal Contraceptives

- Thrombophlebitis or thromboembolic disorder (current or remote)
- Cerebrovascular or coronary artery disease (current or remote)
- Complex migraines
- Diabetes with associated peripheral vascular disease
- Smoker aged ≥35 years

- Known or suspected breast cancer
- History of, or known or suspected, estrogen-dependent neoplasia
- Undiagnosed abnormal genital bleeding
- Benign or malignant liver tumors or liver failure
- Known or suspected pregnancy

Table 5-3 Conditions Requiring Cautions When Prescribing Combined Hormonal Contraceptives

Condition	Explanation/Management Issues
History of thrombophlebitis associated with IV drug use, immobilization, or trauma	Estrogen promotes thromboembolic phenomena; however, COCs and Lunelle are only contraindicated in individuals at risk for future thromboembolic events
Elevated liver function enzymes; history of cholestatic jaundice in pregnancy; hepatitis	COCs and Lunelle are metabolized by the liver and affect liver function; once the liver function has stabilized (e.g., chronic hepatitis with history of elevated liver), a combined contraceptive can be prescribed; confirm liver function remains stable
Migraine; hypertension; diabetes mellitus	Prescribe combined contraception; adjust diabetic, anti-hypertensive, and antimigraine medication as needed
Lactation	Estrogen can decrease the quantity of breast milk if lactation is not well established; COCs and Lunelle can be safely begun 4 weeks postpartum because the amount of hormone received by the infant has not been shown to adversely affect infant growth or development
Gallbladder disease	Estrogen may worsen symptoms
Use of rifampin, barbiturates, and some antiepileptic medication	These medications increase metabolism of COCs and Lunelle and may reduce contraceptive efficacy

Adapted from Hatcher RA, Trussell J, Stewart F, et al. Contraceptive Technology, 17th ed. New York: Ardent Media; 1998; and from Pocket Guide for Family Planning Service Providers. Baltimore: JHPIEGO; 1995.

may be prescribed.* If the woman has experienced specific side effects with a certain pill in the past, the provider should attempt to prescribe a formulation that is unlikely to produce a recurrence of these side effects (Table 5-5). For

---

*An exception in Yasmin, which because of the anti-mineralocorticoid effects of its progestin (drospirenone), may potentially lead to hyperkalemia and thus should be prescribed more selectively. Women taking ACE inhibitors, ACE receptor blockers, potassium-sparing diuretics, heparin, adosterone antagonists, and NSAIDs should not be prescribed this COC.

some women, more than one formulation may need to be tried, each for at least 3 to 6 months, before side effects are mitigated or tolerable. A scheme for managing bleeding/spotting is shown in Figure 5-2 on page 109.

Combined oral contraceptives are packaged in 21-day and 28-day formats, but the latter is generally prescribed to enhance pill-taking compliance. For most 28-day formulations, the last seven pills in the pack are free of hormone, but some brands add minerals or drugs to the placebo pills to replenish nutrients or reduce breakthrough bleeding (e.g., Estrostep Fe contains iron in the 7-day hormone-free stage). Mircette, one of the most recently approved lower dose (20 µg) COCs, contains 10 µg ethinyl estradiol in the last 5 days of the 28-day pack. Biphasic and triphasic regimens of COCs were designed to better mimic the normal endocrinology of the menstrual cycle; however, no clinical superiority has been demonstrated. The original monophasic pills offer the option of electively manipulating the timing of "menses" by taking active pills for longer than 21 days (see Noncontraceptive Benefits section below).

To minimize starting COCs during undiagnosed pregnancy, one usually begins the pill either on the first day of menses, by the fifth day of menses, or on the Sunday following the onset of menses. Alternatively, COCs may be begun at any time during a woman's menstrual cycle as long as pregnancy is not suspected. This approach is often used for amenorrheic women switching from other hormonal methods. In the event that COCs are accidently begun during the first trimester of pregnancy, the woman can be reassured that COCs do not increase teratogenic risk (15-17). When pregnancy is desired, the woman may discontinue the pill and immediately attempt conception. The average return to fertility is approximately 3 months (16,17); however, she may ovulate as soon as 48 hr.

Use in the Setting of Chronic Diseases

Low-dose COCs are safe in the setting of many chronic diseases. Hypertension, diabetes mellitus without vascular complications, connective tissue disorders, migraine, seizure disorders, gallbladder disease, and cholestatic jaundice of pregnancy are not contraindications to low-dose pills (18-31). However, women with these disorders do require additional monitoring of their chronic diseases. One consideration in deeming COCs safe is that, in the face of these chronic conditions, the morbidity and mortality rates associated with pregnancy far exceed those associated with this reliable form of contraception.

Risk of Arterial and Venous Thrombotic Events

The oral contraceptive preparations of the 1960s and early 1970s containing 80 to 150 µg synthetic estrogen were associated with a significant excess risk of arterial and venous thromboembolic events and mortality, especially among smokers (32-35). Reductions in the estrogen dose reduced the risk of

Table 5-4 Combined Oral Contraceptives Available in the United States

Drug	Estrogen (µg)*	Progestin (mg)†	Cost ($)‡
Low Dose Combined			
Monophasic			
Ovcon 35 21, 28 (Warner Chilcott)	Ethinyl estradiol (35)	Norethindrone (0.4)	31.76
Brevicon 21, 28 (Watson)	Ethinyl estradiol (35)	Norethindrone (0.5)	27.63
Modicon 28 (Ortho-McNeil)	Ethinyl estradiol (35)	Norethindrone (0.5)	32.71
Necon 0.5/35E 21, 28 (Watson)	Ethinyl estradiol (35)	Norethindrone (0.5)	27.86
Nelova 10/11 21 (Warner Chilcott)§	Ethinyl estradiol (35)	Norethindrone (0.5, 1)	13.90
Genora 1/35 21, 28 (Physicians Total Care)	Ethinyl estradiol (35)	Norethindrone (1)	8.59
Necon 1/35 21 (Watson)§	Ethinyl estradiol (35)	Norethindrone (1)	25.54
Nelova 1/35 28 (Warner Chilcott)	Ethinyl estradiol (35)	Norethindrone (1)	16.41
Norinyl 1/35 21, 28 (Watson)	Ethinyl estradiol (35)	Norethindrone (1)	29.98
Ortho-Novum 1/35 21, 28 (Ortho-McNeil)	Ethinyl estradiol (35)	Norethindrone (1)	29.98
Ortho-Cyclen 21, 28 (Ortho-McNeil)	Ethinyl estradiol (35)	Norgestimate (0.25)	29.98
Demulen 1/35 21 (Searle)§	Ethinyl estradiol (35)	Ethynodiol diacetate (1)	30.84
Zovia 1/35 E (Watson)§	Ethinyl estradiol (35)	Ethynodiol diacetate (1)	27.60
Loestrin 1.5/30 21, 28 (Parke-Davis)	Ethinyl estradiol (30)	Norethindrone acetate (1.5)	31.15
Levien 21, 28 (Berlex)	Ethinyl estradiol (30)	Levonorgestrel (0.15)	30.83
Levora 21, 28 (Watson)	Ethinyl estradiol (30)	Levonorgestrel (0.15)	26.61
Nordette 21, 28 (Wyeth-Ayerst)	Ethinyl estradiol (30)	Levonorgestrel (0.15)	30.85
Lo/Ovral (Wyeth-Ayerst)§	Ethinyl estradiol (30)	Norgestrel (0.3)	31.96
Low-Ogestrel (Watson)§	Ethinyl estradiol (30)	Norgestrel (0.3)	28.01
Desogen 28 (Organon)	Ethinyl estradiol (30)	Desogestrel (0.15)	26.13
Ortho-Cept 21 (Ortho-McNeil)§	Ethinyl estradiol (30)	Desogestrel (0.15)	29.26
Yasmin 28 (Berlex)**	Ethinyl estradiol (30)	Drospirenone (3)	28.79
Genora 1/50 28 (Physicians Total Care)	Mestranol (50)	Norethindrone (1)	9.25
Necon 1/50 21, 28 (Watson)	Mestranol (50)	Norethindrone (1)	25.54
Nalova 1/50 21, 28 (Warner Chilcott)	Mestranol (50)	Norethindrone (1)	16.41
Norinyl 1/50 21, 28 (Watson)	Mestranol (50)	Norethindrone (1)	28.26
Ortho-Novum 1/50 28 (Ortho-McNeil)	Mestranol (50)	Norethindrone (1)	29.98
Multiphasic			
Tri-Levlen 21, 28 (Berlex)	Ethinyl estradiol (30, 40, 30)	Levonorgestrel (0.05, 0.075, 0.125)	28.02
Triphasil 21 (Wyeth-Ayerst)	Ethinyl estradiol (30, 40, 30)	Levonorgestrel (0.05, 0.075, 0.125)	29.94
Trivora-28 (Watson)	Ethinyl estradiol (30, 40, 30)	Levonorgestrel (0.05, 0.075, 0.125)	25.66
Estrostep 28 (Parke-Davis)	Ethinyl estradiol (20, 30, 35)	Norethindroe acetate (1)	30.85
Ortho Tri-Cyclen (Ortho-McNeil)‖	Ethinyl estradiol (35)	Norgestimate (0.18, 0.215, 0.25)	29.98
Tri-Norinyl 21, 28 (Watson)	Ethinyl estradiol (35)	Norethindrone (0.5, 1, 0.5)	27.01
Ortho-Novum 7/7/7 21 (Ortho-McNeil)§	Ethinyl estradiol (35)	Norethindrone (0.5, 0.75, 1)	29.98
Jenest-28 (Organon)	Ethinyl estradiol (35)	Norethindrone (0.5, 1)	22.39
Necon 10/11 21, 28 (Watson)	Ethinyl estradiol (35)	Norethindrone (0.5, 1)	27.86
Ortho-Novum 10/11 28 (Ortho-McNeil)	Ethinyl estradiol (35)	Norethindrone (0.5, 1)	31.45
Extra Low Dose Combined			
Alesse 21, 28 (Wyeth-Ayerst)	Ethinyl estradiol (20)	Levonorgestrel (0.1)	30.23
Levlite 21, 28 (Berlex)	Ethinyl estradiol (20)	Levonorgestrel (0.1)	29.60
Loestrin 1/20 21, 28 (Parke-Davis)	Ethinyl estradiol (20)	Norethindrone acetate (1)	30.85
Mircette 28 (Organon)	Ethinyl estradiol (20, 0, 10)	Desogestrel (0.15)	28.83

Table 5-4 *(Continued)*

Drug	Estrogen (µg)*	Progestin (mg)†	Cost ($)‡
Higher Dose Combined			
Ovral 21, 28 (Wyeth-Ayerst)	Ethinyl estradiol (50)	Norgestrel (0.5)	48.93
Ogestrel-28 (Watson)	Ethinyl estradiol (50)	Norgestrel (0.5)	41.94
Ovcon 50 28 (Warner Chilcott)	Ethinyl estradiol (50)	Norethindrone (1)	35.05
Zovia 1/50E 21 (Watson)§	Ethinyl estradiol (50)	Ethynodiol diacetate (1)	30.78
Progestin Only			
Ovrette (Wyeth-Ayerst)	None	Norgestrel (0.075)	30.85
Micronor (Ortho-McNeil)	None	Norethindrone (0.35)	34.82
Nor-QD (Watson)	None	Norethindrone (0.35)	31.92

*Ethinyl estradiol and mestranol are not equivalent on a milligram basis; the results of some studies indicate that 30 to 35 µg ethinyl estradiol are equivalent to 50 µg mestranol.
†Different progestins are not equivalent on a milligram basis.
‡Cost to the pharmacist for 28-day use, based on wholesale price (AWP) listings in *Drug Topics Red Book* 2000 and May *Update.*
§Also available in 28-day regimen at slightly different cost.
‖Also FDA-approved for acne.
**Contraindicated in the setting of certain medications (see footnote on page 112).
From Medical Letter. 2000;42:43–4; with permission.

Because estrogen increases the risk of arterial and venous thrombotic events, combined hormonal contraception is contraindicated for some women.

these problems (36,37), but transient ischemic attacks, thrombotic strokes, myocardial infarctions, and deep venous thromboses (with or without pulmonary embolism) can still occur as a result of COC use. Increasing age and cigarette use both increase the risk of arterial events and act synergistically with COCs. This constitutes the reasoning behind the recommendation that smokers aged 35 and older not use COCs.

Some (38-40) but not all (41) studies suggest that other risk factors such as migraine (particularly migraine with aura) and hypertension act independently to increase the risk of stroke in women using COCs. Until the evidence is more solid, however, a reasonable recommendation is to prescribe COCs with caution to women with these medical problems and to follow them more closely. Progression of migraine headaches or worsening of associated aura after beginning COCs is cause for discontinuation. Some authorities consider the risk of stroke too high in women with complex migraines (migraines with associated focal neurologic symptoms), however, and recommend avoiding COCs altogether in this subgroup (40).

Tobacco use also clearly increases the risk of both cerebral and coronary thrombotic events associated with COCs in a dose-dependent manner, with greater than one half pack per day clearly associated with greater risk than

Table 5-5 Management of Combined Oral Contraceptive Side Effects and Health Problems

Side Effect or Problem (May or May Not Be Pill Related)	Assessment	Management
Amenorrhea (absence of bleeding or spotting)	1. Ask patient how often she has been taking her pills. Has she missed any pills in the cycle? 2. Rule out pregnancy by symptoms, physical exam, and pregnancy test. 3. Is she using a low-estrogen pill (≤20–35 µg ethinyl estradiol)?	1. Missed pills or pills taken late increase risk of pregnancy. Obtain a pregnancy test if this has been the case. 2. If intrauterine pregnancy is confirmed, counsel patient regarding options. If patient elects to continue the pregnancy, stop COCs and assure her that the small dose of estrogen and progestin in the COCs to which she was exposed will have no harmful effect on the fetus. 3. If the patient is taking COCs correctly, reassure. Explain that absent menses is most likely due to lack of build-up of uterine lining and that no menstrual bleed is needed. As long as she takes her pill regularly at the same time each day, she can remain confident that she has not become pregnant, even in the absence of withdrawal bleeding. If the patient remains dissatisfied, try a higher dose estrogen pill (50 µg or less) if there are no conditions requiring caution. Alternatively, choose a pill with the same estrogen dose but lower progestin dose.
Breast Fullness or Tenderness (usually improves within three months of starting the COCs)	1. Determine whether patient is pregnant by history, pelvic exam, and/or pregnancy test. 2. Determine whether the woman has breast lumps or nipple discharge suspicious for cancer. 3. Ask patient whether she notices this side effect only at a certain time of the month.	1. If pregnant, manage as per Amenorrhea section above. 2. If physical exam shows lump or discharge suspicious for cancer, refer to appropriate source for diagnosis. If malignancy is discovered, help her make an informed choice of another contraceptive method. 3. Decrease estrogen in pill if not already at lowest level. Advise patient to avoid caffeine, chocolate, etc. If the lowest dose pill is unacceptable and symptomatic management is not helpful, assist patient in making an informed choice of a progestin-only or other method.
Depression	1. Ask patient about potential causes of depression (e.g., family, job, finances, social problems).	1. Counsel, treat, or refer as appropriate. Work with provider treating depression to get it under control. If depression worsens on COCs, help patient make informed choice of another contraception method. If COC has not caused depression to worsen, pills can be continued.
Headaches	1. Are the headaches severe, frequent, or associated with nausea? Has patient had loss of speech, numbness, weakness or tingling, or visual changes associated with the headaches? Have her migraines or migraine auras worsened with COC use?	1. If yes, discontinue COCs. Patients with TIA-type symptoms may require further evaluation. One should assist the patient in choosing a progestin-only or nonhormonal method of contraception. If her migraines or aura have remained stable, or if her headaches are not severe, frequent, or associated with nausea, reassure and treat with nonsteroidal anti-inflammatory agent.

Table 5-5 *(Continued)*

Side Effect or Problem (May or May Not Be Pill Related)	Assessment	Management
Headaches *(continued)*	2. Has she ever had high blood pressure (BP?)	2. Regardless of history, check BP. If elevated, see High Blood Pressure section below.
	3. Have the headaches become worse since patient began the pill?	3. If worse on COCs, switch to progestin-only or nonhormonal contraceptive method. If no worse or better, explore cause of headaches. COCs can be continued unless neurologic symptoms or signs develop or headaches or aura worsen.
	4. Does she have nasal drip or tenderness in area of sinuses?	4. Treat for sinus disease. Continue pills.
High Blood Pressure	1. Clarify whether this is the first time elevated blood pressure has been noted.	1. Continue COCs. Encourage lifestyle changes (e.g., salt reduction, regular exercise, weight loss [if indicated]). Follow BP.
	2. Recheck BP on three visits, one week apart.	2. If blood pressure remains consistently elevated, either continue the COCs and treat the elevated blood pressure or discontinue the COCs and help the patient choose a nonhormonal contraception method.
Nausea/Dizziness/ Vomiting (usually improves during first 3 months)	1. Clarify whether pills are taken in morning or on an empty stomach.	1. Take with evening meal or before bedtime.
	2. Exclude pregnancy.	2. If pregnant, manage as per Amenorrhea section.
	3. None of the above?	3. Counsel that the symptom(s) will probably decrease with time or switch to a lower estrogen pill or a progestin-only method.
Spotting or Bleeding Between Periods (common during first 3 months after starting pill; see Fig. 5-2)	1. Has patient recently begun COCs?	1. Reassure. Spotting and bleeding decrease markedly in most women by the fourth month of use.
	2. Ask if she has missed one or more pills and if she takes them at a different time every day.	2. If yes, provide instructions. If no, and no contraindications, use high-dose COCs (50 µg ethinyl estradiol) for several cycles until spotting resolves. Then return to low-dose COCs.
	3. Exclude gynecologic problems (e.g., tumor, pregnancy, ectopic pregnancy, abortion, pelvic inflammatory disease, vaginitis)	3. Address gynecologic problems or refer for management.
	4. Is client taking new medicine (e.g., antiepileptics, rifampin)?	4. Patient may require a higher dose COC (ethinyl estradiol 50 µg) if no contraindication, or a switch to injectable (Depo-Provera) or nonhormonal method, or use a backup method (e.g., condoms) with COCs.
Melasma (Chloasma)	1. Are the skin changes cosmetically unacceptable?	1. If no, continue COCs and observe for possible worsening. If yes, the COCs should be discontinued because the patchy hyperpigmentation often progresses with continued use and is sometimes permanent. The provider should assist the patient in choosing a contraceptive method that does not contain estrogen.
Alopecia	1. Has hair loss persisted for longer than 3 months?	1. If no, reassure the patient that this rare side effect is usually transient. If yes, discontinue COCs and counsel patient in choosing a nonhormonal contraception method.

Adapted from Pocket Guide for Family Planning Service Providers. Baltimore: JHPIEGO;1995.

less than one half pack per day (39). Studies indicate that in nonsmokers the absolute incidence of stroke is so small that low-dose oral contraceptive use does not increase the risk (32,42-44).

The epidemiology of thrombotic venous events appears to differ from that of arterial events. While increasing age is a risk factor, for example, smoking is not (39). Other factors such as family history of venous thrombotic events, which may point to an inherited hypercoagulable state, may be more helpful in identifying women at risk for venous events with COC use. In addition, evidence points to the possibility that the third-generation progestins may also contribute to venous events. Some studies show a slightly higher risk of venous thromboembolism among users of the oral contraceptives that contain desogestrel or gestodene compared with users of first- or second-generation progestins (45-47). Because previous data have implicated estrogen and not progestins in thrombotic events, this finding is not easily explained. However, rigorous meta-analyses (48) and subsequent cohort studies (49) indicate that these observation studies were fraught with bias, which explains some of the apparent increased risk (50,51). Moreover, even if the relative risk for venous thromboembolism is 1.3 to 1.8 times that of the older progestin levenorgestrel (52,53), the absolute incidence of venous thromboembolism still remains very low (approximately 3/10,000); therefore these COCs may be prescribed to women who would benefit from the less androgenic profile.

Interestingly, among COC users, the third-generation progestins are associated with a *lower* incidence of arterial thrombotic events (38,39). The risk of arterial events is also lower in women using COCs containing the lowest dose of ethinyl estradiol (20 µg) (38,39,41). Although the incidence of arterial events in most reproductive-aged women is so low as to not influence the choice of COC type, it may be a consideration in women at higher risk (e.g., a woman in her 40s who does not smoke but has other cardiac risk factors).

Certain surgical procedures (e.g., pelvic surgery, lower extremity surgery) and prolonged bedrest increase the risk of venous thrombosis. Therefore women who are to undergo elective surgery associated with pelvic dissection or prolonged immobilization should ideally stop COCs 1 month before surgery and not resume them until 2 weeks after surgery. Such a strategy must be individualized, however, because its benefits may be outweighed by the risk of unintended pregnancy with temporary discontinuation of this reliable form of contraception (54).

Cholesterol, Acne, and Carbohydrate Metabolism

Although studies demonstrate a statistically significant lowering of HDL among individuals using low-dose oral contraceptives with usual progestins such as levonorgestrel, these changes do not translate into increased risk for atherosclerotic heart disease among nonsmoking women (32,42,43,55-57). In fact, animal studies using *Cynomolgus* monkeys demonstrate reduced coronary artery plaque formation with oral contraceptive administration (58,59). The third-generation progestins (desogestrel, gestodene, norgestimate) were developed to minimize androgenic side effects (e.g., muscular weight gain, acne, oiliness of the skin, adverse effects on the lipid profile, carbohydrate intolerance); however, data do not demonstrate clinical superiority of these formulations with regard to carbohydrate and lipid clinical outcomes (24-29,60-65). Nonetheless, while all COCs may improve acne, these newer progestin formulations are associated with enhanced improvement and may be selected on this basis.

Noncontraceptive Benefits

Numerous noncontraceptive benefits accrue to pill users. Some benefits relate directly to menstruation: a reduction in the number of "menstrual" bleeding days, blood loss, and dysmenorrhea. There is also evidence that COCs provide protection against pelvic inflammatory disease by inhibiting ascension of organisms through thickening of the cervical mucus (66). However, as with other nonbarrier methods, COCs do not provide protection against lower genital tract sexually transmitted diseases or HIV, and patients should be advised that condom use is required for this purpose. COCs also reduce the incidence and prevalence of benign breast disease and help prevent osteoporosis (66,67).

The noncontraceptive benefits of COCs allow for their therapeutic use in such conditions as primary and secondary dysmenorrhea, endometriosis, mittelschmerz, polycystic ovary syndrome, recurrent functional ovarian cysts, dysfunctional uterine bleeding, iron deficiency anemia from menorrhagia, hypothalamic amenorrhea with associated osteoporosis, and acne (6,9,68,69). Also, monophasic pills may be useful to delay "menstrual bleeding" by taking additional hormonally active pills from a separate pack. Such manipulation of the cycle is not only useful for preventing bleeding on vacations or weekends but may also be therapeutic for patients whose medical conditions are aggravated by menstruation (e.g., some patients with asthma). The patient can be instructed to skip the placebo week and proceed directly to the next pill pack, thereby limiting the number of bleeding episodes. Patient satisfaction has been documented with limiting bleeding episodes to once every 6 to 12 weeks (70), and new COCs will soon be marketed that have 7 to 12 weeks of active pills followed by one week of placebo, thereby inducing a withdrawal bleed every 2 to 3 months.

Cancer

The use of COCs significantly reduces the lifetime risk of endometrial (71,72) and ovarian cancer (73-76) via effects on cell proliferation in these tissues. In fact, a recent case-control study detected a 40% reduction in the risk of ovarian cancer associated with having ever used COCs and a greater than 50% reduction following use for 5 years or longer (76).

In contrast to ovarian and endometrial cancer, the relationship of oral contraceptive use to breast and cervical cancer is less positive. The data for breast cancer have been contradictory, in part due to flawed studies. Subgroup analysis reveals that oral contraceptive users are at slightly increased risk of breast cancer developing before age 45 (odds ratio, 1.4; 95% confidence interval, 1.0–2.1) (17,77-80). However, in part because the incidence of breast cancer among young women is so low, recent well-designed studies have demonstrated that overall the risk of breast cancer is not increased among women who are using or have used oral contraceptives (17,76,81,82).

Controversy continues to surround the possible increased risk of cervical cancer with current and former oral contraceptive use (17,83,84). It is possible that the hormonal effects on the cervix predispose it to neoplastic changes or make it more vulnerable to HPV infection. However, it is also possible that COC use is merely a marker for increased sexual activity or decreased use of barrier contraception, and therefore greater exposure to human papilloma virus. If the risk is increased, the absolute magnitude is small, and certainly a history of cervical dysplasia is not a contraindication to pill use (17).

Use in the Perimenopause

Low-dose combined contraceptive pills can be safely used until menopause in nonsmoking women with no contraindications to oral contraceptive use (8,9,85,86). In fact, during the peri-menopause combined oral contraceptives can provide several therapeutic benefits such as relief from menstrual irregularity, relief of vasomotor symptoms, reduced risk of ovarian and endometrial carcinomas, and protection from osteoporosis (71-73, 85-88).

Because the hormonal content of oral contraceptives is much higher than that necessary for postmenopausal hormonal replacement therapy (HRT), patients should be switched to HRT upon reaching menopause. Of course, because the COCs will usually continue to induce a monthly withdrawal bleed, determining the onset of menopause may present a challenge. One approach is to check the FSH (follicle stimulating hormone) level annually beginning at age 50 or 51. This should be performed during days 5, 6, or 7 of the hormone-free interval. If the FSH is greater than 20 mIU/mL, the patient is menopausal and should be switched to HRT. If the FSH is less than 20 mIU/mL, she should continue COCs. If one suspects the patient may be menopausal and that the FSH is falsely low due to persistent suppression by the exogenous hormones, one can retest after 2 weeks of withholding the COCs. In this situation, patients at risk for pregnancy should use barrier contraception until the result is known and, if found to not be menopausal, until COCs have been resumed for at least 2 weeks. A simpler approach is to just continue the COCs until the woman is 55 years old, at which time COCs can be discontinued and HRT begun. Rationales for this strategy include the demonstrated safety of COCs and the finding that FSH levels can remain unreliable even beyond two weeks following COC discontinuation (89,90).

Counseling

In addition to the usual counseling points, significant patient education should be devoted to how to take the pill and what to do if a pill is missed (Boxes 5-1 and 5-2).

Data indicate that the 1-year continuation rate of oral contraceptives is generally as low as 50%; the most frequently reported reason for discontinuation is side effects (2-5, 6,8,9,91,92). Ideally, therefore, first-time users should be seen

---

Box 5-1 Sunday Start Method for Taking Combined Oral Contraceptives

- COC pills can be started on any day as long as pregnancy is ruled out, but for most women a Sunday start translates into no menses on weekends.
- Advise patient to
  A. Begin the first pill on the Sunday after her period begins. If she has had an abortion, start on the Sunday after the first day of bleeding. If postpartum, start on a Sunday 4 to 6 weeks postpartum.
  B. Try to take the pill at the same time each day.

Box 5-2 Instructions for Missed Pills (Combined Oral Contraceptives)

- If the patient misses 1 pill, she should
  A. Take it as soon as she remembers. If she does not remember until the next day, she should take 2 pills the next day.
- If she misses 2 consecutive pills, she should
  A. Take 2 pills the day she remembers and 2 pills the following day.
  B. Use a back-up method for 7 days.
- If she misses more than 2 consecutive pills the risk of unplanned pregnancy may be substantial. She should
  A. Stop taking the daily pills and use emergency contraception (see text). (Her period will begin within 2–4 weeks, unless she is pregnant.)
  B. Begin a new package of pills on the Sunday after her period begins.
  C. Use a back-up method of birth control (such as condoms) from the time the error was discovered until the 8th day of the new package of pills.

in follow-up 1 to 2 months later by the physician or medical support personnel to assess side effects, compliance, and satisfaction. Alternatively, the patient may follow-up by telephone. She should also be instructed to call before discontinuing the pill; often a different formulation can be prescribed by telephone. Experienced oral contraceptive users require only routine visits for pelvic examination, Pap smear, and sexually transmitted diseases screening as indicated.

Combined Injectable Contraception (Lunelle)

Lunelle, a monthly combined injectable contraceptive approved by the FDA in October 2000, contains both an estrogen (estradiol cypionate 5 mg) and a progestin (medroxyprogesterone acetate 25 mg). Contraceptive efficacy is excellent, comparable to that for Norplant, Depo-Provera, IUDs, and sterilization (93).

The initial injection can be given within 5 days of the onset of a normal menstrual period, within 20 days of a first trimester abortion, or between 4 and 6 weeks postpartum. Subsequent injections should be scheduled for every 28 to 30 days but may be given as early as 23 days and as late as 33 days after the last injection. Thus Lunelle is not as convenient as Depo-Provera (which is administered every 12 weeks); however, the more frequent dosing allows for a lower dose of progestin (approximately half), which results in a lessening of the side effects and a faster return to fertility. In addition, the estrogen component allows for induction of a regular monthly withdrawal bleed lasting 5 to 7 days and helps to prevent irregular bleeding.

Because this method contains estrogen, however, the same contraindications and cautions apply as for COC use (see Tables 5-2 and 5-3). On the other hand, most of the noncontraceptive health benefits associated with COCs remain. Lunelle is appropriate for patients unwilling or unable to comply with taking daily COCs.

Progestin-Only Contraception

Currently available progestin-only contraceptives are the progestin-only pill ("mini-pill"), Depo-Provera, and the Norplant system. Other implantable and injectable forms are under development, and some are already available in other countries. Characteristics of progestin-only contraceptives are summarized in Table 5-6.

Women at risk for thromboembolic disease are appropriate candidates for progestin-only contraceptive methods; in fact, it is commonplace for women who smoke cigarettes to switch from COCs to a progestin-only method upon reaching age 35. Also, because these methods do not contain estrogen they may be initiated immediately postpartum or postabortion. Note, however, that

Table 5-6 Comparison of Progestin-Only Methods

Method	Mechanism	Typical Bleeding Patterns	Advantages	Disadvantages	Special Uses
Progestin-only pills (POPs)	Increases cervical nervous viscosity; also renders endometrium less hospitable; decreases tubal motility	Regular ovulatory menstrual cycles with superimposed spotting, especially initially	Easily reversible; low dose	Higher failure rate (~13%) than other hormonal methods	Women whose fertility is already lowered (e.g., smokers over age 40, lactating women)
Depo-Provera (injectable depot medroxyprogesterone acetate)	Inhibits ovulation; increases cervical mucous viscosity	Usually irregular spotting that progresses to complete amenorrhea after 1–2 years of use	Highly effective; convenient dosing (every 12 weeks)	Delayed return to fertility; side effect profile (especially weight gain)	Women taking antiepileptic drug and other medications that diminish efficacy of less potent methods; patients with sickle cell anemia; women who cannot take COCs reliably
Norplant system (levonorgestrel implants)	Initially inhibits ovulation, but after 3–4 years method more likely dependent on increasing cervical mucous viscosity	Usually irregular spotting for first few years, then regular cycles	Highly effective; user independent; long-term method (5 years)	Requires minor outpatient procedure; expensive (cost-effectiveness improves with duration of use)	Teens; older women who wish to avoid sterilization

Progestin-only contraception is commonly used in smokers age 35 or older, women intolerant of the side effects of estrogen, or those wanting a more user-independent method.

women with *current* thrombophlebitis or active coronary or cerebrovascular disease should generally not use any form of hormonal contraception. Package inserts for progestin-only contraceptives list contraindications identical to those for COCs. However, because the serious thromboembolic disorders associated with combined oral contraceptives are related to the estrogen content of the pill (32-34, 36), many of the listed contraindications are irrelevant for progestin-only methods.

The implantable and injectable methods are fairly user independent and particularly suitable for women who have difficulty remembering to take pills daily. As with other nonbarrier methods, none of the progestin-only contraceptive methods protects against STDs, and this should be carefully communicated to the patient. Simultaneous condom use should be encouraged in appropriate contexts. As with COCs, however, the increased viscosity of the cervical mucus may help prevent ascension of infection and offers some protection against pelvic inflammatory disease (PID).

Progestin-Only Pill ("Mini-Pill")

Progestin-only pills (POPs) available in the United States contain either norethindrone (Micronor 0.35 mg, Nor-QD 0.35 mg) or norgestrel (Ovrette 0.075 mg). The dose of progestational agent is lower than that found in combined oral contraceptives (Table 5-7); this, together with the absence of estrogen, produces inconsistent inhibition of ovulation. Consequently, the contraceptive efficacy of progestin-only pills is inferior to COCs (1-year failure rate of 0.51% with perfect use, but 1.1% to 13% failure rate with typical use). POPs rely on increases in the viscosity of cervical mucus to make sperm penetration unlikely. The progestational effect also reduces ovum transport by decreasing the motility of the fallopian tubes and renders the endometrial lining

Table 5-7 Progestin-Only Pill ("Mini-Pill")

Trade Name	Pharmaceutical Company	Progestin	Dose (mg)
Micronor	Ortho-McNeil	Norethindrone	0.35
Nor-Q D	Syntex	Norethindrone	0.35
Ovrette	Wyeth-Ayerst	Norgestrel	0.075

atrophic, which makes implantation less likely (8,9,94). Maximal contraceptive efficacy is achieved by consistently taking the pill at the same time of day, a point particularly important to communicate to the patient. Ideally pill-taking should be timed so that intercourse occurs when the progestational effect on cervical mucus is maximal (e.g., 3 to 22 hr after administration) (94,95).

In contrast to COCs, there are no placebo pills to trigger a withdrawal bleed; identical hormone doses are taken daily. The patient typically continues to ovulate and menstruate at her usual schedule, but she may also experience superimposed spotting. As with other progestin-only methods, menstrual disturbances are particularly likely to occur in the first few months of use and are a major reason for patient discontinuation (95,96).

In addition to unpredictable bleeding, side effects may include breast tenderness, acne/oily skin, weight gain, and headaches. Like COCs, progestin-only contraceptives have important noncontraceptive benefits that include decreased menstrual flow, improved hematocrit, and diminished dysmenorrhea. Though generally protective against ectopic pregnancy, the rate of ectopic pregnancy in the event of contraceptive failure is estimated to be 2.8 to 4.1 per 100 pregnancies, which is slightly higher than for noncontraceptors (95). This may stem from the mini-pill's suppression of fallopian tube motility. There is no delay in return of fertility or net loss of fertility.

Absolute contraindications to the use of progestin-only contraceptive pills include 1) current coronary artery or cerebrovascular disease, 2) undiagnosed genital bleeding or pregnancy, 3) known or suspected hormone dependent neoplasia, and 4) past or present benign or malignant liver neoplasm. Use of progestin-only pills should also be avoided among women taking rifampin or antiepileptics, because these medications increase the metabolism of the pills and reduce contraceptive efficacy.

Progestin-only pills are sometimes chosen for women who desire the convenience of an oral method but who are intolerant of the estrogenic side effects of COCs, or for whom estrogen is contraindicated (95). Because of the relatively poor efficacy of this method compared with other forms of hormonal contraception, however, POPs may be best suited for women whose fertility is already lowered, such as older women who smoke or women who are lactating (9,97). Other patients seeking a highly reliable method of contraception usually choose another agent. Patient education information on taking POPs and on what to do in the event of a missed pill are shown in Boxes 5-3 and 5-4.

Depot Medroxyprogesterone Acetate (Depo-Provera)

Contraceptive Action and Dosage
Another progestin-only contraceptive option is depot medroxyprogesterone acetate (DMPA; Depo-Provera). This long-acting contraceptive produces con-

---

Box 5-3 Patient Information for Progestin-Only Pills

- Instruct patient to begin the first pill on the Sunday after her period begins. If she has had an abortion or delivery, begin on the Sunday following the procedure.
- Emphasize that risk of pregnancy markedly increases with a missed pill.
- Optimum efficacy of POPs is between 3 and 22 hr after ingestion.
- Pills are to be taken daily. There is no pill-free interval.

Box 5-4 Management of Missed Progestin-Only Pills

If a pill is missed or taken late, the patient is at increased risk for pregnancy and breakthrough bleeding. A missed pill should be taken as soon as remembered. If the pill is more than 3 hr late, a back-up method should be used for 48 hr. If more than 1 pill is missed, advise the woman to

A. Stop taking the pills. Begin emergency contraception. (Her period will begin within 2–3 weeks unless she is pregnant.)

B. Start a new package of pills on the day her period begins.

C. Use a back-up method of birth control (such as condoms) from the time the error is discovered until the 8th day of the new package.

---

sistent and complete ovulatory inhibition. Like other progestational contraceptives it produces increased cervical mucus viscosity that reduces sperm penetration and causes endometrial atrophy, which makes implantation unlikely (98-100). The reliable 14 weeks of anovulation produced by DMPA is responsible for its very low failure rate of 0.3%; its user-independent mode of action contributes to its efficacy even with typical use.

DMPA is available in 150 and 400 mg/DL formulations, but the 150 mg preparation has greater bioavailability and is the only formulation that should be used for contraception (100). It is administered as a deep muscular injection using a $1\frac{1}{2}$-inch needle in the deltoid or gluteal muscle; the area should not be massaged after injection because massage may affect absorption. Ideally, DMPA is initiated within 5 days of the beginning of a normal menses, immediately postabortion, immediately postpartum in nonbreastfeeding women, or 6 weeks postpartum in breastfeeding women (101). This approach provides inhibition of ovulation with the first cycle and avoids inadvertent exposure in early pregnancy. When administered outside this window, a negative pregnancy test and patient counseling regarding the possibility of a very early pregnancy must be documented. If injection inadvertently occurs coincident with early pregnancy, the woman can be reassured that there is no evidence that DMPA is a teratogen (98,102). Thickening of the cervical mucous quickly takes effect in 1 to 2 days, but backup contraception is required for this time if DMPA is initiated outside the first 5 days of menses. Although an injection is protective against pregnancy for a full 14 weeks, repeat injections are generally scheduled every 12 weeks (every 3 months) to enhance compliance and allow for a margin of error. If a woman returns for reinjection more than 14 weeks after the previous injection, pregnancy should first be ruled out using a sensitive urine human chorionic gonadotropin (HCG) test after an appropriate interval of abstinence (usually 2 weeks) from intercourse. Alternatively, the next injection may be administered more expeditiously after a negative urine HCG result and documented discussion regarding the possibility of very early pregnancy that is yet undetectable.

Side Effects
Because DMPA contains moderate doses of progestin yet lacks estrogen, the endometrial lining becomes atrophic and dyssynchronous shedding is inevitable. Patients should be counseled to expect irregular bleeding. Irregular, heavy, and absent menses can all occur, and the patient should be forewarned and reassured. However, when heavy bleeding results from atrophy of the endometrium to the basalis layer, a short course of estrogen is often indicated to restore the functional layer (Table 5-8). With continued use of DMPA most patients develop complete amenorrhea—approximately 50% after 1 year and 80% after 3 years (102). Although some patients remain concerned about the amenorrhea despite reassurance that it is not unhealthy, most patients grow to appreciate this side effect.

Other common side effects include nausea, dizziness, changes in appetite with subsequent weight gain or loss, hair growth or loss, oiliness of the skin, acne, and headaches. As with Norplant (see below), side effects for an individual patient cannot be predicted based on user experience with other hormonal methods or user profile. Fortunately, many side effects are short-lived and can be managed symptomatically.

DMPA may not be ideal for those concerned about maintaining a slender body image because weight gain often results (average 5.4 lb in first year, 8.1 lb after 2 years, and 13.8 lb after 4 years of use) (98,100,102). Additionally, women at risk for bone loss/osteoporosis (e.g., chronic steroid users, amenorrheic elite

Table 5-8 Management of DMPA-Related Bleeding

* Premarin 1.25 mg daily for approximately 14 days *or*
* Ethinyl estradiol 50 µg daily for approximately 14 days (see Ref 102a)

athletes) might consider estrogen-containing contraceptive alternatives. In normal ovulating woman DMPA causes a reversible decrease in bone density (103-105) of no demonstrated clinical significance (112–114). In contrast, athletes with hypothalamic amenorrhea and decreased bone density demonstrate increased bone deposition with progesterone use (109). Nonetheless, such patients may benefit further from the addition of estrogen (Chapter 3).

Like COCs, DMPA has important noncontraceptive health benefits. The most significant is an 80% reduction in the incidence of endometrial carcinoma (110,111). Other noncontraceptive benefits include reduced incidence of iron deficiency anemia, dysmenorrhea, mittelschmerz, and ovarian cysts (112,113). As shown for COCs, epidemiologic data demonstrate that DMPA protects against pelvic inflammatory disease (98,112,113) but not against lower genital tract STDs. Additionally, DMPA may be the contraceptive of choice for women with seizure disorders because its efficacy is not compromised by antiepileptics and the high dose of progesterone may increase the seizure threshold (114-116). In women with sickle cell anemia DMPA has been shown to stabilize the red cell membrane, improve the hematocrit by decreasing menstrual blood loss, and reduce the incidence of painful crises (117,118).

Restoration of Fertility and Contraindications

Because DMPA entails relatively high doses of progestin that accumulate with long-term use, as many as 30% of users may fail to conceive within 12 months after discontinuation. Because return of fertility may sometimes be delayed as long as 22 months, this contraceptive method may not be ideal for women who desire pregnancy within 1 or 2 years.

Long-term use of Depo-Provera can be associated with a delayed return to fertility of nearly 2 years.

Table 5-9 lists the absolute contraindications to DMPA use.

Counseling

In addition to the usual counseling it is important to stress that unpredictable vaginal bleeding is inevitable with the DMPA form of hormonal contraception but that eventually most women become amenorrheic. Abnormal

Table 5-9 Absolute Contraindications to DMPA Use

- Active thrombophlebitis or thromboembolic disorder
- Undiagnosed abnormal genital bleeding
- Known or suspected pregnancy
- Acute liver disease; benign or malignant liver tumors
- Known or suspected malignancy of the breast

Proper patient education helps women anticipate and better tolerate the irregular bleeding that is a frequent cause for discontinuation of progestin-only methods.

bleeding constitutes the most common reason for discontinuation, but adequate patient education before initiating the method can improve continuation rates. Users should be instructed to call or return if side effects cause dissatisfaction and should return at least every 3 months for reinjection.

Implantable Contraception (Norplant)

The Norplant contraceptive system (Wyeth-Ayerst, Philadelphia) is currently the only implantable contraceptive system available for general use in the United States. This highly effective and safe contraceptive method consists of six levonorgestrel-containing Silastic capsules that are inserted subdermally in the upper inner arm of the woman. This office procedure requires only local anesthesia and can be performed by any trained provider. Each capsule, measuring 34 by 2.4 mm, releases levonorgestrel by diffusion. All six capsules are required to ensure contraceptive efficacy of greater than 99% over 5 years. With a 1 year failure rate of 0.09%, Norplant is the most effective reversible hormonal contraceptive method available in the United States.

Safety and Side Effects
Because hormone is continually released, only a very low dose is necessary for efficacy, and serum levels of hormone in Norplant users are lower than those associated with oral or injectable methods (119). This, together with the fact that Norplant contains no estrogen, is responsible for its superior safety profile compared with combined oral contraceptives (119,120).

The absence of estrogen to regulate cycles does result in irregular, unpredictable bleeding. This bleeding is not harmful and, even if prolonged, blood loss is seldom heavy enough to cause anemia. In fact, hemoglobin levels typically rise among Norplant users (119-121). However, when significant or prolonged, bleeding is often best treated with a brief course of estrogen therapy to establish a less atrophic endometrium (as with DMPA) (Table 5-10). With continued Norplant use, serum hormone levels decline, and typically after 3 or 4 years ovulation and normal menstrual cycles resume.

Other potential side effects are those that can occur in users of other hormonal forms of contraception and can include nausea, dizziness, change in appetite with subsequent weight gain or loss, hair growth or loss, oiliness of the skin, acne, and headaches. As with oral contraceptives, many of the side effects associated with Norplant are short-lived; generally, the only side effect

Table 5-10 Management of Abnormal Bleeding in Patient on Norplant

Prolonged or Frequent Bleeding (see Refs 122-124)
Thorough evaluation is required to exclude nonhormonal causes, particularly infection. A history, pelvic examination, gonorrhea and chlamydia testing, saline wet mount/KOH prep, and sometimes hematocrit are indicated. Most commonly, however, the abnormal bleeding results from atrophy of the endometrial lining and to dyssynchronous shedding. Routine transvaginal sonogram or endometrial biopsy is not necessary.

Treatment Regimens
Ibuprofen 800 mg tid × 5 days
Or if no contraindication to estrogen:
   Combined oral contraceptives for 1 cycle (either low dose or 50 µg preparation)* *or*
   Ethinyl estradiol 50 µg q day × 21 days

Amenorrhea
Reassurance
Do not induce bleeding
Obtain an hCG if any of the following:
   Patient is worried about pregnancy
   Insertion was not within 7 days of last menstrual period and patient has persistent
      amenorrhea
   Amenorrhea occurs after the establishment of regular cycles

*When using COCs to treat menorrhagia it is often helpful to explain to the patient that these are prescribed as a convenient method of administering estrogen, not because the contraceptive action of her method is lacking.

that lasts a year or more is the irregular, unpredictable bleeding episodes (119-121, 125). Unfortunately, the side effects that a given patient will experience with Norplant cannot be predicted based on user experience with other progestin-only contraceptive methods, such as the progestin-only pill or DMPA, or with a "trial" of an oral course of medroxyprogesterone. Despite side effect experiences, clinical research documents user satisfaction among both adolescents and adults (126,127). Users who were properly counseled regarding potential side effects before Norplant insertion tend to continue with the method (127-131). It should be emphasized, however, that when a woman desires Norplant removal rather than symptomatic treatment of side effects her decision must be respected. As with insertion, removal is an office procedure performed with local anesthesia by a trained provider.

Contraindications
Absolute contraindications to Norplant use are given in Table 5-11 (8,9,101). A woman with chronic liver disease yet stable liver enzyme levels may be a

Table 5-11 Absolute Contraindications to Norplant Use

- Active thrombophlebitis
- Undiagnosed abnormal genital bleeding
- Acute liver disease or benign or malignant liver tumors
- Known or suspected carcinoma of the breast
- Known or suspected pregnancy

candidate, in part because of the low dose of levonorgestrel released by Norplant. Certainly, a woman with a history of liver disease who now exhibits normal liver function is a candidate. There are no restrictions to using Norplant based on body weight (120). However, medications that enhance the hepatic metabolism of steroids such as rifampin, barbiturates, and antiepileptics (e.g., phenytoin, carbamazepine) reduce the contraceptive efficacy of Norplant, and women using these agents should consider alternative contraception.

Timing of Insertion
Norplant is usually inserted within 7 days of onset of menstruation (101) to lessen the risk of insertion during early, undetected pregnancy. If Norplant is inadvertently inserted during a pregnancy that will be continued, the implants should be removed, yet the woman should be reassured that there is no evidence of teratogenicity associated with Norplant (119). Norplant can be inserted safely immediately postabortion or postpartum (132). Current recommendations are that breastfeeding mothers wait 6 weeks postpartum before having Norplant inserted; however, Norplant does not prevent the milk letdown mechanism and data indicate that Norplant does not affect the health or development of the infant (133-135).

Return to Fertility
Norplant users can be assured there is no delay in return of fertility once the implants are removed (119,136); a couple trying to conceive after Norplant removal has an 85% chance of achieving pregnancy within 1 year. Serum levels of levonorgestrel are undetectable within 2 weeks of removal of all implants. If for technical reasons all six implants cannot be removed, the woman must be advised to use alternative contraception to prevent pregnancy.

Counseling
In addition to the usual counseling points it is of the utmost importance to educate the Norplant patient that for 3 to 4 years she will likely have intermittent, irregular spotting before returning to ovulatory, predictable monthly cycles.

Emergency Contraception

Yuzpe and Progestin-Only Methods

Emergency, or postcoital, contraception refers to those interventions designed to prevent pregnancy after unprotected intercourse. The most commonly used method is that described by Yuzpe in 1974, which relies on the use of combination oral contraceptives administered in high doses. Though its mechanism of action is not completely understood, the Yuzpe method probably works by inhibiting or delaying ovulation (137-140). In addition, because pregnancy is defined as beginning at implantation (and not at fertilization), changes induced in the endometrial lining that make implantation unlikely may also contribute to the efficacy of this method (141). This method has proven effectiveness started within 72 hr after unprotected intercourse; however, the sooner the regimen is started the more effective it is in preventing pregnancy (142). When using commonly available combination oral contraceptive pills (30–35 µg ethinyl estradiol), four pills are administered within 72 hr from the episode of unprotected intercourse, and another four pills are taken 12 hr after the first dose. If a 20-µg pill such as Alesse or Levlite is used, five pills are necessary at each dose, because at least 100 µg of ethinyl estradiol and 0.50 mg of levonorgestrel are required. Preven is a prepackaged emergency contraception kit. It contains four tablets of ethinyl estradiol 50 µg/levonorgestrel 250 µg (to be taken as 2 tablets immediately and then repeated 12 hr later) and a pregnancy test to rule out pregnancy existing before the unprotected intercourse that prompted emergency contraception use. If the patient has no reason to suspect she is already pregnant, she can save the pregnancy test for later use if menses fail to occur within 3 weeks of taking the emergency contraception.

With ideal use the Yuzpe method can be expected to reduce the risk of pregnancy by 75% from the expected incidence resulting from a single act of intercourse (143-145). The technique is ineffective if implantation has already occurred. Nausea is a common side effect of this regimen. When emesis occurs within 2 hr of pill ingestion a repeat dose is necessary. Prophylactic antiemetics, such as prochlorperazine (Compazine) dimenhydrinate (Dramamine), or promethazine hydrochloride (Phenergan), can be used to minimize patient discomfort and improve efficacy.

Recent evidence suggests that the levonorgestrel (progestin-only) method of emergency contraception is superior to the Yuzpe method, both in efficacy and side-effect profile. This postcoital regimen resembles the Yuzpe method except that the hormone consists of 1.5 mg levonorgestrel (or 3.0 mg norgestrel) taken twice. Plan B (Women's Capital Corporation, Seattle) is a blister pack of two pills. A less convenient method consists of using the pills taken from two packages of the progestin-only pill Ovrette (Wyeth-Ayerst Laboratories). Twenty Ovrette tablets are taken together within 72 hr after unprotected sex, then the dose is repeated 12 hr later (142,146). Progestin-only formulations may be particularly useful in lactating women and others unwilling or unable to take estradiol.

The Yuzpe and progestin-only methods have few contraindications. The most important is the presence of a pregnancy existing before the episode of unprotected coitus. However, if emergency contraception is inadvertently administered during early pregnancy or if the method fails, one can reassure the patient that there is no evidence of teratogenicity associated with oral contraceptive exposure (15,17).

A recent study found that making emergency contraception more accessible to patients by giving them a supply of pills to keep at home resulted in a reduced number of unwanted pregnancies. Such availability did not lead to repeated use or decrease the likelihood that patients would use more reliable forms of contraception (147). It should be noted that lack of awareness by physicians and patients and inadequate consumer demand have resulted in many pharmacies not keeping Preven, Plan B, or progestin-only pills in stock. Because emergency contraception requires prompt access to medication, it is important for physicians to be familiar with postcoital regimens that use ordinary combined oral contraceptives. Because of the critical issue of access and in light of the safety of emergency contraceptives, a petition has been filed with the FDA to make them available as an over-the-counter product. Oral methods of emergency contraception are listed in Table 5-12.

Other Postcoital Contraception Methods

A copper intrauterine device (IUD) inserted within 7 days of unprotected intercourse is an important nonhormonal, postcoital contraceptive option. The postcoital IUD can reduce the risk of pregnancy by 99%. This method is an attractive choice for women who also desire long-term contraception. Candidates for this method must be carefully selected (see Intrauterine Devices). The antiprogesterone agent mifepristone (Mifeprex, commonly known as RU 486) has also been shown to be very effective as an emergency contraceptive (94,148). Although approved only for use as an abortifacient, when mifepristone is used earlier and at lower doses its antiprogesterone action prevents pregnancy.

Patient Education

For all emergency contraceptive options (except for emergency IUD insertion), it is important to educate patients regarding the intended episodic use of this technique, particularly because emergency contraceptive techniques

Table 5-12 Oral Methods of Emergency Contraception

Trade Name and Manufacturer	Formulation	Number of Pills Taken With Each Dose*
Progestin Only		
Plan B Women's Capital Corporation Seattle	0.75 mg levonorgestrel	1
Ovrette Wyeth-Ayerst Philadelphia	0.075 mg norgestrel	20
Yuzpe Method		
Preven Gynetics, Inc. Belle Mead, N.J.	0.05 mg ethinyl estradiol 0.25 mg levonorgestrel	2
Lo-Ovral Wyeth-Ayerst	0.03 mg ethinyl estradiol 0.30 mg norgestrel	4
Nordette Wyeth-Ayerst	0.03 mg ethinyl estradiol 0.15 mg levonorgestrel	4
Levlen Berlex Wayne, N.J.	0.03 mg ethinyl estradiol 0.15 mg levonorgestrel	4
Triphasil Wyeth-Ayerst	(Yellow pills only) 0.03 mg ethinyl estradiol 0.125 mg levonorgestrel	4
Trilevlen Berlex	(Yellow pills only) 0.03 mg ethinyl estradiol 0.125 mg levonorgestrel	4
Alesse Wyeth-Ayerst	0.02 mg ethinyl estradiol 0.10 mg levonorgestrel	5
Levlite Berlex	0.02 mg ethinyl estradiol 0.10 mg levonorgestrel	5

*Treatment consists of two doses taken 12 hr apart. Use of anti-emetic agent before taking the medication lessens the risk of nausea and vomiting, common side effects (25).

have reduced efficacy compared with routine contraception. Additionally, the significant incidence of side effects associated with the Yuzpe method makes this contraceptive method unacceptable for frequent use.

First-time users of emergency contraception should follow-up in 3 weeks. A sensitive urine or serum HCG test should be performed if menses has not yet occurred. In the case of undesired pregnancy, the patient should be counseled regarding the options of termination and prenatal care. Patients experienced with this method can be instructed to follow-up only if menses does not occur within 3 weeks. If a routine method of contraception is not chosen when the emergency contraception is provided, a follow-up visit is useful for counseling and method selection.

Intrauterine Devices

Mechanism of Action and Insertion

A device inserted into the uterine cavity for the purpose of preventing pregnancy is termed an *intrauterine device*. Worldwide, the IUD is the most popular method of reversible contraception (149). It has the advantages of being user independent and highly effective. Ideal candidates are monogamous parous, and without any undiagnosed vaginal bleeding (Table 5-13).

Until recently only two IUD products have been available in the United States. The copper IUD (Paragard T380A) is designed for up to 10 years of use and has a failure rate (0.6%–0.8%) comparable to that for surgical sterilization. The progesterone IUD (Progestasert) releases 65 μg/day of progesterone and must be replaced each year. This IUD is less effective (2.9% failure rate)

Table 5-13 Intrauterine Devices Available in the United States

Type of IUD	Components	Duration of Action	Failure Rate	One-Year Continuation Rate
ParaGuard	Copper wire wrapped around the vertical stem and horizontal arms; clear-white monofilament polyethylene string	10 years	Perfect use: 0.6% Typical use: 0.8%	78%
Progestasert	Reservoir releasing progesterone; blue-black monofilament string	1 year	Perfect use: 1.5% Typical use: 2%	81%
Mirena	Silastic rod impregnanted with levonorgestrel; silver-gray string	5 years	<0.5%	94%

but has a more favorable side effect profile. The suppressive effect of the progesterone on the endometrium is associated with reduced dysmenorrhea and menstrual flow (150); however, the same action causes an increased incidence of intermenstrual spotting. The copper IUD has been associated with dysmenorrhea and increased menstrual blood loss, especially for a short time following insertion. Irregular vaginal bleeding and pain have been reported with both devices.

An IUD containing levonorgestrel (Mirena IUS, Berlex) became available in 2001. The most common side effect is irregular breakthrough bleeding, which occurs during the first 6 months after insertion; however, eventually almost half of all users become amenorrheic. Its local hormonal action renders this IUD useful for noncontraceptive indications such as treating menorrhagia. It is effective for at least 5 years after insertion, another distinct advantage for most women (151).

Some IUDs release a progestin and thus may also be therapeutic for conditions such as menorrhagia.

Although the mechanism of action of contraception is not entirely understood, evidence shows that IUDs prevent fertilization and are not abortifacients (8,9,152). It is thought that the chronic sterile foreign body reaction in the endometrial cavity elicited by these devices is spermicidal (152). In addition, copper is known to be sperm toxic. The progesterone- and levonorgesterol-releasing IUDs have the additional actions of decidualizing the endometrium and thickening the cervical mucus, making sperm penetration more difficult.

Intrauterine devices can be inserted any time during the menstrual cycle, as long as pregnancy has been excluded. Many practitioners prefer to perform insertion within 1 to 5 days of the onset of menses because the cervical os may be more open, allowing for easier and more comfortable insertion, and because pregnancy is less likely. First-time users should return to their practitioners after menses and first intercourse has occurred. Correct placement of the IUD should be verified, and the IUD string may be trimmed for patient comfort. The patient must be asked to return upon expiration of their particular device. New IUD insertion can be performed at that time. The user should also be reminded that this contraception method offers no protection against STDs.

Side Effects and Contraindications

The risk of pelvic infection has concerned providers and patients alike since the withdrawal of the Dalkon Shield from the market. However, the increased incidence of PID associated with the Dalkon Shield has been attributed to its multifilament string, which acted as a wick for bacteria to ascend from the vagina. Monofilament strings are now used, and data on current IUDs reveal a remarkable margin of safety (149,153). Reanalysis of international data from the World Health Organization reveals a low risk of PID (<2/1000 patient years) associated with long-term IUD use (154). In a large prospective cohort of American women there was no increased risk of PID among monogamous married or cohabitating women (155). Most infections occur in the first month after insertion and are most likely associated with bacterial contamination during insertion (149,153,154,156).

Absolute contraindications and cautions to IUD use are listed in Tables 5-14 and 5-15.

Counseling

In addition to routine counseling about failure rates, mechanism of action, STD risk, and contraindications, potential IUD users should be advised to periodically feel in the vagina for the string. This helps determine that the IUD has not been inadvertently expelled or dislodged.

Table 5-14 Absolute Contraindications to Intrauterine Device Use

- Active, recent, or recurrent pelvic inflammatory disease
- Multiple sexual partners
- Partner has multiple sexual partners
- Recent history of STD
- HIV infection
- Known or suspected pregnancy

Table 5-15 Conditions Requiring Caution with Intrauterine Device Use

- Untreated/undiagnosed purulent or mucopurulent cervicitis
- Remote history of gonorrhea, chlamydia
- History of pelvic inflammatory disease, postpartum or postabortal endometritis/salpingitis
- Immunocompromised state
- Undiagnosed genital bleeding
- History of ectopic pregnancy
- Previous problems with IUDs
- High-risk category for infective bacterial endocarditis
- Uterine abnormalities that preclude proper insertion
- Nulliparous women who desire future childbearing

Barrier Contraception

Barrier methods function by interposing physical and/or chemical barriers to the passage of sperm into the upper reproductive tract. Currently available barrier methods include male condoms, female condoms, diaphragms, cervical caps, and chemical barriers. All except diaphragms and cervical caps are available over the counter. Barrier methods require that a woman or couple is highly motivated to use this method, and many forms require that both are comfortable with her body. A cooperative partner is therefore a requirement for successful use of these methods. Allergy to material components or the inability to consistently and correctly use these methods is an absolute contraindication.

Couples selecting these methods must be aware that even with theoretically perfect use, a significant number of pregnancies may occur. Efficacy is optimized when used correctly in combination with another method. Patients choosing to use barrier contraception alone benefit from being made aware of the availability of emergency contraception. Giving such patients a prescription for emergency contraception or a package of COCs to keep on hand may be particularly useful in helping to prevent pregnancy in the event of condom breakage or other method failure.

Barrier methods are an option for women who decline hormonal contraception, and those rare individuals who have true contraindications to other methods. Barrier methods provide simultaneous protection against pregnancy and sexually transmitted diseases, and this latter feature may represent an important advantage for some women. The male and female condoms offer good protection against STDs, and other barrier methods do so to a lesser degree.

Male Condoms

Condoms are popular, easily available, nonprescription, single-use contraceptives that serve as a mechanical barrier to sperm, bacteria, and viruses. Although these products are made of a variety of materials and membranes, only latex and, probably, polyurethane and Tactylon (a synthetic latex) condoms are effective in reducing STD transmission (157-159). Some latex condom products are lubricated with spermicide, most commonly nonoxynol-9, which increases contraceptive effectiveness. Nonoxynol-9 was previously thought to also reduce transmission of many STDs (160); however, more recent studies (161,162) demonstrate lack of protection against HIV and cervical infection by chlamydia or gonorrhea.

With perfect use, the 1-year contraceptive failure rate is as low as 1% to 4% (8,9,163). Among typical users, however, failure rates are 10% to 20% (8,9,11). At 1 year of use, the usual continuation rate is approximately 63%.

To ensure correct condom use and protection from both unwanted pregnancy and STDs, patient counseling should be explicit:

1. The condom should be rolled onto the erect penis.
2. After placement a $1/_2$-inch tip of the condom should be pinched to create a reservoir.
3. Withdrawal from the vagina, mouth, or rectum should occur prior to the loss of the erection.
4. The rim of the condom should be held during withdrawal in order to prevent spillage.
5. In the event of condom breakage, intravaginal spermicide should be used immediately and the patient should be instructed to seek post-coital contraception.
6. Only water-based lubricants should be used with latex condoms.
7. Condoms are not reuseable.
8. Condoms should be stored in a cool dry, dark place; they may be kept in a wallet for up to 1 month.

First-time users are encouraged to follow-up with their contraceptive providers if they experience problems with this method. A reassessment of contraceptive needs can occur at that time.

Female Condom

The female condom consists of a polyurethane sheath with a flexible ring at the opening and another at the closed base. The device is lubricated with a nonspermicidal silicone-based gel. The use of this device is contraindicated in individuals with a polyurethane or silicone allergy. With correct and consistent use, failure rates as low as 5.1% have been estimated (164). However, its contraceptive efficacy is comparable to that for the diaphragm and cervical cap, which may have typical use failure rates as high as 23%.

This device may be inserted up to 8 hr before intercourse and should not be used in conjunction with a male latex condom (165). Like the male condom, the female condom offers substantial protection against sexually transmitted bacterial and viral pathogens (166,167) and, in fact, the design of the female condom may offer superior protection of the vulva. This feature, and the fact that the female partner has direct control, are the major advantages of the female condom. Compared to the male condom this one-time use method is relatively expensive, however.

Diaphragm

The diaphragm is a dome-shaped reusable latex rubber device, with a flexible rim. It covers the cervix, providing a physical barrier to sperm entry. The diaphragm is available in four rim types (arching spring, coil spring, flat spring, and wide seal), ranges in size from 50 to 105 mm, and requires fitting by an experienced provider. The largest size that maximally covers the cervix with minimal discomfort is selected for use. Once inserted, a correctly fitted diaphragm should not be noticeable to the patient or her partner. It should be placed at least 30 min but no longer than 6 hr before coitus and must be left in place at least 6 hr afterwards (8,9). Diaphragm use requires spermicidal jelly or cream to facilitate placement as well as maximize contraceptive efficacy. Additional acts of intercourse during a single wear require placement of intravaginal spermicide. If diaphragm placement has occurred more than 2 hr before coitus, it is advisable to insert intravaginal spermicide before the act. With previous use the failure rate can be as low as 2% per year but typically can be as high as 23%. After pregnancy or weight change of more than 10 lb, the fit of the diaphragm should be reassessed. Manual dexterity and coordination is required for correct diaphragm placement. The device should not be used in those who can not demonstrate its correct placement. Individuals with latex rubber allergy should avoid its use.

Regular diaphragm users have been noted to be at increased risk for urinary tract infection (169). It is unclear whether this is a result of urethral obstruction caused by the device or by the lubricating spermicide, or both. In addition, poorly fitting diaphragms and those devices in place for more than 20 to 24 hr can be responsible for vaginal irritation, abrasions, and discomfort (8,9).

Important noncontraceptive benefits are associated with diaphragm use. These include reduced rates of cervical infections, pelvic inflammatory disease, and infertility (170). However, it is unclear to what degree the diaphragm, when used with a spermicide, provides protection against viral STDs.

First-time users should return to their physician shortly after the first few acts of intercourse using the diaphragm. Patient acceptability, comfort, and compliance should be assessed, and alternative forms of contraception may need to be discussed.

Cervical Cap

The cervical cap is a thimble-shaped rubber cup that is designed to fit snugly over the cervix. Like the diaphragm, it requires fitting by an experienced provider. Sizing this device is more problematic because it is available in only four sizes. The size, shape, and position of the cervix may change with time, pregnancy, cervical surgery, and pelvic relaxation; thus the fit of the device should be reassessed periodically. Spermicides facilitate the placement and maximize contraceptive efficacy. Like the diaphragm, insertion is at least 30 min but no longer than 6 hr before intercourse, and removal takes place at least 6 hr after. In contrast to the diaphragm, however, the cervical cap may be left in place for a maximum of 36 to 48 hrs (8,9). Though not yet studied, it probably affords a similar degree of protection against STDs as the diaphragm. Allergy to latex and inability to correctly use the device are the only contraindications. Typical failure rates are as high as 40% (8,9).

Vaginal Contraceptive Sponge

The over-the-counter, vaginal contraceptive sponge (Today, Allendale) was withdrawn from the market because of manufacturing problems but is now being readied for general use. The vaginal contraceptive sponge is a polyurethane barrier containing nonoxynol-9 designed to fit high in the vagina. It is a one-size, single-use device that can be inserted up to 24 hr before intercourse. The first-year failure rate for the sponge is similar to that of the diagram but can rise significantly among parous women.

Chemical Barriers

Spermicides are widely available nonprescription chemical barrier preparations. They consist of either nonoxynol-9 or octoxynol suspended in a carrier (foam, cream, jelly, film, suppository, or tablet). These preparations are detergents that disrupt the cell membranes of sperm in the vagina and prevent sperm entry into the upper reproductive tract. Spermicides are generally applied 10 to 30 min before intercourse, but the timing of intravaginal application varies and package directions should be followed. Spermicides may remain effective for up to 6 to 8 hr after coitus, and for this reason patients should not douche for at least 6 to 8 hr. Reapplication is required with each coital episode. Spermicides are considered fair contraceptives; the failure rates associated with using spermicides alone are estimated to range from 1% to more than 30% (168).

By the same mechanism that enables them to be active against sperm, spermicides have been shown to be effective against bacteria and viruses *in vitro* and thus may afford some degree of protection against STDs (8,9,160). Whether spermicide use leads to a reduction in infections is more difficult to establish (166-168,171,172), but protection against gonorrhea and chlamydia is estimated at 10% to 50% (173,174). Paradoxically, however, use of spermicides by prostitutes has been associated with damage to vaginal mucosal surfaces and increased risk of HIV acquisition (175-177). Based on this information spermicides may afford some protection against STDs for individuals who do not have frequent acts of intercourse in one day. However, even in these women spermicides can cause shifts in the vaginal flora that lead to bacterial vaginosis and possibly urinary tract infection (178).

Sterilization

Female Sterilization (Tubal Ligation)

For women who have completed childbearing and who desire a user-independent nonhormonal method, surgical contraception is an important, permanent option. Various techniques involve occluding, destroying or otherwise interrupting the fallopian tubes, all with the intent to render the individual permanently sterile (Table 5-16). One-year failure rates ranging from 0.2% to 0.4% among experienced providers (168) make this approach very attractive for women who do not desire or cannot risk pregnancy. The absolute contraindications to tubal ligation are given in Table 5-17.

Like any other contraceptive approach, however, tubal ligation is not 100% effective. The 1996 report of the CREST Study indicated that female sterilization failures can occur several years after the procedure, and 10-year cumulative failure rates may be as high as 1.85 pregnancies for every 100 procedures (179). In comparison, vasectomy is by far a superior permanent method, and even the Cu T380 IUD (ParaGard) or two successive insertions of Norplant contraceptive implants are theoretically as effective as female sterilization at 10 years. However, the CREST Study results may not be generally applicable. An unusually high rate of technical failure was observed for women who underwent sterilization at teaching institutions, and some of the procedures performed were techniques that had only recently been developed.

Table 5-16 Tubal Ligation Procedures

Timing	Procedure
<48 hr postpartum	Mini-laparotomy with bilateral occlusion of the fallopian tubes by one of a variety of surgical techniques
Interval (≥6 wk postpartum)	Laparotomy with cauterization, or placement of rings, bands, clips, or endoloops; or mini-laparotomy: 5–7 cm suprapubic incision through which the fallopian tubes are interrupted and occluded through a variety of surgical techniques

Table 5-17 Absolute Contraindications to Tubal Ligation

• Desire for future fertility or ambivalence regarding future fertility
• Acute salpingitis (the procedure is delayed until treatment complete)
• Acute peritonitis (a contraindication to any intra-abdominal surgery)

Health Benefits
Women who have undergone tubal ligation have been consistently noted to have a diminished incidence of ovarian cancer (181,182) (see Chapter 13). Protection against salpingitis is another noncontraceptive health benefit, although patients should be educated that tubal ligation affords no protection against lower-tract STDs. Most evidence indicates that tubal occlusion procedures are not associated with subsequent menstrual irregularity or pain (180) or change in sexual function or satisfaction.

Counseling
It cannot be sufficiently emphasized that individuals must be counseled thoroughly regarding the intended permanence of these procedures. Women expressing ambivalence about future childbearing should be steered toward reversible methods. While tubal reversal techniques have been developed that are successful approximately half of the time, tubal ligation should be considered a permanent procedure. The mortality rate of the procedure is 3/100,000—less than half the mortality risk of pregnancy. Most women who undergo this minor outpatient surgical procedure can resume work within a week. At the postoperative visit (usually 4 wk), the woman should be encouraged to continue schedule routine pelvic examination for cervical cancer screening and tests for STDs as indicated.

Male Sterilization (Vasectomy)

Vasectomy involves bilateral occlusion with partial resection of the vas deferens to render permanent male sterilization. In the United States, this safe, office-based procedure is performed primarily by urologists and family physicians. Compared with female tubal sterilization, the procedure is safer and associated with a lower failure rate—ranging from 0.02% to 6%, depending on surgical technique (8,9,168). Complications are rare, local, and usually easily treated. The incidence of hematomas is 0.1% to 5%, incisional infection, 0 to 4%; congestive epididymitis, 0.4% to 6%; and painful granulomas, 2% to 3% (183-185). The lowest surgical complications tend to be seen with the "no scalpel" technique of vasectomy. The "no scalpel" technique refers to the use of a dissecting clamp (no scalpel) to open the skin and a specialized surgical clamp to isolate the vas deferens (184-186). In 1995, approximately 500,000 vasectomies were performed in the United States; almost one-third of these procedures were performed using the "no scalpel" technique (187).

The vasectomy procedure is not considered effective in prevention of pregnancy until semen analysis demonstrates absence of sperm. Time interval to examining the first semen sample varies and may range from 6 to 12 weeks. Some physicians base the scheduling of the follow-up evaluation on the number of ejaculations (often 15–30) postvasectomy (184). Similarly, the number of required azospermic samples before backup contraception is discontinued varies (187), and the couple should follow the recommendations provided. Vasectomy does not impair libido or sexual function nor does it protect against STDs.

Although intended to be permanent, techniques have been developed to reverse vasectomy. Success rates range from 33% to 75% and depend upon such factors as type of vasectomy procedure, length of time from vasectomy, and skill of the operator performing the reversal (184). Absolute contraindications to vasectomy include desire for, or ambivalence regarding, future fertility, and active balanitis, epididymitis, or orchitis.

Since the late 1980s concern has been expressed about increased risk of prostate and testicular cancer among vasectomized men. Analyses indicate that such an association either does not exist or is very weak (184,188-191). The American Urological Association, the American Cancer Society, and the National Institutes of Health have issued statements that no change in vasectomy or prostate cancer screening practices is warranted (192,193).

Counseling includes discussing the impact of vasectomy on sexual function, explaining the procedure, discussing complications and risks and the possibility of failure, explaining the need for postoperative semen analysis, and emphasizing the permanence of the procedure (194).

Natural Family Planning (Periodic Abstinence)

Natural family planning and *the rhythm method* are terms used to refer to methods of fertility control that rely on the avoidance of intercourse during times of peak fertility. The greatest risk for pregnancy is probably during the six-day period that ends on the day of ovulation (195). Thus knowledge of when ovulation occurs is crucial; this may be estimated by monitoring changes in body temperature and cervical mucus that are associated with the preovulatory surge in progesterone (196). Such methods require very regular menstrual cycles, an exceptionally motivated patient and partner, and an experienced clinician or counselor.

With perfect use the failure rates for the rhythm method may be as high as 10%, and this increases further to between 20% and 86% with typical use. Efficacy is increased by the concomitant use of barrier contraception (197). In addition to compliance issues, problems such as fevers (which interfere with basal body temperature determination) and vaginal infections (which interfere with interpretations of cervical mucous quality) contribute to the high failure rate.

The chief benefits of this technique are that it involves no expense to the couple, increases their awareness and knowledge of reproductive function, and is without side effects. Motivated couples seeking this type of contraception should be referred to counselors or practitioners with expertise in this area.

Lactational Amenorrhea Method

The lactational amenorrhea method (LAM) is short-term contraception that fully or almost fully breastfeeding women can use. Its 98% effective rate only applies during the first 6 months postpartum to women who, after postpartum bleeding ends, remain amenorrheic and provide little (e.g., water only) supplemental feeding to the infant (198-200).

Nipple stimulation results in depression of gonadotropin-releasing hormone secretion, which in turn inhibits pituitary gonadotropin secretion and ovulation. Frequent suckling, including nighttime, is required. It has been estimated that for this method to be effective, the woman must nurse 15 or more times per day for at least 10 min per feeding (198). Any couple using this method should be counseled that LAM is short term; it is necessary to use another method if any one of the three criteria (amenorrhea, fully or almost fully breastfeeding, less than 6 months postpartum) change (200). Follow-up should be frequent enough to permit initiation to another method when efficacy wanes; the woman should be seen before 6 months postpartum.

New Methods

One implantable contraceptive method that has been approved but is not yet available in the United States is Norplant II (Jadelle, Wyeth), which consists of two Silastic rods instead of six, making insertion and removal easier. Like Norplant, it will release levonorgestrel over 5 years. Another implantable contraceptive, Implanon, consists of one Silastic capsule containing desogestrel and is effective for 3 years. Gynefix is a frameless IUD consisting of a non-biodegradable suture thread onto which six small copper tubes are threaded. This IUD is attached to the interior uterine myometrium, and its new design is intended to minimize expulsion and the dysmenorrhea sometimes associated with IUD use.

Vaginal contraceptive rings release either progestins alone or estrogen and progestin; they are designed for 1 to 12 months of use, depending on formulation. In October 2001 the FDA approved NuvaRing, a 1-month vaginal ring that is worn 3 continuous weeks, then removed (and discarded) for 1 week, during which time withdrawal bleeding occurs. In November 2001 Evra, an estrogen/progestin skin patch, received FDA approval. A new patch is worn weekly for 3 out of 4 weeks. The safety and effectiveness of both the ring and the patch are comparable to COCs. Barrier methods under development include easier and more effective diaphragm-like products such as FemCap and LeaShield.

The development of microbicides/spermicides is a relatively new but intense area of research. These substances offer better protection against bacterial and viral STDs and pregnancy. Also in development are reversible hormonal contraception for men, transcervical methods of sterilization, and immunocontraceptives.

Summary

Although virtually no form of contraception is without side effects, with proper guidance most women who wish to prevent pregnancy will ultimately find an acceptable method. Familiarity with the various types of contraception and their advantages allows the primary care physician to assist the patient in choosing her optimal method. In addition, debunking myths regarding the "dangers" of contraceptives, appraising the patient of expected side effects, communicating the noncontraceptive benefits of methods, and arranging appropriate follow-up are all ways the physician can help ensure better compliance with contraception. It is anticipated that such efforts will have an impact on the unusually high rate of unintended pregnancy in the United States.

REFERENCES

1. **Henshaw SK.** Unintended pregnancy in the United States. Fam Plann Persp. 1998;30:24–9.
2. **Zabin LS.** Ambivalent feelings about parenthood may lead to inconsistent contraceptive use—and pregnancy. Fam Plann Perspect. 1999;31:246–7, 260.
3. **Rosoff JI.** Not just teenagers. Fam Plann Persp. 1988;20:52.
4. **Jones EF, Forrest JD, Henshaw SK, et al.** Unintended pregnancy, contraceptive practice and family planning services in developed countries. Fam Plann Persp. 1988;20: 53–76.
5. Basic Principles in Family Planning Service Delivery: Informed Choice. New York: AVSC International, 1999.
5a. **Stewart FH, Harper CC, Ellertson CE, et al.** Clinical breast and pelvic examination requirements for hormonal contraception: current practice versus evidence. JAMA. 2001;285:2232-9.

6. **Piccinino LJ, Mosher WD.** Trends in contraceptive use in the United States: 1982–1995. Fam Plann Persp. 1998;4–10, 46.

7. **Forrest JD, Fordyce RR.** Women's contraceptive attitudes and use in 1992. Fam Plann Perspec. 1993;25:175–9.

8. **Hatcher RA, Trussell J, Stewart F, et al.** Contraceptive Technology, 17th ed. New York: Ardent Media, 1998.

9. **Speroff L, Darney PD.** A Clinical Guide for Contraception, 2nd ed. Baltimore: Williams and Wilkins; 1996.

10. **Foster DC.** Low-dose monophasic and multiphasic oral contraceptives: a review of potency, efficacy, and side effects. Semin Reprod Endocrinol. 1989;7:205–12.

11. **Trussell J, Kost K.** Contraceptive failure in the United States: a critical review of the literature. Stud Fam Plan. 1987;18:237–83.

12. **Jones EF, Forrest JD.** Contraceptive failure rates based on the 1988 NSFG. Fam Plann Persp. 1992;24:12–9.

13. **Moghissi KS, Syner FN, McBride LC.** Contraceptive mechanism of microdose norethindrone. Obstet Gynecol. 1973;41:585–94.

14. **Elstein M, Morris SE, Groom GV, et al.** Studies on low-dose oral contraceptives: cervical mucus and plasma hormone changes in relation to circulating D-norgestrel and 17-ethynyl estradiol concentrations. Steril. 1976;27:892–8.

15. Dialogues in contraception. Contracep Fetal Risk. 1991;3:1–8.

16. **Huggins GR, Cullins VE.** Fertility after contraception or abortion. Fertil Steril. 1990;54:559–73.

17. Hormonal Contraception. ACOG Technical Bulletin No. 198, Oct. 1994.

18. Metabolic effects of oral contraceptives: fact vs. fiction. In: Grimes DA, ed. Contraception Report. 1996;6:4–14.

19. **Klein BE, Moss SE, Klein R.** Oral contraceptives in women with diabetes. Diabetes Care. 1990;13:895–8.

20. **Garg SK, Chase HP, Marshall G, et al.** Oral contraceptives and renal and retinal complications in young women with insulin-dependent diabetes mellitus. JAMA. 1994;271:1099–1102.

21. **Sullivan JM, Lobo RA.** Considerations for contraception in women with cardiovascular disorders. Am J Obstet Gynecol. 1993;168:2006–11.

22. **Stone SC.** Clinical challenge: oral contraceptives and hypertension. Int J Fertil. 1994;39:143–7.

23. **Wild RA.** Clinical challenge: the diabetic on oral contraceptives. Int J Fertil. 1994;39:148–52.

24. **Mestman JH, Schmidt-Sarosi C.** Diabetes mellitus and fertility control: contraception management issues. Am J Obstet Gynecol. 1993;168:2012–20.

25. **Loriaux DL, Wild RA.** Contraceptive choices for women with endocrine complications. Am J Obstet Gynecol. 1993;168:2021-6.

26. **Comp PC, Zacur HA.** Contraceptive choices in women with coagulation disorders. Am J Obstet Gynecol. 1993;168:1990–3.

27. **Knopp RH, LaRosa JC, Burkman RT Jr.** Contraception and dyslipidemia. Am J Obstet Gynecol. 1993;168:1994–2005.

28. **Upton GV.** Lipids, cardiovascular disease, and oral contraceptives: a practical perspective. Fertil Steril. 1990;53:1–12.

29. **Breckwoldt M, Wieacker P, Geisthovel F.** Oral contraception in disease states. Am J Obstet Gynecol. 1990;163:2213–6.

30. **Kyos SL, Shoupe D, Douyan S, et al.** Effect of low-dose oral contraceptives on carbohydrate and lipid metabolism in women with recent gestational diabetes: results of a controlled, randomized, prospective study. Am J Obstet Gynecol. 1990;163:1822–7.

31. **Vessey M, Painter R.** Oral contraceptive use and benign gallbladder disease revisited. Contraception. 1994;50:167–73.

32. **Ramcharan S. Pellegrin FA, Ray RM, Hsu J-P.** A prospective study of the side effects of oral contraceptives. Volume III—an interim report: a comparison of disease occurrence leading to hospitalizations or death in users and nonusers of oral contraceptives. J Reprod Med. 1980;25:345–72.

33. Further analyses of mortality in oral contraceptive users. Royal College of General Practitioners' Oral Contraception Study. Lancet. 1981;1:541–6.

34. **Vessey M, Mant D, Smith A, Yeates D.** Oral contraceptives and venous thromboembolism: findings in a large prospective study. Br Med J. 1986;292:526.

35. **Grodstein F, Stampfer M, Goldhaber SZ, et al.** Prospective study of exogenous hormones and risk of pulmonary embolism in women. Lancet. 1996;348:983–7.

36. **Gerstman BB, Pip JM, Tomita DK, et al.** Oral contraceptive estrogen dose and the risk of deep venous thromboembolic disease. Am J Epidemiol. 1991;133:32–7.

37. **Koster T, Small RA, Rosendaal FR, Helmerhorst FM.** Oral contraceptives and venous thromboembolism: a quantitative discussion of the uncertainties. J Intern Med. 1995;238:31–7.

38. **Lidegaard O, Kreiner S.** Cerebral thrombosis and oral contraceptives: a case-control study. Contraception. 1998;57:303–14.

39. **Lidegaard O, Bygdeman M, Milsom I, et al.** Oral contraceptives and thrombosis; from risk estimates to health impact. Acta Obstet Gynecol Scand. 1999;78:142–9.

40. **Becker WJ.** Use of oral contraceptives in patients with migraine. Neurology. 1999; 53(suppl 1):S19–25.

41. **Gillum LA, Mamidpudi SK, Claiborne JS.** Ischemic stroke risk with oral contraceptives: a meta-analysis. JAMA, 2000;284:72–8.

42. **Porter JB, Jick H, Walker AM.** Mortality among oral contraceptive users. Obstet Gynecol. 1987;70:29–32.

43. **Porter JB, Hunter JR, Jick H, Stergachis A.** Oral contraceptives and nonfatal vascular disease. Obstet Gynecol. 1985;66:1–4.

44. **Petitti DB, Sidney S, Bernstein A. et al.** Stroke in users of low-dose oral contraceptives. N Engl J Med. 1996;335:8–15.

45. Effect of different progestagens in low oestrogen oral contraceptives on venous thromboembolic disease. World Health Organization Collaborative Study of Cardiovascular Disease and Steroid Hormone Contraception. Lancet. 1995;346:1582–8.

46. **Jick H, Jick SS, Gurewich V, et al.** Risk of idiopathic cardiovascular death and nonfatal venous thromboembolism in women using oral contraceptives with differing progestagen components. Lancet. 1995;346:1589–93.

47. Venous thromboembolic disease and combined oral contraceptives; results of an international multicentre case-control study. World Health Organization Collaborative Study of Cardiovascular Disease and Steroid Hormone Contraception. Lancet. 1995; 346:1575–82.

48. **Spitzer WO.** The aftermath of a pill scare: regression to reassurance. Hum Reprod Update. 1999;5:736–45.

49. **Lidegaard O.** Thrombotic diseases in young women and the influence of oral contraceptives. Am J Obstet Gynecol. 1998,179:S62–7.

50. **Lidegaard O, Edstrom B, Kreiner S.** Oral contraceptives and venous thromboembolism: a case-control study. Contraception. 1998,57:291–301.

51. **Suissa S, Spitzer WO, Rainville B, et al.** Recurrent use of newer oral contraceptives and the risk of venous thromboembolism. Hum Reprod. 2000;15:817–21.

52. **Farmer RDT, Lawrenson RA, Thompson CR, et al.** Population-based study of risk of venous thromboembolism associated with various oral contraceptives. Lancet. 1997; 349:83–8.

53. **Farmer RDT, Todd JC, MacRae KD, et al.** Oral contraception was not associated with venous thromboembolic disease in recent study. BMJ. 1998;316:1090–1.

54. **Blumenthal PD, McIntosh N.** Pocket guide for Family Planning Service Providers, 2nd ed. JHPIEGO Corporation, 1996.

55. **Krauss RM, Kurkman RT Jr.** The metabolic impact of oral contraceptives. Am J Obstet Gynecol. 1992;167:1177–84.

56. **Burkman RT, Robinson C, Moran-Kruszon D, et al.** Lipid and lipoprotein changes associated with oral contraceptive use: a randomized clinical trial. Obstet Gynecol. 1988;71:33.

57. **Godsland IF, Crook D, Simpson R, et al.** The effects of different formulations of oral contraceptive agents on lipid and carbohydrate metabolism. N Engl J Med. 1990;323: 1375–81.

58. **Adams MR, Clarkson TB, Koritnik DR, Nash HA.** Contraceptive steroids and coronary artery atherosclerosis in *Cynomolgus* macaques. Fertil Steril. 1987; 47:1010–8.

59. **Clarkson TB, Shively CA, Morgan TM, et al.** Oral contraceptives and coronary artery atherosclerosis of *Cynomolgus* monkeys. Obstet Gynecol. 1990; 75:217–22.

60. **Palatsi R, Hirvensalo E, Liukko P.** Serum total and unbound testosterone and sex hormone binding globulin (SHBG) in female acne patients treated with two different oral contraceptives. Acta Derm Venereol (Stockh). 1984;64:517–23.

61. **Phillips A. Demarest K, Hahn DW, et al.** Progestational and androgenic receptor binding affinities and in vivo activities of norgestimate and other progestins. Contraception. 1990;41:399–410.

62. **Archer DF.** Clinical and metabolic features of desogestrel: a new oral contraceptive preparation. Am J Obstet Gynecol. 1994;170:1550–5.

63. **Gutmann JN, Corson SL.** The new progestins: pharmacologic and clinical aspects. Int J Fertil. 1994;39:163–176.

64. **Derman RJ.** Oral contraceptives: androgenicity and estrogenicity. Int J Fertil. 1994;39(suppl 3):177–82.

65. **Fotherby K, Caldwell ADS.** New progestogens in oral contraception. Contraception. 1994;49:1–32.

66. **Mishell DR Jr.** Noncontraceptive health benefits of oral steroidal contraceptives. Am J Ostet Gynecol. 1982;142:809.

67. **Kost K, Forrest JD, Harlap S.** Comparing the health risks and benefits of contraceptive choices. Fam Plann Perspec. 1991;23:54–61.

68. Dialogues in Contraception 3: Therapeutic Uses of Oral Contraceptives. Vol. 30, No. 3, 1991.

69. **Jones KP, Ravnikar VA, Tulchinsky D, Schif I.** Comparison of bone density in amenorrheic women due to athletics, weight loss, and premature menopause. Obstet Gynecol. 1985,66:5.

70. **Sulak PJ, Cressman BE, Waldrop E, et al.** Extending the duration of active oral contraceptive pills to manage hormone withdrawal symptoms. Obstet Gynecol. 1997; 89:179–183.

71. CDC/NICHD. Oral contraceptives and endometrial cancer: combination oral contraceptive use and the risk of endometrial cancer. JAMA. 1987;257:6.

72. Oral contraceptive use and the risk of endometrial cancer. The Centers for Disease Control Cancer and Steroid Hormone Study. JAMA. 1983;249:1600–4.

73. Oral contraceptive use and the risk of ovarian cancer. The Centers for Disease Control Cancer and Steroid Hormone Study. JAMA. 1983;249:1596–9.

74. **Sanderson M, Williams MA, Weiss NS, et al.** Oral contraceptive and epithelial ovarian cancer: does dose matter? J Reprod Med. 2000;45:720–6.

75. **Siskind V, Green A, Bain C, Purdie D.** Beyond ovulation: oral contraceptives and epithelial ovarian cancer. Epdemiology. 2000;11:106–10.

76. **La Vecchia C, Franceschi S.** Oral contraceptives and ovarian cancer. Eur J Cancer Prev. 1999;8:297–304.

77. **Wingo PA, Lee NC, Ory HW, et al.** Age-specific differences in the relationship between oral contraceptive use and breast cancer. Obstet Gynecol. 1991;78:161–70.

78. **McGonigle KF, Huggins GR.** Oral contraceptives and breast disease. Fertil Steril. 1991,56:799–819.

79. **Wingo PA, Lee NC, Ory HW, et al.** Age-specific differences in the relationship between oral contraceptive use and breast cancer. Cancer. 1993;71(suppl 4):1506–17.

80. **Rookus MA, van Leeuwen FE.** Oral contraceptives and risk of breast cancer in women aged 20–54 years. Lancet. 1994;344:844–51.

81. **Harlap S.** Oral contraceptives and breast cancer: cause and effect? J Reprod Med. 1991;36:374–95.

82. Oral contraceptive use and the risk of breast cancer. The Cancer and Steroid Hormone Study of the Centers for Disease Control and the National Institute of Child Health and Human Development. N Engl J Med. 1986;315:405–11.

83. **Schlesselman JJ.** Cancer of the breast and reproductive tract in relation to use of oral contraceptives. Contraception. 1989;40:1–38.

84. Risk of cervical dysplasia in users of oral contraceptives, intrauterine devices or depot-medroxyprogesterone acetate. The New England Contraception and Health Study Group. Contraception. 1994;50:431–41.

85. **Grimes DA.** Oral contraceptives and your older patient. Dialog Contracept. 1988;2: 1–3.

86. **Connell EB.** Rational use of oral contraceptives in the perimenopausal woman. J Reprod Med. 1993;38:1036–40.

87. **Cambacciani M. Spinetti A, Taponeco F, et al.** Longitudinal evaluation of perimenopausal vertebral bone loss: effects of a low-dose oral contraceptive preparation on bone mineral density and metabolism. Obstet Gynecol. 1994;83:392–6.

88. **Sulak PJ.** Age-related concerns of oral contraceptive use: the perimenopausal patient. Int J Fertil. 1994;39:158–62.

89. **Castracane VD, Gimpel T, Goldzieher JW.** When is it safe to switch from oral contraceptives to hormonal replacement therapy? Contraception. 1995;52:371–6.

90. **Kaunitz AM, Schnare SM.** Contraception and older reproductive-age women. Dialog Contracept. 2000;6:4–8.

91. Preventing Pregnancy, Protecting Health: A New Look at Birth Control Choices in the United States. Chapter 5—Pregnancies Occurring During Contraceptive Use. New York: Alan Guttmacher Institute; 1991;33.

92. **Rosenberg MJ, Waugh MS, Burnhill MS.** Compliance, counseling and satisfaction with oral contraceptives: a prospective evaluation. Fam Plann Persp. 1998;30:89–92.

93. A multicenter phase III comparative study of two hormonal contraceptive preparations given once-a-month by intramuscular injection. I. Contraceptive efficacy and side effects. World Health Organization Special Programme of Research, Development and Research Training in Human Reproduction, Task Force on Long-Acting Systemic Agents for Fertility Regulation. Contraception. 1988;37:1–20.

94. **McCann MF, Lotter LS.** Progestin-only oral contraception: a comprehensive review. Contraception. 1994;50(suppl I):SI-195.

95. **Chi IC.** The progestin-only pills and the levonorgestrel-releasing IUD: two progestin-only contraceptives [Review] [71 refs]. Clin Obstet Gynecol. 1995;38:872–89.

96. **Broome M, Fotherby K.** Clinical experience with the progestogen-only pill as a contraceptive method. Br J Fam Plann. 1990;16–84.

97. **Tankeyoon M, Dusitsin N, Chalapati S, et al.** Effects of hormonal contraceptives on milk volume and infant growth. WHO Special Programme of Research, Development and Research Training in Human Reproduction Task Force on Oral Contraceptives. Contraception. 1984;30;505–22.

98. **Kaunitz AM.** Injectable contraception. Clin Obstet Gynecol. 1989;356–68.

99. **Rosenfield A, Maine D, Rochat R, et al.** The Food and Drug Administration and medroxyprogesterone acetate. JAMA. 1983;249:2922–8.

100. **Kaunitz AM.** Long-acting injectable contraception with depot medroxyprogesterone acetate. Am J Obstet Gynecol. 1994:170:1543–9.

101. Physicians' Desk Reference, 52nd ed. Montuale, NJ: Medical Economics; 1998; 3085–7,2079–83.

102. **Kaunitz AM, Mishell DR.** Progestin-only contraceptives: current perspectives and future directions. Dialog Contracept. 1994;4(2).

102a. **Said S, Sadek W, Rocca M, et al.** Clinical evaluation of the therapeutic effectiveness of ethinyl oestradiol and oestrone sulphate on prolonged bleeding in women using depot medroxyprogesterone acetate for contraception. World Health Organization, Special Programme of Research, Development and Research Training in Human Reproduction, Task Force on Long-acting Systemic Agents for Fertility Regulation. Hum Reprod. 1996;11(suppl 2):1–13.

103. **Cundy T, Evans M, Roberts H, et al.** Bone density in women receiving depot medroxyprogesterone acetate for contraception. BMJ. 1991;303:13–6.

104. **Cundy T, Farquhar CM, Cornish J, Reid IR.** Short-term effects of high dose oral medroxyprogesterone acetate on bone density in premenopausal women [see Comments]. J Clin Endocrinol Metab. 1996;81:1014–7.

105. **Cromer BA, Blair JM, Mahan JD, et al.** A prospective comparison of bone density in adolescent girls receiving depot medroxyprogesterone acetate (Depo-Provera), levonorgestrel (Norplant), or oral contraceptives. J Pediatr. 1996;129:671–6.

106. **Taneepanichskul S, Intaraprasert S, Theppisai U, Chaturachinda K.** Bone mineral density in long-term depot medroxyprogesterone acetate acceptors. Contraception. 1997;56:1–3.

107. **Taneepanichskul S, Intaraprasert S, Theppisai U, Chaturachinda K.** Bone mineral density during long-term treatment with Norplant implants and depot medroxyprogesterone acetate: a cross-sectional study of Thai women. Contraception. 1997;56: 153–55.

108. **Gbolade B, Ellis S, Murby B, et al.** Bone density in long term users of depot medroxyprogesterone acetate. Br J Obstet Gynaecol. 1998;105:790–4.

109. **Prior J. Vigne YM, Barr SL, et al.** Cyclic medroxyprogesterone treatment increases bone density: a controlled trial in active women with menstrual cycle disturbances. Am J Med. 1994;521–96.

110. Depot medroxyprogesterone acetate (DMPA) and risk of endometrial cancer. WHO Collaborative Study of Neoplasia and Steroid Contraceptives. Inter J Cancer. 1991;49: 186–90.

111. Depot-medroxyprogesterone acetate (DMPA) and cancer: memorandum from a WHO meeting. Bull WHO. 1993;71:669–76.

112. **Cullins VE.** Noncontraceptive benefits and therapeutic uses of depot medroxyprogesterone acetate [review] [57 refs]. J Reprod Med. 1996;41:428–33.

113. **Kaunitz AM.** Injectable depot medroxyprogesterone acetate contraception: an update for U.S. clinicians [Review] (55 refs]. Int J Fertil Womens Med. 1998;43:73–83.

114. **Mattson RH, Cramer JA, Caldwell BV, Siconolfi BC.** Treatment of seizures with medroxyprogesterone acetate: preliminary report. Neurology. 1984;34:1255–8.

115. **Blackham A, Spencer PSJ.** Response of female mice to anticonvulsants after pretreatment with sex steroids [Letter to the Editor]. J Pharm Pharmacol. 1970;22:304–5.

116. **Zimmerman AW, Holden KR, Reiter EO, Dekaban AS.** Medroxyprogesterone acetate in the treatment of seizures associated with menstruation. J Pediatr. 1973;83:959–63.

117. **Isaacs WA, Hayhoe FGJ.** Steroid hormones in sickle-cell disease. Nature. 1967;215: 1139–42.

118. **DeCeulaer K, Hayes R, Gruber C, Serjeant GR.** Medroxyprogesterone acetate and homozygous sickle-cell disease. Lancet. 1982,2:229–31.

119. Norplant Levonorgestrel Implants: A Summary of Scientific Data. New York: Population Council; 1990:1–30.

120. Sivin I. International experience with Norplant and Norplant-2 contraceptives. Stud Fam Plann. 19:81–94.

121. Injectables and Implants. Hormonal contraception: new long-acting methods. Popul Rep. March-April 1987.

122. **Diaz S, Croxatto HB, Panez M, et al.** Clinical assessment of treatments for prolonged bleeding in users of Norplant implants. Contraception. 1990;42:97–109.

123. **Alvarez-Sanchez F, Brache V, Thevein F, et al.** Hormonal treatment for bleeding irregularities in Norplant implant users. Am J Obstet Gynecol. 1996;174:919–22.

124. **Witjaksono J, Lau JM, Affandi B, Rogers SAW.** Oestrogen treatment for increased bleeding in Norplant users: preliminary results. Hum Reprod. 1996;11:109–14.

125. **Darney PD.** Hormonal implants: contraception for a new century. Am J Obstet Gynecol. 1994;170:1536–43.

126. **Darney PD, Atkinson E, Tanner S, et al.** Acceptance and perceptions of Norplant among users in San Francisco, USA. Stud Fam Plann. 1990;21:152–60.

127. **Cullins VE, Remsburg RE, Blumenthal PD, Huggins GR.** Comparison of adolescent and adult experiences with Norplant levonorgestrel contraceptive implants. Obstet Gynecol. 1994;83:1026–32.

128. **Haugen MM, Evans CB, Kim MH.** Patient satisfaction with a levonorgestrel-releasing contraceptive implant: reasons for and patterns of removal. J Reprod Med. 1996;41: 849–54.

129. **Berenson AB, Wiemann CM.** Patient satisfaction and side effects with levonorgestrel implant (Norplant) use in adolescents 18 years of age or younger. Pediatr. 1993;92: 257–60.

130. **Hinkel LT.** Education and counseling for Norplant users [Review]. J Obstet Gynecol Neonatal Nurs. 1994;23:387–91.

131. **Klaisle CM, Wysocki S.** Innovations in contraception: the Norplant system. NAACOGS Clin Issues Perinat Womens Health Nurs. 1992;3:267–9.

132. **Phemister DA, Laurent S, Harrison FNH Jr.** Obstetrics: use of Norplant contraceptive implants in the immediate postpartum period: safety and tolerance. Am J Obstet Gynecol. 1995;172:175–9.

133. Progestogen-only contraceptives during lactation. II Infant development. World Health Organization, Task Force for Epidemiological Research on Reproductive Health; Special Programme of Research, Development, and Research Training in Human Reproduction. Contraception. 1994;50:55–68.

134. **Affandi B, Karmadibrata S, Prihartono J, et al.** Effect of Norplant on mothers and infants in the postpartum period. Adv Contracept. 1986;2:371–80.

135. **Visness CM, Rivera R.** Progestin-only pill use and pill switching during breastfeeding [Editorial]. Contraception. 1995;51:279–81.

136. **Croxatto HB, Diaz S, Pavez M, et al.** Clearance of levonorgestrel from the circulation following removal of Norplant subdermal implants. Contraception. 1988;38:509–23.

137. **Yuzpe AA, Lanier WJ.** Ethinyl estradiol and dl-norgestrel as a postcoital contraceptive. Fertil Steril. 1977;28:932–6.

138. Emergency oral contraception. ACOG Pract Patterns. 1996;31:1–8.

139. **Van Hertzen H, Van Look PFA.** Research on new methods of emergency contraception. Fam Plann Perspect. 1996;28:52–88.

140. **Swahn ML, Westlund P, Johannisson E, Bygdeman M.** Effect of post-coital contraceptive methods on the endometrium and the menstrual cycle. Acta Obstet Gynecol Scand. 1996;75:738–44.

141. **Young DC, Wehle RD, Joshi SG, Pinderster AN.** Emergency contraception alters progesterone associated endometrial protein in serum and uterine luminal fluid. Obstet Gynecol. 1994;84:266.

142. Randomised controlled trial of levonorgestrel versus the Yuzpe regiment of combined oral contraceptives for emergency contraception. Task Force on Postovulatory Methods of Fertility Regulation. Lancet. 1998;352:428–33.

143. **Grou F, Rodrigues I.** The morning-after pill: how long after? Am J Obstet Gynecol. 1995;171:1529–34.

144. **Trussell J, Rodriguez G, Ellertson C.** New estimates of the effectiveness of the Yuzpe regimen of emergency contraception. Contraception. 1998;5:363–9.

145. **Creinin MD.** A reassessment of efficacy of the Yuzpe regimen of emergency contraception. Hum Reprod. 1997;12:496–8.

146. **Ho PC, Kwan MS.** A prospective randomized comparison of levonorgestrel with the Yuzpe regimen in post-coital contraception. Hum Reprod. 1993;8:389–92.

147. **Glasier A, Baird D.** The effects of self-administering emergency contraception. N Engl J Med. 1998;339:1–4.

148. **Webb AM.** Intrauterine contraceptive devices and antigestagens as emergency contraception. Eur J Contracept Reprod Health Care. 1997;2:243–6.

149. **Treiman K, Liskin L, Kols A, Rinehart W.** IUDs: a new look. Popul Rep B. March 1989, No. 5.

150. **Anderson J, Rybog.** Levonorgestrel-releasing IUD in the treatment of menorrhagia. Br J Obstet Gynecol. 1990; 97:1–36.

151. **Dardano KL, Burkman RT.** The intrauterine contraceptive device: an often-forgotten and maligned method of contraception. Am J Obstet Gynecol. 1999,181:1–5.

152. **Sivan I.** IUDs are contraceptives, not abortifacients: a comment on research and belief. Stud Fam Plan. 1989;20:355–9.

153. **Burkman RT.** Intrauterine devices and pelvic inflammatory disease: evolving perspectives on the data [IUDs: a state-of-the art conference]. Obstet Gynecol Surv. 1996; 51:35S–41S.

154. **Lee NC, Robin GL, Boruck R.** The IUD and pelvic inflammatory disease's: new results from the Women's Health Study. Obstet Gynecol. 1988;72:1–6.

155. **Lee NC, Rubin GL, Borucki R.** The intrauterine device and pelvic inflammatory disease revisited: new results from the Women's Health Study. Obstet Gynecol. 1988;72:1–6.

156. **Grimes DA.** Intrauterine devices and pelvic inflammatory disease: recent developments. Contraception. 1987;36:97–109.

157. **Donovan B.** Condoms and the prevention of sexually transmissible diseases [Review] [18 refs]. Br J Med Hosp. 1995;54:575–8.

158. **Lytle CD, Routson LB, Seahorn GB, et al.** An in vitro evaluation of condoms as barriers to a small virus. Sex Transm Dis. 1997;24:161–4.

159. **Bounds W.** Female condoms. Eur J Contracept Reprod Health Care. 1997;2:113–6.

160. **Cook RL, Rosenberg MJ.** Do spermicides containing nonoxynol-9 prevent sexually transmitted infections? A meta-analysis. Sex Transm Dis. 1998;25:144–50.

161. **Roddy RE, Zekeng L, Ryan KA, et al.** A controlled trial of nonoxynol-9 film to reduce male-to-female transmission of sexually transmitted diseases. N Engl J Med. 1998; 339:504–10.

162. **Roddy RE, Schulz KF, Cates W.** Microbicides, meta-analysis and the N-9 question: where's the research [Editorial]? Sex Transm Dis. 1998;25:151–3.

163. **Schirm AL, Trussell J, Menken J, Grady WR.** Contraceptive failure in the United States: the impact of social, economic, and demographic factors. Fam Plann Perspect. 1982;14:68–75.

164. **Trussell J, Sturgen K, Strickler J, et al.** Comparative efficacy of the female condom and other barrier methods. Fam Plann Persp. 1994;16:66–72.

165. **Grimes DA, Wallach M, eds.** Modern Contraception. Totowa, NJ: Euron; 1997.

166. **Drew WL, Blan M, Miner RC, Conant E.** Evaluation of the virus permeability of a new condom for women. Sex Transm Dis. 1990;17:110.

167. **Soper DE, Shoupe D, Shangold GA, et al.** Prevention of vaginal trichomoniasis by compliant use of the female condom. Sex Transm Dis. 1993;20:137–9.

168. **Trussel J, Hatcher RA, Cates W.** Contraceptive failure in the United States: an update. Stud Fam Plann. 1990;21:51–4.

169. **Fihn SD, Latham RH, Roberts P, et al.** Association between diaphragm use and urinary tract infection. JAMA 1985;254:240–5.

170. **Kost K, Forrest JD, Harlap S.** Comparing the health risks and benefits of contraceptive choices. Fam Plann Perspect. 1991;23:54.

171. **Niruthisard S, Roddy RE, Chutvongse S.** Use of nonoxynol-9 and reduction in rate of gonococcal and chlamydial cervical infections. Lancet. 1992;339:1371.

172. **Kreiss J, Ngugi E, Holmes K, et al.** Efficacy of nonoxynol-9 contraceptive sponge use in preventing heterosexual acquisition of HIV in Nairobi prostitutes. JAMA. 1992; 268:477-82.

173. **Roddy Re, Schulz KF, Cates W Jr.** Microbicides, meta-analysis, and the N-9 question: where's the research? Sex Transm Dis. 1998;25:151–3.

174. **Cook RI, Rosenberg MJ.** Do spermicides containing nonoxynol-9 prevent sexually transmitted infections? A meta-analysis. Sex Transm Dis. 1998;25:144–50.

175. **Niruthsard S, Roddy RE, Chutivonge S.** The effects of frequent nonoxynol-9 use on vaginal and cervical mucosa. Sex Transm Dis. 1991;268:176-9.

176. **Roddy RE, Zekeng K, Ryan KA, et al.** A controlled trial of nonoxynol-9 film to reduce male-to-female transmissions of sexually transmitted diseases. N Engl J Med. 1998; 339:504–10.

177. **Van Damme L, Masse B, Laga M, et al.** Vaginal microbicides: an update. Thirteenth World Conference on HIV/AIDS. Durban, South Africa, July 12, 2000.

178. **Horton TM, Miller S, Johnson C, et al.** *E. coli* bacteria and contraceptive method. JAMA. 1991;265:64.

179. **Peterson HB, Xia Z, Hughes JM, et al.** The risk of pregnancy after tubal sterilization: findings from the U.S. Collaborative Review of Sterilization. Am J Obstet Gynecol. 1996;174:1161–70.

180. **Pati S, Carignan C, Pollack AE.** What's new with female sterilization: an update. Contemporary OB/GYN. 1991:117.

181. **Irwin KL, Weiss NS, Lee NC, et al.** Tubal sterilization, hysterectomy and the subsequent occurrence of epithelial ovarian cancer. Am J Epidemiol. 1991;134:362–9.

182. **Hankinson SE, Hunter DJ, Golditz GA, et al.** Tubal ligation, hysterectomy, and the risk of ovarian cancer: a prospective study. JAMA. 1993;270:2813–8.

183. **Raspa FR.** Complications of vasectomy. Am Fam Phys. 1993;48:1264–8.

184. **Pollack Am, Rarone M.** Male sterilization in gynecology and obstetrics. In: Sciarra J, ed. Philadelphia: Lippincott-Raven; 1999.

185. **Davis LE, Stockton MD.** No-scapel vasectomy. Prim Care. 1997;24:433–61.

186. **Reynolds RD.** Vas deferens occlusion during no-scalpel vasectomy. J Fam Pract. 1994;39:577–82.

187. **Haws JM, Morgan GT, Pollack AE, et al.** Clinical aspects of vasectomies performed in the United States in 1995. Urology. 1998;52:685–91.

188. **Pollack AE.** Vasectomy and prostate cancer. Adv Contracept. 1993; 9:181–6.

189. **Farley TMM, Meirik O, Mehta S. Waites GMH.** The safety of vasectomy: recent concerns. Bull WHO. 1993;71:413–9.

190. **Møller H, Knudsen LB, Lynge E.** Risk of testicular cancer after vasectomy: cohort study of over 73,000 men. BMJ. 1994;309:295–9.

191. **John EM, Whittemore AS, Wu AH, et al.** Vasectomy and prostate cancer: results from a multiethnic case-control study. J Natl Cancer Inst. 1995;87:662–9.

192. **Howards SJ.** American Urological Association response to two articles on the relationship of vasectomy to prostate cancer. Oncology. 1991;5:78–80.

193. National Institutes of Health. Does vasectomy cause prostate cancer? JAMA. 1993;169: 2620.

194. **Haws JM, Feigin J.** Vasectomy counseling. Am Fam Physician. 1995;52:1395.

195. **Wilcox AJ, Weinberg CR, Baird DD.** Timing of sexual intercourse in relation to ovulation: effects on the probability of conception, survival of the pregnancy, and sex of the baby [see Comments]. N Eng J Med. 1995;333:1517–21.

196. **Ryder B, Campbell H.** Natural family planning in the 1990s [see Comments] [Review] [33 refs]. Lancet. 1995;346:233–4.

197. **Geerling JH.** Natural family planning. Am Fam Physician. 1995;52:1749–56.

198. **Grimes DA, Wallach M, eds.** Modern Contraception: Updates from the Contraceptive Report. Wayne, NJ: Emron; 244–7.

199. **Ramos R, Kennedy KI, Visness CM.** Effectiveness of lactational amenorroea in prevention of pregnancy in Manila, the Philippines: a noncomparative prospective trial. BMJ. 1996;313:909–12.

200. **Hight-Laukaran V, Labbok MH, Peterson AE, et al.** Multicenter study of the lactational amenorrhea method (LAM). II Acceptability, utility, and policy implications. Contraception. 1997;55:337–46.

CHAPTER 6

Spontaneous and Induced Abortion

LAURA D. CASTLEMAN, MD, MPH
PAUL D. BLUMENTHAL, MD, MPH

A bortion is defined as the termination of pregnancy before viability. Usually this term is applied to a pregnancy lost or terminated before 24 weeks gestation or before the fetus weighs 500 g, as, for the past several decades, these milestones have been linked to fetal viability. Beyond 24 weeks other obstetric terms for the termination of pregnancy are appropriate such as *intrauterine fetal demise* or, in the setting of delivery, *stillbirth*.

Abortion occurs through one of two mechanisms: 1) some pathologic process (spontaneous abortion), or 2) induced by medical or surgical means (induced abortion). The following sections review the epidemiology, physiology, and clinical management of these two categories of abortion.

Spontaneous Abortion

Definitions

There are many types of spontaneous abortions. The accurate classification of the physiologic process provides prognostic information.

Threatened Abortion—vaginal bleeding that occurs in a patient with a closed cervical os and a viable intrauterine pregnancy. Such bleeding occurs in about 30% to 40% of pregnancies and, of these, 20% to 50% will eventually abort (1).

Inevitable Abortion—all products of conception remain intrauterine, though the os is open and fetal expulsion is deemed inevitable. Usually the patient seeks care for symptoms of bleeding and cramping.

Incomplete Abortion—similar to an inevitable abortion, except some products of conception have already been expelled from the uterus. Depending on the gestational age, patients may have brisk bleeding and, if untreated, may become infected.

Complete Abortion—all products of conception are expelled from the uterus and the os is closed. Bleeding is minimal and likelihood of infection is low.

Missed Abortion—loss of fetal viability but no expulsion of conception products for at least 8 weeks. The cervical os is closed, and there is little or no bleeding. This term is commonly used to indicate any early pregnancy with nonviable products of conception. Sometimes *missed abortion* is used interchangeably (though not correctly) with the term *blighted ovum*.

> *Spontaneous abortion can be classified as threatened, inevitable, incomplete, complete, missed, and septic.*

Blighted Ovum—ultrasound reveals a gestational sac without a fetus in a pregnancy greater than 7 weeks gestation. Usually, these patients have minimal bleeding and cramping. In clinical practice, this term is often used before 7 weeks gestation.

Septic Abortion—infection that occurs at any stage of spontaneous or induced abortion. Signs and symptoms include fever, fundal tenderness, foul-smelling discharge, and leukocytosis.

Epidemiology and Etiology

Although the true incidence is unknown, as many as 40% to 50% of all conceptions and approximately 15% to 20% of clinically documented pregnancies end in spontaneous abortion (2,3). Reproductive history is the most important predictor of future pregnancy outcome. A woman whose last pregnancy ended in a live birth has only a 5% chance of spontaneous abortion, whereas a woman whose previous pregnancy miscarried has a 20% chance of recurrence. Recurrence rate after two previous abortions is 35%. This climbs to 47% after three previous losses with no live births.

In the first trimester, 50% to 70% of spontaneous abortions are the result of chromosomal abnormalities (4). Other important risk factors include high parity (greater than 4) and increasing maternal and paternal age (5,6). Although the ultimate cause of a specific patient's pregnancy loss is often unknown, several different factors frequently contribute to first or second trimester spontaneous abortions.

Box 6-1   Causes of First Trimester Abortion*

- Chromosomal causes/abnormal embryo (>50% of first trimester losses)
- Infections (syphilis, tuberculosis)
- Systemic illness (e.g., diabetes mellitus, lupus, hypothyroidism, sickle cell anemia)
- Hormonal causes (progesterone deficiency)
- Environmental toxins (smoking, cocaine, alcohol, radiation, work exposures such as silicon)
- Anatomic abnormalities (intrauterine polyp, fibroids, adhesions)
- Intrauterine device
- Lupus anticoagulant activity and antiphospholipid antibody
- Advanced maternal age

*Data from Refs 7 to 11.

First Trimester

Eighty percent of spontaneous abortions occur before the 12th week of gestation. Many etiologies have been identified (Box 6-1), but by far the commonest cause is fetal chromosomal abnormalities. Trisomy syndromes make up approximately 50% of this group, especially trisomy 13, 16, 18, 21, and 22. Turner's syndrome (monosomy 46, X) accounts for 15% to 20% of chromosomally abnormal abortions. The rate of chromosomal anomalies clearly increases with advancing maternal age (Fig. 6-1). Maternal age has a strong impact on both a woman's ability to conceive and her ability to maintain a pregnancy. For instance, 80% of conceptions in women over age 47 end in miscarriage, approximately two to four times higher than the rate for women under 30 years old (2,6). Advancing maternal age increases the rate of abortion even in the chromosomally normal conceptus; possible mechanisms include interference with implantation and structural changes in the aging uterus (12).

Many maternal systemic diseases, such as diabetes mellitus and sickle cell anemia, are associated with increased rates of spontaneous abortion at every gestational age. For instance, in women with diabetes, hyperglycemia even at the time of conception appears to increase rates of fetal loss (13). Undiagnosed or inadequately treated hypothyroidism has also been shown to increase the risk of spontaneous abortion. Other causes of spontaneous abortion in the first trimester include infections (syphilis and tuberculosis), anatomic abnormalities (intrauterine polyp, fibroids, and adhesions), and antiphospholipid antibody. Maternal factors that are controversial include the contribution (if any) of progesterone deficiency to pregnancy loss as well as

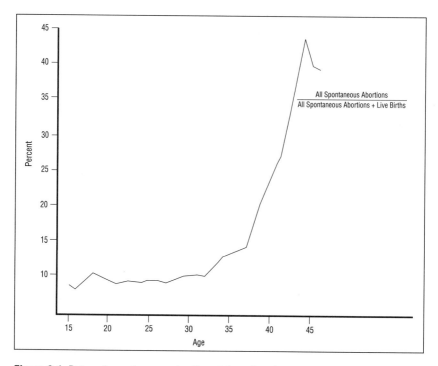

Figure 6-1 Rates of spontaneous abortion at three hospitals in New York City over a period spanning approximately 4 years. Note that the rate of spontaneous abortion increases with advancing age. (From Stein ZA. A woman's age: childbearing and child rearing. J Epidemiol. 1985;121:327; with permission.)

the effects of pelvic infections on pregnancy. No prospective, controlled studies have been able to document an association between gonorrhea or chlamydia and spontaneous abortion.

Many environmental factors have been associated with an increased risk of spontaneous abortion. For instance, drug exposures including cocaine and possibly alcohol may increase the risk for pregnancy loss at any gestational age (14,15). Heavy caffeine intake (>300 mg/day) has been reported to be associated with late first or early second trimester miscarriages (16,17), though the effect of smaller quantities is less clear. Chapter 19 further discusses environmental factors in pregnancy.

Second Trimester

While many of the factors linked to miscarriage in the first trimester can also precipitate a second trimester loss, maternal anatomic or physiologic problems are more commonly responsible. Both maternal and fetal anomalies can cause spontaneous midtrimester abortion (Box 6-2). For instance, fetal anom-

---

Box 6-2 Causes of Second Trimester Spontaneous Abortion*

Maternal anomalies
  Uterine
    Fibroids (also cause first trimester losses)
    Bicornuate or unicornuate uterus
    Maternal diethylstilbestrol (DES) exposure (T-shaped uterus)
  Cervical
    Incompetent cervix
  Maternal systemic disease (e.g., hypertension, sickle cell anemia,
  hypoparathyroidism)
  Maternal sepsis
    Infection (e.g., syphilis, measles, *Listeria*)
    Group B streptococci
  Fetal anomalies (e.g., holoprosencephaly, congenital cardiac defects,
  abdominal wall defects, neurologic defects)

---

*Data from Refs 18 to 23.

---

alies such as abdominal wall and neurologic defects are found at an increased incidence in fetuses miscarried in the second trimester (24). In addition, maternal uterine anomalies may create an environment that is inhospitable to gestation. For example, uterine defects that decrease intraluminal volume, such as a bicornuate uterus, can be associated with fetal loss in both the first and the second trimester (25). Both fever and systemic illness are associated with increased spontaneous abortion in both trimesters (26).

Cervical incompetence is defined as painless dilatation of the cervix with resultant fetal expulsion, usually between 16 to 24 weeks. In the past, this has been an enigmatic problem of uncertain etiology. In addition to primary cervical incompetence, a retrospective, case-control WHO study suggested that iatrogenic causes, such as previous rapid cervical dilatation to greater than 12 to 14 mm (such as may occur during an induced abortion), are important in subsequent cervical incompetence (27). However, these results were inconsistent within the WHO study and have not been replicated in subsequent studies (28). More recently, cervical conization and electrosurgical ablative procedures performed on the cervix, such as the loop electrocautery excision procedure (LEEP), have been associated with spontaneous abortion, most likely due to cervical incompetence (29). Fortunately, most women who undergo such cervical procedures will have completely normal subsequent pregnancies. An actual causal relationship has not been proven, but this etiology should be considered for patients who suffer a midtrimester loss and have this history.

Infections such as bacterial vaginosis, group B streptococci, mycoplasma, and *Ureaplasma urealyticum* have been associated with preterm labor and delivery (30,31). These may also contribute to midtrimester losses.

Clinical Assessment

History

Depending on the condition of the patient at the time she presents, a thorough medical, obstetric, and gynecologic history should be obtained. Specifically, the physician should try to establish gestational age and the duration and extent of vaginal bleeding, cramps, and abdominal pain. Often a completed abortion will be suggested by the patient noting the passage of tissue followed by the definite termination of cramps and bleeding. Symptoms of potential hemodynamic problems, such as weakness or dizziness, should be investigated as well as symptoms of infection, such as fevers and chills. The patient should be asked whether her current pregnancy is desired, because this might influence interventions that could result in pregnancy termination if the fetus is still viable.

The signs and symptoms of spontaneous abortion, particularly in the first trimester, often overlap with those of ectopic pregnancy and warrant its inclusion in the differential diagnosis. Refer to Chapter 9 for further discussion of ectopic pregnancies.

Physical Examination

Physical examination includes vital signs with orthostatic indices (both blood pressure and pulse), especially if the patient has significant bleeding. The abdomen should be assessed for tenderness, bowel sounds, and uterine size. Usually the fundus is palpable abdominally after 12 weeks gestation, depending on habitus. The pelvic examination must include a speculum examination to assess the degree of bleeding. If bleeding is minimal, it is often helpful to wipe the blood from the os and observe how long it takes to reaccumulate. Any foul odor or purulence in the vaginal discharge should be noted, as well as any cervical lacerations that may indicate attempts at self-induced abortion with sharp, contaminated instruments. Any products of conception that are visible at the os and therefore partially extruded should be

Physical examination in a patient undergoing a spontaneous miscarriage must include evaluation of hemodynamic stability, speculum examination to assess the rate of bleeding, and a bimanual vaginal examination to assess fundal tenderness and cervical dilatation.

removed. This is easily accomplished either digitally or with ring forceps and gentle traction on the tissue.

Bimanual examination should then be performed. The internal os should be examined for dilatation and tenderness. If a finger can be placed through the internal os, the cervix is "open" and an incomplete or inevitable abortion is likely present. Uterine tenderness and cervical motion tenderness suggest peritoneal irritation, usually from infection and/or blood. The uterine size should be assessed to obtain an estimate of gestational age independent of patient history.

Laboratory Assessment

URGENT CLINICAL SETTING

Immediate laboratory assessment for patients who appear hemodynamically unstable due to an ongoing spontaneous abortion should include hemoglobin (or hematocrit) and Rh status. The hemoglobin helps gauge the patient's volume status, thereby influencing the decision whether to observe the patient or to intervene surgically. Patients whose Rh status is negative should receive Rh-immune globulin (Rhogam) within 72 hr to prevent sensitization that could complicate subsequent pregnancies.

> *The Rh status of any woman undergoing either spontaneous or induced abortion should be determined, and all Rh-negative patients should receive Rh-immune globulin.*

NONURGENT CLINICAL SETTING

For patients who appear hemodynamically stable, screening should be performed for infectious causes of spontaneous abortion such as chlamydia, gonorrhea, and group B streptococci. Testing for mycoplasma and *Ureaplasma* has also been advocated, especially in cases of repeated loss (32). Because bacterial vaginosis is commonly associated with spontaneous abortion, a wet prep should be performed if clinically feasible. In addition, Rh status should be documented and Rhogam given to Rh-negative patients.

Management

Patients experiencing a spontaneous abortion should be triaged in relation to their hemodynamic stability. Patients with an incomplete or inevitable abortion require uterine evacuation; hemodynamic stability determines whether this must be done emergently. The patient with bleeding significant enough to cause hemodynamic changes or with evidence of infection needs immediate uterine evacuation. Untreated, such cases can result in significant hemorrhage, sepsis, and death. Methods of evacuation are exactly the same for both elective and spontaneous abortions. See Induced Abortion Procedures section later in this chapter.

Patients with a septic abortion require immediate uterine evacuation. Because such infections are likely to be polymicrobial, broad-spectrum IV antibiotics should be started as soon as possible after the diagnosis of septic abortion is made. Preferably, these should be given before any suction evacuation is performed and continued until the patient has been afebrile for 48 hr. Because septic, incomplete abortions can be a dangerous clinical entity, patients should be monitored closely for signs of septic shock (33). For specific procedure-related complications, refer to the section on Complications of Induced Abortions below.

Patients who report a completed abortion at home or who are diagnosed as such should be managed so as to confirm that their pregnancy has ended. This can be done by following the patient's symptoms and examination findings and by obtaining serial pregnancy tests as indicated. A serum HCG can remain detectable for over 2 weeks after a complete abortion (2). Patients having already completed a spontaneous abortion must also undergo Rh testing so that Rh-negative women may be identified and treated.

Patients with a septic, incomplete, or inevitable abortion require uterine evacuation.

Threatened abortions are best managed by observation, as long as the patient is hemodynamically stable. Because patients with ectopic pregnancies also may present with vaginal bleeding, a closed cervical os, and a positive pregnancy test, this diagnosis must also be considered (see Chapter 9). Once threatened abortion has been established as the working diagnosis, the patient should have intrauterine viability confirmed either by visualizing fetal heart motion on ultrasound or by following appropriate rises in the β-hCG (beta-human chorionic gonadotropin) level. In a viable pregnancy, β-hCG should double approximately every 48 to 72 hr. In addition, once fetal heart motion is seen (usually visible on transvaginal ultrasound by 7 weeks gestation), the patient can be reassured that she has more than a 90% chance of having a normal, term pregnancy (34,35). For a patient with a threatened abortion, bed rest, pelvic rest, and oral hydration are commonly advised, though scant literature exists to validate these practices. Increased bleeding or cramping mandates reevaluation.

A patient with a threatened abortion and an apparently nonviable gestation can be offered conservative management, waiting for either spontaneous expulsion or resolution of cramping or bleeding. If conservative management is unacceptable or clinically inappropriate, an evacuation should be performed (see Induced Abortion section).

Couples with recurrent pregnancy loss, defined as three or more spontaneous abortions, should be referred to a specialist who can perform studies to differentiate the causes. Patients who are somewhat older with respect to reproductive capacity (approximately over age 35) should be referred for evaluation after two losses.

All patients with a spontaneous abortion should receive contraceptive counseling. While it is physically safe for a patient to conceive again immediately following a fetal loss, often the patient requires time for emotional healing. These patients may require considerable psychological and emotional support. They should be reassured that the loss is not their fault, for even if not acknowledged, the patient often feels guilty and responsible (2).

Induced Abortion

Definition

Abortion is defined as induced when surgical or medical means are used to terminate a pregnancy and ensure that the products of conception are removed or expelled from the uterine cavity.

Epidemiology

In the United States, approximately 11% of reproductive aged women become pregnant annually, resulting in approximately 6 million pregnancies per year. Half of these pregnancies are unplanned (36,39); of these, 43% are contraceptive failures. Half of these unplanned pregnancies end in abortion, making it one of the most common surgical procedures in the United States. The number of abortions in the U.S. peaked at 1.4 million in 1990 (37), but by 1997 had declined slightly to 1,180,000 abortions (38). Among women requesting abortion, teenagers and women over 39 years old have the highest age-specific rates, although the absolute number of abortions in these groups is lower than in the intervening ages (Fig. 6-2). Approximately 43% of women will have at least one abortion by the time they reach age 45 (39).

Worldwide, approximately 50 million abortions are performed annually, of which approximately 20 million occur under unsafe conditions (40). Globally, abortion is the third leading cause of maternal death and accounts for 15% of maternal mortality; this figure escalates to 60% in some areas (41). Unsafe abortions result in a daily global death rate of 500 women and an annual death rate of 70,000 to 80,000 women.

As legal abortions have become available in the United States over the past 30 years, the complications due to illegal abortions (hemorrhage, infection,

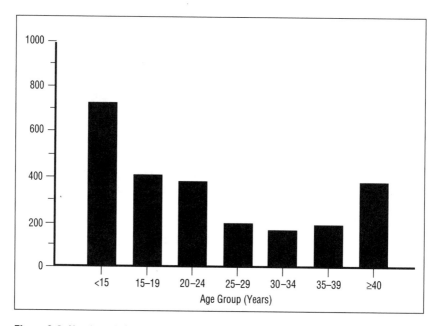

Figure 6-2 Number of abortions in the United States per 1000 live births, 1996. The highest ratio is for teenagers, followed by women over age 39. (From the Centers for Disease Control and Prevention. MMWR. 1999;48(SS-4):14.)

and death) have substantially decreased and now mainly affect women with problems of access secondary to geography, age (minors), or economics. The mortality rate of legal abortions in the United States has dropped to less than 1 in 100,000 procedures, making it one of the safest procedures performed. The risk of death from childbirth is approximately ten times greater than that from abortion (39).

Approximately 88% of induced abortions in the United States are performed in the first trimester; only 5% take place after 16 weeks, and 1.4% after 20 weeks (38).

History and Physical Examination

A focused but thorough history and physical should be performed, similar to a preoperative evaluation. Questions should focus on menstrual history, particularly the date and certainty of the last menstrual period, contraceptive history, including any methods used at time of conception, and a complete gynecologic and obstetric history.

Preprocedure assessment also should focus on medical conditions that may affect a safe outcome. Early induced abortions usually require only local anesthesia, whereas later procedures are often longer and may be associated with greater sympathetic activity. Identification of previously undiagnosed cardiac, pulmonary, and thyroid conditions, and control of known conditions, are appropriate but should not delay the abortion procedure if possible. Prior problems with anesthesia or a family history of deaths related to anesthesia should be elicited.

In addition to evaluating the overall health of the patient, the physical examination must include an assessment of uterine size and position. A wet prep should be performed for symptoms or objective evidence of malodorous discharge and any active infection treated, because there is evidence that active *Trichomonas* infection at the time of an abortion procedure increases perioperative morbidity (42). Evidence also supports screening and treating women for asymptomatic bacterial vaginosis, because treatment with metronidazole before the procedure can substantially lower the risk of postabortion pelvic inflammatory disease (43).

Patient evaluation should include counseling that focuses on the decision to have an abortion and alternative options for the pregnancy such as adoption and parenting. Issues that should be discussed include the types of procedures available, what to expect, and the risks involved. Psychological and emotional support often is best provided by staff from several disciplines, including doctors, nurses, social workers, and specially trained staff. The practitioner must be familiar with state laws regarding the content of counseling, parental notification, and informed consent relating to minors.

Before the Procedure

Either at or before the procedure, hemoglobin level, Rh status, and a positive pregnancy test should be documented. All Rh-negative patients should receive Rh-immune globulin at the time of the abortion. Ideally, cervical testing for gonorrhea and chlamydia should have been recently obtained, though this is not always possible, and the results are not always available at the time of the procedure. In the first trimester, especially after 8 weeks gestation, ultrasound need only be obtained for any patient with an uncertain last menstrual period, or where a large discrepancy exists such that the uterine size is considerably larger than the patient's dates would indicate. When a termination procedure is planned for a patient pregnant less than 7 weeks, some authorities recommend that an ultrasound be obtained to document the presence of an intrauterine pregnancy. However, in general, a patient in the first trimester whose dates agree with her examination does not need an ultrasound before an elective abortion. Sonographic confirmation of gestational age is advised for all pregnancies greater than 12 weeks.

Procedures

Both first and second trimester procedures can be performed on an outpatient basis with access to a facility where complications requiring operative intervention can be effectively managed. Prophylactic antibiotics are recommended. Commonly a course of doxycyline is provided and started either the day before or the day of the procedure. Recently, a well-designed, prospective, randomized clinical trial demonstrated that a 3-day course of doxycycline 100 mg bid is as effective as a 7-day course (44). Cervical preparation before a suction procedure, particularly for gestations over 10 weeks, may help reduce patient discomfort during the procedure. In addition, cervical preparation decreases the risk of perforation, cervical laceration, the need for intravenous analgesia, and, possibly, reduces the chance of a subsequent incompetent cervix (45,46). Methods of cervical preparation include placement of osmotic dilators such as laminaria tents or Dilapan 12 to 24 hr before the procedure, or intravaginal placement of the prostaglandin analog misoprostol (Cytotec) several hours before the procedure. Alternatively, the antiprogesterone agent mifepristone (Mifeprex, previously known as "RU 486") can be taken orally 36 hr before the procedure to help prepare the cervix (47).

For abortion procedures over 10 weeks gestation, cervical preparation is recommended.

First Trimester

In the first trimester, induced abortions can be performed either surgically or medically. Surgical abortions in the first trimester are most commonly performed in outpatient settings using local anesthesia alone or in combination with intravenous sedation. Technical considerations relating to induced abortion procedures are discussed below.

Recall that spontaneous abortions can be managed surgically, medically (with misoprostol, see below), or expectantly. In the first trimester, surgical management consists of either dilatation and curettage (D&C) or manual vacuum aspiration; both techniques are performed identically for spontaneous and induced abortions.

Vacuum Aspiration

Used between 5 and 14 weeks, a suction cannula is attached to either a handheld syringe (for gestations less than 12 weeks from LMP) or a machine that electrically generates suction (Fig. 6-3). The cannula is inserted through the cervix into the uterus. Suction is then generated to evacuate the uterine contents. Products of conception almost always can be readily identified either

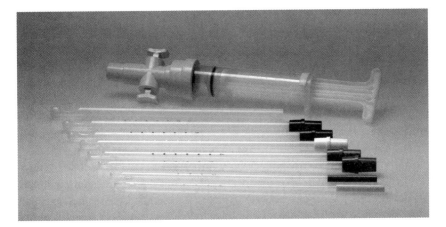

Figure 6-3 Manual vacuum aspirator. This hand-held device consists of a syringe and plunger, used to create a vacuum, attached to plastic cannulae. The cannulae are available in different sizes, with the larger ones used for more advanced gestational ages. The cannulae is inserted through the cervical os into the uterus, and the products of conception are aspirated into the syringe. (Courtesy IPAS, Chapel Hill, N.C.)

grossly or with a dissecting microscope, effectively ruling out ectopic pregnancy. Gentle curettage with either the suction cannula or, if necessary, a metal curette is performed until the uterus feels gritty and contracts substantially around the suction cannula or curette, indicating complete evacuation. Effectiveness exceeds 98% (48).

The principal contraindication to such simple suction procedures is duration of pregnancy greater than 14 weeks. Also, elective procedures should not be performed during an active infection. Women with large fibroids, bleeding disorders, or significant medical problems such as severe cardiac disease should be referred to a center where they can be appropriately monitored.

MEDICAL ABORTIONS

Both mifepristone (Mifeprex) and methotrexate are safe and effective means of achieving terminations in early pregnancy (49). In the United States, these methods have been used up to 49 days (methotrexate) and 63 days (mifepristone) from the last menstrual period (50). In either case the regimen consists of two sequential medications, the first of which terminates the pregnancy (mifepristone or methotrexate), and the second, a prostaglandin (misoprostol, or Cytotec), which induces uterine contractions and eventual expulsion of the conceptus. Essentially, therefore, women experience symptoms similar to a miscarriage.

Mifepristone is an antiprogesterone that blocks corpus luteum support (progesterone), causing termination of the early pregnancy. It has been used in millions of women worldwide to induce an abortion, and in September 2000 the FDA approved mifepristone combined with misoprostol for use in terminating pregnancies up to 49 days.

Despite demonstrated safety and efficacy in France and other countries, mifepristone remained unavailable in the United States during the 1990s, largely due to political controversy. Consequently, investigators pursued early medical abortion using other drugs. The folic acid antagonist methotrexate, typically administered intramuscularly, interferes with dihydrofolate reductase, thereby blocking DNA synthesis and resulting in pregnancy demise. Clinically, the differences between mifepristone and methotrexate are that mifepristone works much faster and has generally been shown to have higher efficacy at later gestational ages than methotrexate. Mifepristone-induced abortions are usually completed within a couple days, whereas methotrexate-induced abortions require at least a week, and several weeks may pass before the process is completed.

Studies demonstrate high rates of success (defined as pregnancy termination after medications without need for surgical evacuation) for these medical abortion regimens. The mifepristone/misoprostol combination is over 95% effective and is usually completed in 2 days, though it can take up to 14 days (51). Earlier trials found its effectiveness to decline with advancing pregnancy, with a success rate of 89.1% for pregnancies between 50 and 56 days gestation, and only 84.4% for pregnancies from 57 to 63 days gestation (52,53). However, subsequent research in the United States has improved these regimens. When misoprostol is administered intravaginally and in higher doses, a success rate of 96% to 97% has been observed, even in pregnancies up to 63 days (54,55). Importantly, worldwide experience indicates that, independent of the regimen, as provider experience increases, so does effectiveness.

The methotrexate/misoprostol combination was shown in one study to be 90.6% effective at gestations 49 days and under (56), whereas other studies show its effectiveness to be at least 95% (57). The efficacy rate falls to 80% to 90% for gestations between 50 to 56 days. Seventy percent of abortions were completed in 2 weeks, though some women required up to 4 weeks before the process was completed.

FDA labelling describes three visits for mifepristone/misoprostol abortions. At the first visit the patient receives counseling and is assessed to determine her eligibility. Often a pelvic ultrasound is used to confirm that the pregnancy is not beyond 49 days. Mifepristone is given on site. Two days later the patient returns and the misoprostol is administered orally. She can then choose to stay in the office or go home, as expulsion of the conceptus usually occurs within hours of having taken the misoprostol. Two weeks after the initial visit the patient makes a third visit to confirm that the abortion is complete. Often a pelvic exam is adequate to make this assessment, but pelvic ultrasound may also be used.

Side effects of both the methotrexate and mifepristone regimens include cramping and bleeding in all patients. Most commonly, women compare it to a very uncomfortable and/or heavy menses. A minority of women will experience nausea and vomiting. Side effects are correlated with the type and route of administration of the prostaglandin, with vaginal administration of misoprostol producing fewer side effects than oral dosing. Side effects are also minimized in women with earlier gestations compared to women who are over 49 days gestation. In United States mifepristone trials, only 4 patients out of 2480 required blood transfusions.

Typically, a medical abortion costs approximately the same as a surgical one, mostly due to the expense of the mifepristone (57a). However, medical abortion may likely improve access to abortion for many women, because it is anticipated that many physicians unwilling or untrained to provide surgical abortions will offer these medications (57b). On the other hand, the three visits required for a medical abortion (as opposed to one or two for a surgical one) may pose a hardship for women who must travel a great distance or suffer economic losses. One possible evidence-based alternative to the FDA-approved regimen entails eliminating the second office visit and allowing the patient to self-administer the misoprostol at home (57c). Others include the use of a lower dose of mifepristone (100–200 mg) in combination with intravaginal misoprostol (800 µg) (57c), more flexible timing of the misoprostol administration (i.e., 1, 2, or 3 days after mifepristone [57d]), and the use of medical abortion for slightly later gestational ages (57e). These alternatives have been shown safe and effective and are associated with fewer side effects, lower cost, and more convenience than the regimen approved in the original FDA labelling.

Second Trimester

In the second trimester, the closed cervix should be prepared before an induced abortion. Cervical preparation may involve osmotic or hygroscopic devices placed in the cervix for at least 6 hr, intravaginal application of prostaglandins, or oral administration of mifepristone. The abortion is then performed by one of two general methods: surgical evacuation or medical induction.

Surgical Evacuation of the Uterus

Dilatation and evacuation (D&E) is conceptually similar to techniques performed at earlier gestations. Like earlier procedures, a vacuum is used to evacuate uterine contents. However, whereas in earlier procedures vacuum alone is usually sufficient after 14 weeks, here the vacuum serves primarily to empty amniotic fluid. Specialized forceps are used to remove the fetal parts and placental tissue. Cervical preparation to soften and open the cervix before D&E is very important to help prevent complications, especially in later gestational ages.

MEDICAL INDUCTION

Uterotonic drugs, such as oxytocin, or prostaglandin compounds, such as PGF2-α, PGE2, or PGE1, are used to evacuate the uterus in gestations over 14 weeks, most commonly over 18 weeks. These medications cause the uterus to contract and put the patient into labor. This type of abortion relies on establishing uterine contractions sufficient to expel the fetus and placenta. Induction abortions usually take less than 10 hr, though they can require up to 3 days. They can be performed either in a hospital or in a clinic. Disposal of the fetus depends upon parental wishes and state law.

Post-Procedure Management

After any type of surgical abortion, the patient is observed for one to several hours before discharge to monitor levels of pain and vaginal bleeding. All Rh-negative patients should receive anti-Rh (D) gamma globulin (Rhogam) 300 μg IM. Gestations prior to 12 weeks require only 50 μg of anti-Rh (D) gamma globulin.

Ibuprofen usually suffices for pain control after discharge. Patients should be instructed to expect vaginal bleeding similar to menstrual flow for the next several days. Increases in pain, bleeding, or development of fever are indicative of potential complications, and the patient should be instructed to contact the provider.

The need for post-abortion contraception should always be addressed, because ovulation can occur as early as 11 days after termination of a pregnancy. Patients may be instructed to begin using their chosen contraceptive method either immediately or as early as possible within 2 weeks of the procedure. Oral contraceptives may be started on the same day, DMPA injections may be given immediately, and contraceptive implants can be inserted before the patient is discharged. In the setting of a clean, safe, induced abortion, IUDs can also be inserted immediately post-abortion. Barrier methods can be used when the patient resumes intercourse. In general, to reduce the risk of infection, patients should be counseled to abstain from intercourse and avoid tampons and douching for at least 1 week after the procedure.

Complications

When performed by competent providers, abortion is statistically a safer procedure than childbirth. Mortality rates in the United States for first trimester abortions are approximately 0.5 for every 100,000 procedures performed (58).

Mortality rates increase with duration of gestation. In the second trimester, overall mortality rates are 4 to 8 per 100,000 procedures. After 18 weeks gestation, mortality approximates that of childbirth. Complications are directly related to the experience of the operator, particularly in the case of surgical abortions (46). Unfortunately, the current socio-political climate has adversely affected the availability of experienced providers in this country. When performed in the proper setting, morbidity due to infection, bleeding, and incomplete procedures is less than 1%. Major complications include unintended surgery, hemorrhage requiring a blood transfusion, and infection requiring hospitalization. For vacuum aspiration these complications occur in less than 0.4% of cases (48).

Acute Complications

In the immediate post-abortion setting, bleeding is the most commonly encountered problem. After the abortion, patients are generally told to expect bleeding up to the amount of a menses; this should decrease over time. The clinician should evaluate any patient who experiences bleeding that is worrisome to her or who reports physical changes such as lightheadedness or tachycardia.

Bleeding may result from atony or retained products of conception. When atony is diagnosed in the presence of bleeding, uterotonic agents such as oxytocin, misoprostol, or an ergot alkyloid should be administered. If retained products of conception are suspected, a repeat evacuation should be performed or misoprostol provided to effect expulsion of retained tissue. Although uncommon, uterine or cervical perforation must always be considered. In the case of possible uterine perforation, the patient must be monitored closely and may require laparoscopy or laparotomy. If there is evidence of injury to peritoneal organs, such as the appearance of fat in the evacuate, surgical evaluation of the abdomen is mandatory (59). With a cervical laceration, bleeding often can be controlled with pressure or an agent such as silver nitrate; otherwise, surgical repair may be required.

Other procedure- and anesthetic-related problems include air embolism (very unusual with current suction devices), arrhythmias, vagal reaction, and anaphylaxis. Occasionally hematometra occurs (also called *post-abortion syndrome*), which is retained blood inside the uterus and which causes intense cramping hours after the abortion. Repeat evacuation generally relieves the cramping and resolves the problem.

Delayed Complications

VAGINAL BLEEDING

Within 24 hr after uterine evacuation, vaginal bleeding should decrease to levels similar to menstrual flow. The patient who presents with increased bleeding should have a thorough physical exam, which can be helpful in differentiating between the causes listed in Table 6-1. Cervical lacerations can occur during dilatation or from traction with a tenaculum. Usually, they occur during second trimester procedures and can be seen on careful speculum exam. An abnormally tender uterus or abdomen may indicate perforation and intraperitoneal injury. A boggy uterus or bleeding not attributable to any other etiology suggests atony, which is the most common cause of post-abortal bleeding. Continued cramping suggests retained products, especially if accompanied by fever.

While overall problems are few, one of the more frequently seen complications is retained products of conception. Patients with this complication present with continued cramping and bleeding and often the os remains open. Surgical evacuation remains the standard approach. In situations where the patient is stable, however, misoprostol can be administered to attempt expulsion. If the uterus becomes infected from retained products, the patient will likely have a fever and a tender uterus. These patients are treated like those described earlier with a septic abortion. First, a course of broad-spectrum antibiotics should be administered. In conjunction with antibiotics, emergent uterine evacuation with suction and curettage usually results in resolution of the infection. Curettage performed on an infected, pregnant uterus can easily result in perforation, and the practitioner must proceed with caution.

ASHERMAN'S SYNDROME

Over-vigorous uterine curettage can cause intrauterine synechiae to form. Clinically, this manifests as a history of diminishing menstrual flow over time, which may eventually result in amenorrhea. Often cyclic cramping indicative of menses is present, but no menstrual flow occurs. Most commonly,

Table 6-1 Causes and Treatment of Increased Vaginal Bleeding Within 24 Hours after Abortion

Cause	Treatment
Uterine atony	Uterotonic agent (oxytocin 10–30 U IM or mixed with crystalloid and given IV); or methyl ergotamine in patients without a history of hypertension, given 0.2 mg po q 4–8 hr for 1–2 days; or misoprostol 400 μg orally or 800 μg vaginally/rectally
Uterine hematometra (uterine overdistention with blood)	Repeat evacuation/suction
Uterine perforation	Laparoscopy or laparotomy; in selected cases, observation can be considered if the patient is hemodynamically stable
Retained products	Repeat uterine evacuation
Cervical laceration	Repair

the patient presents with amenorrhea and/or infertility. Such a pattern is especially common in a woman who has a pregnant and/or infected uterus and undergoes a vigorous curettage. Adhesions result from the removal of the basalis layer of the endometrium. Whenever myometrium is seen on a pathology specimen of a suction curettage, the clinician should be watchful for the development of this syndrome.

Guilt and Regret

Studies of long-term psychological sequelae have not demonstrated significant problems relating to induced abortions. Most studies reveal that no long-term emotional problems develop (60). The large majority of women feel relieved, although some women do feel guilty and, rarely, depressed. Nonjudgmental preabortion counseling is important to help identify women who may experience a negative reaction afterwards. Those with poor social support or a previous history of psychiatric problems are most at risk for negative reactions after abortion, although even most of these women have no psychological problems afterwards (61).

Infertility

With the exception of Asherman's syndrome, induced abortions properly performed do not appear to affect future fertility.

Breast Cancer

Recently, the media have cited studies suggesting that young women who undergo elective abortion have an increased risk of breast cancer. However, these retrospective studies have been sharply criticized, and no good prospective studies have been able to document this link. Several large meta-analyses and case-control studies have found no association between abortion and breast cancer (62,63).

Summary

Abortion refers to pregnancy loss prior to fetal viability, usually defined as occurring before 24 weeks gestation or when the fetus weighs less than 500 g. Approximately 20% of all clinically documented pregnancies end in spontaneous abortion. Eighty percent of these occur in the first trimester and, of these, over half are due to fetal chromosomal anomalies. Risk factors for spontaneous abortion include advancing maternal and paternal age, previous pregnancy losses (especially if more than one loss has occurred), and maternal systemic diseases such as poorly controlled diabetes mellitus. Second trimester losses are often related to maternal anatomic anomalies, such as a bicornuate uterus, and physiologic anomalies such as cervical incompetence. In the United States approximately 1.2 million induced abortions are performed annually, while worldwide the figure is approximately 50 million. Globally, unsafe abortion is the third leading cause of maternal mortality and results in 70,000 to 80,000 maternal deaths per year. In the United States, however, abortion mortality is extremely rare, occurring in less than 1 in 100,000 procedures, with the rate increasing with increasing gestational age. With an experienced provider, complication rates are under 1% but include infection, hemorrhage, incomplete procedures, and unintended surgery.

Abortions can also be induced by medical means. Methotrexate and mifepristone have been used in conjunction with a prostaglandin to induce an abortion.

REFERENCES

1. **Adelusi B, Dada OA.** Prognosis of pregnancy after threatened abortion. Int J Gynaecol Obstet. 1980;18:444-7.

2. **McBride WZ.** Spontaneous abortion. Am Fam Physician. 1991;43:175-82.

3. **Herbst AL, Mishell DR Jr, Stenchever MA, Droegemueller W.** Comprehensive Gynecology, 2nd ed. St Louis: Mosby-Year Book; 1992:426-7.

4. **Speroff L, Glass RH, Kase NG.** Clinical Gynecologic Endocrinology and Infertility, 5th ed. Baltimore: Williams and Wilkins; 1994:842.

5. **Smith KE, Buyalos RP.** The profound impact of patient age on pregnancy outcome after early detection of fetal cardiac activity. Fertil Steril. 1996;65:35-40.

6. **Cunningham FG, MacDonald PC, Grant NF, et al.** Williams Obstetrics. Norwalk, CT: Appleton and Lange; 1993:666.

7. **Armstrong BG, McDonald AD, Sloan M, et al.** Cigarette, alcohol, and coffee consumption and spontaneous abortion. Am J Public Health. 1992;82:85-7.

8. **Temmerman M, Lopita MI, Sanghvi HC, et al.** The role of maternal syphilis, gonorrhea, and HIV-1 infections in spontaneous abortions. Intl J STD AIDS. 1992;3:418-22.

9. **Schulz KF, Cates W Jr, O'Mara PR.** Pregnancy loss, infant death, and suffering: legacy of syphilis and gonorrhea in Africa. Genitourin Med. 1987;63:320-5.

10. **Schenker MB, Gold EB, Beaumont JJ, et al.** Association of spontaneous abortion and other reproductive effects with work in the semiconductor industry. Am J Ind Med. 1995;28:639-59.

11. **Scarselli G, Garguilo A, Branconi FD, Tommaso M.** Post-conception failures in reproduction: infectious diseases and immunization problems. Acta Eur Fertil. 1984; 15:363-7.

12. **Jones EE.** In: Reece EA, ed. Medicine of the Fetus and Mother. Philadelphia: JB Lippincott; 1992.

13. **Miodovnik M, Mimouni F, Tsang RC, et al.** Glycemic control and spontaneous abortion in insulin dependent diabetic women. Obstet Gynecol. 1986;68:366-9.

14. **Singer L, Arendt R, Song LY, et al.** Direct and indirect interactions of cocaine with childbirth outcomes. Arch Pediatr Adolesc Med. 1994;148:959-64.

15. **Blume SB.** Is social drinking during pregnancy harmless? There is reason to think not. Adv Alcohol Subst Abuse. 1986;5:209-19.

16. **Srisuphan W, Bracken MB.** Caffeine consumption during pregnancy and association with late spontaneous abortion. Am J Obstet Gynecol. 1986;154:14-20.

17. **Klebanoff MA, Levine RJ, DerSimonian R, et al.** Maternal serum paraxanthine, a caffeine metabolite, and the risk of spontaneous abortion. N Engl J Med. 1999:341:1639-44.

18. **Lindstrand A, Bergstrom S, Bugalho A, et al.** Prevalence of syphilis infection in Mozambican women with second trimester miscarriage and women attending antenatal care in second trimester. Genitourin Med. 1993;69:431-3.

19. **Fliegner JR.** Can anything be done about mid-trimester fetal wastage? Aust N Z J Obstet Gynaecol. 1987;27:205-9.

20. **Gabbe S, Niebyl JR, Simpson JL.** Obstetrics: Normal and Problem Pregnancies, 2nd ed. New York: Churchill Livingstone; 1999:1140.

21. **Selvaggi L, Loverro G, Schena FP, et al.** Long term follow-up of women with hypertension in pregnancy. Int J Gynaecol Obstet. 1988;27:45-9.

22. **Eberhart-Phillips JE, Frederick PD, Baron RC, Mascola L.** Measles in pregnancy: a descriptive study of 58 cases. Obstet Gynecol. 1993;82:797-801.

23. **Daugaard HO, Thomsen AC, Henriques U, Ostergaard A.** Group B streptococci in the lower urogenital tract and late abortions. Am J Obstet Gynecol. 1988;158:28-31.

24. **Eurenius K, Axelsson O.** Outcome for fetuses with abdominal wall defects detected by routine second trimester ultrasound. Acta Obstet Gynecol Scand. 1994;73:25-9.

25. **Copeland LJ.** Textbook of Gynecology. Philadelphia: WB Saunders; 1993:221.

26. **Kline J, Stein Z, Susser M, Warburton D.** Fever during pregnancy and spontaneous abortion. Am J Epidemiol. 1985;121:832-42.

27. **WHO: Excessive dilatation may affect later pregnancy.** Fam Plann Perspect. 1977; 9:134-5.

28. **Hogue CJ, Cates W Jr., Tietze C.** Impact of vacuum aspiration abortion on future childbearing: a review. Fam Plann Perspect. 1983;15:119-26.

29. **Moinian M, Andersch B.** Does cervix conization increase the risk of complications in subsequent pregnancies? Acta Obstet Gynecol Scand. 1982;61:101-3.

30. **Llahi-Camp JM, Rai R, Ison C, et al.** Association of bacterial vaginosis with a history of second trimester miscarriage. Hum Reprod. 1996;11:1575-8.

31. **Horowitz S, Mazor M, Romero R, et al.** Infection of the amniotic cavity with *Ureaplasma urealyticum* in the midtrimester of pregnancy. J Reprod Med. 1995;40:375-9.

32. **Quinn PA, Shewchuk AB, Shuber J, et al.** Efficacy of antibiotic therapy in preventing spontaneous pregnancy loss among couples colonized with genital mycoplasmas. Am J Obstet Gynecol. 1983;145:239-44.

33. Safe Motherhood: Clinical Management of Abortion Complications—A Practical Guide. Geneva: World Health Organization; 1994.

34. **Molo MW, Kelly M, Balos R, et al.** Incidence of fetal loss in infertility patients after detection of fetal heart activity with early transvaginal ultrasound. J Reprod Med. 1993; 38:804-6.

35. **Rempen A.** The incidence of abortions in viable pregnancies in the first trimester. Zentralbl Gynakol. 1993;115:249-57.

36. **Winikoff B.** "RU-486": a luncheon speech. Ann N Y Acad Sci. 1994;736:87-101.

37. **Koonin LM, Smith JC, Ramick M, et al.** Abortion surveillance: United States, 1993 and 1994. MMWR. 1997;46:57.

38. Abortion surveillance: preliminary analysis—United States. MMWR. 1997;48;51.

39. **Alan Guttmacher Institute.** Facts in Brief: Induced Abortion; 2/2000.

40. **Van Look P.** Maternal Mortality: A Global Factbook. Geneva: World Health Organization; 1991.

41. **Winkler J.** Unpublished report; 1994.

42. **Morton K, Regan L, Spring J, Houang E.** A further look at infection at the time of therapeutic abortion. Eur J Obstet Gynecol Reprod Biol. 1990;37:231-6.

43. **Centers for Disease Control and Prevention.** 1998 guidelines for treatment of sexually transmitted diseases. MMWR. 1998;47(No. RR-1):71.

44. **Lichtenberg SE.** Randomized double-blind, placebo-controlled trial of 7 versus 3 day oral doxycycline prophylaxis following elective first trimester abortion. Presented to National Abortion Federation, 21st Annual Meeting, Boston; 4-6 May 1997.

45. **Blumenthal PD.** Prospective comparison of Dilapan and Laminaria for pretreatment of the cervix in second-trimester induction abortion. Obstet Gynecol. 1988;72:243.

46. **Grimes DA, Schulz KF, Cates WJ Jr.** Prevention of uterine perforation during curettage abortion. JAMA. 1984;251:2108-11.

47. **Henshaw R, Norman J, Norman SB, et al, for the World Health Organization.** Cervical ripening with mifepristone (RU 486) in late first trimester abortion. Contraception. 1994;50:461-73.

48. **Winkler J, Blumenthal PD, Greenslade FC.** Early abortion services: new choices for providers and women. Advances in Abortion Care. 1996;5.

49. **Hausknecht RU.** Methotrexate and misoprostol to terminate early pregnancy. N Engl J Med. 1995;333:537-40.

50. **Creinin MD.** Methotrexate and misoprostol for abortion at 57-63 days gestation. Contraception. 1994;50:511-5.

51. **Peyron R, Aubeny E, Targosz V, et al.** Early termination of pregnancy with mifepristone (RU 486) and the orally active prostaglandin misoprostol. N Engl J Med. 1993; 328:1509-13.

52. **Aubeny E, Peyron R, Turpin CL, et al.** Termination of early pregnancy (up to 63 days of amenorrhea) with mifepristone and increasing doses of misoprostol. Int J Fertil Menopausal Stud. 1995;40(suppl 2): 85-91.

53. New drug application for the use of mifepristone for interruption of early pregnancy. Gaithersburg, MD: FDA Reproductive Health Advisory Committee, Center for Drug Evaluation and Research; 19 July 1996.

54. **Schaff EA, Eisinger SH, Stadalius LS, et al.** Low-dose mifepristone 200 mg and vaginal misoprostol for abortion. Contraception. 1999;59:1-6.

55. **Ashok P, Penney G, Flett G, Templeton A.** An effective regimen for early medical abortion: a report of 2000 consecutive cases. Hum Reprod. 1998;13:2962-5.

56. **Creinin MD, Vittinghoff E, Keder L, et al.** Methotrexate and misoprostol for early abortion: a multicenter trial. Contraception. 1996;53:321-7.

57. **Creinin MD, Vittinghoff E, Schaff E, et al.** Medical abortion with oral methotrexate and vaginal misoprostol. Obstet Gynecol. 1997;90:611-6.

57a. **Breitbart V, Rogers MK, Vanderhei D.** Medical abortion service delivery. Am J Obstet Gynecol. 2000;183(2 suppl):S16-25.

57b. **Koenig JD, Tapias MP, Hoff T, et al.** Are U.S. health professionals likely to prescribe mifepristone or methotrexate? J Am Med Womens Assoc. 2000;53(3 suppl):155-60.

57c. **Schaff EA, Fielding SL, Eisinger SH, et al.** Low dose mifepristone followed by vaginal misoprostol at 48 hours for abortion up to 63 days. Contraception. 2000;61:41-6.

57d. **Schaff EA, Fielding SL, Westhoff C, et al.** Vaginal misoprostol administered 1, 2, or 3 days after mifepristone for early medical abortions: a rnadomized trial. JAMA. 2000; 284:1948-53.

57e. **Newhall EP, Winikoff B.** Abortion with mifepristone and misoprostol: regimens, efficacy, acceptability, and future directions. Am J Obstet Gynecol. 2000;183(2 suppl): 544-53.

58. **Munsick RA.** In: Copeland LJ, ed. Textbook of Gynecology. Philadelphia: WB Saunders; 1993:189-90.

59. **Darney PD, Atkinson E, Hirabayashi K.** Uterine perforation during second trimester abortion and cervical dilation and instrumental extraction: a review of 15 cases. Obstet Gynecol. 1990;75:441-4.

60. **Baker A, Beresford T, Halvorson-Boyd G, Garrity J.** Informed consent, counseling, and patient preparation. In: Paul M, Lichtenberg ES, Borgotta L, Grimes D, eds. National Abortion Federation's A Clinician's Guide to Medical and Surgical Abortion. New York: Churchill Livingstone; 1999:28.

61. **Zolese B, Blacker CV.** The psychological complications of therapeutic abortion. Br J Psychiatry. 1992;160:742-9.

62. **Wingo PA, Newsome K, Marks JS, et al.** The risk of breast cancer following spontaneous or induced abortion. Cancer Causes Control. 1997;8:93-108.

63. **Tavani A, La Vecchia C, Francesci S, et al.** Abortion and breast cancer risk. Int J Cancer. 1996;65:401-5.

CHAPTER 7

Cervical Cancer Screening and Initial Management of Abnormal Pap Smears

RICHARD H. BAKER, MD

n many ways cervical cancer screening is the greatest success story of all cancer screening programs. Though prospective randomized clinical trials assessing cytological screening are lacking, historical and case control studies have documented the effectiveness of such screening. Case control studies have repeatedly shown that Pap smear screening reduces the risk of cervical cancer by more than 70% (1). Numerous studies have demonstrated that as screening coverage increases, the mortality from cervical cancer in a population falls. In countries where screening is not established, cervical cancer remains the most common cancer killer of women, whereas in the United States the annual mortality has fallen to fewer than 5000 women (2). It is reasonable to assume that screening is largely responsible for this reduction in cervical cancer.

Thoughtful use of Pap smears requires several points be kept in mind:

- *For a woman at risk the maximum benefit per test is obtained in the first smear performed.* The proportion of the population screened is more important than the frequency of screening, because most cervical cancer occurs in women who have not been screened.
- *Cervical cancer screening detects vastly more dysplasia than outright carcinoma.* Histologically, dysplasia is a failure of the epithelial cells to fully mature and can be a step in the development of cancer. The great majority of cases of cervical intraepithelial neoplasia will not progress to cancer, but it is difficult to distinguish cases that will from those that will not.

- *Cervical cancer is generally slow to develop.* Years to decades are generally required for the progression from normal to dysplasia to invasive cancer. Thus a new lesion missed on one Pap smear is unlikely to progress to cancer before the next routine screening.

Screening for Cervical Cancer

Standard of Practice versus Evidence-Based Medicine

The issue of screening frequency for cervical cancer presents a challenge for the clinician practicing evidence-based medicine. Physicians in the United States are more aggressive in screening for cervical cancer than those in other countries with national screening programs (2,3). Evaluation of the epidemiologic evidence indicates that American physicians could reduce the intensity of screening with significant improvements in cost effectiveness and only minimal increases in morbidity and mortality (4). Unfortunately, the cervical smear is not a perfect test (5), and with either an aggressive or conservative screening program some women will still die of cervical cancer. The clinician must consider practice standards of the community as well as the scientific evidence in setting his or her personal practice style.

Frequency

Traditionally gynecologists in the United States have recommended yearly Pap smears on all women and to a large extent this has become the standard of care. However, there is good evidence that yearly examinations add little screening benefit to one performed every three years and serve to triple the cost and increase the likelihood of false-positive findings. Because so few extra cancers are found in yearly examinations versus an examination conducted every three years (a difference of 12 cancers per 10,000 women followed over 55 years), the cost per extra year of life saved is estimated at over $500,000 (6). Based in part on models developed by David Eddy, the American College of Physicians-American Society of Internal Medicine offers a general recommendation to perform Pap smears every three years for women aged 20 to 65 and every two years for women at higher risk (6).

The U.S. Preventive Services Task Force (USPSTF) uses an evidence-based approach to recommend that Pap smears be done at least every three years on women who have been sexually active and who have a cervix. They found little evidence to indicate screening on an annual basis. In contrast to the consensus recommendation cited below, they do not favor screening women who have not become sexually active, unless the sexual history is thought to be unreliable and the patient is at least 18 years old (2).

A more commonly cited recommendation is the consensus guideline adopted by the American Cancer Society, the National Cancer Institute, the American College of Obstetrics and Gynecology, and the American Medical Association, among others (7). This guideline recommends that women receive annual Pap smears starting at age 18 or at the onset of sexual activity, whichever is first. After three negative Pap smears the frequency can be decreased at the discretion of the physician. This recommendation allows the physician to continue annual Pap smears out of concern for the patient's risk factors or because of personal preference. An every three to five year screening program is common in most of the rest of the Western world, without significant differences in the incidence of cervical cancer in screened women.

The "yearly exam" practice standard that now exists may have an indirect benefit as a reason for a woman to see her doctor, permitting her to achieve other benefits from the encounter. Annual screening, while often the standard of practice, cannot be supported on its screening benefits alone but may be justifiable if additional benefits of the patient-clinician contact are realized. The following sections address decision points in the use of Pap smears and only consider their impact on preventing cervical cancer death.

When To Start

The age at which to commence cervical screening should ideally be just before the occurrence of the earliest or youngest cases of cervical cancer. The first cases of cervical cancer appear in women in their early 20's (Fig. 7-1); it is virtually unheard of in teenagers. Despite this fact, most U.S. guidelines recommend beginning screening after the patient has begun having intercourse or at age eighteen. These early Pap smears can offer some secondary benefits: detecting premalignant changes in high-risk women, establishing a pattern of health care at a formative age, and providing a means of contact between a young woman and a doctor so that issues of sexuality, contraception, and communicable disease can be addressed. The incidence of cervical cancer in women who have never had sexual intercourse is exceedingly low to nonexistent. The recommendation to begin at age eighteen without a history of sexual intercourse is probably best justified by the high rate of sexual intercourse by this age in association with a possible reluctance of patients to reveal their true experiences. In a woman with a reliable history of abstinence or an intact hymen, this concern would not be justified and screening is not indicated, as per the USPSTF recommendation (2). For a woman planning her first sexual encounter, the examination will be less uncomfortable if delayed until after sexual activity has started.

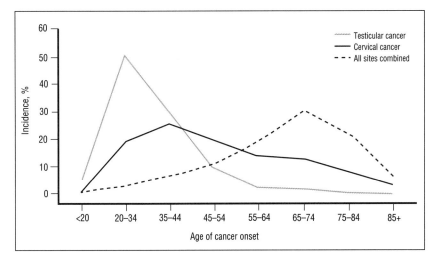

Figure 7-1 Like testicular cancer, cervical cancer is unusual in that it is not a disease of aging. Though the peak incidence of all other cancers combined is between the ages of 65 and 74, cervical cancer incidence peaks between the ages of 35 and 44. (From Hall D. J Natl Cancer Inst. 1998;90:1864; with permission.)

When To Stop

The consensus recommendation on cervical cancer screening adopted by the American Cancer Society, the National Cancer Institute, the American College of Obstetrics and Gynecology, and the American Medical Association, among others, does not address an age at which to discontinue Pap testing (7). Other recommendations, including those of the USPSTF, advise discontinuing Pap smears in women over 65 who have had consistently normal smears (2). This recommendation to discontinue screening should only be applied to women who have been carefully screened over the preceding decades, because close to half of the deaths from cervical cancer in the United States occur in women over the age of 65. Most cancer patients in this age group have not undergone any recent screening, and many have never had any screening. Women over 65 years of age who have not been previously screened achieve a benefit from screening and should receive Pap smears. In a low-risk woman over age 65 who had not previously been screened, it would be reasonable to discontinue screening after three annual negative smears.

Women with Risk Factors

Several risk factors have been linked to cervical cancer. These include genital human papilloma virus (HPV) infection, low socioeconomic status, multiple sexual partners,* early onset of sexual intercourse, cigarette smoking, and heredity. These common risk factors are generally cited as indications for annual testing. However, there are no data to support more frequent than triennial testing in women having risk factors but with previous, normal smears. Sound arguments can be made that screening frequency should be based on the sensitivity of the test and the rate of disease progression, not on risk factors (8). Still, the predictive value of the test is likely to improve in the presence of risk factors, and it is a common standard of practice to follow women with one or more risk factors on an annual basis. The recommendation for more frequent screening in these women arises from expert opinion and from a sense of caution rather than solid epidemiologic evidence. If previous screening has revealed atypical cells on Pap smear, at least annual follow-up is indicated. Women with HPV infections often have cellular changes on Pap smear and warrant aggressive follow-up. A concern that HIV is highly associated with HPV infection and a worry that HIV infected women may be at higher risk for rapidly developing cervical cancer have led to a recommendation that HIV-positive women receive screening every six months (9,10).

Risk factors for cervical cancer include genital HPV infection, low socioeconomic status, multiple sexual partners, early onset of sexual intercourse, cigarette smoking, and heredity.

Diethylstilbestrol

Diethylstilbestrol (DES) was used from 1940 until 1971 to manage high-risk pregnancies. Women exposed *in utero* to this drug have a 45% chance of having glandular columnar epithelium appear ectopically in the vagina, a condition referred to as *vaginal adenosis*. Rarely, DES exposure *in utero* is associated with the subsequent development of clear-cell adenocarcinoma of the vagina or cervix (fewer than 0.15% of exposed women). This cancer occurs in the second decade of life, with a peak at age 19. A woman with known *in utero* exposure to this drug should be referred to a gynecologist with experience with this condition. Since DES-induced adenocarcinoma is a disease of young women and use of the drug in pregnancy ended in 1971, this association will soon be mostly of historical interest (11).

---

*Risk of cervical cancer increases continuously with the number of sexual partners. There is no agreement on how many sexual partners over what time frame constitutes a clinically significant risk. The clinician needs to use his or her judgment to decide which women warrant more frequent testing.

Post-Hysterectomy

In women who have undergone a hysterectomy for a cervical neoplasm the appropriate duration and interval for follow-up screening are unclear. There are cohort reports that reveal potential for vaginal recurrence or a higher than normal incidence of vaginal cuff dysplasia in women who have undergone hysterectomies for preinvasive carcinoma of the cervix (12,13). Vaginal disease is most likely to occur in the first 20 months after the hysterectomy, and the incidence declines over years. Annual screening in the first ten years after an operation is probably wise; however, the effectiveness of the Pap smear to screen for vaginal cancer has not been demonstrated.

In women who have undergone a complete hysterectomy for benign disease, continued screening has been performed by many, ostensibly to screen for vaginal cuff cancer. Vaginal cancer is rare and fails to meet many of the criteria required for a disease to warrant screening. Moreover, vaginal smears are not a routine part of gynecologic screening in women who have not undergone hysterectomies, so it is inconsistent to perform them only on a woman without a cervix. Two recent analyses demonstrate that following a hysterectomy performed for benign causes, screening is not indicated (14,15).

The exception to this rule would be women who have had a hysterectomy without removal of the cervix. Hysterectomy without removal of the cervix was more commonly performed before the 1960s but has had a moderate resurgence recently due to the advent of laparoscopic hysterectomy, the lower complication rate associated with supracervical hysterectomy, and a belief held by some that retention of the cervix offers better sexual function following surgery (16). Before discontinuing screening, a speculum exam to check for a cervix is indicated in patients who do not have clear documentation of removal of the cervix.

Pap smears are unnecessary for women who have undergone hysterectomy for benign causes. A speculum exam to confirm that the cervix was removed is sometimes warranted, however.

Performing a Pap Smear

To achieve the maximum benefit of a Pap smear the clinician needs to develop a meticulous technique. The patient should ideally be advised to avoid coitus or douching for 24 hr before the exam, to avoid tampon use for 48 hr before the exam, and to avoid the use of intravaginal medications for a week before the exam. A small amount of blood will not prevent viewing and interpretation of cellular morphology, but if a woman is having full menstrual flow the blood will completely obscure the cells and the exam should be rescheduled.

Since the Pap smear requires sampling the cells of the squamo-columnar junction, it is important to obtain the Pap smear at the beginning of the gynecologic exam, before any other component of the exam disturbs the epithelial layer. Thus the Pap smear should precede both the bimanual exam and any endocervical cultures.

In obtaining the Pap smear:

1. The vaginal speculum should be placed carefully to reveal the entire cervix. Copious secretions or mucous should be gently removed with a proctoswab. Any unexpected abnormality of the cervical epithelium should be noted. Even if the cytology is normal, referral for colposcopy or a second opinion is indicated if the clinician is not certain of the reason for the abnormal appearance. Nabothian cysts and ectopy of the endocervix are two common normal variants that should be learned and recognized (see Chapter 1).

2. The ectocervix should be scraped with an Ayres spatula that is placed firmly into the cervical os. It should be rotated 360 deg to ensure sampling from the entire ectocervix. In some young patients the red endocervical lining extends to the ectocervix. An additional circumferential scraping of the outside edge of this tissue is necessary to ensure that the squamo-columnar junction has been sampled. The scraping should be smeared on a glass slide so that it is too thick to read newsprint through.

3. Place the cytobrush firmly in the cervical os and rotate it 360 deg. Then roll the resultant scrapings on a slide, ensuring that all 360 deg of the cytobrush are applied to the slide. The endocervical component is usually obtained after the ectocervical component. Most dysplasia arises at the squamo-columnar junction, and for many women this resides in the anatomic endocervix. The presence of columnar endocervical cells is important because it assures that the squamo-columnar junction, the area of highest risk, has been sampled. Because cytobrushes have a better retrieval rate for the endocervical component, they are now recommended. The alternative is to use a cotton applicator, which needs to be moistened in normal saline to prevent desiccation of the cells.

4. It is essential to spray the slide with fixative immediately after application of the smears because the cells may become dried and desiccated within seconds. Because the amount of material obtained is smaller with the endocervical component and it is thus at increased risk of desiccation, and because the cytobrush has a tendency to cause bleeding, the spatula should be used before the cytobrush. The samplings from the cytobrush and spatula can be combined on one slide or placed on two separate slides. Using two separate slides allows for fixation of the spatula sample immediately but requires two slides to be reviewed.

5. Vaginal spotting is expected after the cytobrush is used, so patients should be warned and reassured that this does not indicate a problem.

Screening Analysis

Sources of Error

There are basically two sources of error that lead to false-negative reports (5):

1. *Sampling Error*—inadequate preparation of the slide (e.g., neoplastic cells are present on the cervix but are not present on the slide).
2. *Screening Error*—errors in interpretation of the slide (e.g., neoplastic cells are on the slide but are not seen on review or are seen but misinterpreted).

These errors account for an estimated sensitivity of 45% to 80%, with recent meta-analyses indicating the average sensitivity of the Pap smear to be 50% (17). Even in the best-run laboratories 80% is often considered the standard true positive rate. Thus at least 20% of the patients with dysplasia have their diagnosis missed on the smear for one of the above two reasons.

The specificity of the smear is much higher, 70% to 85% (2). Because the Pap smear screens for dysplasia as well as cancer, however, the vast majority of "positive" Pap smears are not indicative of a diagnosis of cancer.

Interpreting the Report

The internist frequently faces difficulty in deciding what to do with an abnormal Pap smear result. This difficulty is further complicated by recent revisions in the classification system. Papanicolaou's original five-point numerical grading scale or the World Health Organization's descriptive scale was commonly used until the early 1990s (Table 7-1). Great difficulty arose in interpreting abnormal results, and the clinician was often left without clear guidance as to what the result truly meant.

Bethesda System

With the purpose of fostering a more consultative role for the cytologist, the Bethesda System was proposed in 1988 (18) and revised in 1991 (19) to provide greater information to the clinician. This new system gives a description of the adequacy of the smear as well as possible causes of atypia (Fig. 7-2). The following is a review of the Bethesda System and the appropriate response of the internist to each report.

Table 7-1. Papanicolaou's Original Five-Point Scale and the World Health Organization's Descriptive Scale*

Papanicolaou Scale	WHO Scale
Class I	Normal
Class II	Atypical
Class III	Dysplasia
	Mild
	Moderate
	Severe
Class IV	Carcinoma *in situ*
Class V	Adenocarcinoma

*Neither scale is now in common use.

Statement of Adequacy of Specimen for Interpretation

One of three general responses should be given: *satisfactory, satisfactory but limited by . . . ,* and *unsatisfactory*. A *satisfactory* sample can be interpreted without any qualification. If a sample is less than optimal (*satisfactory but limited*) it can still provide information, but that information may be limited. The cytologist should indicate the reason for the limitation (e.g., inadequate endocervical component, partially obscured by inflammation). If the sample is unacceptable for evaluation, the cytologist should call the specimen *unsatisfactory*.

A frequent report is *satisfactory, but limited by inadequate endocervical component*. This indicates that one has failed to obtain endocervical cells, which suggests that one may have failed to adequately sample the squamocolumnar junction. The possibility of sampling error leading to a false-negative is greater in these patients than in those with completely satisfactory smears. If previous smears have been negative and the woman's risk is perceived to be low, one can accept a limited but otherwise normal finding and repeat the smear in a year. If the woman has a history of abnormal smears or is felt to be at high risk, a repeat exam within the next few months would be appropriate. This same guideline applies to smears that are read as satisfactory but limited by some other confounding feature.

General Categorization

This categorization divides the specimens into those "within normal limits" and "others". This is meant to facilitate sorting of reports for review and consideration of further action.

Descriptive Diagnosis

INFECTIONS

The cytologist will often specify an organism present on the slide. If the organism identified (generally *Candida* or *Gardnerella*) is not a sexually trans-

THE
BAYVIEW MEDICAL
CENTER

CYTOPATHOLOGY

Patient: DOE, JANE   Path # C00-2
History # 098-79-87   Accessed: 03/03/2000
Birthdate: 02/18/1947 (Age 53)   Location: A2W
Gender: F   Race: W   Specimen Taken: 03/03/2000
FSK Physician: RICHARD BAKER, MD

CLINICAL INFORMATION
Routine Annual Exam: Yes
L.M.P.: 2/25/00
Contraception: No
Pregnant: No
History of Gynecologic Disorder or Malignancy: No
Chief Complaint: Not Stated

SPECIMEN INFORMATION
Specimen 1 COMBINED: VAG. POOL/ECTOCERVICAL/ENDOCERVICAL
1 Smear

INTERPRETATION AND DIAGNOSIS: (sxg) 03/03/2000
1) COMBINED: VAG. POOL/ECTOCERVICAL/ENDOCERVICAL:

General Categorization

FINAL DIAGNOSIS: ATYPICAL SQUAMOUS CELLS OF
UNDETERMINED SIGNIFICANCE; FAVOR A REACTIVE
PROCESS.

Descriptive Diagnosis

SMEAR CHARACTERISTICS: PREDOMINANCE OF
COCCOBACILLI CONSISTENT WITH SHIFT IN
VAGINAL FLORA.

Statement of Adequacy of Specimen for Interpretation

ADEQUACY: SPECIMEN IS SATISFACTORY FOR
EVALUATION; ENDOCERVICAL CELLS ARE PRESENT.

RECOMMEND: CLEAR INFLAMMATION AND REPEAT SMEAR.

SUSAN GEDDES, CT(ASCP), XSG

Other Cytopathology Specimens Known to the Computer: C00-1

Figure 7-2 Sample Pap smear report using the Bethesda system.

mitted disease, the patient is asymptomatic, and the sample is satisfactory, the patient does not require any further treatment because these organisms often colonize the vagina. The exception to this rule would be a pregnant or soon-to-be-pregnant woman, or a woman for whom gynecologic surgery is planned. Recent studies have shown that bacterial vaginosis is associated with an increased risk of preterm labor, miscarriage, and postoperative infection. One should therefore consider treatment in these select patients, even if asymptomatic (see Chapter 8).

If the inflammation associated with an infection has significantly interfered with the adequacy of the Pap smear specimen, the patient should be tested for cervical and vaginal infections (if not performed at the time of the Pap smear) and treated appropriately. If no infection is diagnosed, an empiric one-week course of topical (or oral) metronidazole (or oral doxycycline) is commonly prescribed to help clear the inflammation to allow a satisfactory repeat specimen. There are no data to support this practice, however, and many experts discourage empiric treatment. The Pap smear should be repeated 2 to 4 months following treatment.

Trichomoniasis

The diagnosis of trichomoniasis on cervical cytology is problematic. Though the sensitivity of the Pap smear in diagnosing trichomoniasis (56% to 63%) is approximately that of the wet mount, the specificity of the Pap smear (70% to 85%) means the positive predictive value in a population with a normal prevalence (<5%) may only be 50% (20). Considering the social implications of the diagnosis for many women, a 50% false-positive rate is unacceptable. A confirmatory test by wet mount is prudent for women at low risk for *Trichomonas* infection and whenever diagnostic certainty is important to the clinician or patient. While the disease is usually sexually transmitted, asymptomatic cases do not result in morbidity, so a delay in treatment or a falsely negative follow-up wet mount should not cause great concern for the clinician (see Chapter 8).

> *Because of the high false-positive rate, the finding of Trichomonas on a Pap smear should be confirmed by wet mount. This is particularly important for women at low risk for the infection or who may suffer significant psychosocial consequences.*

Human Papilloma Virus

Human papilloma virus (HPV) is known to be the principal cause of cervical cancer. While certain types of HPV (16,18) are oncogenic and others usually only cause condyloma (6,11), the routine use of HPV typing procedures in cervical cancer screening has not yet been accepted. Because HPV subtypes cannot be distinguished cytologically, women with HPV on a Pap smear should be considered high risk and followed on a yearly basis. Such a finding, however, does not indicate the presence of a lesion requiring treatment. Recently, however, it has been shown that HPV cannot be reliably diagnosed on Pap smear, and it has therefore been merged with CIN I in the Low Grade Squamous Intraepithelial Lesion (LGSIL) category.

REACTIVE CHANGES

A reactive change is not a premalignant condition but a normal reaction to some cervical challenge. Inflammation, atrophy, IUDs, and radiation are all potential causes of these reactive or reparative changes. The underlying problem should be addressed if the patient is symptomatic, and the patient should be followed in the usual manner. If the specimen is within normal limits and satisfactory, nothing else need be done.

BENIGN FINDINGS

From a cancer screening perspective, findings of mild inflammation not interfering with specimen adequacy, parakeratosis, benign cellular changes, squamous metaplasia, and cervicitis should be considered benign findings and ignored. Cervicitis may be associated with gonorrhea or chlamydia but can also be a nonspecific finding. Patients not screened for these infections at the time of their Pap smear are often asked to return for this testing; however, this practice may be influenced by the prevalence of these STDs in the given patient population and the manner in which the local cytopathology laboratory uses the term.

Mild inflammation, benign cellular changes, parakeratosis, squamous metaplasia, and cervicitis are benign Pap smear findings that do not affect cancer screening.

ATYPICAL SQUAMOUS CELLS OF UNCERTAIN SIGNIFICANCE

The finding of atypical squamous cells of uncertain significance (ASCUS) should be distinct from other findings. Atypical cells should truly be of uncertain significance; thus this classification should be used only rarely (<5% of all smears). Because this is such a gray zone and studies are still ongoing, its implication for management is not clearly defined. Many cytopathologists qualify this category by stating an impression that the atypical cells originate from reactive changes, as in "ASCUS, favor reactive". In these patients any underlying infection should be treated and the Pap smear repeated in 4 to 6 months, with recent data demonstrating the longer interval to be adequate (4). If the abnormality is present on the repeat Pap smear, referral for colposcopy is indicated. In all other forms of ASCUS (i.e., unspecified ASCUS and "ASCUS, favor dysplasia") the management plan has often been to refer all patients to colposcopy with an expectation that they will be seen within a few months. Alternatively, a less intensive but acceptable plan would be to repeat the Pap smear in 4 to 6 months and only refer for colposcopy if a subsequent report shows either persistent ASCUS or higher-grade lesion. However, it should be emphasized that this plan is appropriate only for women who are expected to be extremely compliant with follow-up. This less intensive plan has been favored by the interim guidelines proposed by the 1992 National Cancer Institute Workshop (21).

In postmenopausal women estrogen deficiency is a common cause of ASCUS and can often be reversed with a course of vaginal estrogen cream.

In postmenopausal women, atrophy from estrogen deficiency can lead to an ASCUS finding. Prescribing a brief course of intravaginal estrogen cream for 1 to 2 months may reverse the abnormality, and the repeat smear performed a few weeks thereafter is often normal. If ASCUS persists after topical estrogen therapy, then referral for colposcopy is appropriate.

LOW-GRADE SQUAMOUS INTRAEPITHELIAL LESIONS
Low-grade squamous intraepithelial lesions (LGSIL) make up a class that encompasses the former stages CIN I, mild dysplasia, and "cellular changes secondary to (HPV) infection"; the new classification is clearer because distinguishing between the older classes had been both difficult and unreliable. Moreover, the natural history of these conditions is similar. Most LGSIL of the cervix will revert to normal spontaneously, but about 15% will progress to more severe lesions, with a minority of these progressing to cancer (22,23). The interim guidelines proposed by the National Cancer Institute Workshop (21) suggest that compliant patients can be followed initially by Pap smears every 4 to 6 months, returning to a normal screening interval if the next three smears are normal. Patients with repeatedly abnormal smears must be referred for colposcopy. Despite these recommendations, most gynecologists still recommend colposcopic evaluation on all patients with LGSIL.

HIGH-GRADE SQUAMOUS INTRAEPITHELIAL LESIONS
Any patient with a smear revealing high-grade squamous intraepithelial lesions (HGSIL) should be referred to a gynecologist or other trained clinician

for colposcopy within the next few weeks. Depending on these results, an excisional biopsy may be indicated.

GLANDULAR CELL ABNORMALITIES

Atypical glandular cells may indicate an endometrial or endocervical process, including cancer. Their interpretation and management are difficult and best left to the expert. A retrospective 5-year study showed almost a third of patients with atypical glandular cells of undetermined significance (AGUS) will have preinvasive or invasive lesions, the majority of which are SIL (24). Women with AGUS must be referred for colposcopy and endocervical curettage. Referral to a gynecologist with experience in managing these findings is appropriate.

Because AGUS may sometimes reflect disease as significant as adenocarcinoma, it is managed much more aggressively than ASCUS. Women with AGUS must be referred for colposcopy and endocervical curettage.

Thin-Layer Smears, Computerized Cytological Review, Visual Inspection, and HPV Testing

Recently, several new modalities have been proposed to augment or replace conventional Pap smear screening (25). Thin-layer smears (ThinPrep and others) are prepared by immersing the spatula and cytobrush into a liquid, followed by submitting the liquid sample to a semiautomated slide preparation process. The process yields a more even distribution of cells from all parts of the cervix, reducing sampling error, and results in easier viewing due to a more even dispersion of cells on the slide, reducing screening error. According to some studies, the ThinPrep slide demonstrates a 93% sensitivity for significant disease versus up to 80% for conventional smears. However, it is unclear whether this technique has any effect on reducing the morbidity or mortality from cervical cancer beyond what the conventional Pap smear provides (26).

Papnet and AutoPap systems combine automated microscopy and computer analysis of standard smears to reduce screening errors and reportedly improve the sensitivity to 95% and 97% respectively. Analysis of cost effectiveness suggests these automated systems may be more economical than ThinPrep. Additionally, though all three methods add cost to the screening process, they can offer improvements in overall cost effectiveness if their greater sensitivity encourages physicians to adopt a less frequent screening regimen.

An alternative to cytologic screening is visually inspecting the cervix with the naked eye after an acetic acid wash. A number of studies (27-29) have demonstrated this procedure to be more sensitive but less specific than cytology for the detection of clinically significant squamous cervical lesions. A major advantage of the technique is that it offers immediate results compared with the delay of days to weeks required of other methods. In the United States this method could be used as an adjunct to other tests (particularly HPV testing) to reduce the number of false-negative results associated with Pap smears (30). In developing countries where Pap smears are often not feasible, visual inspection may emerge as a principal means of cervical cancer screening. In fact, data from South Africa and Thailand demonstrate that visual inspection followed by an offer of immediate treatment with cryotherapy may represent the most cost-effective cervical cancer prevention strategy (31,32).

Because HPV infection is necessary but not sufficient for the development of cervical cancer, HPV screening by self-collected swabs has been proposed as a supplementary method of improving cancer screening in at-risk patients (33). All patients testing positive for HPV would then undergo colposcopic examination. This method offers similar sensitivity but reduced specificity compared with cytologic screening, because many women with HPV never develop dysplasia.

Although all of the foregoing methods may improve the effectiveness of the screening process, by far the greatest potential gains in cervical cancer prevention remain to be found not in improving the test process but in increasing the penetration of screening into the population of at-risk women.

"The Angst Factor"

Even the most benign of atypical findings has the potential to carry a huge emotional cost to the woman. Careful communication and sensitivity to the risks of possible misinterpretation by the patient are an essential part of the compassionate management of an abnormal Pap smear. Most abnormalities seen on Pap smear will regress spontaneously and reassurance is justified.

Colposcopy

Cervical colposcopy is the magnified examination of the vaginal and cervix. Application of 3% to 5% acetic acid to the cervix removes mucus and causes intracellular swelling of the abnormal epithelial cells. Consequently, the abnormal epithelium changes from red to white, highlighting areas for further examination and biopsy. After the acetic acid examination, the Schiller test may be performed by pouring Lugol's iodine solution into the vagina. Iodine stains normal glycogen-containing squamous epithelium a deep chocolate brown while leaving the columnar epithelium pink. Atypical epithelia, which are free of glycogen, will stain a deep yellow, clearly distinguishing these areas for further inspection and biopsy.

Treatment

Colposcopically visualized, biopsy-proven squamous intraepithelial lesions are often treated by excisional biopsy. One method of accomplishing this is a therapeutic conization, a surgical procedure in which a cone shaped core containing the lesion is cut from the center of the cervix. The loop electrodiathermy excision procedure (LEEP) uses a loop cautery wire to remove a cone of tissue. The LEEP has the advantage of being an office procedure and having an acceptable safety profile. Cryotherapy is also safe and effective for precancerous lesions but is less so if the lesion is large (i.e., occupying four quadrants or more than 70% of the cervical surface) (34).

Cervical cancer is treated by radical hysterectomy and/or radiation therapy. Surgery alone is only appropriate in stage I and stage IIa disease, whereas radiation may be used in all stages of the disease. In stage Ib and IIa cancers, surgery and radiation each achieve an 85% survival rate. Chemotherapy has an adjuvant role in association with these two treatments and only a limited response rate when used alone.

Summary

The challenges in treating cervical cancer reinforce the importance of consistent and widespread screening. The slow progression to cervical cancer and the ease of detection of several well-defined premalignant stages make this disease an ideal opportunity for primary prevention. With consistent screening of all eligible women and thoughtful reaction to test results, most cervical cancer can be prevented. Although cervical cancer screening remains imperfect, the greatest progress in cervical cancer prevention will come not from improving the testing but from ensuring that more women undergo screening.

REFERENCES

1. **Dewar MA, Hall K, Perchalski J.** Cervical cancer screening: past success and future challenge. Prim Care. 1992;19:589-606.

2. **United States Preventive Services Task Force.** Screening for cervical cancer. In: Guide to Clinical Preventive Services. Baltimore: William & Wilkins; 1996:57-61.

3. **Paul C, Bagshaw S, Bonita R, et al.** Cancer screening: 1991 cervical screening recommendations. A Working Group Report. N Z Med J. 1999:104:291-5.

4. **Sawaya GF, Kerlikowske K, Lee NC, et al.** Frequency of cervical smear abnormalities within three years of normal cytology. Obstet Gynecol. 2000;96:219-23.

5. **DeMay RM.** Common problems in Papanciolau smear interpretation. Arch Pathol Lab Med. 1997;121:229-38.

6. **Eddy DM.** Screening for cervical cancer. Ann Intern Med. 1990;113:214-26.

7. **American College of Obstetrics and Gynecology.** Cervical cytology: evaluation and management of abnormalities. ACOG Technical Bulletin. 1993;183:1-8.

8. **Frame PS, Frame JS.** Determinants of cancer screening frequency: the example of screening for cervical cancer. J Am Board Fam Pract. 1998;11:87-95.

9. **Bartlett JG.** Medical Management of HIV Infection. Baltimore: Williams & Wilkins; 1997:27-9.

10. **Goldie SJ, Weinstein MC, Kuntz, KM, Freedberg KA.** The costs, clinical benefit, and cost effectiveness of screening for cervical cancer in HIV-infected women. Ann Intern Med. 1999;130:97-107.

11. **Berek JS, Hacker NF.** Practical Gynecologic Oncology. Baltimore: Williams & Wilkins; 1994:243-83.

12. **Fawdry RDS.** Carnicoma *in situ* of the cervix: is post-hysterectomy cytology worthwhile? Br J Obstet Gynaecol. 1984;91:67-72.

13. **Weiner JJ, Sweetnam PM, Jones JM.** Long-term follow up of women after hysterectomy with a history of pre-invasive cancer of the cervix. Br J Obstet Gynaecol. 1992;99:907-10.

14. **Pearce KF, Haefner HK, Sarwar SF, Nolan TE.** Cytopathological findings on vaginal Papanicolaou smears after hysterectomy for benign gynecologic disease. N Engl J Med. 1996;335:1559-62.

15. **Fetters MD, Fischer G, Reed BD.** Effectiveness of vaginal Papanicolaou smear screening after total hysterectomy for benign disease. JAMA. 1996;275:940-7.

16. **Hasson HM.** Cervical removal at hysterectomy for benign disease: risks and benefits. J Reprod Med. 1993;38:781-90.

17. **Fahey MT, Irwig L, Macaskill P.** Meta-analysis of Pap test accuracy. Am J Epidemiol. 1995;141:680-9.

18. The 1988 Bethesda system for reporting cervical/vaginal cytological diagnoses. JAMA. 1989;262:931-4.

19. The revised Bethesda system for reporting cervical/vaginal cytological diagnoses: report of the 1991 Bethesda workshop. Acta Cytologica. 1992;36:273-5.

20. **Kreiger JN, Tam MR, Stevens MA, et al.** Diagnosis of trichomoniasis: comparison of conventional wet-mount examination with cytologic studies, culture, and monoclonal antibody staining of direct specimens. JAMA. 1988;259:1223-7.

21. **Kurman RJ, Henson DE, Herbst AL, et al.** Interim guidelines for management of abnormal cervical cytology. The 1992 National Cancer Institute Workshop. JAMA. 1994; 271:1866-9.

22. **Montz FJ, Monk BJ, Fowler JM, Nguyen L.** Natural history of the minimally abnormal Papanicolaou smear. Obstet Gynecol. 1992;80:385-8.

23. **Nasiell K, Roger V, Nasiell M.** Behavior of mild cervical dysplasia during long-term follow-up. Obstet Gynecol. 1986;67:665-9.

24. **Veljovich DS, Stoler MH, Anderson WA, et al.** Atypical glandular cells of undetermined significance: a five-year retrospective histopathologic study. Am J Obstet Gynecol. 1998;179:382-90.

25. **Brown AD, Garber AM.** Cost-effectiveness of three methods to enhance the sensitivity of Papanicolaou testing. JAMA. 1999;281:347-53.

26. **Sawaya GF, Grimes DA.** New technologies in cervical cytology screening: a word of caution. Obstet Gynecol. 1999;94:307-10.

27. **Megevand E, Denny L, Dehaeck K, et al.** Acetic acid visualization of the cervix: an alternative to cytologic screening. Obstet Gyencol. 1996;88:383-6.

28. Visual inspection with acetic acid for cervical-cancer screening: test qualities in a primary-care setting. University of Zimbabwe/JHPIEGO Cervical Cancer Project. Lancet. 1999;353:869-73.

29. **Belinson JL, Pretorius RG, Zhang WH, et al.** Cervical cancer screening by simple visual inspection after acetic acid. Obstet Gynecol. 2001;98:441-4.

30. **Blumenthal PD, Gaffikin L, Chireuje ZM, et al.** Adjunctive testing for cervical cancer in low-resource settings with visual inspection, HPV, and the Pap smear. Int J Gynaecol Obstet. 2001;72:47-53.

31. **Goldie SJ, Kuhn L, Denny L, et al.** Policy analysis of cervical cancer screening strategies in low-resource settings: clinical benefits and cost-effectiveness. JAMA. 2001; 285:3107-15.

32. **Mandelblett J, Lawrence W, Gaffikin L, et al.** Benefits and costs of alternative strategies to screening for cervical cancer in less developed countries. J Natl Cancer Inst. In press.

33. **Wright TC, Denny L, Kuhn L, et al.** HPV DNA testing of self-collected vaginal samples compared with cytologic screening to detect cervical cancer. JAMA. 2000;283:81-6.

34. **Mitchell MF, Tortolero-Luna G, Cook E, et al.** A randomized clinical trial of cryotherapy, laser vaporization, and loop electrosurgical excision for treatment of squamous intraepithelial lesions of the cervix. Obstet Gynecol. 1998;92:737-44.

CHAPTER 8

Vaginitis and Sexually Transmitted Diseases

L. CHESNEY THOMPSON, MD
JANICE RYDEN, MD
JAMES A. McGREGOR, MD, CM

Vaginitis

Vaginitis is one of the most common gynecologic problems and is responsible for more than 10 million office visits annually in the United States and billions of dollars spent on diagnosis and cure (1). At least one third of all premenopausal women will experience an episode of some type of vaginitis (2).

By definition, vaginitis is an inflammatory process involving the vaginal mucosa and/or vulvar skin. Symptoms include discharge, odor, burning, itching, and even pain. In addition to the vagina and vulva, symptoms may involve the urinary tract and perianal skin.

There are many possible etiologies for vaginitis, including physiologic and pathologic bacteria, fungal organisms, parasitic protozoa, and viral processes. In addition, atrophy, inflammatory responses, and certain hygiene practices may cause vaginitis. Fortunately, vaginitis symptoms are only rarely caused by cancer. Nevertheless, vaginitis has profound relationships to other important health problems such as preterm labor and birth, premature rupture of the membranes, infertility, and chronic pelvic pain, as well as increasing the likelihood of HIV acquisition and transmission.

Ecosystem of Normal Vagina

The vulva and vagina are normally colonized by a variety of bacteria, with the predominant vaginal organism being hydrogen peroxide producing strains of

Lactobacillus. In the patient of reproductive age, estrogen stimulates the vaginal epithelial cells to produce glycogen, which the lactobacilli ferment to lactic acid, yielding a remarkably acidic environment (pH ≤ 4.5). Together the hydrogen peroxide and low vaginal pH serve as nonspecific antimicrobial defenses and are of paramount importance in maintaining the delicate ecosystem of the vagina. Conditions that lead to reduction of the normal lactobacilli or that alter the pH of the vagina may allow overgrowth of other flora or permit invasion. Even seemingly innocuous processes such as the introduction of alkaline-buffered semen from intercourse, douching, blood from menses, pregnancy, estrogen deprivation from menopause, or hormonal manipulation may disturb the normal vaginal flora and contribute to vulvovaginitis.

The normal vagina has a physiologic discharge that appears clear, white, or greyish in color, and is flocculent, meaning it is a liquid base containing small flecks of solid material. The normal discharge does not adhere to the vaginal walls but rather pools in the posterior fornix when the patient is recumbent. The pH range of the normal discharge is 3.8 to 4.5 and does not cause any symptoms of irritation, pruritus, disagreeable odor, or dysuria.

Evaluation of Vaginitis

The evaluation of vulvovaginitis is frequently straightforward; however, it should always be methodical and thorough. This is important because there can be significant variation and overlap in clinical presentations, and simultaneous co-infection is common. The proper evaluation of vaginitis includes four elements: clinical history, physical examination, pH and amine testing, and microscopic evaluation of the discharge. The history should include a detailed account of the symptoms, including duration, timing, and relation to sexual activities. If a discharge is present, characteristics such as the volume, color, and presence of pruritus or a disagreeable odor should be elicited. Other points to be covered include potential exposure to sexually transmitted infections, sexual habits, number of partners, methods of contraception, and hygiene habits. More general medical issues that can affect the diagnosis are age, symptoms of menopause, surgical history, systemic illnesses such as diabetes or immunosuppression, and recent or current medication use (in particular, corticosteroids and antibiotics).

After the history, one proceeds with a physical examination. An abdominal exam is performed first, noting any masses, tenderness, or peritoneal signs. The presence of CVA tenderness should also be assessed. Palpation of the inguinal area may reveal lymphadenopathy. The vulva should be carefully inspected for erythema, dystrophy, edema, warts, erosions, or other skin changes or masses. A vaginal speculum is then placed so that one can first note the appearance of the cervix. It is wise to carefully inspect the cervical os for possible emanating discharge because patients complaining of "vaginitis" are sometimes found to have cervicitis or upper reproductive tract infection. Next, one evaluates the vaginal walls for color, the appearance of the rugae, and the presence of any odor or discharge. If a discharge is present, one should note the texture, volume, color, and location.

Using cotton swabs, one next collects three samples from the lateral wall of the proximal (deep) aspect of the vagina. One swab is applied to nitrazine paper to test pH, one swab is mixed in a drop or two of normal saline on a slide and then covered with a cover slip, and the third swab is similarly mixed with a slide containing one to two drops of 10% KOH solution. The "whiff test" is performed by taking note of the presence of an amine ("fishy") odor when introducing the cotton swab contents into the KOH.

Although the posterior fornix often harbors the largest volume of discharge, any vaginal discharge at this location is mixed with cervical secretions and possibly semen and blood, all of which could alter the pH reading and microscopy findings. Therefore the optimal site for sampling is the lateral wall of the proximal vagina. An abnormally elevated pH (>4.5) is typical of bacterial vaginosis, *Trichomonas vaginalis*, or atrophic vaginitis. A normal pH (<4.5) is found in the setting of a candidal infection or irritant vaginitis.

Cultures or DNA probes for gonorrhea and chlamydia are typically collected from the endocervix at this point. If subsequent bimanual examination and microscopic evaluation fail to raise suspicion for the presence of any sexually transmitted diseases, these specimens may sometimes be discarded. It should be noted that routine culturing of vaginal discharge has not been proven to be useful, partly because of the polymicrobial environment of the vagina and partly because many of the pathogens are also normal vaginal colonizers that can be cultured from asymptomatic women. Aerobic vaginal cultures are obtained in such rare situations as a patient suffering recurrent bouts or a prolonged course of vaginitis that cannot be diagnosed with confidence using the standard approach.

A bimanual exam is next carefully performed, noting in particular any evidence of cervical motion tenderness or uterine or adnexal masses or tenderness (see Chapter 1).

The saline slide and KOH slides are essential in the evaluation of vaginitis. The wet mount slide is examined carefully for clue cells and motile trichomonads. In addition, the presence of increased leukocytes (approximately >10/hpf) may be helpful in distinguishing possible etiologies. Assessment of the volume of cytoplasm in the vaginal epithelial cells gives the degree of estrogen effect and helps make the diagnosis of atrophic vaginitis. The KOH slide is used to identify the hyphal and budding forms of yeast.

The Three Common Vaginitides: Bacterial Vaginosis, Yeast Vaginitis, and *Trichomonas vaginalis*

Ninety percent of patients presenting to a primary care office with symptoms of vaginitis will be diagnosed with bacterial vaginosis, yeast vaginitis (vaginal candidiasis), or *Trichomonas vaginalis*. This tends to simplify the workup. However, a thorough evaluation will allow accurate diagnosis for the reasons stated previously, including the observation that 35% of the time there may be multiple pathogens (2).

Bacterial Vaginosis

Bacterial vaginosis is the leading cause of abnormal or offensive vaginal discharge. In fact, 30% to 50% of women with complaints of vaginitis are diagnosed with this entity (2). When originally described by Gardner and Dukes, bacterial vaginosis was felt to be caused by *Haemophilus vaginalis* (since reclassified as *Gardnerella vaginalis*). Subsequent investigation has revealed that numerous other bacteria contribute to bacterial vaginosis, in particular, the anaerobes. The derangement in the normal vaginal flora is accompanied by a concomitant reduction in lactobacillus growth. Consequently, there is a decrease in lactic acid and hydrogen peroxide production and thereby loss of the normally acidic vaginal environment and host defenses.

DIAGNOSIS

The patient with bacterial vaginosis often complains of an amine or "fishy" odor. If she is observant, she may report that the odor is exacerbated by exposure to alkaline substances (such as soap or semen), because such contact increases volatization of the amines. Other complaints include a discharge of variable volume that is sometimes but not always accompanied by pruritus and irritation of the vagina.

On examination the vaginal walls appear normal, lacking signs of inflammation. A homogenous gray/white discharge clings abnormally to the vaginal walls and may emit an amine odor even before instillation in KOH. The volume of discharge may vary widely, but its thin, homogeneous (i.e., nonflocculent) appearance has earned the description "cup of milk".

The pH will be more alkaline than normal (>4.5). Microscopic evaluation of the wet mount slide reveals the presence of "clue cells", vaginal epithelial cells whose borders appear studded because of adherent bacteria (Fig. 8-1). If such clue cells comprise at least 20% of the epithelial cells, the microscopic appearance is considered pathognomonic for bacterial vaginosis. Further careful examination of the saline slide demonstrates an excess number of epithelial cells, fewer of the normal lactobacilli and a lack of increased leuko-

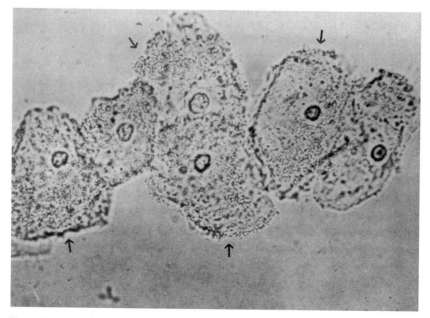

Figure 8-1 Bacterial vaginosis. Microscopic evidence of bacterial vaginosis is the "clue cell", an epithelial cell whose borders are studded with bacteria (*arrows*) rather than appearing smooth. Diagnostic criteria require that clue cells comprise at least 20% of the epithelial cells. Lack of increased leukocytes attests to the noninflammatory nature of this condition. (Courtesy of Jean R. Anderson, MD, Department of Gynecology and Obstetrics, Johns Hopkins University School of Medicine.)

cytes. Another compelling, but not required, finding is the presence of curved motile rods, which suggests *Mobiluncus* species.

Immediately upon preparation of the KOH slide the vaginal discharge produces a fishy odor because of the release of aromatic amines (positive "whiff test"). The KOH slide is also examined for co-existing yeast. It should be noted that vaginal culture for bacterial vaginosis is not used in making the diagnosis because the organism *G. vaginalis* is a normal colonizer and has been recovered in 60% of asymptomatic women (3).

TREATMENT
The mainstay of therapy consists of metronidazole 500 mg PO bid for 7 days or metronidazole 0.75% vaginal gel used nightly for 5 days. These two regimens are equally efficacious. The oral metronidazole regimen entails systemic side effects (primarily a transient altering of taste and risk of Antabuse-like reaction if alcohol is consumed); however, it is significantly less expensive. The vaginal clindamycin regimen appears somewhat less effica-

cious. Also, the clindamycin cream is oil-based and may weaken latex condoms and diaphragms. Finally, although oral clindamycin 300 mg PO bid for 7 days has been prescribed, it may be associated with diarrhea and/or colitis and is not FDA-approved for this indication (Table 8-1). After treatment for bacterial vaginosis, 20% to 30% of women will have a recurrence within 3

Table 8-1 Treatment of the Three Common Infectious Vaginitides

Bacterial Vaginosis	Candidiasis	Trichomoniasis
Metronidazole (Flagyl) 500 mg PO bid × 7 days	**Miconazole (Monistat)** 2% cream qhs × 7 days 100 mg supp qhs × 7 days 200 mg supp qhs × 3 days	**Metronidazole (Flagyl)** 2 g PO × 1 *Alternative regimen:* 500 mg PO bid × 7 days
Metronidazole (Metrogel) **0.75% vaginal cream** 1 applicatorful per vagina qhs (or bid) × 5 days	**Clotrimazole (Gyne-Lotrimin, Mycelex)** 1% cream qhs × 7–14 days 100 mg supp qhs × 7 days 2 × 100 mg supp qhs × 3 days 500 mg supp × 1	N.B. Treat partners also.
Clindamycin (Cleocin) **2% vaginal cream** Qhs × 7 days		
	Butaconazole (Femstat) 2% cream qhs × 3 days 2% cream, 5 g SR, single application	
	Tioconazole (Vagistat) 6.5% ointment, 5 g, single application	
Alternatives: **Clindamycin** 300 mg PO tid × 7 days *(not FDA approved for this indication)*	*Prescription requiring:* **Terconazole (Terazole)** 5 g 0.4% cream qhs × 7 days 80 mg supp qhs × 3 days 0.8% cream qhs × 3 days	
Metronidazole (Flagyl) 2 g PO × 1 *(less effective)*	**Fluconazole (Diflucan)** 150 mg PO × 1	
	Alternative: **Nystatin vaginal tablet (Mycostatin)** 100,000 U tablet qhs × 14 days	

months, which often responds to a repeat 7-day course of oral metronidazole (4). Multiple recurrences require re-evaluation to confirm the diagnosis.

Routine treatment of sexual partners is not advocated because more than one controlled trial has shown lack of efficacy in preventing relapse by treating the male partner (5,6). This is despite the fact that experimental studies have shown that cultures from the male partner's genitalia can yield many of the bacteria associated with bacterial vaginosis. The role of sexual transmission is unclear, for while demographics implicate sexual activity as a possible mode of transmission, bacterial vaginosis has also been diagnosed in virgins. The lack of a male counterpart to bacterial vaginosis makes this question difficult to elucidate. However, one recent study of 21 monogamous lesbians and their partners supports sexual transmissability (7). The study revealed a high concordance rate for infection because of the 11 index patients who had bacterial vaginosis, 8 (73%) had affected partners, whereas of the 10 control patients, only one (10%) of the partners was found to have bacterial vaginosis.

ASSOCIATION WITH OTHER DISEASES

Recent studies link bacterial vaginosis with many serious sequelae. In the susceptible pregnant patient bacterial vaginosis may be associated with such adverse outcomes as premature rupture of the membranes, preterm labor and birth, chorioamionitis, and postpartum endometritis. Therefore, to ensure adequate treatment of the upper genital tract, bacterial vaginosis diagnosed during pregnancy is preferably managed with oral rather than topical medications. Although long feared to be mutagenic, recent meta-analyses have found metronidazole to have no adverse affect on the human fetus (8-10), and the drug can be safely prescribed in pregnancy, particularly after the first trimester. Issues relating to the management of asymptomatic bacterial vaginosis during pregnancy remain controversial.

Bacterial vaginosis has also been implicated in contributing to other pathology. Studies suggest that it may be associated with abnormal cells (generally ASCUS) on Pap smears as well as greater susceptibility to HIV infection because of the more neutral pH of the vagina being more hospitable to the target CD4 cells (11). Bacterial vaginosis may also contribute to upper genital tract infection such as plasma cell endometritis, post-abortion pelvic inflammatory disease, and surgical wound cellulitis after pelvic surgery. For this reason, patients who are to undergo abortions or other pelvic procedures are now often screened for asymptomatic bacterial vaginosis. Those who meet Amsel's criteria for bacterial vaginosis (i.e., those women who have at least three of the four following criteria: homogeneous vaginal discharge, presence of positive "whiff test," vaginal pH > 4.5, and clue cells > 20%) are offered treatment before surgery, even in the absence of symptoms.

Yeast Vaginitis

Yeast infections are the second most common cause of vulvovaginitis, representing 20% to 40% of symptomatic office presentations (2). Fully 75% of women may experience an episode of vulvovaginal candidiasis during their lifetime (12). Fungal infections are responsible for an estimated 13 million cases of vulvovaginitis per year in the United States, which reflects a 50% increase in the number of diagnoses from 1980 to 1990 (13). It is uncertain whether the incidence has truly increased or whether this reflects detection bias or overdiagnosis.

Candida albicans is the responsible strain for approximately 80% to 92% of the episodes of vulvovaginitis; however, the relative incidence of *C. tropicalis* and *glabrata* infections has been increasing. The cause for this is unknown but may reflect selection for these more resistant strains through widespread use of over-the-counter antifungal medications, shorter courses of treatment, or chronic use of oral antifungals in immunocompromised patients (14).

Candida is a constituent of the normal vaginal flora, and the progression from colonization to infection is not completely understood. Episodic cases are usually without identifiable precipitants; however, some cases are easily related to recent antibiotic use. Also, although the infection is not traditionally considered sexually transmitted, there is also an increase in frequency at the time women first begin regular sexual activity, and orogenital sex may be a risk factor (14).

Diagnosis

Symptoms of yeast vaginitis most commonly include itching and/or burning in both vaginal and vulvar tissues, sometimes accompanied by dysuria, sometimes accompanied by a thick discharge. Pelvic examination reveals that even the external genitalia to be irritated and diffusely erythematous, although sometimes it may be so edematous as to appear pale. Excoriations and papular satellite lesions can sometimes be noted. The vaginal walls are also diffusely erythematous with an adherent thick, white or yellowish "cottage cheese" vaginal discharge. However, approximately 25% of the time the presentation is less classic, with a thin discharge noted.

The pH of the vaginal secretions is normal (<4.5), and the whiff test is negative. The saline wet mount is notable for an increased number of leukocytes because an inflammatory response accompanies the condition. The KOH slide is examined carefully and thoroughly for hyphae, and further close inspection may sometimes reveal numerous tiny spores (Fig. 8-2). Unfortunately, even with careful scrutiny of 10 to 20 high-power fields, the sensitivity of the KOH slide is only 50% to 60%. The diagnostic yield may be increased by taking a large sample of the vaginal discharge and by gently warming the KOH slide to

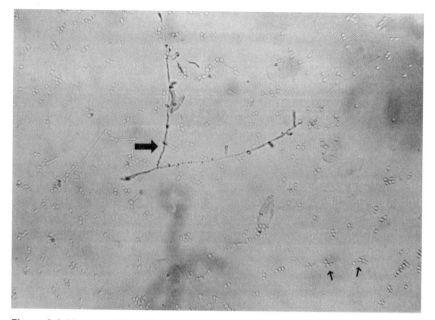

Figure 8-2 Yeast vaginitis. Microscopic examination of the KOH slide reveals a large hypha (*large arrow*). Close inspection of the background also reveals numerous small, round spores scattered throughout (*small arrows*). Even with careful scrutiny of 20× high-power fields, approximately half of cases will lack these microscopic findings, and the diagnosis must be made using other clinical criteria. (From Sexually Transmitted Genital Tract Infections Slide Set. Baltimore: JHPIEGO; 1991; with permission.)

maximally lyse the surrounding cellular elements. Some have also advocated the use of methylene blue stain, which highlights the hyphal elements. Patients are often treated empirically when microscopy fails to confirm the diagnosis, but such a situation warrants close follow-up because other conditions such as hypersensitivity or allergic reactions may mimic the classic findings of yeast vaginitis.

TREATMENT

The most recent CDC treatment recommendations state no preference for any of the various regimens for yeast vaginitis. However, many authors have suggested that first-line therapy should be over-the-counter topical azole agents (butoconazole, clotrimazole, or miconazole), using a 7-day regimen in order to help lower the risk of recurrence. Relapses are fairly common and may require a repeat course of longer duration (10 to 14 days). The resistant organisms are typically *C. tropicalis* and *glabrata* strains; although they are not always responsive to the over-the-counter agents or to oral medications, they currently remain susceptible to the prescription topical agent tercona-zole (Terazole).

Alternative treatments for yeast vaginitis include single-dose treatment with the oral medication fluconazole 150 mg. However, some have argued that topical agents should be used to treat a focal infection. An older but less well tolerated treatment is for the practitioner to paint the vagina with gentian violet dye. Intravaginal boric acid suppositories are highly effective and have generated much excitement in the research literature; however, these are not commercially available, and most pharmacists are currently unfamiliar with formulating these gelatin capsules.

RECURRENT YEAST VAGINITIS

Recurrent yeast vaginitis is defined as four or more infections per year; unlike the patient with the single isolated episode, a work-up for these patients is indicated. Women should generally be tested for HIV because this is sometimes the presenting sign of the disease, and they might also be evaluated for possible diabetes. Review of the patient's medical history, medications, and habits may reveal a predisposing cause and potential area for intervention. Hormonal conditions that increase the risk of symptomatic yeast vulvovaginitis include pregnancy and high-dose (≥50 µg estrogen) oral contraceptive use. Any cause of immunosuppression, including systemic steroid use, is implicated. Antibiotic use may also be the culprit. The presence of foreign bodies such as an IUD and the contraceptive sponge have also been associated with an increased prevalence, as have obesity, tight-fitting garments, and diets high in refined sugar.

The treatment for recurrent yeast infections should be individually tailored. Those who suffer monthly symptoms can be treated with monthly use of over-the-counter topical medications daily or twice weekly during the luteal phase. Those with more continuous symptoms may require ketoconazole 100 mg orally daily for 6 months (note the risk of hepatotoxicity, gastrointestinal side effects, and potential drug interactions) or fluconazole 150 mg orally taken once weekly or once monthly. Prophylactic use of one intravaginal boric acid 600 mg suppository daily for one week each month (usually during menstruation) has been shown to be effective and well tolerated in research trials. One small study also suggested possible benefit from the daily ingestion of yogurt containing live lactobacilli cultures (15).

Trichomonas vaginalis

Trichomonas vaginalis is a flagellated protozoon, which, worldwide, is the most common sexually transmitted infection. However, its incidence in the United States has decreased greatly since the introduction of metronidazole in the 1960s so that it now represents only 10% to 25% of vaginitis cases.

Studies clearly demonstrate the sexual transmissibility of this infection (2). However, the protozoon can also be spread through such fomites as shared moist towels and bathing suits as well as lubricating jelly at physicians' offices. In addition, the organism has been shown to survive tap water, chlorinated pools, and even hot tubs.

DIAGNOSIS

After an incubation period of 5 to 28 days, most women report a vaginal discharge, sometimes accompanied by a disagreeable odor. Some also note vulvovaginal soreness or irritation. Up to half note urinary symptoms, and a small minority report abdominal pain. On examination, copious amounts of a thin discharge are typically seen pooling in the posterior fornix. The "classic" green or yellowish color is present less than half the time. Bubbles, when noted, are fairly specific; however, the discharge may alternatively be thick. Patchy erythema of the vaginal walls and cervix ("strawberry cervix") is rarely visible with the naked eye but easily seen with the colposcope and results from injury to the epithelium induced by the whipping action of the flagella. The pH is generally markedly elevated; values range from 5 to 6. The "whiff test" is sometimes positive because of the overgrowth of anaerobes resulting from the consumption of oxygen by the trichomonads. Microscopy demonstrates an influx of leukocytes; however, the hallmark of diagnosis is the observation of motile trichomonads, which are easily identified as wriggling flagellated oval organisms slightly larger than the surrounding white blood cells (Fig. 8-3). Tapping the microscope stage may stimulate the trichomonads to move and make them more apparent. Identifying trichomonads is 100% specific, but the wet mount is only 60% to 90% sensitive.

TREATMENT

The CDC-recommended treatment regimen is metronidazole 2 g PO in a single dose (with the alternative regimen 250 mg PO bid for 7 days) for the patient and all sexual partners. Patients should be instructed to avoid alcohol during and for 2 days after completion of therapy. Because there is no effective alternative, those allergic to the drug require desensitization. Also, unlike bacterial vaginosis, infection with *Trichomonas* involves the urethra and paraurethral glands; consequently, topical metronidazole is not an option. Until they are beyond the first trimester, pregnant women are commonly treated with palliative medication, such as topical clotrimazole, then treated definitively with oral metronidazole; however, the CDC has approved first-trimester use of metronidazole for symptomatic women.

Unfortunately, treatment failures are becoming increasingly common. Once re-infection has been excluded, the patient should be retreated with a longer course such as metronidazole 500 mg PO bid for 7 days. If resistance is

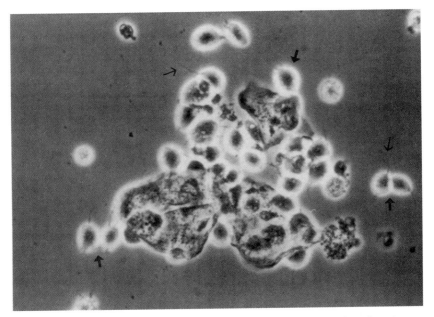

Figure 8-3 *Trichomonas vaginalis*. *Trichomonas vaginalis* is a pear-shaped protozoon (*thick arrows*) usually slightly larger in size than the surrounding leukocytes. Detecting this organism on the wet mount is facilitated by its wriggling motion and the rotatory whipping action of the flagellae (*thin arrows*). (From Sexually Transmitted Genital Tract Infections Slide Set. Baltimore: JHPIEGO; 1991; with permission.)

suspected, the organism can ultimately be cultured on Diamond's media so that sensitivities can be obtained. The CDC can provide expert consultation for treating resistant organisms.

ASSOCIATION WITH OTHER DISEASE

Because *Trichomonas* is sexually transmitted, the patient should be screened for other sexually transmitted diseases, including chlamydia, gonorrhea, syphilis, HIV, and hepatitis B. Education regarding safe sex should be provided, and adults presenting with a sexually transmitted disease have been identified as a target group for vaccination against hepatitis B. Some evidence suggests that *Trichomonas* may

Because Trichomonas is sexually transmitted, infected patients should be screened for other sexually transmitted diseases, including chlamydia and gonorrhea, and offered serologic screening for syphilis, hepatitis B, and HIV at a scheduled follow-up visit.

possibly be associated with pelvic inflammatory disease, perhaps via its motion promoting ascension of bacteria into the upper genital tract, as well as increased HIV acquisition because of the increased number of target lymphocytes in the vagina. Sometimes the finding of *Trichomonas* is reported on a Pap smear; however, it should be noted that this test has an unacceptably high false-positive rate for diagnosing *Trichomonas*, and the patient should return for a confirmatory wet mount before being told of the possibility of having a sexually transmitted disease.

Less Common Infectious Vaginitides

The less common causes of infectious vulvovaginitis should be considered if the patient's presentation fails to meet the diagnostic criteria of the three common infections. These infections are rare even in tertiary referral centers, and consultation with gynecologists is often appropriate.

Desquamative Inflammatory Vaginitis

Desquamative inflammatory vaginitis is a rare and challenging diagnosis of unknown etiology. The symptoms involve dyspareunia, a malodorous purulent discharge, burning, and a dystrophic-like rash of the vulva. Examination discloses raw patchy inflammatory areas of the vagina, usually in the upper one third. The pH is elevated above 5. Evaluation of the discharge demonstrates numerous polymorphonuclear neutrophil leukocytes, few if any lactobacilli, and immature basal and parabasal cells. Interestingly, although many of these criteria mimic atrophic vaginitis, the condition is found in premenopausal women or women on hormone replacement therapy. Attempts to correlate the condition with bacterial infection or immunologic processes have been unsuccessful. The diagnosis is essentially one of exclusion once no clear pathogen can be identified and the presence of adequate estrogen confirmed. Treatment is controversial; regimens vary from intravaginal hydrocortisone suppositories to 2% clindamycin cream.

Vaginitis Emphysematosa

Vaginitis emphysematosa is an unusual form of vaginitis of elusive cause. On examination, the vaginal epithelium, particularly in the upper vagina, is lined with tiny cystic structures. They may be appreciated by their bumpy presentation on palpation or by small shiny vesicular mounds. Patients may note a discharge, spotting, or even complain of a popping sound during intercourse or manipulation. The cysts are actually carbon dioxide-filled bubbles that burst producing the noise. The treatment regimen for vaginitis emphysematosa remains controversial, but fortunately intervention is often unnecessary.

Noninfectious Vaginitis

Atrophic Vaginitis

At the time of menopause, falling estrogen levels induce numerous changes in the vagina. The vaginal epithelium becomes thin and loses its lubricating qualities. The superficial epithelial cells decrease in number and produce less glycogen. As a consequence, the vaginal population of lactobacilli falls, with a concomitant decline in lactic acid production. The vaginal pH consequently rises to 5 to 7, rendering the vagina more hospitable to fecal flora.

Despite these dramatic changes, most women are asymptomatic. When symptoms do occur, they are often most prominent in the perimenopausal transition and wane over time. In fact, vaginal soreness sometimes may be the presenting sign of menopause, preceding hot flashes and menstrual aberrations. In addition to menopause, atrophic vaginitis can occur in the setting of other hypoestrogenic states, such as lactation, treatment with GnRH agonists, use of injectable depot medroxyprogesterone acetate (Depo-Provera) and, rarely, with oral contraceptives.

In addition to menopause, atrophic vaginitis may occur in the setting of other hypoestrogenic states, such as lactation, use of Depo-Provera, treatment with GnRH agonists, and, rarely, with oral contraceptive use.

The symptoms of atrophy may be referable to either the vagina or urinary tract and include vaginal dryness, soreness, pruritus, burning leukorrhea, spotting, and dyspareunia, as well as dysuria, urgency, frequency, infection, and incontinence.

Inspection of the vulva may reveal perivaginal irritation from urinary incontinence, a urethral caruncle, and friability of the labia minora. The vagina may appear pale, dry, atrophic, and lacking the normal rugae, and possibly stenotic. Sometimes petechiae and ecchymoses are seen. Also, if there is inflammation resulting from changes in the vaginal flora, there may be a serosanguinous or watery discharge. The vaginal pH is more than 5, and microscopy often reveals increased numbers of leukocytes. A more diagnostic wet mount finding is the replacement of the usual large flat epithelial cells containing abundant cytoplasm with small rounded parabasal and intermediate cells.

Atrophic vaginitis is best treated with topical estrogen. It should be noted that even women already taking systemic hormone replacement therapy can suffer symptoms of urogenital atrophy and require the addition of topical therapy. Dosing is flexible but typically one applicatorful of conjugated estrogen (Premarin) cream or estradiol (Estrace) cream is placed intravaginally at bedtime for 1 to 2 weeks, then the dose is reduced to one-half tube for the same length of time (Table 8-2). Thereafter, a maintenance dose of one-half applicatorful once or twice weekly is generally adequate. An intravaginal estrogen ring that releases a low dose of estrogen continuously for 3 months has recently become available (Estring) and has been preferred by trial subjects as being less messy (16). (For further discussion of this and other postmenopausal hormone therapies, see Chapter 16.)

Alternatives for the rare patient who is not a candidate for topical estrogen include vaginal lubricants. A recent comparison trial demonstrated that when a moisturizing vaginal gel (Replens) was applied vaginally three times per week, both symptoms and signs of atrophic vaginitis improved nearly as well as with treatment with estrogen cream (17).

Contact Vulvovaginitis

Contact vulvovaginitis, or irritant vaginitis, is a fairly common cause of vulvovaginitis. The patient usually complains of burning and itching and, occasionally, discharge. Careful history taking can usually uncover the likely culprit. Common causes include soaps and perfumes, detergents, formaldehyde (in new fabric), rubber, sanitary napkins, spermicides, and latex condoms. Certain medications such as benzocaine, topical diphenhydramine, povidone-iodine, and antimycotic creams can also cause irritation.

On examination, typically the vulva is inflamed as well as the vagina, and the clinical presentation may resemble that of *Candida* vaginitis. Moreover, the condition may predispose the patient to infection with *Candida*, confounding the diagnosis. The pH is normal, and the wet mount and KOH fail to reveal abnormal organisms.

The primary treatment strategy consists of identifying and eliminating the offending agent. Symptomatic relief may be aided by cool baths and compresses with mild drying astringents such as Burrow's solution; if the skin is cracked and fissured, lubrication with vegetable oils may be helpful. In severe cases, hydrocortisone 1% ointment may be necessary. Antihista-

Table 8-2 Treatment of Noninfectious Vulvovaginitis

Atrophic vaginitis	Estrogen cream $1/_2$–1 applicatorful per vagina q 3–7 days @ HS *or* estrogen vaginal ring q 90 days
Contact vulvovaginitis	Identification and elimination of offending agent Burrow's solution diluted 1:20 applied topically Hydrocortisone 1% ointment Oral antihistamines or low-dose TCA (e.g., desimpramine 10–25 mg qhs)

mines or desipramine in low doses (i.e., 10 to 25 mg) at bedtime may also be a useful adjunct.

Sexually Transmitted Diseases

Although the preceding sections included pathogens that may relate to sexual activity, the following section describes those organisms clearly spread by sexual contact, namely *Chlamydia trachomatis, Neisseria gonorrhea*, herpes simplex virus (HSV), syphilis, HIV, hepatitis B, and human papilloma virus (HPV). The less common sexually transmitted infections also are discussed.

Sexually transmitted diseases vary in their seriousness, but some may be acutely life-threatening (e.g., pelvic inflammatory disease) or have ultimately fatal consequences (e.g., HIV). Other sequelae include chronic pelvic pain, ectopic pregnancies, infertility, obstetric complications, and chronic hepatitis. Some infections at first appear to cause only local problems, such as genital ulcers, warts, or vaginitis. However, even these seemingly limited infections may have far-reaching consequences. For example, certain serotypes of human papilloma virus cause cervical cancer, and recent studies indicate that both ulcerative and nonulcerative sexually transmitted diseases may facilitate HIV transmission and susceptibility (18).

Some general principles apply to sexually transmitted diseases. When a sexually transmitted infection is identified, the patient is encouraged to notify her partner(s) so he/they can be evaluated and treated. Exposed partners are assumed to be infected and are treated empirically, but typically diagnostic testing is performed beforehand to allow definitive diagnosis. This allows for tracking and subsequent notification of their respective partners. It should be noted that syphilis, gonorrhea, and AIDS are reportable diseases in every state, and chlamydia is in most states. Clinicians unfamiliar with reporting requirements should contact their local health department.

Sexual partners of those diagnosed with a sexually transmitted disease are treated presumptively, yet are also tested to allow definitive diagnosis and notification of their respective partners.

Often patients presenting with a sexually transmitted disease harbor a second sexually transmitted disease. Therefore, in addition to obtaining specimens from the cervix, women should also be offered serologic testing for syphilis, HIV, and hepatitis B at an appropriately timed follow-up visit (usually at least 3 to 4 weeks after exposure). Of the patients who are seronegative, many should undergo repeat testing, and unvaccinated persons who are

Adults diagnosed with a sexually transmitted disease have been identified as a target group for the hepatitis B vaccination series. One should first clarify vaccination history and, if negative, verify lack of natural immunity with anti-hepatitis B core antibody testing.

seronegative for hepatitis B core antibody should be offered the hepatitis B vaccine series.

Physicians should seize opportunities to review safe-sex practices. After eliciting the patient's sexual history in a nonjudgmental manner, a prevention message can be specifically tailored to the patient's behaviors, taking care to convey compassion and respect, and using understandable language. Condoms have been shown to prevent most sexually transmitted diseases. Female condoms have not been well studied; however, these are an alternative when the male condom cannot be used. In addition, the CDC recommends both partners be tested for sexually transmitted diseases, including HIV, before initiating intercourse.

Chlamydia trachomatis

Chlamydia trachomatis is an intracellular bacteria causing one of the most common sexually transmitted diseases in the United States, with estimates indicating about 4 million cases annually (Fig. 8-4). Infection is clearly related to sexual activity and to risk factors associated with other sexually transmitted diseases, such as unmarried and lower socioeconomic status, age less than 25, and an increased number of partners. The presence of chlamydia is also linked to gonorrhea transmission, so that an individual diagnosed with gonorrhea should also be empirically treated for chlamydia. The transmission rate is probably only 25% from a single sexual encounter, with an incubation period ranging from a few days to weeks.

Diagnosis
The columnar cells of the urethra and endocervix are the sites of chlamydia infection. This may result in mild vaginal discharge or frank urinary tract infection symptoms. It is therefore important to include chlamydia in the differential diagnosis when patients present with symptoms of vaginitis or dysuria. However, in at least 50% percent of cases, chlamydia infections in women are either asymptomatic or produce symptoms so mild in nature that they remain untreated. Unfortunately, this not only fosters further spread of the epidemic, but also can allow the infection to silently ascend to cause pelvic inflammatory disease. If the infection has already progressed to pelvic inflammatory disease, the patient may still be asymptomatic or report symptoms as fulminant as peritonitis.

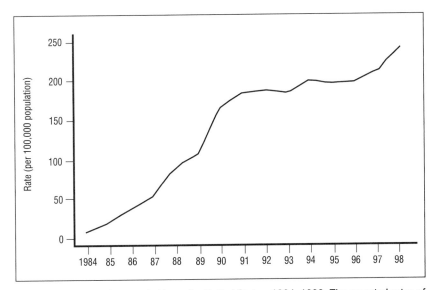

Figure 8-4 Reported rates of chlamydia: United States, 1984–1998. The reported rates of chlamydia denote more than simply the prevalence of infection. The rise also reflects the increase in the number of states designating chlamydia a reportable disease as well as increased detection through greater screening efforts. Screening for chlamydia can reduce the incidence of pelvic inflammatory disease by as much as 60%. (From the Centers for Disease Control and Prevention.)

Examination of patients with uncomplicated chlamydia infections can reveal a completely normal pelvic exam, mere friability of the endocervix (i.e., excessive bleeding with specimen procurement), or at other times a purulent exudate emanating from the cervical os ("mucopurulent cervicitis"). If examination of the infected patient reveals cervical motion tenderness, and/or adnexal or significant uterine tenderness, the infection has ascended to involve the endometrium and/or salpinges. Such a chlamydia infection is no longer considered "uncomplicated" because such findings suggest progression to pelvic inflammatory disease, which requires different evaluation and management (see Pelvic Inflammatory Disease section below and Chapter 9).

Uncomplicated chlamydia cervicitis may be diagnosed at the time of presentation on the basis of history, examination, and wet mount of the cervical discharge revealing greater than 10 PMNs per high power field. However, definitive diagnosis is necessary to enable notification and treatment of partners. Chlamydia DNA probe and culture are currently the most commonly used tests. In either of these two tests, the sample must be carefully collected from the endocervix (or from the urethra in an infected woman who has previously undergone hysterectomy) using special swabs. Chlamydia testing by DNA-amplification of urine specimens is now also available. Although more expensive than traditional nonculture tests, this testing eliminates the need for pelvic or genital examination and may be particularly well suited for mass screening programs (19).

Treatment

Treatment of uncomplicated chlamydia infection is usually either doxycycline or azithromycin (Table 8-3). The two drugs are equally efficacious, but for nonpregnant patients doxycycline has been used more extensively and is less expensive. Azithromycin is preferred when patient compliance may be an issue because it has the advantage of being administered in a single dose and ideally can be dispensed on-site and administration directly observed. Newer regimens include ofloxacin 300 mg twice daily for 7 days and levofloxacin 500 mg daily for 7 days. The quinolones have the advantage of simultaneously treating uncomplicated gonorrhea infection. Because studies of immature animals demonstrate arthropathy from fluoroquinolone exposure, however, these drugs are avoided in pregnancy, lactation, and in the patient under 18 years, although in the latter host single-dose regimens have been used. Patients should be instructed to promptly notify their partner(s) for evaluation and empiric treatment and should avoid sexual contact until both partners

Table 8-3 Treatment Regimens for Chlamydia and Gonorrhea*

Uncomplicated chlamydia infection	Azithromycin 1 g PO × 1 dose Doxycycline 100 mg PO bid × 7 days *Alternative regimens:* Erythromycin base 500 mg PO qid × 7 days Erythromycin ethylsuccinate 800 mg PO qid × 7 days Ofloxacin 300 mg PO bid × 7 days Levofloxacin 500 mg qid × 7 days
Chlamydia in pregnancy	Erythromycin base 500 mg PO qid × 7 days Amoxicillin 500 mg PO tid × 7 days
Uncomplicated gonorrhea infection	Ceftriaxone 250 mg IM × 1 Ciprofloxacin 500 mg PO × 1 Ofloxacin 400 mg PO × 1 Levofloxacin 250 mg PO × 1 *Plus empiric treatment for chlamydia with:* Azithromycin 1 g PO × 1 *or* Doxycycline 100 mg PO bid × 7 days
Pelvic inflammatory disease (PID)	(See Boxes 9-3 & 9-5 in Chapter 9)

*Tetracyclines and fluoroquinolones are contraindicated for pregnant and lactating women; erythromycin estolate is contraindicated in pregnancy.
Adapted from Centers for Disease Control and Prevention. 2002 Guidelines for treatment of sexually transmitted diseases. MMWR. In press.

have completed treatment. In the case of a single-dose regimen, they should abstain for 1 week after treatment. Treatment of pelvic inflammatory disease differs from that for uncomplicated cervicitis and is discussed below.

Follow-up visits for test-of-cure are no longer recommended for compliant and asymptomatic patients with uncomplicated infections because the aforementioned antimicrobial agents are highly effective. Current strategy calls instead for scheduling a follow-up appointment several months later to screen for re-acquisition of infection. A possible exception is when erythromycin is used, because a test-of-cure might be considered three weeks following completion of therapy (23). However, in all patients diagnosed with chlamydia, a close follow-up visit might be used for serologic testing for other sexually transmitted diseases (e.g., syphilis, HIV, hepatitis B).

Screening

Screening programs play an important role in helping to control the sexually transmitted disease epidemic, particularly because the majority of women with chlamydia infection lack either symptoms or mucopurulent cervicitis. The U.S. Public Health Service recommends annual screening of sexually active adolescents and women under age 25. Other considerations to prompt screening include new sex partner or more than one sex partner during the past 90 days, lack of consistent barrier contraception use, and pregnancy. An analysis of patients attending family planning clinics in Baltimore determined that expanding chlamydia screening to include all women under 30 years of age would miss fewer cases and therefore be more cost-effective (20). This is in part because the average cost of acute care of pelvic inflammatory disease is estimated at $843 (1998 U.S. dollars) (21), which does not include the indirect costs associated with chlamydia infection related to possible subsequent infertility, ectopic pregnancy, and chronic pelvic pain. Recent cost analysis of various health practices has determined that screening for chlamydia infection by any criterion is one of the few health care interventions that yield a net savings to society, even when only direct costs are considered (22).

Neisseria gonorrhoeae

Neisseria gonorrhoeae is a gram-negative diplococci that remains a common cause of sexually transmitted disease in the United States, with teenagers claiming a disproportionate number of cases. The prevalence of gonorrhea varies according to the patient population, ranging from less than 1% in private practices to 25% in sexually transmitted disease clinics. Gonorrhea is usually limited to lower genital tract infection such as either asymptomatic cervicitis or mucopurulent cervicitis, but nearly 20% of infections will ascend to the upper genital tract and cause pelvic inflammatory disease.

The organism has an affinity for columnar epithelium and therefore infects the endocervical canal. Concurrent infection of the rectum may occur half of the time, and involvement of the urethra, Skene's, and Bartholin's glands is not uncommon. In addition, it can infect the pharynx (3% to 20% of infected individuals). The transmission rate is dependent on sexual practices but generally is approximately 80% for a single male-to-female exposure and 20% to 35% in female-to-male encounters. The incubation period for gonorrhea is 2 to 10 days.

Diagnosis

Ninety percent of men with gonorrhea develop a urethral discharge, with or without dysuria; however, women are commonly asymptomatic. When women develop symptoms, they may note a vaginal discharge and, if the infection ascends beyond the cervix, may report abdominal pain, abnormal vaginal bleeding, or fever. Laboratory diagnosis requires bacterial culture or DNA probe. When sampling the endocervix, the swab should be placed in the endocervical canal and rotated for 5 to 10 seconds. Less commonly, specimens can be obtained from women who have previously undergone hysterectomy by milking the purulent discharge from the urethra onto a cotton tip applicator. Anal and pharyngeal cultures can be collected when indicated. The enzyme-linked immunosorbent assay (ELISA) detects bacterial antigen from swab specimens and is now in common use. When culture is used instead, the sample needs to be immediately applied to the agar (that is then covered with a CO_2 tablet if available) and kept at room temperature because *Neisseria* is very susceptible to cold.

Treatment

Uncomplicated gonorrhea is easily treated with ceftriaxone 125 mg IM, given as a single dose. Alternatively, oral regimens using one-time doses of fluoroquinolones are options (see Table 8-3). However, because of the prevalence of resistant organisms, quinolones should not be used for infections acquired in Asia or the Pacific, including Hawaii. Patients diagnosed with gonorrhea should receive empiric treatment for chlamydia (usually either azithromycin or doxycycline) as well because chlamydia is a common co-infection (23). Patients should also undergo serologic screening for other sexually transmitted pathogens, such as syphilis, HIV, and hepatitis B. The patient should be made aware of the importance of encouraging her partner(s) to be tested and empirically treated, even if they remain asymptomatic. A test-of-cure can be performed 2 weeks after treatment; however, as with the case of chlamydia, some authorities have argued to delay re-testing for several months and screen for reacquisition instead.

Disseminated Gonococcal Infection

Disseminated gonococcal infection is a rare but serious complication of gonorrheal infection, occurring in only 1% of cases. Patients present with fever, petechial or pustular acral skin lesions, asymmetric arthralgias, and tenosynovitis or septic arthritis. Both gonoccocal meningitis and endocarditis must be excluded and, if present, warrant expert consultation. The diagnosis of disseminated gonoccal infection relies on blood cultures as well as gram stain and culture obtained from the affected areas by swab or aspiration. Treatment includes initial hospitalization and parenteral ceftriaxone until 24 to 48 hr after symptoms resolve, followed by oral cefixime, ciprofloxacin, or ofloxacin to complete a week of therapy. As with other gonococcal infections, empiric treatment for chlamydia and of sexual partners is indicated. Vertical transmission of gonorrhea can also occur via delivery through a colonized birth canal, resulting in conjunctivitis and ophthalmitis in the offspring.

Pelvic Inflammatory Disease

Pelvic inflammatory disease is an infectious process that results from the ascent of organisms through the cervix to the upper reproductive tract. This entity may include endometritis, salpingitis, and tubo-ovarian abscess, as well as peritonitis and perihepatitis (Fitz-Hugh–Curtis syndrome).

Pelvic inflammatory disease is usually initiated by sexually transmitted infection of the lower tract with *Neisseria gonorrhea* or chlamydia, or both. When these organisms ascend to infect the upper genital tract, they disturb host defenses and alter the environment such that aerobic and anaerobic bacteria endogenous to the lower genital and gastrointestinal tract (e.g., *Bacteroides, Prevotella*, anaerobic streptococci) can then flourish. Thus antibiotic coverage must be broad in order to treat this polymicrobial infection. In addition, the course of antibiotic therapy is longer (usually 14 days) than that for uncomplicated cervicitis. (See Chapter 9 for further discussion and specific regimens.)

Pelvic inflammatory disease is primarily a disease of adolescents and young women. This age group not only has the highest incidence of sexually transmitted diseases but also is at greater risk for ascension of infection after cervical colonization by chlamydia. Two proposed explanations include the larger zone of cervical ectopy in this age group, and the relative lack of antibody protection against chlamydia. Other risk factors for pelvic inflammatory disease include those that predispose a patient to sexually transmitted disease exposure, such as multiple sexual partners, substance abuse, and living in an area with a high local prevalence of sexually transmitted diseases.

In addition, frequent vaginal douching appears to predispose to pelvic inflammatory disease, possibly by altering the vaginal flora (24). IUD use is a risk factor, but mainly in the first 4 months after insertion. Recent menses is also a risk for the onset of pelvic inflammatory disease, with proposed explanations being interruption of the cervical mucous barrier or a cyclic decline in systemic immune function (25). Previous pelvic inflammatory disease also predisposes to recurrent episodes, possibly because of microscopic tubal damage that may facilitate repeat infection, but often because of reinfection caused by failure to treat sexual partner(s) for chlamydia and gonorrhea at the time of diagnosis. Episodes of pelvic inflammatory disease that are unrelated to sexually transmitted diseases are typically iatrogenic and follow gynecologic procedures that break the cervical mucous barrier, such as endometrial biopsy, induced abortion and other curettage procedures, IUD insertion, and hysteroscopy.

Barrier contraception can protect against sexually transmitted diseases and pelvic inflammatory disease. Although oral contraceptive pills may be associated with a slightly increased risk of sexually transmitted disease infection, they appear to decrease the chance of ascension to pelvic inflammatory disease, possibly by thickening the cervical mucous, decreasing uterine or tubal motility, or by shortening the duration of menstrual flow. Women who have previously undergone tubal ligation may develop pelvic inflammatory disease in the proximal stump of the ligated fallopian tube, but this is unusual. In general, pelvic inflammatory disease is rare in women who are amenorrheic, and, because of the cervical mucous plug, it is rare during the second and third trimesters of pregnancy.

The diagnosis of pelvic inflammatory disease is made on clinical grounds; however, it must be recognized that the clinical presentation varies widely, and the use of overly strict criteria results in underdiagnosis and failure to treat. Most patients with pelvic inflammatory disease report lower abdominal pain that at times may be severe, but in some instances the pain may be mild and in others isolated to dyspareunia. "Silent" or painless pelvic inflammatory disease can also occur. Other symptoms of pelvic inflammatory disease may include intermenstrual spotting, abnormal vaginal discharge, and dysuria.

On examination almost all patients with pelvic inflammatory disease are found to have lower abdominal and adnexal tenderness as well as cervical motion tenderness. These findings are very helpful in distinguishing pelvic inflammatory disease from uncomplicated cervicitis. However, although the presence of these findings is fairly reliable, it must be noted that they may also signify another pelvic process (see Chapter 9). Some patients with pelvic inflammatory disease have a palpable tubo-ovarian abscess. Some but not all patients have a purulent discharge either in the vagina or on the cervix. Fever and leukocytosis are inconsistently present, and sometimes even testing of the cervix fails to detect chlamydia or gonorrhea.

Because pelvic inflammatory disease is an extensive polymicrobial infection, the treatment consists of broad-spectrum antibiotics for 14 days. The shorter and more focused drug regimens used to treat uncomplicated cervicitis are inadequate for pelvic inflammatory disease. Established criteria are used to determine whether the patient with pelvic inflammatory disease requires inpatient treatment. (For details of the diagnosis and management of pelvic inflammatory disease, see the section on PID in Chapter 9, pages 253–257.)

The management of pelvic inflammatory disease differs from uncomplicated cervicitis in its expanded antimicrobial coverage, longer course of treatment, more thorough assessment, and closer follow-up.

Sexually Transmitted Diseases That Cause Genital Ulcers

The causes of genital ulcers vary worldwide. In the United States, most are caused by genital herpes or syphilis or, in certain areas, occasionally chancroid (23). Less common causes of genital ulcers include granuloma inguinale (donovanosis) and lymphogranuloma venereum. Because the clinical appearance of these ulcers may vary widely and overlap, laboratory testing for herpes simplex virus (HSV) and syphilis should ideally be performed for all patients presenting with genital ulcers. Even after laboratory testing, however, more than 25% of patients will not have a definitive diagnosis. Thus, unless the lesions are classic for genital herpes, patients are often treated empirically for syphilis (or both syphilis and chancroid in some communities) while awaiting laboratory results (23).

Genital ulcers may be associated with HSV, syphilis, chancroid, granuloma inguinale, and lymphogranuloma venereum. Because the clinical diagnosis of these ulcers is often challenging, it is recommended that the most common etiologies in the United States, HSV and syphilis, both be excluded as the cause of any genital ulcer.

Each of these diseases is associated with an increased likelihood of HIV. HIV testing is recommended for patients diagnosed with syphilis and chancroid, and it should also be considered for those with herpes (23). With the exception of herpes, partners of patients with genital ulcers should be examined, tested when possible, then presumptively treated.

HSV

HSV is a DNA virus that causes oral (usually HSV type 1) and genital (usually HSV type 2) ulcerative lesions. However, the biological differences between the two types are subtle; as many as 30% of genital lesions may be caused by type 1, and type 2 can infect the mouth. Herpes infection of the genital tract is the now the most common cause of genital ulcers in the United States. Its prevalence has increased ten-fold in the past three decades such that nearly 22% of adults demonstrate seropositivity to HSV-2. Transmission to a seronegative person may occur in 70% of sexual encounters with a sympto-matic individual, but it is now understood that even in the absence of an out-break infected patients may transmit HSV, the rate of which is unknown.

The virus invades mucosal surfaces or open skin lesions. It has an affinity for nerve roots, where it remains dormant until activation, causing the char-acteristic recurrent lesions of the genital skin or mucosa. The incubation pe-riod from exposure to symptoms is typically 3 to 7 days but may be as long as 3 weeks. The classic presentation of primary genital herpes infection is a clus-ter of painful vesicles on an erythematous base, accompanied by systemic symptoms of low-grade fever and malaise. The vesicles then crust over and clear in 10 to 14 days. Symptoms may be milder if the patient is seropositive to the other viral type. Also, it should be noted that women may sometimes develop genital herpes on the buttock or thigh.

The diagnosis is usually made at the time of presentation by recognition of the painful vesicular lesions and supportive history. However, it should be noted that approximately one-third of patients with clinically symptomatic HSV infection will have a less classic presentation, with findings such as fis-sures, cervicitis, or dysuria (26).

Diagnosis

Laboratory testing should be performed on all suspected cases to confirm the diagnosis. Swab specimens from a de-roofed vesicle can be sent for either vi-ral culture or HSV antigen testing. Although viral culture may require 5 days, it has the advantage of allowing for typing of the isolate as HSV-1 or HSV-2. The Tzank prep is a stained cytologic smear that is examined for the presence of multinucleated giant cells but is too insensitive to be helpful. If needed, fol-low-up studies may include recently developed serologic assays that can now distinguish between HSV-1 and HSV-2. As stated earlier, testing for syphilis should also be routinely performed.

Treatment

Antiviral therapy is recommended for all patients with clinical evidence of pri-mary genital herpes infection (Table 8-4). Although such treatment does not

Table 8-4 Treatment Regimens for Sexually Transmitted Diseases Causing Genital Ulcers*

Syphilis

Less than 1 yr	Benzathine penicillin 2.4 million U IM × 1 *For penicillin-allergic patients:* Tetracycline 500 mg PO qid × 2 wk Doxycycline 100 mg PO bid × 2 wk
Greater than 1 yr or of unknown duration	Benzathine penicillin 2.4 million U IM q wk × 3 wk *For penicillin-allergic patients (minimal evidence to support these regimens):* Tetracycline 500 mg PO qid × 4 wk Doxycycline 100 mg PO bid × 4 wk
Neurosyphilis	Aqueous crystalline penicillin 18–24 million U q day IV × 10–14 days (administered as 3–4 million U IV q 4 h × 10–14 days) *Alternative regimen:* Procaine penicillin 2.4 million U IM q day × 10–14 days with probenecid 500 mg PO qid × 10–14 days
In pregnancy	Treat per stage as above using penicillin only; penicillin-allergic patients require testing and desensitization

Herpes simplex virus

Primary outbreak	Acyclovir 400 mg PO tid 7–10 days or 200 mg PO 5 × daily × 7–10 days Famciclovir 250 mg PO tid × 7–10 days Valacyclovir 1 g PO bid × 7–10 days
Recurrent outbreaks	Acyclovir 400 mg PO tid × 5 days or 800 mg PO bid × 5 days Famciclovir 125 mg PO bid × 5 days Valacyclovir 500 mg PO bid × 3–5 days Valacyclovir 1 g PO q day × 5 days
Suppressive therapy	Acyclovir 200–400 mg PO bid Famciclovir 250 mg PO bid Valacyclovir 500 mg PO q day Valacyclovir 1000 mg PO q day

Chancroid	Azithromycin 1 g PO × 1 Ceftriaxone 250 mg IM × 1 Ciprofloxacin 500 mg PO bid × 3 days Erythromycin base 500 mg PO tid × 7 days
Lymphogranuloma venereum (LGV)	Doxycycline 100 mg PO × 21 days *Alternative regimen:* Erythromycin base 500 mg PO qid × 21 days
Granuloma inguinale	Trimethoprim-sulfamethoxazole-DS 1 bid × ≥21 days Doxycycline 100 mg bid × ≥21 days *Alternative regimens:* Ciprofoxacin 750 mg bid × ≥21 days Erythromycin base 500 mg PO qid × ≥21 days Azithromycin 1 g PO q week × ≥3 wk *(Pregnant and lactating women should be treated with the erythromycin regimen, and the addition of a parenteral aminoglycoside should be strongly considered—which should also be added for HIV-infected persons.)*

*Tetracyclines and fluoroquinolones are contraindicated for pregnant and lactating women; fluoroquinolones are contraindicated for patients under 18 years. Erythromycin estolate is contraindicated in pregnancy.
Adapted from Centers for Disease Control and Prevention. 2002 Guidelines for treatment of sexually transmitted diseases. MMWR. In press.

eradicate the latent virus and has no impact on preventing subsequent recurrences, it can shorten the duration of systemic symptoms, diminish the extent and duration of local symptoms, and limit viral shedding, thereby decreasing the risk of transmission to others. Sometimes supplemental therapy is required in the form of intravenous fluids, potent analgesics, and Foley catheter if spontaneous voiding is painful.

Recurrences of genital herpes are associated with fewer and less painful vesicles that resolve more quickly, and minimal, if any, systemic effects. Often the patient can sense a prodrome of itching, burning, or mild swelling at the site of the outbreaks. Most patients with HSV-2 and some patients with HSV-1 will suffer recurrent episodes. The frequency of recurrent bouts is unpredictable and can vary widely, but it may be as often as monthly. Factors that suppress immune function, such as physical or emotional stress, sleep deprivation, and illness contribute to recurrences.

Recurrent episodes cannot altogether be prevented, but two pharmacologic strategies may help limit the severity and/or number of recurrences: episodic and suppressive therapy. Patients who suffer frequent recurrences (>6 per year) may opt to take daily suppressive therapy. After 2 years, the patient can be offered a trial of discontinuing suppressive therapy because a recent study confirmed that outbreaks decrease in frequency over time (27). The alternative strategy is episodic treatment, whereby the patient starts a 3- to 5-day course of antiviral medication at the first sign of prodromal symptoms in order to shorten the course and severity of lesions. The patient should be instructed to keep a ready supply of medication on hand so treatment can begin promptly. Headache and nausea are commonly reported side effects of acyclovir and valacyclovir. It should be noted that topical acyclovir cream appears to have no therapeutic value.

Counseling is an important component of treating patients with genital herpes, but because palliation of symptoms is the focus for patients presenting with primary infection, this is best accomplished at a scheduled follow-up visit. The diagnosis of an incurable and recurrent sexually transmitted disease is often associated with significant psychosocial distress, and the clinician should take interest in the patient's emotional response. It is important to reassure the patient that she will continue to be able to engage in intimate relationships. One must also educate the patient about the highly variable nature of recurrences, the risk of transmission to sex partners, and the occurrence of subclinical shedding. She should be encouraged to tell potential sex partners of the infection, abstain from intercourse during recurrences, and use condoms at other times. The options of episodic or suppressive therapy can be discussed, and decisions guided by disease severity and frequency and the individual's preference (26). Unless future childbearing is unlikely, she should also be reassured that transmission to neonates during vaginal delivery is rare, but that in the event of pregnancy she should inform her obstetrician of the infection. This allows for careful inspection during labor for evidence of active recurrence (which if present might necessitate cesarean delivery) and/or the option of suppressive therapy during the last month of pregnancy.

Syphilis

Syphilis is a potentially chronic infection with many possible clinical manifestations caused by the spirochete *Treponema pallidum*. The incidence of new cases of syphilis in the United States has waxed and waned for the past five decades, with an abrupt decline after the advent of penicillin and a subsequent resurgence of cases during the past three decades (Fig. 8-5). In the 1970s and 1980s, syphilis was maintained primarily by the gay male population, but today the majority of new infections are associated with heterosexual activity. Two important causes of this shift are the adoption of safer sexual practices in the gay community and the emergence of new, highly promiscuous behavior related to exchanging sex for drugs (28).

Treponema pallidum is a long spiral-shaped bacterium that is spread only by direct contact because it will not survive outside of a moist environment. The bacterium enters the host by passing through breaches in the integument such as small abrasions in mucosal surfaces. The risk of transmission is approximately 30% per sexual act. In addition to sexual transmission, the infection can be acquired by kissing, accidental direct innoculation (usually of medical personnel), transplacentally, during vaginal delivery, and transfusion of fresh (but not stored) blood products. The treponemes multiply at the point of entry and, after an average incubation period of 3 weeks (range 10 to 90 days), produce the chancre of primary syphilis. Subsequent regional lymphadenopathy and bacteremia can then occur

Primary syphilis in the classic form presents as a painless ulcer with firm raised borders that is sometimes tender to palpation. The appearance may vary, however. For instance, occasionally the papule fails to ulcerate, sometimes no skin lesion develops, and at other times multiple ulcers may be present, a fairly common occurrence in HIV-infected patients (29). In females the chancre may be obscured within the vagina or on the cervix and go unnoticed. Other locations associated with sexual activity include oral and anal or rectal ulcers. The chancre usually heals spontaneously in 2 to 8 weeks.

Secondary syphilis is a systemic infection resulting from bacteremic spread of the treponemes and occurs 1 to 6 months after initial infection. Outward manifestations include lymphadenopathy and a maculopapular rash, typically involving the palms and soles. In moist intertrigonous areas, the rash forms condyloma lata and pustules. As with the case of the primary chancre, *T. pallidum* has been cultured from the rash, so caution must be ex-

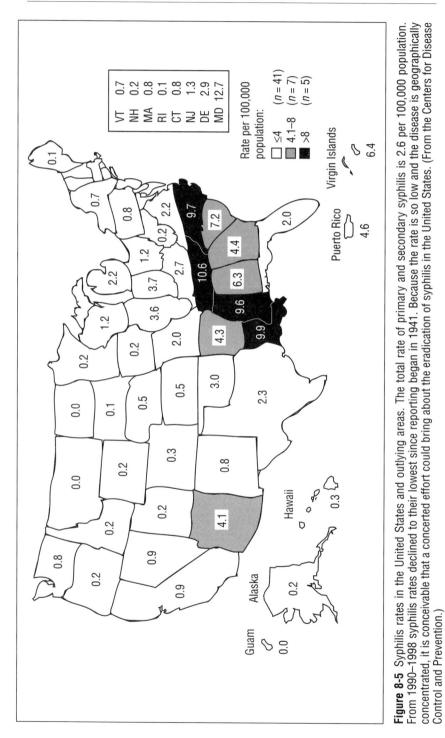

Figure 8-5 Syphilis rates in the United States and outlying areas. The total rate of primary and secondary syphilis is 2.6 per 100,000 population. From 1990–1998 syphilis rates declined to their lowest since reporting began in 1941. Because the rate is so low and the disease is geographically concentrated, it is conceivable that a concerted effort could bring about the eradication of syphilis in the United States. (From the Centers for Disease Control and Prevention.)

ercised in examining these patients. Evidence of other organ system involvement may include glomerulonephritis, hepatitis, arthritis, central nervous system symptoms, and fever or malaise.

Latent syphilis is the quiescent period following the spontaneous resolution of the secondary symptoms, divided into early and late latent syphilis, for infection less than or greater than 1 year, respectively. This distinction appears important for treatment considerations and in obstetrics because the risk of a recurrent bacteremia and subsequent transplacental passage of bacteria is greater in the early latent phase. Twenty-five to thirty-five percent of untreated individuals will progress to a tertiary stage represented by cardiovascular or neurologic symptoms, including aneurysms, cardiomyopathy, vasculitis, muscular weakness, tabes dorsalis, and Argyll Robertson pupil. This process may take 5 to 20 years to evolve and is less likely to occur in females.

Diagnosis

The laboratory diagnosis of syphilis differs depending on the stage at presentation. In cases of primary syphilis, scraping from a chancre followed by visualization of *T. pallidum* by dark-field microscopy confirms the diagnosis. Serum screening tests include Venereal Disease Research Laboratory (VDRL) and rapid plasma reagin (RPR) tests, which are nonspecific tests to detect the presence of antibody. These tests are initially used qualitatively for screening purposes, but because of the high incidence of false-positive tests, confirmation with a specific marker is necessary before treatment, using either a fluorescent treponemal antibody (FTA) detection or *Treponema pallidum* particle agglutin assay (TP-PA). The latter specific tests will remain positive after treatment, whereas the screening tests (i.e., RPR) can be measured in titers that decline after treatment (sometimes returning to a negative status), and are often used quantitatively to measure treatment efficacy.

Because all of these tests detect an immune response, they are not 100% reliable in an early primary infection because the chancre may precede an adequate host response. Therefore, in suspicious cases where dark-field microscopy is unavailable or negative and initial serology is negative, repeat serology is indicated in 2 to 3 weeks. Immunocompromised individuals may have a false-negative or delayed antibody response; therefore empiric therapy must often be considered. In secondary and latent syphilis, however, the serologic tests are essentially 100% sensitive. False-positive results of VDRL or RPR results are not uncommon in the elderly, intravenous drug users, recipients of multiple blood transfusions, or in the settings of autoimmune disease, pregnancy, hepatitis, other infections, and recent vaccinations. Subsequent testing with the treponemal tests (TP-PA and FTA-Abs) usually identifies those that are false-positive, but, unfortunately, occasionally the same conditions may affect these tests also.

Lumbar puncture for cerebrospinal fluid (CSF) examination is indicated for any patient diagnosed with syphilis who has central nervous system symptoms. In addition, some authors feel that CSF examination should be performed for those whose syphilis infection is of greater than 1 year's duration and for patients with concomitant HIV or other immunocompromised state.

Treatment

Penicillin is the preferred treatment for syphilis, with tetracycline and doxycycline being alternative therapies (see Table 8-4 for inclusive recommendations). When there is central nervous system involvement, either parenteral procaine or aqueous penicillin is necessary because benzathine penicillin and other antibiotics fail to penetrate the central nervous system. Penicillin is also the only option in the setting of pregnancy because it reliably crosses the placenta and treats the fetus. Therefore, in cases of penicillin allergy, skin testing and, if necessary, in-patient desensitization of the pregnant woman is warranted.

Before treatment, all patients should be forewarned of the possibility of a Jarisch-Herxheimer reaction, which may be treated with aspirin or prevented with prednisone. After treatment the patient should be followed for development of signs or symptoms of syphilis, and a quantitative nontreponemal serologic test (i.e., RPR or VDRL) should be repeated (using the same serologic test and laboratory) at 6, 12, and 24 months to monitor response. Titers that are initially high normally decline at least four-fold (e.g., 1:32 to 1:8) within 12 to 24 months, and those that fail to do so should be evaluated for neurosyphilis and treated if appropriate (23).

Screening and Prevention

Current guidelines recommend screening patients for syphilis at the first prenatal visit, screening patients who present with other sexually transmitted diseases, and screening partners of people with sexually transmitted diseases. All patients diagnosed with syphilis should be tested for HIV infection, and patients who have risk factors for HIV but test negative should be re-tested 3 months later (23). Condoms are successful at limiting the spread of syphilis.

Chancroid

Chancroid is caused by the bacteria *Haemophilus ducreyi*. Worldwide it is an extremely common sexually transmitted disease, and in some areas of the United States it is endemic; nonetheless, it is only rarely diagnosed in women. In this country, chancroid is associated with poor hygiene and low socioeconomic status and is most frequently diagnosed in nonwhite uncircumcised men. Chancroid has been implicated in facilitating the transmission of HIV, and high rates of HIV infection have been noted in patients who present with chancroid. Syphilis and herpes are also common co-infections.

The bacteria invade via small defects in the mucosa of the genital tract and propagate. After an incubation period ranging from 1 to 35 days, one or a few tender papules develop which erode within a few days to form purulent ulcers. The ulcers typically have a ragged edge that is soft and pliable, and tender when squeezed. They are usually painful, unless located in the vagina or on the cervix, and last a couple of weeks. Unilateral or bilateral inguinal lymphadenopathy commonly appears 1 week after onset of the ulcers and classically is very tender. At times large buboes develop, which makes the diagnosis easy; at other times the nodes may be barely palpable and nontender.

Diagnosis

Reliable laboratory testing for chancroid is lacking. Gram stain of a scraping from the ulcer base might reveal the gram negative rods in a "school of fish" pattern, but superinfection with multiple bacteria makes this evaluation difficult. Culture methods are not readily available; immunologic and molecular techniques are currently being investigated. Therefore the diagnosis must be made on clinical grounds and by excluding other causes. The presence of one or more genital ulcers with associated inguinal lymphadenopathy warrants the inclusion of chancroid in the differential diagnosis. Granuloma inguinale and lymphogranuloma venereum can produce similar ulcerative lesions, as can herpes and syphilis, and because herpes and syphilis are by far more common, routine testing for should be conducted (as stated previously). In addition, because of the association of HIV with chancroid, HIV screening is prudent.

Treatment

Treatment for chancroid includes erythromycin, ceftriaxone, azithromycin, or ciprofloxacin (see Table 8-4). Patients should be re-examined 3 to 7 days after initiation of therapy. Lack of resolution at follow-up suggests incorrect diagnosis, co-infection with another sexually transmitted disease, underlying HIV, noncompliance, or a resistant strain. However, large ulcers may require 2 or more weeks to heal. Fluctuant lymphadenopathy may require needle aspiration or incision and drainage. Partners having had contact with patients within 10 days of onset of symptoms should be examined and empirically treated (23).

Lymphogranuloma Venereum

Lymphogranuloma venereum (LGV) is a rare infection in the United States caused by the invasive L serotypes of *Chlamydia trachomatis*. Patients with

LGV may present with systemic symptoms such as malaise and fever, a wide spectrum of destructive anogenital lesions, and painful lymphadenopathy. Usually the self-limited painless ulcer that appears at the innoculation site goes unnoticed and has already resolved by the time of presentation. The inguinal lymphadenopathy may be either unilateral or bilateral, and with time the nodes become matted together and adhere to the overlying skin, which may become discolored. If the femoral nodes are affected as well, the inguinal ligament between the two groups creates the "groove sign", which is pathognomonic for LGV. If allowed to progress, hypertrophic ulceration, fistulas, stricture formation, and elephantiasis of the genitalia may occur.

The most commonly used laboratory test is the serologic antibody titer. Chlamydial complement fixation titers greater than 1:64 are considered diagnostic because, although other chlamydial subgroups will cause positive titers, these are usually lower.

LGV responds to the same medications as other chlamydia infections but requires an extended course of 21 days (see Table 8-4). Fluctuant inguinal nodes should be aspirated. It should be emphasized, though, that incision and drainage of nodes is contraindicated. Sexual contacts within 30 days before onset of symptoms should be examined, tested for urethral or cervical chlamydial infection, and empirically treated (23).

Granuloma Inguinale (Donovanosis)

Granuloma inguinale is a slowly progressive and destructive infection of the genitalia caused by *Calymmatobacterium granulomatis*. It is rare in temperate climates, and the relatively few cases in the United States are limited to the Southeast.

Although nonvenereal spread can probably occur, the infection is usually transmitted with repeated sexual contact. The incubation period ranges from 2 weeks to 3 months, at which point a painless ulcer develops at the site of innoculation. Heaped-up granulomatous tissue may follow and via subcutaneous extension to the inguinal area may form "pseudo-buboes"; however, the absence of true lymphadenopathy is a hallmark of this infection. Untreated, the infection can progress to cause fibrosis and deformity of the genitalia.

Laboratory diagnosis consists of histopathology of tissue crush preparation or biopsy. Wright's or Giemsa's stain is used to identify Donovan bodies (hence the alias "donovanosis"), which are accumulations of bacterial rods in the cytoplasm of macrophages. Again, as in the case of LGV and chancroid, exclusion of the more common ulcerative diseases, herpes and syphilis, is necessary.

Treatment includes doxycycline or trimethoprim-sulfamethoxazole (see Table 8-4 for details and alternative regimens) and should continue until lesions heal, which may require 2 to 5 weeks. Continued follow-up is important because the infection tends to relapse. Partners having contact within 60 days before the onset of symptoms should be examined and treated if they have evidence of disease (23).

Other Sexually Transmitted Diseases

Human Papilloma Virus

Human papilloma virus (HPV) is a double-stranded DNA virus that is rapidly gaining recognition as an extremely common sexually transmitted disease, with new evidence indicating that the virus may be ubiquitous in the sexually active population. HPV is responsible for venereal warts and most cases of squamous and some adenosquamous lower genital tract carcinomas. The virus subtypes have been grouped according to their likelihood to cause condylomata (types 6 and 11), low-grade cytologic changes, or high-grade cytologic changes, with types 16, 18, and 31 linked to cervical cancer. This association is not steadfast, however.

HPV is most frequently transmitted by direct skin-to-skin contact during sexual encounters, but vertical transmission and spread via fomites (i.e., shared sex toys) have also been reported. Most HPV infections resolve spontaneously, but some may persist as latent infections of the squamous cells of the vulva, vagina, and cervix. A very small subset of these persistent infections will manifest as visible condyloma. Another subset of persistent infection will manifest as cellular changes on Pap smear cytology (LGSIL or HGSIL) or progression to cervical cancer. It is now felt that HPV is responsible for over 90% of the cases of squamous cell cancer of the cervix.

Expression of HPV infection is extremely labile and may be affected by the patient's nutritional status, sexual activity, smoking, alcohol or other drug intake, and the status of the immune system. Modification of lifestyle factors may therefore impact profoundly on the infection. Likewise, HPV expression is also facilitated by pregnancy, and subsequent spontaneous resolution is typically seen in the postpartum period.

HPV infection may manifest as genital warts, which can be a variety of colors and assume four different appearances: "cauliflower" warts, keratotic warts, dome-shaped papules, and flat-topped papules.

The warts may assume four different appearances: 1) condyloma acuminata, which are soft and fleshy "cauliflower" warts that are pink-to-gray in color and vary widely in size; 2) dome-shaped papules measuring 1 to 4 mm; 3) flat-topped papules; and 4) keratotic genital warts having a thick horny layer resembling common warts or seborrheic keratoses (30). Most warts are asymptomatic, although some may be pruritic, friable, or, rarely, painful. Lesions often appear first at the posterior fourchette and labia, then may emerge on other parts of the vulva. Less commonly, the vagina may be involved. When the cervix is involved, the warts appear flat and usually can only be seen only after the application of acetic acid or with the aid of a colposcope. Most genital warts are easily diagnosed on clinical grounds; however, when necessary they should be differentiated from the condyloma lata of secondary syphilis. Also, lesions larger than 1 cm, atypical lesions (e.g., those that are pigmented, ulcerated, fixed to underlying structures, or indurated), and lesions that fail to respond to a few months of therapy should be biopsied to exclude other diagnoses such as bowenoid dysplasia and squamous cell carcinoma.

The rationale for removing genital warts differs from that for treating most other sexually transmitted diseases because the purpose of removal is alleviation of physical or emotional distress. Although with treatment some patients can be rendered wart-free, there is no evidence that doing so lowers their infectivity, because HPV infection is likely still present (23). Consequently, recurrences are common. Treatment options for external genital warts include patient-applied and provider-administered therapies (Table 8-5). Patient-applied agents include podofilox (Condylox) and imiquimod (Aldara). Provider administered techniques include fine-scissors excision, curettage, cryotherapy, and electrosurgery, as well as tricholoracetic acid (TCA), bichloroacetic acid (BCA), 5-FU, and podophyllin resin. Laser therapy and intralesional interferon are more complex modalities reserved for refractory cases. Side effects of treatment are common and can lead to chronic vulvodynia or hypoesthesia. Patients should be counseled and monitored closely to ensure that the treatment is not worse than the disease (30).

Table 8-5 Treatment Regimens for External Genital Warts

External genital warts (human papilloma virus)	*Physician-provided regimens:** Surgical removal × 1 or cryotherapy of lesion q 1–2 wk 25%–80% Trichloroacetic acid topically q wk (the only medication safe in pregnancy) 25% Podophyllin in benzoin topically q wk *Patient-applied regimens:* Podofilox 0.5% topically bid × 3 wk (use × 4 days, drug holiday × 3 days) 5-Fluorouracil 5% cream topically 2 × q wk Imiquimod 5% cream topically 3 × wk

*Alternative treatments: intralesional interferon or laser surgery.

The second type of lesion association with HPV infection is abnormalities detected on Pap smear. If the Pap smear reports evidence of HPV but no cytological abnormalities, no treatment is offered. Any abnormal cervical cytology or pathology is managed in standard fashion. Management may change in the future, however, as the various subtypes and their varying degrees of malignant potential are better understood. The presence of external genital warts does not alter the standard recommendations for screening Pap smears (23).

Prevention of HPV presents challenges. Barrier contraceptive methods offer incomplete protection because the virus lives in the vulvar and perianal regions, and total prevention of skin-to-skin contact is probably impossible. Screening is not performed, and asymptomatic partners of affected individuals are not presently evaluated or treated. Studies are underway to evaluate partner "screen and treat" strategies.

Human Immunodeficiency Virus

As of December 1998, as many as 1.5 million individuals living in the United States were infected with the HIV virus. Women and children represent the fastest growing segment of this population. Women of color are particularly affected. Currently 1 in 160 African American women in the United States are infected with HIV (31). Although the virus continues to be highly prevalent in the homosexual population, particularly in urban African American men, behaviors related to substance abuse (needle sharing and trading sex for drugs) are playing increasingly important roles in the epidemic of the United States. In addition to sexual activity and needle sharing, HIV can be spread via vertical transmission, parenteral exposure to blood or blood products (needlestick injuries and transfusions), and very rarely by artificial insemination devoid of sexual activity. The risk of transmission per episode of unprotected receptive vaginal intercourse is 0.1% to 0.2%, whereas that for anal intercourse is higher at 0.1% to 3% (32). The risk of contracting HIV through receptive oral sex is lower but facilitated by oral problems such as bleeding gums. Overall, the risk of transmission is greater with higher viral loads; heterosexual transmission by persons having viral loads less than 1500 copies/mL appears to be rare (33).

After an incubation time of 1 to 6 weeks, approximately one-half of infected individuals report suffering the acute retroviral syndrome (fever, malaise, lymphadenopathy, and skin rash). Later manifestations of HIV disease include such gynecologic findings as an increased incidence of precancerous changes and cervical cancer (which may relate to the patients' sexual exposures rather than immunosuppression by HIV), painful vulvovaginal ulcers, and recurrent vaginal candidiasis in women with AIDS.

Standard serologic testing includes enzyme-linked immunosorbent assay (ELISA), followed by a confirmatory Western blot assay (over 99% sensitive and specific). However, patients presenting with acute retroviral syndrome will be antibody negative, and some individuals will remain seronegative for up to 6 months after infection, in which case detecting the HIV RNA by PCR is helpful. In cases of repeatedly equivocable Western blot testing, PCR testing or blood cultures for HIV are definitive.

Testing requires informed consent in all 50 states and should be offered to all persons whose behavior puts them at risk for the disease, to those who present for evaluation for possible sexually transmitted diseases, or to anyone who requests testing. All pregnant women should be offered HIV testing at the first prenatal visit (23). Women with possible findings of HIV infection should also be offered testing and if persistently negative be considered for testing for HIV-2 virus, which, although still extremely rare in the United States, is prevalent in parts of Africa, France, and Portugal (23). All patients found to be HIV-positive are encouraged to notify their partners themselves, but the physician or health department can assist them with confidential notification when necessary.

The recent decline in the growth rate of the HIV epidemic has been attributed to various interventions, of which widespread education efforts leading to behavior modification appear most important. Pre-test and post-test counseling are important educational components that primary care physicians should provide. In addition, identification and appropriate management of HIV-infected pregnant women has led to dramatic reductions in the rate of vertical transmission, from approximately 21% to 8% (34). HIV-infected women living in the United States should also be advised to not breastfeed. Recognition of the acute retroviral syndrome on clinical grounds may be challenging, but confirmation with RNA testing followed by immediate intervention with two nucleoside reverse transcriptase inhibitors and a protease inhibitor may favorably influence long-term prognosis.

Physicians should also be familiar with HIV post-exposure prophylaxis (PEP) (Box 8-1) (35). Support for this practice is derived from a case-control study of percutaneous exposures endured by health care workers wherein PEP decreased the risk of HIV infection by 79% (36). Studies using macaques also demonstrate that after intravaginal exposure, PEP can limit local propagation of the virus and thereby allow for total eradication by host immune defenses. These studies show that treatment is most effective when started within hours and is not likely to be effective after 24 to 36 hr. The CDC offers no formal recommendations for nonoccupational exposures and notes that the effectiveness of such therapy is unproven and carries some risks. Some authors have also expressed concern that providing PEP may result in a "disinhibition" of sexual behaviors, leading to an increased incidence of new HIV infections. Others have argued that the expense of preventing one HIV infection ($136,500) could be better invested in effective behavioral HIV prevention strategies.

Box 8-1   Post-Exposure Prophylaxis for HIV*

Zidovudine 300 mg PO tid
plus
Lamivudine 150 mg PO bid for 4 wk

- CBC and renal and hepatic studies should be obtained at baseline and again at 2 wk.
- Note that the cost of a 28-day supply of both medications is about $500 and not always covered by insurers.

*This regimen was developed for occupational exposures; the CDC has yet to establish recommendations for nonoccupational HIV exposure. For exposures of greater risk (such as unprotected receptive anal intercourse or needle sharing with an HIV-infected partner having a high viral load), the protease inhibitor indinavir is often added to the regimen. From 1998 Guidelines for treatment of sexually transmitted diseases. MWWR. 1998;47:RR-17.

PEP should be considered on an individual basis for unanticipated sporadic exposures and prescribed only when the probability of HIV infection is high, when therapy can be initiated promptly, and when adherence to the 28-day drug regimen is likely. One might consider offering PEP when the exposure carries an estimated risk of infection of 0.30% or greater. (For further discussion of PEP, see the Sexual Assault section in Chapter 9, pages 263–268.)

Development of highly active antiretroviral treatment (HAART) regimens has resulted in dramatic reductions in opportunistic infections and may also reduce infectiousness. Primary care physicians can access current treatment recommendations from resources such as the CDC (*www.cdc.gov/hiv*); however, because of the complexity of current regimens, most now refer HIV-infected patients to specialists for antiretroviral therapy and comprehensive care. Nonetheless, the primary care physician plays other important roles in slowing the HIV epidemic. Because the presence of other sexually transmitted diseases facilitates acquisition and transmission of HIV, routine screening and treatment of these other infections will reduce the incidence of new HIV infections. Also, identification and treatment of substance abuse (including alcohol) leads to modification of behaviors that are closely tied to the spread of HIV.

Hepatitis B

Hepatitis B is a double-stranded DNA virus that replicates in hepatocytes and is responsible for one of the world's major causes of liver disease. In the United States, approximately one-half of cases are transmitted through sexual contact, with the remainder through contaminated needles, vertical trans-mission, or blood products.

Of those individuals that contract hepatitis, only 20% to 40% will demon-strate clinical manifestations of acute infection (i.e., nausea, emesis, jaundice, fever, malaise, right upper quadrant tenderness). If measured, liver function tests will be elevated. Treatment of the acute infection is limited to supportive therapy with hydration, anti-emetics, and bowel rest. Although most individ-uals suffer only a self-limited infection, 1% to 6% of those infected as adults will develop chronic infection. Such persons remain infectious to others and are at risk for developing hepatocellular carcinoma or cirrhosis. Treatment of chronic infection includes alpha-interferon and antiretroviral agents such as lamivudine, but it is often unsuccessful.

The diagnosis is confirmed with serologic studies. In contrast to many other infections, acute infection with hepatitis B is associated with measur-able antibody production (anti-hepatitis B core antibody) before the develop-ment of clinical symptoms. Sometimes, but not always, hepatitis B surface antigen will also be detectable. The presence of e antigen may indicate in-creased infective potential. The subsequent development of surface antibody usually heralds resolution of the disease and protective immunity.

Because infected neonates fare much worse than adults (up to 90% develop chronic infection) (23), significant effort has been devoted to decreas-ing vertical transmission. Recommendations for pregnant women include early universal screening with repeat testing throughout the pregnancy for high-risk individuals. Infants born to surface antigen positive mothers should promptly receive hepatitis B immunoglobulin and initiate the vaccine series (see Chapter 19). For the past decade, pediatricians have been vaccinating children against this sexually transmitted disease. However, most adults re-main at risk for hepatitis B infection, and those unvaccinated persons who are diagnosed with a sexually transmitted disease and have no evidence of previ-ous infection (i.e., who are hepatitis B core antibody negative) have been identified by the CDC as a target group for the vaccination series (23). Hepati-tis B surface antibody can be used to confirm adequate antibody response to vaccination. Future directions may include liberalized use of the vaccine.

Molluscum Contagiosum

Molluscum contagiosum is a benign sexually transmitted infection that is also transmitted by skin-to-skin contact in children and athletes. The incuba-tion period for this DNA poxvirus is 2 to 3 months. The diagnosis is made upon recognition of multiple small, flesh-colored, and smooth wart-like papules with central depressions located in the genital area. Diagnosis can be aided by squeezing the lesion and extruding caseous material from the umbil-ication. If necessary, one can confirm the diagnosis by crushing a curetted papule between two slides, applying fixative and requesting cytologic examination for intracytoplasmic inclusions.

In the immunocompetent adult host the lesions are usually self-limited and spontaneously resolve in weeks to months. In contrast, patients with HIV infection may suffer increasing size and number of lesions that may recur after treatment. Ablation focuses on cosmetically objectionable or persistent lesions, and one can employ simple curettage, cautery, cryotherapy, or laser excision (37).

Ectoparasites

SCABIES

Although usually not sexually a transmitted infestation in children, scabies are sometimes transmitted by this means in adults. Thus a patient presenting with complaints of pruritus and found to have papules and excoriations in the pelvic girdle area should prompt consideration of this diagnosis.

The itch mite *Sarcoptes scabiei* burrows into the skin and causes severe itching that intensifies at night. The first time a person becomes infected several weeks may be required for sensitization to occur, but with subsequent re-infestation symptoms may develop within 1 day. In addition to the pelvic area, the interdigital web spaces, wrists, ankles, periumbilical skin, buttocks, knees, and elbows are common sites of infection. The diagnosis may be aided by drawing over a suspected burrow with an ink pen followed by removal of excess superficial ink with an alcohol swab, which will leave the burrow highlighted (38).

The treatment of choice for nonpregnant patients is prescription strength permethrin 5% (Elimite), which must be applied as directed and repeated 1 week later, together with simultaneous decontamination of clothing and bedding by washing in hot water or dry cleaning. Patients should trim fingernails and reapply medication to hands after handwashing. Because of retained mite parts, pruritus may persist for up to 2 weeks after successful treatment and can be alleviated with oral antihistamines and soothing lotions containing 0.5% menthol and camphor.

PUBIC LICE

Phthirus pubis, also called "crabs" because of the organism's microscopic appearance, is transmitted by sexual or close body contact and less often through shared bedding or clothing. Lice attach to pubic hair and other body hair of similar diameter and thus may also be found on eyelashes, axillary hair, and coarse truncal hair. The patient typically complains of pruritus and presents with erythematous macules, papules, and excoriations. Examination with a magnifying glass often reveals the 0.5 mm ovoid nits attached to the pubic hair shafts and occasionally a few gray-brown adult lice climbing on the hairs or burrowing into the skin (39). Preferred treatment includes either prescription or over-the-counter strength permethrin and treatment of partners.

Summary

Vaginal symptoms are common in the primary care setting. Those physicians adept at managing vaginitis will earn their patients' favor because such conditions are typically readily diagnosed and successfully reversed within a week's time. Physician familiarity with appropriate treatment of sexually transmitted diseases may have profound implications for the health of not only the patients but their contacts and families as well.

Acknowledgments
The authors wish to acknowledge the critical review and expert input of Kimberly A. Workowski, MD, Chief, Guidelines Unit, Division of STD Prevention, Centers for Disease Control and Prevention.

REFERENCES

1. **Kent HL.** Epidemiology of vaginitis. Am J Obstet Gynecol. 1991;165:1168.
2. **Chantigian PDM.** Vaginitis: a common malady. Prim Care. 1988;15:517.
3. **Hill LV.** Anaerobes and *Gardnerella vaginalis* in non-specific vaginitis. Genitourin Med. 1985;61:114-9.
4. **Carr PL, Felsenstein D, Friedman RH.** Evaluation and management of vaginitis. J Gen Intern Med. 1998;13:335-46.
5. **Mengel MB, Berg AO, Waver CH, et al.** The effectiveness of single-dose metronidazole therapy for patients and their partners with bacterial vaginosis. J Fam Pract. 1989; 28:163-71.
6. **Moi H. Erkkola R, Jerve F et al.** Should male consorts of women with bacterial vaginosis be treated? Genitourin Med. 1989;65:263-8.
7. **Berger BJ, Kolton S, Zenilman JM, et al.** Bacterial vaginosis in lesbians: a sexually transmitted disease. Clin Infect Dis. 1995;21:1402-5.
8. **Burtin P, Taddio A, Ariburnu O, et al.** Safety of metronidazole in pregnancy: a meta-analysis. Am J Obstet Gynecol. 1995;172(2 Pt 1):525-9.
9. **Schwebke JR.** Metronidazole: utilization in the obstetric and gynecologic patient. Sex Transm Dis. 1995;22:370-6.
10. **Piper JM, Mitchel EF, Fay WA.** Prenatal use of metronidazole and birth defects: no association. Obstet Gynecol. 1993;82:348-52.
11. **Taha ET, Hoover DR, Dallabetta GA, et al.** Bacterial vaginosis and disturbances of vaginal flora: association with increased acquisition of HIV. AIDS. 1998;12:1699-1706.
12. **Sobel JD.** Vulvovaginitis. Dermatol Clin. 1992;10:339.

13. **Horowitz BJ.** Vulvovaginitis: Causes and Therapies. National Institute of Health Symposium. Bethesda, Maryland; 4-5 February 1991.

14. **Sobel JD.** Vaginitis. N Engl J Med. 1997;26:1896-1903.

15. **Hilton E, Isenberg HD, Alperstein P, et al.** Ingestion of yogurt containing *Lactobacillus acidophilus* as prophylaxis for candidal vaginitis. Ann Intern Med. 1992;116:353-7.

16. **Nachtigall LE.** Clinical trial of the estrodiol vaginal ring in the U.S. Maturitas. 1995;22(Suppl):S43-7.

17. **Bygdeman M, Swahn ML.** Replens versus dienoestrol cream in the symptomatic treatment of vaginal atrophy in postmenopausal women. Maturitas. 1996;23:259-63.

18. **Fleming DT, Wasserheit JN.** From epidemiological synergy to public health policy and practice: the contribution of other sexually transmitted diseases to sexual transmission of HIV infection. Sex Transm Infect. 1999;75:3-17.

19. **Gaydos CA, Howell MR, Pare B, et al.** *Chlamydia trachomatis* infections in female military recruits. N Engl J Med. 1998;339:739-44.

20. **Howell MR, Quinn TC, Gaydos CA.** Screening for *Chlamydia trachomatis* in asymptomatic women attending family planning clinics: a cost-effectiveness analysis of three strategies. Ann Intern Med. 1998;128:277-84.

21. **Rein DB, Kassler WJ, Irwin KL, Rabiee L.** Direct medical cost of pelvic inflammatory disease and its sequelae: decreasing, but still substantial.Obstet Gynecol. 2000;95:397-402.

22. **Tengs TO, Adams ME, Pliskin JS, et al.** Five hundred life-saving interventions and their cost-effectiveness. Risk Anal. 1995;15:369-90.

23. **Centers for Disease Control and Prevention.** 1998 Guidelines for treatment of sexually transmitted diseases. MMWR. 1998;47(No. RR-1):1-111.

24. **Zhang J, Thomas AG, Leybovich E.** Vaginal douching and adverse health effects: a meta-analysis. Am J Public Health. 1997;87:1207-11.

25. **Korn AP, Hessol NA, Padian NS, et al.** Risk factors for plasma cell endometritis among women with cervical *Neisseria gonorrhoeae*, cervical *Chlamydia trachomatis*, or bacterial vaginosis. Am J Obstet Gynecol. 1998;178:987-90.

26. **Wald A.** New therapies and prevention strategies for genital herpes. Clin Infect Dis. 1999;28(Suppl 1):S4-13.

27. **Benedetti JK, Zeh J, Corey L.** Clinical reactivation of genital herpes simplex virus infection decreases in frequency over time. Ann Intern Med. 1999;131:14-20.

28. **Siegal HA, Carlson RG, Falck R, et al.** High-risk behavior for transmission of syphilis and human immunodeficiency virus among crack cocaine-using women: a case study from the Midwest. Sex Transm Dis. 1992;19;5:266-71.

29. **Tramont EC.** *Treponema pallidum* (syphilis). In: Mandell GL, Bennett JE, Dolin R (eds). Principles and Practice of Infectious Diseases, 4th ed. New York: Churchill Livingstone; 1995.

30. **Beutner KR, Wiley DR, Douglas JM, et al.** Genital warts and their treatment. Clin Infect Dis. 1999(Suppl 1);S37-56.

31. **Centers for Disease Control and Prevention.** CDC Fact Sheet. www.cdc.gov, Aug. 1999.

32. **Mastro TD, de Vincenzi I.** Probabilities of sexual HIV-1 transmission. AIDS. 1996;10 (Suppl A):S75-82.

33. **Quinn TC, Wawer MJ, Sewankambo N, et al.** Viral load and heterosexual transmission of human immundodeficiency virus type 1. N Engl J Med. 2000;342:921-9.

34. **Connor EM, Sperling RS, Gelber R, et al.** Reduction of maternal-infant transmission of human immunodeficiency virus type 1 with zidovudine treatment. Pediatric AIDS Clinical Trials Group Protocol 076 Study Group. N Engl J Med. 1994;331:1173-80.

35. **U.S. Public Health Service.** Updated U.S. Public Health Service Guidelines for the management of occupational exposures to HBV, HCV and HIV and recommendations for postexposure prophylaxis. MMWR. 2001;50(RR-11):1-52.

36. **Cardo DM, Culver DH, Ciesielski CA, et al, and the Needlestick Surveillance Group.** A case-control study of HIV seroconversion in health care workers after percutaneous exposure. N Engl J Med. 1997;337:1485-90.

37. **Neff JM.** Parapoxviruses and molluscum contagiosum and tanapox viruses. In: Mandell GL, Douglas Jr G, Bennett JE (eds). Principles and Practice of Infectious Diseases, 3rd ed. New York: Churchill Livingstone; 1990.

38. **Wilson BB, Weary PE.** Scabies. In: Mandell GL, Bennett JE, Dolin R (eds). Principles and Practice of Infectious Diseases, 4th ed. New York: Churchill Livingstone; 1995.

39. **Wilson BB.** Lice (pediculosis). In: Mandell GL, Bennett JE, Dolin R (eds). Principles and Practice of Infectious Diseases, 4th ed. New York: Churchill Livingstone; 1995.

CHAPTER 9

Gynecologic Emergencies

Dee E. Fenner, MD
Janice Ryden, MD

Gynecologic emergencies can be divided into four groups: emergencies related to pregnancy; emergencies that present as pelvic pain secondary to pathology of the reproductive organs or other pelvic viscera; trauma; and hemorrhage (unrelated to pregnancy or sexual assault). This chapter reviews the approach to patients with common gynecologic emergencies, including essential aspects of the history, important physical findings, and standard use of laboratory and radiologic studies. A solid knowledge of this topic will facilitate the diagnosis and appropriate management or referral of the patient.

When initially evaluating the patient, one must remember that there are many possible causes of pelvic pain and not all are of gynecologic origin. Abnormalities of all organ systems found in the abdomen and pelvis must be considered as potential sources of pain. Appendicitis, diverticulitis, colitis, nephrolithiasis, pyelonephritis, cholecystitis, cholelithiasis, and pancreatitis are often in the differential diagnosis. In addition, neurologic and myofascial causes are sometimes considerations (Boxes 9-1 and 9-2). Notwithstanding the wide range of possibilities, it is often critical to make the correct diagnosis because certain conditions (e.g., ectopic pregnancy, tubo-ovarian abscess) can be life-threatening. Therefore it is important to conduct an efficient but thorough evaluation.

Box 9-1 Gynecologic Sources of Pelvic Pain

- Ectopic pregnancy
- Pelvic inflammatory disease
- Ruptured ovarian cyst
- Ovarian torsion
- Degenerating myoma
- Endometriosis
- Dysmenorrhea
- Sexual abuse/trauma
- Septic or incomplete abortion
- Ovarian tumor
- Hematometria

Box 9-2 Nongynecologic Sources of Pelvic Pain

- Gastroenteritis
- Inflammatory bowel disease
- Bowel obstruction
- Appendicitis
- Irritable bowel syndrome
- Diverticulitis
- Urinary tract infection
- Renal lithiasis
- Interstitial cystitis
- Myofascial pain

Acute Pelvic Pain and Abnormal Vaginal Bleeding

Gynecologic emergencies are generally associated with bleeding, infection, or injury to or twisting of a pelvic organ. Consequently, typical symptom complaints are pelvic pain or abnormal vaginal bleeding, with pelvic pain being the most common reason for presentation.

Relatively common gynecologic emergencies that present with acute pelvic pain include ectopic pregnancy (a diagnosis to be excluded in all women of childbearing age), septic abortion, pelvic inflammatory disease (PID), ovarian cyst rupture, and ovarian torsion. Any of these conditions can present with an acute abdomen. Figure 9-1 is a simple flow chart to follow when evaluating a patient with pelvic pain.

Abnormal vaginal bleeding is the second most common presentation of gynecologic emergencies. Bleeding may be considered abnormal based on its timing or its volume. In addition to vaginal bleeding, intra-abdominal hemorrhage may occur, as in the case of ectopic pregnancy or ruptured ovarian cyst. If intraperitoneal bleeding is the etiology or if the patient is hemodynamically unstable from vaginal loss of blood, the treating physician must act quickly to stabilize the patient. Standard bloodwork (including type and crossmatch) should be done as one or two large-bore IV catheters are inserted, and volume depletion corrected, initially with Ringer's lactate solution. The patient should be given supplemental oxygen, placed in Trendelenburg's position and

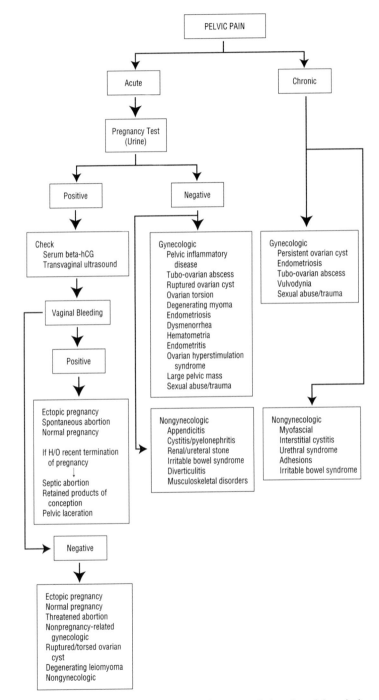

Figure 9-1 Algorithm of common etiologies of acute and chronic pelvic pain based on pregnancy testing.

referred to an emergency room. Urgent gynecologic consultation should be obtained because surgery is often necessary.

As with pelvic pain, abnormal vaginal bleeding requires one to establish pregnancy status. Vaginal bleeding in early pregnancy can result from ectopic pregnancy or septic abortion—two gynecologic emergencies to be excluded—as well as incomplete abortion, threatened abortion, molar pregnancy, and other nonemergent etiologies. A normal pregnancy can also be a nonemergent cause of abnormal vaginal bleeding, beginning approximately one week after conception.

Pelvic pain in a reproductive-age female is an ectopic pregnancy until proven otherwise.

History

A focused but thorough history should be elicited. One should inquire about vaginal bleeding or spotting and abnormal vaginal discharge, itching, or odor. Gynecologic history should include last normal menstrual period, sexual history, contraceptive history, reproductive history, and any history of prior infections. The presence of dysuria, changes in bowel habits, and other symptoms related to nongynecologic abdominal and pelvic etiologies should be queried. Changes in appetite, nausea and vomiting, fevers and chills, medication use, and a brief review of systems should be elicited. Of course, medical and surgical history (including office gynecologic procedures) should also be obtained.

A detailed description of the pelvic pain is important. In the case of ovarian torsion the pain is markedly abrupt in onset, unilateral (often radiating to the anterior and medial thigh), and constant in nature but exacerbated by movement. Ovarian cyst rupture may be spontaneous but is more often seen in the setting of coital trauma. However, overlap in presentation can occur because rupture of ectopic pregnancy may be triggered by the same activity, or by straining at stool, or it may be spontaneous.

Vital Signs

Vital signs in a patient presenting with acute pelvic pain or abnormal vaginal bleeding should always include temperature and orthostatic blood pressure and pulse measurement. Orthostatic vital signs are often the first clue that a young patient who otherwise appears stable has lost significant blood volume.

Physical Examination

When examining a patient with abdominal or pelvic pain, the first goal is to assess whether the patient has peritonitis. The peritoneum may be painfully stimulated by leakage of purulent matter into the peritoneal cavity, by intraperitoneal bleeding or inflammation, or from necrosis of an intra-abdominal structure.

Examination begins with noting the patient's position, because patients with peritonitis are very sensitive to position change and stretching of the peritoneum and often assume the semi-fetal position. Next, one must inspect the abdominal wall for any visible masses, distension, irregularities, suggestion of ascites, and prior incisions. The abdomen is then auscultated for the absence or presence and quality of bowel sounds. One should assess for masses and organomegaly. Guarding and rebound on abdominal palpation are useful in localizing the area of greatest peritoneal irritation. Gentle and superficial palpation of the abdominal wall should also be performed to determine if the pain is originating from the rectus muscles or myofascial sheath. A complete, thorough, but not forceful, pelvic examination must be performed (see Chapter 1).

Vaginal bleeding can originate from the uterus, cervix, or vaginal walls, and careful inspection should identify the source. The cervix should also be inspected for emanating discharge, whether the os is open or closed, and, if open, for retained products of conception. Cultures or appropriate specimens for gonorrhea or chlamydia are typically obtained next, and the walls of the vagina should be carefully inspected as the speculum is removed. The bimanual examination should assess for cervical motion tenderness, uterine or adnexal tenderness, and any abnormal masses. In a patient with pelvic complaints a rectovaginal examination should always be performed, because pelvic masses or other pathology in the cul-de-sac are sometimes only palpable on rectal examination. Hemoccult testing of the stool should be performed when possible.

Laboratory Studies

Laboratory studies for women with pelvic pain or abnormal vaginal bleeding should include a CBC and rapid urine pregnancy test, and for those complaining of acute pelvic pain, a urinalysis as well. Rapid and inexpensive qualitative urine hCG assays should be available in any office or clinic that cares for reproductive-age women, because these assays are essential to the evaluation. All patients of childbearing age presenting with pelvic symptoms or abdominal pain should undergo pregnancy testing, even in situations where pregnancy is unlikely (e.g., reported history of sexual abstinence, prior tubal ligation). If the qualitative pregnancy test is positive, a quantitative beta-hCG should be obtained as soon as possible.

The hematocrit is often helpful, although serial testing is often necessary to detect ongoing bleeding. A white blood cell count is routinely obtained, although leukocytosis rarely directs one to the diagnosis, because it may be present in conditions such as ovarian torsion and ectopic pregnancy, yet sometimes is lacking in infectious processes such as PID.

Radiologic Studies

Ultrasound may be particularly helpful because it can often detect adnexal masses, uterine fibroids, retained products of conception, and free fluid in the peritoneal cavity, and distinguish ectopic from intrauterine pregnancies. Although plain radiography is more commonly available in the primary care setting, it is generally not as useful in the evaluation of gynecologic emergencies. X-rays of the abdomen (performed on nonpregnant women) are helpful in identifying bowel obstructions and renal stones but detect gynecologic pathology in only rare instances such as free air secondary to uterine perforation (following pregnancy termination or other instrumentation) or calcifications in dermoid cysts.

Ectopic Pregnancy

CASE 9-1

Ms Anderson presents to your office complaining of lower abdominal pain for 12 hr. She is 23 years old, gravida 3, para 0, whose last normal menstrual period was 8 weeks ago but who had some spotting yesterday. She reports that she has been sexually active with the same partner for 3 years and is not using any contraception. She has had one induced abortion and two first-trimester spontaneous abortions. Her medical history is significant for one episode of chlamydia 6 years ago; she was treated as an outpatient. She describes the pain as sharp, stabbing, intermittent, and in the right-lower quadrant. The pain is relieved with rest and exacerbated by activity. She had nausea and emesis once yesterday. She denies fever, chills, or change in bowel habits.

An ectopic pregnancy is defined as any gestational implantation outside the uterine cavity. More than 99% of ectopic pregnancies occur in the fallopian tube; other sites include the abdominal cavity, ovary, and cervix. It is important to make this diagnosis, because ectopic pregnancy is the leading cause of maternal death in the first half of pregnancy (1). Also, timely detection and management before rupture may significantly affect the patient's subsequent fertility.

There has been a steady increase in the diagnosis of ectopic pregnancies over the past few decades, such that now in some populations approximately 2% of all clinically recognized pregnancies are ectopic (2). This has been attributed to the greater prevalence of sexually transmitted diseases and the resulting tubal damage, greater utilization of infertility services, increased attempts at tubal ligation reversal, and detection bias secondary to more sensitive tests. The most important risk factor for ectopic pregnancy is prior pelvic inflammatory disease. Prior tubal surgery, prior ectopic pregnancy, infertility, and ovulation-induction medications are also important risk factors. There is some evidence that smoking at the time of conception may contribute to ectopic pregnancy (3). It should be clarified that use of the IUD and tubal ligation do not predispose to ectopic pregnancy; however, should such a patient become pregnant then ectopic is more likely than intrauterine pregnancy. Most importantly, women with ectopic pregnancy do not always have risk factors; in one study nearly 44% of women reported none (4).

The primary mechanism felt to lead to most ectopic pregnancies is impaired motility of the fallopian tube such that the fertilized egg fails to reach the uterine body for implantation. Abnormalities of the egg or the hormonal environment may also affect migration or implantation. An important aspect of an ectopic pregnancy is the tissue's lack of resistance to embryo implantation. The trophoblasts invade the underlying tissue, generally the endosalpinx of the fallopian tube and the blood vessels, leading to bleeding and hematoma formation. As the ectopic pregnancy grows, the bleeding increases and the hematoma expands, causing increases in pressure so that rupture occurs. The pregnancy can either rupture through the serosa of the tube or be expelled through the fimbriated end of the tube. In rare but celebrated cases the pregnancy may survive in the intraperitoneal cavity. Importantly, the ectopic pregnancy can many times involute, or its growth can arrest and the pregnancy resorb without treatment (5). Very rarely and usually in the setting of infertility treatment, one may confront a heterotopic pregnancy (i.e., an ectopic pregnancy in the setting of a simultaneous intrauterine pregnancy), which may pose a diagnostic challenge.

An ectopic pregnancy can mimic almost any pathology that occurs in the pelvis or abdomen. The conditions it most closely resembles are normal pregnancy with ruptured corpus luteal cyst, missed spontaneous abortion, appendicitis, salpingitis, ovarian torsion, renal lithiasis, or a normal pregnancy with another intra-abdominal process. When the diagnosis of ectopic pregnancy is missed it is often because the symptoms have been attributed to a gastrointestinal process and a pregnancy test was not obtained. Pelvic pain in a reproductive-age woman should be considered an ectopic pregnancy until proven otherwise.

History

The patient's history should include her last menstrual period (LMP) and complete gynecologic history, including history of unprotected intercourse, contraception use, and reproductive history. A history of PID, prior ectopic pregnancy, pelvic surgery, or history of infertility—in particular, use of assisted reproductive techniques—should be noted. The patient should be queried for symptoms of pregnancy (such as breast tenderness and nausea), which can be variably present.

The classic triad for ectopic pregnancy is abdominal pain and scanty vaginal bleeding following a period of amenorrhea lasting typically 4 to 12 weeks. However, these three elements are inconsistently present and therefore unreliable. In one study quantifying symptoms, chart review of patients with unruptured ectopic pregnancy found that only 30% reported abdominal or pelvic pain (4). Abnormal bleeding is generally reported in 75% of ectopic pregnancies, and secondary amenorrhea is found in about 68% of cases (6).

If the ectopic has ruptured, a higher proportion of patients will have abdominal pain, usually unilateral, but again this is not universal. Patients with ruptured ectopic pregnancy sometimes report shoulder pain from diaphragmatic irritation by blood. Symptoms of dizziness, urge to defecate, or syncope (one-third of patients) may accompany rupture (6).

Vital Signs

Orthostatic vital sign changes suggest rupture, early shock, and need for immediate surgical intervention. Tachycardia and hypotension signify a surgical emergency. One must also be aware, however, that a relative bradycardia may occur secondary to vagal stimulation by intraperitoneal blood. Most patients with ectopic pregnancy are afebrile, even following rupture.

Physical Examination

As with the history, no single physical finding is diagnostic of an ectopic pregnancy; however, 91% of patients will have abdominal tenderness. In addition to a complete abdominal examination, a thorough pelvic examination should be performed. The latter sometimes reveals bluish discoloration of the cervix (Chadwick's sign) and scant bleeding from the cervical os. Uterine enlargement may occur from hormonal stimulation; therefore this finding does not necessarily signify a normal intrauterine pregnancy. Cervical motion tenderness is sometimes elicited, but adnexal tenderness is more common. An adnexal mass is palpable in only 30% to 50% of cases, depending on the study and examiner (6). Many times a mass in the cul-de-sac can be palpated only on rectal exam. However, in addition to not being a sensitive finding, palpating a mass is also not specific, because the corpus luteum can often be palpated in the setting of a normal intrauterine pregnancy.

Laboratory and Ultrasound Findings

A rapid qualitative urine pregnancy test should be performed. If the patient is found to be pregnant and suspected to possibly have an ectopic pregnancy, she is often best managed by urgent referral to an emergency room or a gynecologist's office (if stable). Quantitative serum beta-hCG (human chorionic gonadotropin) hormone assays and ultrasound can help allow for accurate and early diagnosis of ectopic pregnancy.

A single beta-hCG level does not discriminate normal pregnancy or recent or ongoing miscarriage from an ectopic pregnancy; however, serial measurements obtained two days apart are helpful. In the setting of a normal intrauterine pregnancy, the level of beta-hCG should increase by 1.5- to 2-fold in 48 hr. Failure for the beta-hCG to increase appropriately suggests the possibility of an abnormal pregnancy—either a miscarriage or an ectopic pregnancy. Declining beta-hCG levels suggest miscarriage or a spontaneously absorbing ectopic. The differentiation between an ectopic pregnancy and an abnormal intrauterine pregnancy cannot be made on beta-hCG levels alone but in conjunction with ultrasound findings.

In the setting of a normal intrauterine pregnancy transabdominal ultrasound should visualize contents in the uterus once the beta-hCG exceeds 6000 mIU/mL. Transvaginal ultrasound is capable of detecting an intrauterine pregnancy even earlier, when the beta-hCG is >2500 mIU/mL, or at 4 to 5 weeks gestation (7). When ultrasound fails to demonstrate an intrauterine pregnancy at these beta-hCG levels (and little evidence exists for ongoing or recently completed miscarriage), there is high suspicion for an ectopic pregnancy. Although ultrasound can occasionally detect a mass or embryo in the adnexa, it is primarily by providing information regarding the absence of an intrauterine pregnancy that makes ultrasound so valuable.

In rare instances an ectopic pregnancy may be present despite a negative pregnancy test. In such cases the pregnancy has typically failed, but can nonetheless cause pain and bleeding and may occasionally rupture.

Management

Emergency Treatment
Rupture of an ectopic pregnancy with hemorrhage warrants immediate surgery. Sixteen percent of ectopic pregnancies will present as surgical emergencies from hemorrhagic shock. The patient should be stabilized with intravenous flu-

Sixteen percent of ectopic pregnancies will present as surgical emergencies from hemorrhagic shock.

ids and, if necessary, blood transfusions. Laparotomy or laparoscopy should be performed to control hemorrhage as fast as possible. A salpingectomy is generally performed to rapidly stop the bleeding.

Management of Stable Patients

Until recently all ectopic pregnancies were managed surgically. As medical management options have become more prevalent it is clear that stable patients meeting certain criteria can be managed medically.

MEDICAL MANAGEMENT

Medical management with intramuscular methotrexate is a safe alternative to surgery for stable patients who meet the following criteria:

1. The patient is medically stable and reliable for follow-up.
2. The ectopic pregnancy is unruptured.
3. The ectopic pregnancy is <4 cm by ultrasound.
4. The β-hCG is <10,000 mIU/mL.
5. There is no concomitant intrauterine pregnancy.
6. The patient has normal renal and liver function.

A recent analysis demonstrated that, when used in selected patients, single-dose methotrexate is effective (resolution rate of 87% compared with 91% for fallopian tube-sparing laparoscopic surgery) and can result in a savings of more than $3000 (8). Following methotrexate therapy, the patient is seen at weekly intervals to follow falling beta-hCG levels. If the beta-hCG does not decrease by at least 15% from day 4 to day 7 after methotrexate administration, an additional dose of methotrexate or surgery is indicated (9).

SURGICAL MANAGEMENT

If the patient is stable and the surgeon is skilled, most ectopic pregnancies can be managed through the laparoscope or by mini-laparotomy. Either a salpingectomy (removal of the tube) or salpingostomy (incision in the tube and removal of the ectopic) can be performed. If the ectopic pregnancy has not ruptured, a salpingostomy is preferred to preserve the tube for future fertility if the patient desires. It is important to elicit the patient's plans for future childbearing before taking her to the operating room, because decisions that affect her future fertility must frequently be made intra-operatively.

OBSERVATION-ONLY MANAGEMENT

Although currently uncommon practice in the United States, it is possible to manage stable patients without symptoms with close observation alone, with close monitoring of serial beta-hCG levels. Most ectopic pregnancies can be expected to resolve spontaneously. It should be emphasized, however, that all patients with ectopic pregnancy should be referred for management by a gynecologist.

SUMMARY

Regardless of management, at the time of discharge, the patient should be counseled that she is at significant increased risk (15% to 50%) for a subsequent ectopic pregnancy (10), and that she should see her physician promptly for close monitoring if she becomes pregnant in the future. Contraception options should also be discussed.

Septic Abortion

CASE 9-2

A 22-year-old female presents to the emergency room complaining of severe midline abdominal pain that increases with movement. She reports an elective termination of pregnancy 2 days ago at an outside facility. She has had profuse vaginal bleeding, saturating one pad per hour for the last 6 hr. Pelvic examination reveals an open cervical os with bright red blood emanating vigorously and visible placental tissue. Her uterus is enlarged at 12-week size, soft, and very tender.

Septic (or "infected") abortion can occur following an elective termination of pregnancy or, much less commonly, after a spontaneous abortion (miscarriage). (See Chapter 6 for all other complications of abortion.) Overall, the incidence of septic abortion and related fatalities in the United States has fallen in recent decades, a result of the availability of safe abortion following the legalization of pregnancy termination in the 1970s.

An infected abortion is generally secondary to retained products of conception, or may be secondary to existing cervicitis at the time of termination, or rarely, secondary to nonsterile instruments. Polymicrobial infection may be limited to the pelvis or the patient may present with true sepsis. The differential diagnosis often includes spontaneous, incomplete, or threatened abortion; post-abortion syndrome; ruptured ectopic pregnancy; molar pregnancy; or trauma to the cervix or uterus.

History

The patient will present with abdominal pain, vaginal bleeding, subjective fevers and, sometimes, foul-smelling discharge. On questioning, the patient typically reports being in the first trimester of pregnancy or having recent spontaneous or induced abortion.

Physical Examination

A fever is generally present. A complete examination should be performed, including thorough abdominal and pelvic examination. The cervix must be carefully assessed for products of conception visible in the os and for any lacerations that may be responsible for the bleeding. The os may be open or closed. If the patient has had a recent procedure for elective termination or to complete a spontaneous miscarriage, the os will be open. A threatened abortion rarely becomes infected, but in such instances the os will be closed. Next, cultures of the cervical discharge are taken for aerobic and anaerobic bacteria in addition to *Chlamydia* and gonorrhea.

Bimanual exam is performed to determine the size, consistency, and tenderness of the uterus. Cervical motion tenderness is often present, resembling the presentation of PID. The uterine is usually soft and enlarged, and fundal tenderness is always present. If the uterus is not tender, the diagnosis of septic abortion is questionable.

Laboratory and Radiologic Studies

In addition to the cervical cultures, pregnancy test, CBC, chemistries, and urinalysis should be obtained. The pregnancy test will remain positive for approximately 2 weeks following any spontaneous or elective termination of pregnancy. Leukocytosis is generally present in patients with septic abortion. If the patient appears ill, blood cultures and coagulation tests should also be performed. If the patient is stable, upright abdominal radiography should be performed to exclude the presence of free air under the diaphragm, which would indicate probable uterine perforation and possibly bowel perforation from recent surgical abortion. The finding of gas inside the uterus on x-ray suggests that *Clostridia* may be the causative bacteria, necessitating hysterectomy.

Pelvic ultrasound is generally not useful in this setting, especially if the patient is bleeding—an indication for vacuum aspiration or dilation and curettage. If other diagnoses are being entertained (e.g., tubo-ovarian abscess, appendicitis), an ultrasound may be helpful.

Management

Intravenous antibiotics should be given immediately along with fluids and blood products as indicated. The cornerstone of treatment, however, is uterine evacuation, which is performed promptly, generally within 2 hr after starting antibiotics. Pitocin or intravaginal misoprostol (Cytotec) may also be used to help contract the uterus. Abdominal hysterectomy is generally indicated if there is evidence of infection with *Clostridium perfringens*, or if the sepsis is severe and for some reason the uterus cannot be evacuated via the cervix.

Septic abortion should always be treated with evacuation of the uterus and IV antibiotics.

The patient's vital signs and urine output must be carefully monitored, because septic shock is possible. Antibiotic coverage must be broad and include treatment for gram-negative bacteria and, when the patient is septic, anaerobic organisms, particularly *B. fragilis*, as well.

Pelvic Inflammatory Disease

CASE 9-3

An 18-year-old patient presents to your office with a 2-day history of vague, dull, and constant left lower quadrant pain that she describes as a "pulling sensation", which is exacerbated by walking. She has been sexually active with one partner for the past 2 months and usually uses condoms although not consistently. She denies vaginal discharge, fever, or any previous sexually transmitted diseases. Her LMP began 5 days ago and was slightly heavier than usual but on time.

Pelvic inflammatory disease denotes infection in the upper genital tract (i.e., endometrium, oviducts, ovaries, uterine wall) and may be complicated by extension to the pelvic peritoneum and perihepatic area. PID is usually initiated by a sexually transmitted infection, generally *Chlamydia* or *Neisseria gonorrhoeae* or both; however, the ascending infection quickly becomes

Acute PID is usually initiated by ascending Chlamydia or gonorrhea infection or both. Because the infection quickly becomes polymicrobial, however, its treatment requires a longer course with broader antibiotic coverage compared with acute uncomplicated cervicitis.

polymicrobial, involving normal endogenous aerobic and anaerobic bacteria of the vagina. Less commonly, PID can be a consequence of a recent gynecologic procedure that interrupts the normal cervical mucous barrier (i.e., induced abortion, endometrial biopsy). In these settings latent *Chlamydia* infection or the bacteria associated with bacterial vaginosis are usually responsible. Because of the varying presentations of PID, the differential diagnosis is wide and includes acute appendicitis, ectopic pregnancy, torsion or rupture of an adnexal mass, and endometriosis. Acute PID should be diagnosed with the knowledge that overtreatment is preferable to a missed diagnosis. Table 9-1 lists the diagnostic criteria for PID.

History

Risk factors for PID include multiple sexual partners, recent new sexual partners, intercourse without barrier contraception, history of prior episode of PID, and living in a setting where STD rates are high. A recent invasive gynecologic procedure is another risk factor.

Patients with PID can report pelvic pain symptoms of a wide spectrum of severity, ranging from the classic severe bilateral lower abdominal pain to merely a dull or cramping discom-

Acute PID should be diagnosed with the knowledge that overtreatment is preferable to missed diagnosis.

fort or simply mild dyspareunia. When acute, the pain usually begins shortly after completing menses. Some patients may report a vaginal discharge, abnormal vaginal bleeding or fever. It should be noted, however, that some cases of PID are virtually or completely asymptomatic.

Physical Examination

A documented temperature >101°F (>38.3°C) is supportive of the diagnosis but is often absent. Abdominal examination usually detects bilateral lower abdominal tenderness, and in rare instances detects spread of the inflammation to the perihepatic area (Fitz-Hugh-Curtis syndrome). Findings on pelvic exam may or may not include vaginal discharge emanating from the endo-

Table 9-1   Clinical Criteria for Diagnosis of Pelvic Inflammatory Disease

Criteria	
Abdominal direct tenderness, with or without rebound tenderness Tenderness with motion of cervix and uterus Adnexal tenderness	All 3 necessary for diagnosis*
PLUS	
Gram stain of endocervix (positive for gram-negative, intracellular diplococci) Temperature (> 38°C) Leukocytosis (>10,000) Purulent material (white blood cells present) from peritoneal cavity by culdocentesis or laparoscopy Pelvic abscess or inflammatory complex on bimanual examination or on sonography	One or more necessary for diagnosis

*Note that many cases of PID are mild. The CDC recognizes both the difficulty of diagnosing PID and its potential damage to the reproductive health of women, and therefore recommends empiric treatment of PID be initiated in sexually active women if the first three criteria are present and no other cause for the illness can be identified (12).
From Hager WD, Eschenbach DA, Spence MR, et al. Obstet Gynecol 1983;61:114; with permission.

cervix. Cervical motion tenderness secondary to peritoneal irritation, and uterine and adnexal tenderness upon bimanual examination are usually noted. If a tubo-ovarian abscess is present, an adnexal mass or fullness is often palpable. In severe cases peritoneal signs may be present.

Laboratory and Ultrasound Studies

A CBC is typically obtained to look for leukocytosis, but one should bear in mind that this finding is nevertheless absent in half of all patients with PID, and is a poor predictor of illness severity or need for hospitalization. Cervical cultures (or DNA antigen testing) for gonorrhea and *Chlamydia* should be obtained at the time of the pelvic exam, but again it should be noted that negative studies do not preclude infection by these organisms in the upper reproductive tract. Ultrasound can be helpful to exclude tubo-ovarian abscess in situations where it is suggested on exam, and for patients too uncomfortable to tolerate adequate pelvic exam. Some have recommended ultrasound for all hospitalized patients in order to best guide therapy (11).

Management

Laparoscopy may be indicated if an acute abdomen is present or if the diagnosis is uncertain. Laparoscopy can confirm the diagnosis of PID with such findings as erythema and edema of the oviducts, and exudates on the tubal surface and fimbriae. Sometimes the procedure will identify an alternative diagnosis such as ovarian torsion or appendicitis. Laparoscopy can also allow for operative drainage of tubo-ovarian abscess, which alternatively can be drained percutaneously using ultrasound guidance or, in select situations, be treated with parenteral antibiotics alone with close inpatient monitoring (11).

At present, 80% of patients diagnosed with PID are treated in the outpatient setting (see Box 9-3 for regimens). Note that oupatient treatment regimens for PID are longer than those for uncomplicated cervicitis and include anaerobic coverage. Patients should be seen for follow-up examination within 3 days of initiation of therapy. Those who fail to either defervesce or demonstrate improvement in tenderness are referred for immediate diagnostic testing or surgical intervention or both.

Certain criteria indicate that inpatient treatment of PID is warranted (Box 9-4). Although PID is now rarely fatal, mortality is usually associated with ruptured tubo-ovarian abscess, a true surgical emergency. Therefore patients

---

Box 9-3 Outpatient Regimens for Pelvic Inflammatory Disease

Regimen A
Ofloxacin 400 mg PO bid × 14 days
  plus
Metronidazole 500 mg PO bid × 14 days

Regimen B
Ceftriaxone 250 mg IM*
  plus
Doxycycline 100 mg PO bid × 14 days

*May substitute for ceftriaxone: cefoxitin 2 g IM administered with probenecid 1 g PO in a single dose concurrently.
From Centers for Disease Control and Prevention. 2002 Guidelines for treatment of sexually transmitted diseases. MMWR. In press.

Box 9-4 Criteria for Hospital Admission for Patients with Pelvic Inflammatory Disease

- Tubo-ovarian abscess
- Significant peritoneal signs
- Uncertain diagnosis
- Nausea and vomiting
- Unable to tolerate oral therapy

- Unreliable for oral antibiotics use
    or for follow-up examination in 72 hr
- Pregnant
- Immunosuppression
- Future childbearing concerns

with either tubo-ovarian abscess or significant peritoneal signs are admitted and managed as inpatients. Patients with nausea and vomiting, high fever, or white blood count are usually treated likewise. Other criteria for admission include uncertain diagnosis, pregnancy, and immunosuppression (due to HIV, other illness, or chronic corticosteroid use). In addition, a patient who is unable to tolerate oral therapy or is deemed unlikely to comply with either oral antibiotics or outpatient follow-up is often admitted. Lastly, despite the fact that no comparison trials have been conducted to demonstrate superior long-term fertility outcome with parenteral PID regimens (12), future childbearing concerns sometimes lead to a decision to hospitalize.

Parenteral regimens are listed in Box 9-5. Typically, 24 hr after the hospitalized patient has demonstrated clinical improvement she can be discharged on an oral regimen to complete a 14-day course. However, patients with tubo-ovarian abscess usually complete parenteral antibiotics at home. Note that if an IUD is present it is removed once adequate serum levels of antibiotics are attained.

Box 9-5 CDC Parenteral Pelvic Inflammatory Disease Treatment Recommendations (2002)

Regimen A*
Cefoxitin 2 g IV q 6 hr (or cefotetan 2 g IV q 12 hr)
plus
Doxycycline 100 mg q 12 h[†]

Regimen B
Clindamycin 900 mg IV q 8 hr
plus
Gentamicin 2 mg/kg IV, then 1.5 mg/kg IV q 8 hr

Other Regimens
Ofloxacin 400 mg IV q 12 hr or Levofloxacin 500 mg IV q day *with or without*
   metronidazole 500 mg IV q 8 hr
   or
Ampicillin/Sulbactam 3 g IV q 6 hr *plus* doxycycline 100 mg q 12 hr

*When tubo-ovarian abscess is present, many physicians add clindamycin or metronidazole to extend anaerobic coverage.
[†]Because of the pain associated with intravenous infusion, doxycycline is usually administered orally whenever possible, even in hospitalized patients.
From Centers for Disease Control and Prevention. 2002 Guidelines for treatment of sexually transmitted diseases. MMWR. In press.

Ruptured Ovarian Cyst

A 21-year-old single woman in a monogamous relationship presents to your office with right lower quadrant pelvic pain that began abruptly while having intercourse 2 hr ago. She uses Norplant for contraception and has regular menstrual cycles, the last being 3 weeks ago.

Each month the ovary forms a cyst that ruptures upon ovulation. For most women, there is some slight and brief midcycle discomfort called *mittelschmerz*. Patients rarely present for evaluation or therapy for this phenomenon. However, other, larger ovarian cysts can also rupture that, while usually not life-threatening, can cause significant pain when their contents spill into the peritoneal cavity. Such cysts commonly include hemorrhagic corpus luteal cysts, benign ovarian neoplasms (e.g., dermoids, cystadenomas), and endometriomas.

Most ruptured ovarian cysts will stop bleeding spontaneously, but this should be confirmed by checking orthostatic vital signs and serial hematocrits. If these findings become abnormal or if the patient is anticoagulated, laparoscopic intervention is usually necessary.

History

The patient usually describes a relatively sudden onset of acute abdominal discomfort that may be severe. Rupture may occur at any time in the menstrual cycle, particularly in women with irregular menses. Physiologic cysts can even sometimes occur in women on combined oral contraceptives (especially the lowest dose pills), progestin-only pills, and Norplant. A history of chronic dysmenorrhea, dyspareunia, or infertility may suggest the presence of endometriosis and increase the likelihood of a ruptured endometrioma. An endometrioma is a benign cyst that forms on the ovary and contains dark, old blood that is responsible for the name "chocolate cyst". This fluid can be very irritative to the peritoneum and mimic the signs and symptoms of an acute abdominal process.

Vital Signs

Orthostatic vital signs should be checked. If abnormal, fluid rescusitation should be administered. If the woman continues to have signs of shock, a laparoscopy is indicated.

Physical Examination

Examination of the abdomen sometimes reveals lower quadrant tenderness, typically unilateral, that can range from mild to acute, with guarding and rebound tenderness evident. The vaginal examination is normal; however, cervical motion tenderness is present if there is a significant degree of peritoneal irritation by the ovarian cystic fluid. Adnexal tenderness is generally present, and an adnexal mass is sometimes still palpable following rupture.

Laboratory and Ultrasound Studies

A CBC is typically obtained, which occasionally demonstrates mild leukocytosis if peritoneal irritation is present. If significant ovarian hemorrhage has occurred, anemia or a falling hematocrit will become evident on serial labs. Transabdominal and transvaginal ultrasound studies typically demonstrate free fluid in the cul-de-sac and sometimes a persistent adnexal mass.

Management

If there is no adnexal mass and the patient is stable, the patient may be followed as an outpatient with pain medication as needed. If the diagnosis is uncertain or the pain requires IV medications, then the patient should be admitted to hospital for observation. For any patient who has an acute abdomen on examination, a diagnostic laparoscopy should be considered. Laparoscopy should also be performed if the diagnosis is uncertain or if there is an adnexal mass that could have undergone torsion. If the ovarian cyst is possibly malignant, appropriate consultation with a gynecologic oncologist or general surgeon familiar with ovarian cancer staging should be undertaken.

Ovarian Torsion

CASE 9-5

A 19-year-old college student is participating in dance class. As she jumps into the air, she suddenly feels a sharp pain in her right lower quadrant. The pain persists and she is unable to stand. She is brought to the emergency room by ambulance. Her last menstrual period was 2 weeks ago, and she is not sexually active. CBC and urinalysis are normal.

History

The classic presentation of ovarian torsion is abrupt onset of severe abdominal pain that is constant but exacerbated by movement. The pain may radiate to the flank, which is the embryologic origin of the ovary, or to the anterior and medial thigh. The presence of an ovarian cyst or mass is a risk factor for ovarian torsion, and sometimes this history can be elicited.

Physical Examination

The abdominal exam usually demonstrates unilateral lower quadrant tenderness, which may include guarding and rebound. The vaginal examination is generally normal; however, bimanual exam often reveals a tender, palpable adnexal mass.

Laboratory and Ultrasound Studies

Laboratory testing is usually normal but there may be a mild leukocytosis. Ultrasound reveals a pelvic mass, possibly with reduced Doppler blood flow.

Management

The patient should be taken to the operating room urgently for surgical management, or for diagnostic laparascopy if the diagnosis is unclear. Laparotomy may be indicated depending on the patient's size, prior surgical history, and if there is any concern for malignancy. If the ovary is necrotic, it must be removed. If the ovary appears viable, the pedicle can be "untwisted". An ovarian cyst is likely to be present and should be removed. The ovary may then be sutured to the pelvic sidewall to prevent recurrent torsion.

Toxic Shock Syndrome

CASE 9-6

An 18-year-old women presents to your office with the complaint of abrupt onset of high fever, intense myalgias, diarrhea and vomiting, headache, and sore throat. Her temperature is measured at 104°F (40°C), and she is hypotensive with a blood pressure of 85/50. She appears listless and slow to respond to questions. Her examination is notable for an obvious diffuse blanch-

ing erythroderma. Emergency medical services are contacted to transport the patient to the emergency room; in the meantime IV fluid resuscitation is begun in the office. Further history reveals that her LMP began 2 days ago, and, on questioning, the patient reports the current use of a tampon, which you remove.

Toxic shock syndrome (TSS) is a rare, potentially fatal, multisystem infection that is caused by bacterial exotoxin produced by *Staphylococcus aureus*. Most reported cases of TSS are diagnosed in healthy, young, menstruating females. In the general population 8% to 10% of women have *S. aureus* colonization of the vagina; susceptible hosts appear to be those who also lack antibody protection to the TSST-1 toxin.

Most of the infections are related to tampon use, and the syndrome was most prevalent in the United States in 1980-81 with the introduction of hyperabsorbable tampons, which were consequently removed from the market. Tampons favor bacterial production of the toxin by altering oxygen and carbon dioxide tension and by absorbing magnesium. Cases of TSS have also been associated with diaphragms, vaginal contraceptive sponges, cervical caps, and following episiotomies and cesarean deliveries. Rarely, cases occur in other postoperative wound infections in both men and women, and recent cases have been reported secondary to nasal packing and piercing.

The exotoxin produced by *S. aureus* causes vascular permeability and thus profuse leaking of capillary fluid. Depletion of the intravascular compartment leads to profound loss of vasomotor tone, decreased peripheral resistance, and effects on multiple organ systems. The diagnosis of toxic shock is based on strict criteria established by the CDC (Box 9-6).

History

The TSS patient typically reports sudden onset of myalgias, diarrhea and vomiting, and fevers followed by a diffuse red rash that resembles a sunburn. Sometimes headache, sore throat, and confusion are also present. The patient is usually young (between the ages of 15 and 25), because susceptible hosts usually manifest the disease early. In most cases the woman is in the midst of her menstrual period or has been using a tampon.

Physical Examination

Diffuse blanching erythematous rash and shock are the hallmarks of TSS presentation. Vaginal exam reveals hyperemia and often a discharge. Mucous membrane inflammation can also occur at other sites, namely the conjunc-

Box 9-6 Case Definition of Toxic Shock Syndrome

Fever (temperature 38.9°C [102°F])

Rash characterized by diffuse macular erythroderma

Desquamation occurring 1–2 weeks after onset of illness (in survivors)

Hypotension (systolic blood pressure ≤ 90 mm Hg in adults) or orthostatic syncope

Involvement of three or more of the following organ systems:

Gastrointestinal (vomiting or diarrhea at onset of illness)

Muscular (myalgia or creatine phosphokinase level twice normal)

Mucous membrane (vaginal, oropharyngeal, or conjunctival hyperemia)

Renal (BUN or creatine level ≥ twice normal or ≥ 5 WBC per HPF in absence of urinary tract infection)

Hepatic (total bilirubin, SGOT, or SGPT twice normal level)

Hematologic (platelets ≤ 100,000/mm^3)

Central nervous system (disorientation or alterations in consciousness without focal neurologic signs when fever and hyoptension absent)

Cardiopulmonary (adult respiratory distress syndrome, pulmonary edema, new onset of second- or third-degree heart block, myocarditis)

Negative throat and cerebrospinal fluid cultures (a positive blood culture for *S. aureus* does not exclude a case)

Negative serologic tests for Rocky Mountain spotted fever, leptospirosis, rubeola

From Toxic shock syndrome—United States, 1970–1982. MMWR. 1982; 31:201.

tiva and pharynx. When confusion is present it is unaccompanied by meningeal or focal neurologic signs.

Laboratory Testing

Laboratory abnormalities associated with TSS are listed in Box 9-6.

Management

Acute management typically requires immediate IV fluid resuscitation for shock. Any foreign bodies such as tampons, vaginal sponges, or nose rings should next be removed. Cultures for *S. aureus* should be taken from both the vagina and cervix as well as the blood, then treatment with a beta-lactamase-resistant antistaphylococcal antibiotic begun and continued for 10 to 14 days. Any open wounds should be extensively debrided and irrigated. The patient should be admitted and closely monitored, using the intensive care setting when appropriate.

Mortality is estimated at 2% to 8% of cases. Early recognition of the syndrome is extremely important in the prognosis, because most deaths from TSS are related to missed diagnosis and attribution of symptoms to conditions of less severity, such as gastroenteritis and "the flu". Despite the multiorgan system involvement of the syndrome, if adequate supportive and specific antibiotic therapy is instituted early, full recovery can be expected.

Some women appear to suffer milder cases of TSS and may have regular recurrences, generally on the same day of menses. Usually these are women who were never treated with appropriate antibiotics. Permanent sequelae may result nonetheless and include mild renal insufficiency and neurologic deficits such as memory loss (13).

Once a woman has been diagnosed with TSS she is advised to avoid all use of tampons in the future as well as other intravaginal devices such as the diaphragm. As a general precaution, all menstruating women are advised to change their tampons frequently (at least every 4 to 6 hr) during the day, choose the least absorbent tampon required, and are encouraged to use pads at night.

Sexual Assault

CASE 9-7

A 19-year-old woman presents to your office reporting that she was raped by a new acquaintance just hours earlier. She states she does not plan to press legal charges but desires STD testing and antibiotic prophylaxis.

Sexual assault may be defined as any sexual act performed by one person on another without the person's consent. Legal definitions may vary from state to state, but the term is often defined as nonconsensual genital, anal, or oral penetration by a part of the assailant's body or an object.

In 1994 the U.S. Department of Justice reported the annual incidence of sexual assault as 200 per 100,000 persons, which accounted for 6% of all violent crimes. It has been reported that as many as 44% of women have been victims of actual or attempted sexual assault at some time in their life (14). Sexual assault occurs in all age, racial, and socio-economic groups. The very young, the mentally and physically handicapped, and the very old are at particular risk.

Physician's Role

The physician evaluating the sexual assault victim has a number of responsibilities, both medical and legal. Specific responsibilities may vary depending on the patient's needs and state law. Box 9-7 lists the physician's role in caring for the assault victim. Most states or clinics have developed a sexual assault assessment kit, which outlines the appropriate steps for management and the items needed for medical and forensic purposes. Because of the special legal requirements, rape victims are often best evaluated and treated in settings that are accustomed to doing so rather than in a primary care office. In addition, many clinics and emergency rooms have the advantage of specially trained nurses and rape crisis counselors.

> *The physician evaluating a sexual assault victim has many responsibilities: legal documentation and reporting obligations, immediate medical needs, accurate performance and documentation of history and physical, screening tests and prophylactic treatment, and arranging appropriate counseling and follow-up.*

History

Informed consent should first be obtained, and a chaperone should be present during the entire history and physical. A complete history of the event should be recorded from the patient's own words. It is important to record what acts were performed in detail. *Rape* and *sexual assault* are legal terms that should not be used in medical records. It is the responsibility of the police, not the physician, to obtain a description of the assailant; however, if the patient wants to describe her attacker, the physician should document the description. In addition, a complete gynecologic history should be obtained, including contraceptive use, last menstrual period, and prior history of sexually transmitted diseases.

The history should be written verbatim, and the patient's emotions should be noted. Even if the patient states that she will not press charges, the process of obtaining information and performing the complete history and physical, along with obtaining the evidence, should be completed, because she may later change her mind.

Box 9-7 Physician's Role in Caring for the Victim of Sexual Assault

Medical

Obtain informed consent from patient to conduct history, physical examination, and procurement of samples and specimens

Obtain accurate gynecologic history

Assess and treat physical injuries

Obtain appropriate cultures and treat any existing infections

Provide prophylactic antibiotic therapy and offer immunizations for hepatitis B

Provide emergency contraception

Consider appropriateness of offering HIV postexposure prophylaxis

Offer baseline serologic tests for hepatitis B virus, HIV, and syphilis

Provide counseling

Arrange for follow-up medical care and counseling

Legal

Provide accurate recording of events

Document injuries

Collect samples (pubic hair, fingernail scrapings, vaginal secretions, saliva, blood-stained clothing)

Report to authorities as required

Assure chain of evidence (orderly and unbroken progress of specimens to legal authorities)

Physical Examination

Consent should be obtained before examining a sexual assault victim. The physical examination should begin with careful inspection of the patient's entire body for abrasions, contusions, lacerations, or other signs of trauma. The physician should report findings as "consistent with force" if the examination indicates such, and accurately describe each injury in detail. Diagrams or pictures should be drawn and photographs obtained if possible. Up to 40% of victims who are sexually assaulted will sustain injuries (15). Following assessment the injuries should be treated.

Pelvic examination should carefully note any lacerations or discharge. Specimens for gonorrhea and chlamydia testing are collected from any sites of penetration, and vaginal secretions are sampled for wet mount examination for trichomoniasis and other infections.

In addition, required forensic samples of the patient's pubic hair, nail scrapings, and body fluids are collected (see Box 9-7). Detailed instructions for procurement are described in rape evaluation kits. Also, serologic testing is needed to screen for other sexually transmitted diseases (HIV, hepatitis B, and syphilis) as recommended by the CDC (Box 9-8).

Initial Treatment for Infection and Unwanted Pregnancy

Infections most likely detected following sexual assault are trichomoniasis, gonorrhea, and chlamydia, and screening followed by empiric antibiotic prophylaxis for these three infections are recommended. Patients should be advised to abstain from sexual intercourse for one week to allow completion of

---

Box 9-8 Initial Screening and Treatment for Infection and Unwanted Pregnancy Following Sexual Assault

Screening

Test for *N. gonorrhoeae* and *C. trachomatis* with specimens from any sites of penetration or attempted penetration

Wet mount and culture, if available, or a vaginal swab specimen for *T. vaginalis* infection (and bacterial vaginosis and yeast if malodor or discharge is present)

Collection of serum sample for baseline serologic analysis for HIV, hepatitis B, and syphilis

Pregnancy Prevention

Screen for existing pregnancy first

If negative, prescribe Preven or Plan B as per package directions, or Lo-Ovral, 4 tablets taken immediately and repeated 12 hr later*

Infection Prophylaxis

Initiate hepatitis B virus vaccination series

Empiric recommended antimicrobial therapy (covers chlamydia, gonorrhea, and trichomoniasis plus bacterial vaginosis)

    Ceftriaxone 125 mg IM *plus*

    Metronidazole 2 g orally in a single dose *plus*

    Azithromycin 1 g PO × single dose (alternative: doxycycline 100 mg PO bid × 7 days)

---

*Use of an antiemetic agent before taking the medication will lessen the risk of nausea, a common side effect. For a listing of other oral contraceptive brands and further description of emergency contraception methods, see Chapter 5.

Adapted from Centers for Disease Control and Prevention. 2002 Guidelines for treatment of sexually transmitted diseases. MMWR. In press.

STD treatment. Also, hepatitis B transmission can be effectively prevented with immediate initiation of the vaccine series, and this is recommended for unvaccinated persons.

If the patient is at risk for pregnancy, emergency contraception using Preven, Plan B, or high doses of ordinary contraceptive pills should be provided (after laboratory testing documents absence of existing pregnancy). The risk of pregnancy after a sexual assault is estimated at 2% to 4% in victims who were not protected by some form of contraception at the time of the attack (see Box 9-8 for specific recommended antibiotic prophylaxis and emergency contraception).

The probability of HIV transmission is thought to be low (0.05% to 0.15%) from a single act of unprotected vaginal intercourse, with higher rates (0.8% to 3.2%) for unprotected receptive anal intercourse. Nevertheless, seroconversion has been documented to occur in women as a result of sexual assault.

The CDC notes a lack of data regarding post-exposure prophylaxis (PEP) against HIV following sexual exposure and therefore makes no specific recommendation. However, the effectiveness of PEP in preventing HIV infection has been documented following occupational percutaneous injuries in health care workers (16) and after intravaginal exposure in animal studies (17). Treatment is most effective when started within hours, and most do not recommend initiating therapy more than 72 hr after the exposure (18). If the circumstances of the assault suggest empiric post-exposure prophylaxis against HIV should be offered, discussion with the patient should include the average risk of transmission, the efficacy and side effects of the antiretrovirals, and the need for immediate initiation of, and strict compliance with, therapy for 4 weeks (see Box 9-9 for example of one regimen).

Box 9-9 Postexposure Prophylaxis for HIV*

Zidovudine 300 mg PO tid
   plus
Lamivudine 150 mg PO bid × 4 wk

CBC and renal and hepatic studies should be done at baseline and at 2 wk.

*If the assailant is known to be HIV-positive, a more aggressive regimen may be undertaken upon consultation with an HIV specialist.
Adapted from an occupational exposure regimen from the Centers for Disease Control and Prevention. 1998 Guidelines for treatment of sexually transmitted diseases. MMWR 1998;47:(RR-17). Regimens for sexual PEP are under development.

Psychological Symptoms and Counseling

A woman who is sexually assaulted loses control over her life during the period of the assault. After the assault, a "rape-trauma syndrome" often occurs (18). The *immediate response or acute phase* may last for hours or days. The outward response may range from loss of emotion to complete hysteria. Somatic complaints such as itching, aching, headache, and eating and sleeping disorders may occur. Emotional complaints such as depression, anxiety, and mood swings may also be noted. The next phase, the *delayed or organizational phase*, is characterized by flashbacks, nightmares, and phobias, as well as by gynecologic complaints. This phase may occur months or years after the assault. The rape-trauma syndrome is similar to a grief reaction in some respects. As such, it can only be resolved when the victim has emotionally worked through the trauma and loss.

The physician should discuss the need for counseling and follow-up with the patient. Most emergency rooms and police departments have counselors, both legal and psychological, in place to assist the victims. Names, numbers, and emergency contacts should be provided. The victim may appear calm and in control initially only to become emotionally labile later; thus the protocol should be followed regardless of her current state.

Follow-up

The patient should be seen in follow-up 2 weeks after the assault for repeat evaluation (Box 9-10). If she declined prophylactic antibiotic treatment at the initial visit, screening for chlamydia, gonorrhea, and trichomoniasis should be repeated, because there may have been an inadequate number of organisms present at the initial evaluation for accurate testing. Her psychological condition should also be assessed and counseling should again be offered.

Follow-up is then recommended at 6, 12, and 24 weeks for repeated serologic testing for syphilis and HIV (and hepatitis B if the patient declined the vaccination series). The visits at 6 and 24 weeks are also used for the administration of the second and third hepatitis B vaccinations.

Summary

Gynecologic emergencies often first present for evaluation at the office of the primary care physician. Sometimes the presentation is acute and dramatic; at other times the clinical features may be subtle and the correct diagnosis easily overlooked. Through careful assessment of vital signs, directed but thorough history and examination, and immediate use of office pregnancy testing, gynecologic emergencies can be appropriately identified and referred for treatment.

Box 9-10 Follow-up Care of the Sexual Assault Victim

Follow-up Examination (2 weeks)

Repeat cultures for *N. gonorrhoeae* and *C. trachomatis*, and wet mount (plus culture, if available) for *T. vaginalis* if patient declined prophylactic antibiotics at initial visit

Assess psychological condition

Encourage utilization of counseling (again)

Follow-up Examination (6 weeks)

Repeat serologic testing (if initial test negative) for HIV, hepatitis B, and syphilis

Second hepatitis B vaccination

Follow-up Examinations (12 and 24 weeks)

Repeat serologic testing (if initial tests negative) for HIV and syphilis (and hepatitis B if patient declined vaccination series)

Third hepatitis B vaccination (at 24 weeks)

Adapted from Centers for Disease Control and Prevention. 2002 Guidelines for treatment of sexually transmitted diseases. MMWR. In press.

REFERENCES

1. **Goldner TE, Lawson Hw, Xia Z, Atraxh HK.** Surveillance of ectopic pregnancy: United States, 1970-89. Centers for Disease Control. MMWR. 1993;42(suppl 6):73.

2. **Tay JI, Moore J, Walker JJ.** Ectopic pregnancy. BMJ. 2000;320:916-9.

3. **Saraiya M, Berg CJ, Kendrick JS, et al.** Cigarette smoking as a risk factor for ectopic pregnancy. Am J Obstet Gynecol. 1998;178:493-8.

4. **Stovall TG, Kellerman AL, Ling FW, Buster JE.** Emergency department diagnosis of ectopic pregnancy. Ann Emerg Med. 1990;19:1098-1103.

5. **Atri M, Bret PM, Tulandi T.** Spontaneous resolution of ectopic pregnancy: initial appearance and evolution at transvaginal ultrasound. Radiology. 1993;186:83-6.

6. **Weckstein LN, Boucher AR, Tucker H, et al.** Accurate diagnosis of ectopic pregnancy. Obstet Gynecol. 1985;65:393.

7. **Kadar N, Bohrer M, Kemmann E, Shelden R.** The discriminatory human chorionic gonadotropin zone for endovaginal sonography: a prospective, randomized study. Fertil Steril. 1994;61:1016.

8. **Morlock RJ, Lafata JE, Eisenstein D.** Cost-effectiveness of single-dose methotrexate compared with laparoscopic treatment of ectopic pregnancy. Obstet Gynecol. 2000;95: 407-12.

9. **Lipscomb GH, Bran D, McCord ML, et al.** Analysis of 315 ectopic pregnancies treated with single-dose methotrexate. Am J Obstet Gynecol. 1998;178:1354-8.

10. **Sherman D, Langer R, Sadovsky G, et al.** Improved fertility following ectopic pregnancy. Fertil Steril. 1982;37;497.

11. **McNeeley SG, Hendrix SL, Mazzoni MM, et al.** Medically sound, cost-effective treatment for pelvic inflammatory disease and tubo-ovarian abscess. Am J Obstet Gynecol. 1998;178:1272-8.

12. **Centers for Disease Control and Prevention.** 1998 Guidelines for treatment of sexually transmitted diseases. MMWR. 1998;47 (No. RR-1):80.

13. **Waldvogel FA.** *Staphylococcus aureus* (including toxic shock syndrome. In: Mandell GL, Douglas RG, Bennett JE, eds. Principles and Practice of Infectious Diseases. New York: Churchill Livingstone; 1990.

14. **American Medical Association.** Strategies for Treatment and Prevention of Sexual Assault. Chicago: American Medical Association; 1995.

15. **Marchbanks PA, Lui K-J, Mercy JA.** Risk of injury from resisting rape. Am J Epidemiol. 1990;132:540-9.

16. **Centers for Disease Control and Prevention.** Case-control study of HIV seroconversion in health care workers after percutaneous exposure to HIV-infected blood: France, United Kingdom, and United states, January 1988-August 1994. MMWR. 1995;44:929-33.

17. **Tsai CC, Follis KE, Sabo A, et al.** Prevention of SIV infection in macaques by R-9-2-phosphonylmethoxypropyl adenine. Science. 1995;270:1197-9.

18. **Burgess AW, Holmstom LL.** Rape trauma syndrome. In: Burgess AW, Holmstrom LL, eds. Rape: Victims of Crisis. Bowie, MD: Robert J. Brady; 1974:37-50.

CHAPTER 10

Urinary Incontinence

DELBERT J. KWAN, MD

TAMARA G. BAVENDAM, MD

U rinary incontinence is a common condition in women, one that is associated with significant economic, psychosocial, and physical consequences. One study of community-dwelling women determined the prevalence of urinary incontinence in women over 60 to be 38% (1). Urinary incontinence is a frequently cited reason for relatives placing a family member in long-term care (2); in fact, 50% to 60% of patients in institutionalized settings are incontinent of urine (3,4). However, urinary incontinence is not limited to older women, because one study found that 50% of 4211 healthy, nulliparous women from 18 to 25 years of age reported having experienced involuntary loss of urine with activity, 16% on a daily basis (5).

An estimated 10 billion dollars is spent yearly as a result of urinary incontinence (6). One third of feminine sanitary pads are used for urinary incontinence rather than management of menses (7). The impact on quality of life is less easily quantified, because behavioral changes to minimize urine leakage (e.g., restricting activity and fluid intake, staying near bathrooms) wreak havoc on the affected individual's independence.

Early identification of urinary incontinence can preserve a woman's quality of life and allow for nonsurgical interventions. Unfortunately, however, patients are often reluctant to reveal their incontinence to their physician due to embarrassment or to such mistaken beliefs that it is a normal consequence of aging or that surgery is the only option. Consequently, the physician should take the initiative and include questions about bladder control as part

271

of every complete history. Also, evaluation of the patient's strength and ability to contract the pelvic floor muscles adds only seconds to the routine vaginal exam and can be used to educate women about appropriate preventive exercises before a problem develops.

Diagnosis of any one of the types of urinary incontinence rests upon a careful history and physical examination, urinalysis and simple office testing of bladder function. Some cases may require additional complex testing and referral. Appropriate management can then lead to improvement of the incontinence. It should be noted that many nongenitourinary factors, such as certain medical conditions and medications, can cause or exacerbate urinary incontinence, thereby rendering the well-educated primary care physician the optimal person to initially evaluate and treat incontinent patients.

Anatomy and Physiology of Continence

Urinary continence is the result of normal bladder storage of urine and a competent bladder outlet. Neurologically, this requires coordination between the cerebral cortex, the sensory and motor spinal tracts, and the autonomic and somatic nervous systems. Anatomically, the structure and function of the urethra and the muscular and fascial supports of the bladder neck, proximal urethra, and vagina are critical in providing urinary continence, as is a compliant, normal capacity bladder.

The bladder is composed of three layers of smooth muscle and is innervated by both sympathetic and parasympathetic fibers. Sympathetic stimulation (from segments T10 to L2) promotes urine storage, while stimulation of pelvic parasympathetic fibers (S2 to S4) leads to detrusor muscle contraction, causing bladder emptying.

In the adult female, the urethra is a muscular tube 3 to 4 cm in length. Urethral mucosal coaptation, or "seal", is an important part of the continence mechanism, and normal estrogen levels are important for maintaining the urethral mucosal folds and the vascular network. The muscular components of the outlet mechanism are the internal and external sphincters. The internal urethral sphincter mechanism is composed of involuntary smooth muscle and begins at the vesicourethral junction, while the external urethral sphincter, composed of striated muscle, surrounds the middle third of the urethra and is innervated by the pudendal nerve (S2 to S4).

The pelvic floor muscles (pubococcygeus muscles) are an additional part of the striated muscle component of the continence mechanism. This muscle group, which extends front to back (symphysis pubis to coccyx) and from pelvic sidewall to pelvic sidewall, supports the bladder base, bladder neck, and urethra (Fig. 10-1) (8). The endopelvic fascia is the fascial layer that covers

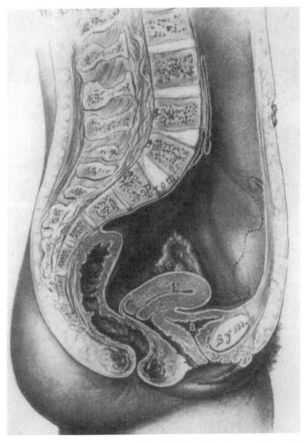

Figure 10-1 Normal relative positions of the bladder (*B*), uterus (*U*), urethra symphysis pubis (*Sym*), and pelvic floor musculature. Note that the bladder normally sits anteriorly and forms an acute angle with the urethra at the vesico-urethral junction. Weakening of the anterior vaginal wall or pelvic floor musculature can lead to prolapse of the bladder or urethral hypermobility and cause stress urinary incontinence. (From DeLancey LOL. Pelvic organ prolapse. In: Scott JR, et al, eds. Danforth's Obstetrics and Gynecology, 7th ed. Philadelphia: Lippincott-Raven; 1997:804; with permission.)

the pubococcygeus muscles and is important in the support and stabilization of the urethra and anterior vaginal wall via its attachment to the pubic bone.

The lower urinary tract has two functions: storage of urine and expulsion of urine. Urinary continence requires a compliant bladder of normal capacity and a competent bladder outlet. When the bladder neck and proximal urethra are well supported in the retropubic position, the angle of the vesico-urethral junction helps contribute to the maintenance of a watertight seal. When bladder capacity is reached, volitional voiding is initiated with relaxation of the external urethral sphincter, followed by a detrusor muscle contraction, which is normally sustained until the bladder is empty.

Incontinence

Definitions

The most common types of incontinence are *stress incontinence, urge incontinence, overflow incontinence,* and *mixed incontinence.* In a study of women 60 years and older, the mixed type of stress and urge incontinence was the most prevalent (55.3%), followed by pure stress incontinence (26.7%), urge incontinence (9.1%), and other forms of incontinence (8.9%) (1). These various types may be distinguished by their differing presentations.

Stress Urinary Incontinence
Stress urinary incontinence is defined as urine leakage secondary to a sudden increase in intra-abdominal pressure secondary to such acts as coughing, laughing, lifting, and sneezing. The increase in intra-abdominal pressure is transmitted to the bladder, raising the intravesical pressure without a concomitant rise in intraurethral pressure. Stress incontinence occurs in the absence of a detrusor contraction and typically involves a small volume of urine.

Urge Incontinence
With urge incontinence, the patient perceives the sudden onset of the sensation to void (the "urge") but is unable suppress it. Leakage of a variable amount of urine results.

Overflow Incontinence
Overflow incontinence occurs when the bladder is already at maximal capacity and the intravesical pressure exceeds bladder outlet pressure.

Mixed Urinary Incontinence
Mixed urinary incontinence occurs when more than one type of incontinence is present in the same patient. The term commonly refers to the combination of stress and urge urinary incontinence.

Other Types of Urinary Incontinence
Less common forms of urinary incontinence include *total* or *continuous incontinence* (the patient is constantly wet, both at rest and during stress maneuvers), *spontaneous* or *"unaware" incontinence* (episodes of urinary leakage that occur without a perceived urge or stress-related activity), *post-*

void dribbling (leakage of small amounts of urine after completion of voiding), and *nocturnal enuresis* (urinary incontinence occurring while the patient is asleep—"bed-wetting").

Pathophysiology

Urinary incontinence occurs any time bladder pressure exceeds bladder outlet resistance and may result from problems with bladder storage, bladder emptying, or the urinary sphincter mechanism (Table 10-1). Importantly, extraurethral and nongenitourinary causes of urinary incontinence may also be responsible for urinary incontinence (Tables 10-1 and 10-2).

Stress Urinary Incontinence

Stress urinary incontinence (SUI) most commonly stems from urethral hypermobility but may arise from other conditions that affect either the function of the sphincteric unit (bladder neck, internal urethral sphincter, and urethra) or the anatomic support of the bladder neck and proximal urethra (see Table 10-1). In normal women, stress maneuvers (coughing, sneezing, heavy lifting) that result in increased intra-abdominal pressure also cause a reflex contraction of the pelvic floor muscles and therefore a simultaneous increase in intra-urethral pressure. Moreover, in a well-supported female ure-

Table 10-1 Urinary Incontinence: Diagnosis and Predisposing Conditions

Diagnosis	Predisposing Condition(s)
Sphincter hypermobility	Pelvic-floor relaxation
Detrusor overactivity	Idiopathic
	Congenital
	Neurogenic
	Bladder outlet obstruction
	Bladder cancer
	Urinary tract infection
	Fibrosis
Sphincter abnormality	Atrophic urethritis/vaginitis
	Idiopathic
	Neurogenic
	Previous urethral, bladder, or pelvic surgery
Impaired detrusor contractility	Neurogenic (e.g., diabetes, multiple sclerosis, spinal cord lesions)
	Previous urethral, bladder, or pelvic surgery
Extra-urethral incontinence	Ectopic ureter
	Urinary-vaginal fistula from trauma (surgical or obstetrical)
Post-void dribbling	Urethral diverticulum
	Vaginal pooling of urine

Table 10-2 Common Nongenitourinary Causes of Incontinence

- *Medications*—diuretics, antipsychotics, anticholinergics, alpha-adrenergic antagonists, calcium-channel blockers, sedatives
- *Endocrine*—hyperglycemia, hypercalcemia
- *Pulmonary*—chronic cough
- *Gastrointestinal*—stool impaction
- *Psychiatric*—psychogenic polydipsia, depression
- *Cognitive*—especially delirium, other confusional states
- *Restricted mobility*—especially by arthritis, weakness, impaired vision, fear of falling
- *Habits/behaviors*—excessive fluid intake or fluid restriction, heavy lifting or straining

thra, the transmission of increased abdominal pressure is to the bladder base and not the bladder neck. In the presence of anterior vaginal wall prolapse, hypermobility of the vesicourethral junction is permitted. Consequently, the bladder neck becomes dependent during stress maneuvers, leading to stress urinary incontinence.

Urge Incontinence

Urge incontinence, which falls under the more general grouping "overactive bladder", is generally related to dysfunction of the bladder, including abnormalities with detrusor function, bladder sensation, bladder capacity, or compliance. Involuntary detrusor contractions are also referred to as *detrusor instability* or *detrusor overactivity*, or, in the setting of a known neurologic abnormality, *detrusor hyperreflexia*. These involuntary detrusor contractions manifest clinically as urgency and, when not successfully inhibited by the woman, as urge incontinence. The cause of the instability may be idiopathic, congenital, or psychosomatic, or may be related to infection, inflammation, or obstruction (see Table 10-1). Interestingly, in women with stress urinary incontinence secondary to urethral hypermobility, detrusor instability may be a concomitant finding 10% to 65% of the time. Stretching of the pelvic nerves may account for this coexistence of stress and urge incontinence (9,10), especially as surgical treatment of urethral hypermobility leads to resolution of the detrusor instability in 80% of patients (11).

Detrusor-related incontinence can also result from reduced bladder capacity secondary to fibrosis. Such fibrosis can be due to surgery, radiation, chemotherapy, inflammation, chronic neuropathy, or infection. As bladder volume increases, the pressure rises due to poor compliance. Consequently, patients must void frequently or risk leaking urine.

Overflow Incontinence

Overflow incontinence in women can be due to a diminished or absent detrusor contraction or, less commonly, to outlet obstruction. Incomplete bladder emptying occurs when the detrusor contraction is insufficient in duration or magnitude or both. The patient may complain of hesitancy, straining to urinate, urinary frequency, sensation of incomplete emptying, and postvoid urinary dribbling, in addition to the symptoms of stress and urge incontinence. A distended bladder may be noted on physical examination. Medications, radical pelvic surgery causing bladder denervation, and neurologic diseases such as diabetes, multiple sclerosis, and spinal cord lesions may result in a weakened detrusor contraction. Fecal impaction is another common cause of overflow incontinence. The mechanism for this is unclear, but it appears not to be related to a simple mechanical obstruction; rather, there is evidence that distension of the rectum alters neural reflexes and inhibits adequate detrusor function. Less commonly, mechanical bladder outlet obstruction may result from urethral kinking in the setting of severe pelvic organ prolapse or from urethral obstruction as an unintended consequence of surgical procedures for incontinence. Primary bladder outlet obstruction is rare in women but can occur at the bladder neck or the urethral meatus (12,13).

Total Urinary Incontinence

Total urinary incontinence is usually caused by a urinary fistula secondary to iatrogenic injury, carcinoma, obstetric trauma, radiation, or inflammatory processes. Vesicovaginal fistulas may be diagnosed by visualizing or palpating a hole in the anterior vaginal wall or vaginal cuff, by observing fluid accumulating in the vagina on pelvic exam, or by infusing methylene blue solution into the bladder with a tampon in the vagina. A voiding cystourethrogram (VCUG) can also facilitate the diagnosis. A ureterovaginal fistula can be diagnosed with the help of a retrograde ureteropyelogram. An undiagnosed ectopic ureter (with an opening in the vagina, distal urethra, or perineum) or type 3 stress urinary incontinence (severe intrinsic urethral deficiency or "stove-pipe" urethra) may also be responsible for total incontinence (14,15). Because ectopic ureters often drain segments of kidneys that do not function well, the volume of the urinary incontinence is not necessarily large.

Spontaneous or "Unaware" Incontinence

Spontaneous or "unaware" incontinence includes nocturnal enuresis. Nocturnal enuresis may be idiopathic or a consequence of either bladder outlet obstruction or neurologic disease. It may also result from detrusor instability, sphincter abnormality, or extra-urethral incontinence and therefore may be associated with other forms of incontinence.

Urethral diverticula are another cause of "unaware" incontinence. They may be congenital or may result from childbirth trauma, infection, or instrumentation of the urogenital tract (16-18). The classic symptoms include the "3 D's": dysuria, dyspareunia, and dribbling (18,19). A history of chronic urinary tract infections along with stress or urge incontinence is commonly elicited.

Physical examination may reveal a tender vaginal mass with urethral discharge or merely some slight fullness to palpation of the anterior vaginal wall.

Nongenitourinary Causes

Nongenitourinary causes of urinary leakage must be considered in the differential diagnosis (see Table 10-2). Depression and delirium can cloud the sensorium and lead to incontinence. The high urine output related to hypercalcemia and hyperglycemia may contribute to incontinence. Excessive water intake must also be considered, particularly for patients taking lithium. As mentioned earlier, stool impaction can lead to urinary retention and predispose to overflow incontinence. In the elderly, restricted mobility that limits timely access to the bathroom often leads to incontinence. Such mobility problems may stem from visual impairment, muscle deconditioning, arthritis, orthostatic hypotension, physical restraints, or a fear of falling (20,21).

Certain pharmacologic agents can also be associated with urinary incontinence (Table 10-3) (20–22). Sedative/hypnotics can increase the risk of confusion and precipitate incontinence. Diuretics increase urinary output and exacerbate urinary frequency and urge incontinence. Alpha-adrenergic antagonists decrease bladder neck closure and urethral pressures. Calcium-chan-

Table 10-3 Medications That Can Cause Urinary Incontinence

Drug Class	Drug Name	Mechanism
Sedatives/hypnotics	Diazepam etc.	Decrease sensorium
Diuretics	Loop diuretics	Increase urine output
	Thiazides	
	Alcohol	
Alpha-adrenergic antagonists	Prazosin	Relax internal sphincter
	Terazosin	(bladder neck mechanism),
	Methyldopa	leading to stress
	Reserpine	incontinence
	Guanethidine	
Calcium-channel blockers	Verapamil etc.	Detrusor relaxation may lead to urinary retention and overflow incontinence
Drugs with anticholinergic effects	Antidepressants (tricyclics)	Detrusor relaxation may lead to urinary retention and overflow incontinence
	Antipsychotics	
	Antihistamines	
	Antispasmodics	
	Antiarrhythmics	
	Opiates	

nel blockers and drugs with anticholinergic effects lead to detrusor relaxation and can precipitate urinary retention and overflow incontinence.

Clinical Evaluation

History

It should be noted that because the patient with urinary incontinence may suffer shame and low self-esteem because of her problem, she may likely be revealing her incontinence for the first time in the clinical setting. It is therefore of utmost importance to conduct the history in a comfortable, informed, and empathic manner.

One should first elicit a description of the circumstances of the incontinence and, in particular, what provokes it. A patient reporting incontinence associated with a strong desire to void typically has urge incontinence. Such a patient may also report the inability to reach the bathroom "in time", needing to urinate frequently, and the sensation of incomplete voiding.

In contrast, the patient with stress incontinence reports leakage of urine when engaging in activity that increases intra-abdominal pressure, such as coughing, sneezing, laughing, and physical exertion such as heavy lifting. The volume of urine is small, and thus the distinction must be made from "pseudo" stress incontinence (a presentation of urge incontinence), in which a large volume of urine is lost from an involuntary bladder contraction stimulated by increases in intra-abdominal pressure.

Symptoms of overflow incontinence may present as stress or urge incontinence, but careful history will also reveal complaints of hesitancy, straining to urinate, the sensation of incomplete emptying, and post-void dribbling.

It is also important to elicit a sexual history, including whether there is any pain, discomfort, or loss of urine with intercourse or climax. In a study of 324 sexually active women, 24% experienced urinary incontinence with intercourse, two thirds with vaginal penetration, and one third with orgasm (23). Loss of urine associated with intercourse is typically secondary to loss of anatomic support, whereas incontinence with orgasm can result from either a triggered detrusor contraction or loss of anatomic support (24).

One should query how often the incontinence occurs, and the type and amount of protection a patient uses. Such information provides only limited insight into the severity of incontinence, however. Further questioning on the patient's self-imposed limitations in fluid intake, and on physical and sexual activities, helps to more fully assess the impact of incontinence on the woman's life. Most patients with urinary incontinence describe an insidious onset of symptoms (Table 10-4). Symptoms of more acute onset (i.e., usually less than 2 months) can suggest a possible infectious or pharmacologic etiology. However, once these easily reversible factors have been excluded, patients

Table 10-4 Urinary Symptoms in the Incontinent Patient

Type of Incontinence	Symptom
Stress incontinence	Urine leakage following sudden increases in intra-abdominal pressure
Urge incontinence	Loss of urine associated with the sudden urge to void
Overflow incontinence	Hesitancy
	Intermittent stream
	Strain to void
	Decreased force of urinary stream
	Sensation of incomplete bladder emptying
	Post-void dribbling
	Urinary frequency

with abrupt onset of incontinence should be evaluated for tumor, stone, foreign body, or neurogenic causes.

The most common medical factors contributing to the development of urinary incontinence in women include advancing age, estrogen deficiency, constipation, obesity, and conditions causing chronic cough. Prior vaginal delivery can also lead to urinary incontinence, because it may cause stretching and compression of pelvic nerves and lead to neuromuscular damage of the pelvic floor (25,26). Stretching of pudendal nerves can also affect the innervation of the bladder neck and proximal urethra (25,26). In addition, childbirth may cause breaks in the endopelvic fascia and detachment of the pubocervical fascia, leading to prolapse and stress incontinence. Because incontinence is often not clinically evident until many years after the childbirth injury, it appears that aging and estrogen deficiency exacerbate existing neuromuscular deficits. Also, superimposed conditions such as constipation, obesity, chronic coughing from smoking or pulmonary disease, and occupations requiring heavy lifting can cause chronic increases in intra-abdominal pressure, aggravate pelvic floor disorders, and stretch already damaged tissues. Even in the absence of childbirth injury, estrogen deficiency (particularly after menopause) can lead to a decrease in urethral pressures and consequently incontinence; thus the patient's estrogen status should always be determined.

Once easily reversible factors (e.g., infections, medications) have been excluded, patients with abrupt onset of incontinence should be evaluated for tumor, stone, foreign body, or neurogenic causes.

A surgical history should be elicited, because prior pelvic surgery or radiation may result in denervation of the pelvic floor, bladder, or urethra. Gynecologic and anti-incontinence surgery with dissection around the bladder and urethra can cause urethral obstruction with urinary dribbling or urethral denervation and subsequent stress urinary incontinence. Repeated urethral dilations or prior internal urethrotomy can lead to urethral scarring and a poorly contractile urethra.

The patient's medical history should also be reviewed, because neurologic disorders resulting from spina bifida, Parkinson's disease, cerebral vascular accidents, and multiple sclerosis can affect bladder and urethral function. Also, visual disturbances, arthritis, neurologic diseases, and other conditions restricting mobility can exacerbate incontinence. The patient's medications should also be carefully evaluated for, as previously mentioned, a number of medications can aggravate incontinence.

When evaluating an incontinent patient, a voiding diary may be of considerable value. A voiding diary records the daily fluid intake, number and amount of voids, and the number of incontinent episodes in a 24-hr period. Incontinent episodes are recorded along with any triggering activity or accompanying sensation of urge. In general, a voiding diary provides insight into the pattern of the incontinence, and occasionally allows the initiation of such conservative therapies as fluid restriction and other behavior modification.

Physical Examination
When evaluating a patient for urinary incontinence, the physical examination should focus on the lower abdomen and pelvis and a brief neurologic assessment of the lower extremities and pelvic reflexes. Palpation of the lower abdomen is performed to determine the presence of a distended bladder. The bulbo-cavernosus reflex is performed by lightly pinching over the clitoris and observing for contraction of the bulbocavernosus muscle (around the introitus), upward movement of the urethral meatus, or contraction of the anal sphincter. Absence of this reflex suggests a neurologic deficit at the S2-S4 levels, although this may be a normal finding in older women (27,28).

The pelvic exam must be carefully performed. The external genitalia are inspected for lesions, discharge, evidence of hypoestrogenism (such as thinning of the perineal skin), and severe pelvic organ prolapse (tissue observed at or protruding through the introitus when the patient is relaxed on the exam table). A urethral caruncle, which is partial prolapse of hyperplastic urethral mucosa, is most typically noted as a red protrusion at the 6 o'clock position, but circumferential prolapse of the urethral mucosa may also occur. The urethral caruncle signifies atrophy and can be a benign source of spotting (29). An atrophic introitus is often very small externally and can limit the use of a vaginal speculum. When significant atrophic changes are observed, gentle introduction of one lubricated finger can first assess the level of discomfort and the width, depth, and angle of the vaginal vault, leading to a gentle, well-tolerated speculum examination.

The speculum is next introduced to expose the cervix (or vaginal cuff when post-hysterectomy). Prolapse of tissue between the blades at rest or with Valsalva maneuver suggests uterine prolapse, enterocele, or prolapse of apical vaginal tissue itself.

It is of utmost importance to next carefully evaluate the pelvic floor support. The Graves speculum is separated into its two blades, and a single blade is introduced and depressed against the posterior vaginal wall so that the "resting" position of the urethra, bladder, and uterus can be assessed. The anterior vaginal wall of nulliparous women is barely visible; it is supported "behind" the pubic symphysis. *Mild relaxation* is present when the bladder base is partially visible high up in the upper half of the vagina; *moderate relaxation* when the bladder base is in the lower half of the vagina; and *severe relaxation* when the bladder is through the introitus. The woman is asked to cough and perform the Valsalva maneuver (i.e., "bear down") to assess the maximum extent of movement of the anterior vaginal wall in response to increased intra-abdominal pressure. When it moves a considerable distance (more than 2 cm) from its resting position, the bladder or urethra or both are considered "hypermobile". With such maneuvers even a well-supported urethra "at rest" can be shown to be hypermobile and associated with stress incontinence. The maximum extent of the movement of the bladder and urethra that is well-supported during provocative maneuvers more closely reproduces the position of the bladder in the standing position. Paradoxically, a severe cystocele at rest may not be associated with stress urinary incontinence. When the bladder base is more dependent than the bladder neck, a rise in intra-abdominal pressure increases the amount of descent of the bladder base and actually acts to protect the vesicourethral junction and prevent incontinence.

Once the anterior vaginal wall has been evaluated, the other blade is lifted against the anterior vaginal wall so that the posterior wall is observed both at rest and with Valsalva to assess for the presence of a rectocele and thinning or inadequate repair of the perineal body after childbirth. At the time of the speculum examination, the vagina is also inspected for signs of hypoestrogenism, such as dryness, lack of rugae, and either pallor or hyperemia of the vaginal mucosa.

After completion of the speculum exam, the anterior vaginal wall tissues are palpated. The urethra should be a "spongy" tube resting in the midline. There should be a palpable "gutter" on either side of the urethra. Fullness, fluctuance, or tenderness in this area suggests the possibility of a urethral diverticulum. The pelvic floor muscles are assessed by circumferentially palpating the levator muscles from the margin of the sacrum to the fibromuscular attachment to the superior margin of the pubic symphysis. Muscles should be supple and nontender throughout.

With one or two of the examiner's gloved fingers in the vagina, the woman is then asked to "tighten" the muscles she "would use to stop the flow of urine" in order to assess the patient's control and strength of her pelvic floor muscles. The ability to isolate the pelvic floor muscles from the gluteal, inner thigh, and lower abdominal muscles is lacking in some women. A woman who cannot voluntarily contract the pelvic floor muscles is a poor candidate for a self-directed program of pelvic muscle exercises and may require a program of formal instruction. Many women can more easily isolate the anal muscle rather than the pelvic floor muscles, and it is sometimes necessary to give the patient several different verbal clues to enable her to successfully isolate the pelvic floor.

During the course of the examination the patient is observed for loss of urine, particularly when she is asked to cough and perform the Valsalva maneuver. Leakage of urine with such activity suggests stress urinary incontinence. These provocative maneuvers can also be repeated in the standing position if the incontinence is not reproduced in the supine position. Leakage that is slightly delayed after a cough suggests "stress-induced" involuntary contractions of the bladder (actually a form of urge incontinence). Loss of urine observed at rest or with minimal increase in intra-abdominal pressure (position change, deep inhalation) is consistent with intrinsic urethral deficiency.

Distinguishing Urinary Incontinence from Vaginal Discharge
Occasionally, vaginal discharge is misinterpreted as urinary leakage, and sometimes distinguishing between the two can be difficult. In such cases, the patient can be instructed to take phenazopyridine hydrochloride (Pyridium) 200 mg orally three times a day; she must wear sanitary napkins because the phenazopyridine stains clothing. If no orange color appears on the sanitary napkins yet wetness occurs, vaginal discharge and not urinary leakage is presumed. However, it must be noted that in addition to urinary incontinence, orange staining may represent vaginal pooling of urine that occurs during the act of urination and then leaks onto the pad at a later time. Vaginal pooling is fairly common in women who are overweight or whose body habitus creates a distance of several centimeters between the external vulva and the urethral meatus. Widely spreading the legs during urination and meticulous post-urination hygiene can help minimize this problem. This phenazopyridine test may also detect a urethral-vaginal fistula, which can be further investigated with the tampon test (as described earlier in the Total Urinary Incontinence section).

Post-Void Residual Volume and Urinalysis

After collection of a voided urine specimen, a post-void residual volume (PVR) can be measured by catheterization, ultrasound determination, or approximated on bimanual examination. A normal post-void residual volume is less than 50 cc, but 50 to 100 cc is considered borderline. A post-void residual volume greater than 100 cc suggests incomplete emptying.

The urine specimen should be examined to help identify conditions that can cause or contribute to urinary incontinence such as tumor, urinary tract infection, or diabetes. Microscopic examination may detect hematuria (> 5 to 8 RBCs/hpf) and pyuria (> 5 to 10 WBCs/hpf). A urine culture should be done to confirm infection in women with pyuria and, if positive, should be treated with 3 to 5 days of appropriate antibiotic. Close follow-up should then be arranged to determine if there was any improvement in the urinary incontinence during or immediately after the antibiotics, because older women especially can experience difficulty remembering whether a specific treatment had any positive impact. When hematuria is present, patients should undergo a hematuria work-up before incontinence is addressed. A hematuria evaluation may include urine cytology, upper tract evaluation (intravenous pyelogram [IVP] or CT scan), and cystoscopy.

Urodynamic Testing

Urodynamics refers to three tests that evaluate urethral and bladder function: cystometry, uroflowmetry, and voiding cystourethrography. The tests may be conducted separately or together. Filling, storage, and emptying phases of lower urinary tract function are studied to examine the activity of the bladder, outlet, and pelvic floor. Information yielded from a urodynamic study is valid only if the clinical symptomatology is reproduced during the study. Referral to a specialist for formal urodynamics testing is recommended in certain clinical situations (Table 10-5).

CYSTOMETRY

Simple cystometry requires no sophisticated equipment and can be performed by trained nursing personnel in a primary care setting. It measures bladder pressure in response to filling and emptying and therefore evaluates bladder sensation, capacity, and compliance. Cystometry is helpful for confirming 1) the diagnosis of urge incontinence when the history and physical are inconclusive and 2) the presence of a sensory neuropathy.

Simple cystometry is performed with the patient either in the lithotomy or standing position. A Foley catheter is inserted and the PVR is measured and discarded. A 60-mL catheter tip syringe (without the plunger) is then connected to the Foley and held above the level of the pubic symphysis to the extent the catheter will allow (approximately 15 cm). Sterile water or saline is

Table 10-5 Indications for Formal Urodynamic Evaluation in the Incontinent Patient

1. Abrupt onset of incontinence (to rule out tumor, stone, foreign body)
2. History of relapsing or recurrent symptomatic urinary tract infections (to exclude a urinary tract abnormality that predisposes to infection)
3. Gross hematuria or microhematuria occurring in the absence of urinary infection (tumor must be excluded by means of cystoscopy, urine cytology, and IVP or CT)
4. Severe hesitancy, straining to begin voiding (may reflect bladder hypersensitivity, bladder outlet obstruction, or decreased detrusor activity)
5. Increased post-void residual (>100 mL) (to rule out bladder outlet obstruction or decreased detrusor activity)
6. Difficulty catheterizing with a 14-Fr catheter (may reflect anatomic blockage of bladder neck or urethra)
7. History of neurologic disease, injury, or related surgery (to evaluate neurologic function)
8. Complicated incontinence: spontaneous or continuous incontinence, new onset enuresis, mixed urge and stress incontinence (for formal evaluation)
9. Recent lower urinary tract or pelvic surgery/irradiation (to rule out structural or functional abnormality related to the procedure)
10. Previous anti-incontinence surgery (to evaluate for complications)
11. Stress incontinence that has not responded to conservative treatment (patient may be suitable candidate for bladder neck suspension or periurethral injection)

poured through the open end of the syringe in measured increments (usually 50 cc initially, then 25 cc). The patient is instructed to report her first sensation of bladder filling, normal urge to void, and strong urge to void, and the total volumes at which these events occur are noted.

The fluid meniscus in the syringe represents the relative intravesical pressure; therefore an increase in intravesical pressure is detected as a rise in the level of the fluid meniscus. The presence of involuntary detrusor contractions and any associated leakage of "urine" from the syringe can therefore be noted as can the total volume at which this occurred. Confounding factors such as abdominal straining, rapid rate of bladder filling, and performing the test in the least provocative position can lead to misinterpretation. Also, it should be noted that when surgery is considered, formal testing is required to provide specific anatomic and functional information.

Single-channel cystometry provides similar information as simple cystometry but uses electronic equipment.

UROFLOWMETRY

Uroflowmetry measures urinary flow rate and reflects the coordinated actions of the bladder, bladder neck opening, and urethra. The normal urinary flow rate is >25 mL/s for women under 50 and >18 mL/s for women 50 and older.

An abnormally low rate raises suspicion for bladder outlet obstruction or a poorly contractile bladder. A normal rate does not exclude obstruction, however, because a sufficiently strong detrusor contraction may compensate.

VOIDING CYSTOURETHROGRAPHY
Voiding cystourethrography provides anatomic correlation to the functional study. The bladder is filled with radiopaque contrast with the patient in the sitting and upright positions. Films are taken with the patient relaxed, then with coughing, straining, and movement. The positions of the contrast-filled bladder reflect pelvic floor muscle support. Voiding cystourethrography can also help in the diagnosis of vesicovaginal fistulae.

Complex Evaluation
Referral to a specialist is recommended for certain patients with incontinence such as women with abrupt onset urinary incontinence, gross or microhematuria, recurrent symptomatic urinary tract infections, neurologic disease, increased post-void residuals, or symptoms of overflow incontinence (see Table 10-5 for a more complete list). In these settings, evaluation must exclude such concerns as tumor, bladder outlet obstruction, decreased detrusor activity, or complications related to prior surgery or irradiation. Also, patients failing conservative treatment for stress incontinence are often referred for consideration of anti-incontinence surgery.

CYSTOSCOPY
Cystoscopy may be recommended by the specialist in order to evaluate the urethra, urethrovesical junction, bladder walls, and ureteral orifices. In addition, information regarding lower urinary tract function can be obtained during the evaluation, including 1) amount of residual urine, 2) bladder volume at the initial urge to urinate, 3) bladder capacity, 4) competence of bladder neck, 5) mobility of the bladder neck and urethra, and 6) ability to elevate and close the urethra with pelvic muscle contractions. In women with continuous incontinence, especially following a cesarean section or hysterectomy, cystoscopy is useful in establishing the presence and location of a fistula.

MULTI-CHANNEL VIDEOURODYNAMICS
Multi-channel videourodynamics offers the most comprehensive means to evaluate voiding dysfunction and incontinence. It permits the synchronous measurement of intra-abdominal pressure, intravesical pressure, detrusor pressure, pelvic floor activity, uroflow curve, and cystourethrogram. It can determine the Valsalva leak point pressure. A study that is properly performed and able to reproduce the patient's symptoms can identify urinary storage and voiding disorders with anatomical correlation.

Treatment

Treatment options for incontinence may be divided into nonsurgical and surgical categories. Nonsurgical treatments include behavioral therapies, medications, and devices. The Agency for Health Care Policy and Research has recommended behavioral treatment as first-line therapy for urinary incontinence (30). Moreover, a recent randomized clinical controlled trial comparing behavioral treatment (i.e., pelvic muscle training and exercise) with drug treatment for urge and mixed incontinence found the former to be more efficacious and better tolerated (31).

Nonsurgical Treatment
KEGEL EXERCISES
Pelvic floor muscle exercises (or "Kegel exercises") utilize techniques to properly identify, contract, and relax the pelvic floor muscles, thereby strengthening the pelvic floor musculature and alleviating or eliminating urinary stress incontinence (Fig. 10-2) (32,33). Studies have shown that these exercises can treat urge incontinence as well, because learned pelvic muscle contractions can also inhibit and abort involuntary de-

All incontinent patients should be offered pelvic floor exercises because they supplement all forms of incontinence treatment and have no adverse side effects.

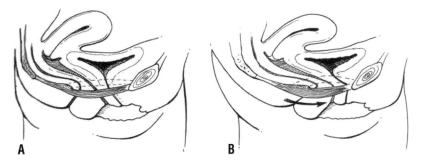

A   **B**

Figure 10-2 *A*, The pubovisceral muscle at rest. *B*, Contraction of the pubovisceral muscle constricting the lumens of the urethra, vagina, and rectum. The pelvic floor muscles, often referred to collectively as the "levator ani muscle", support the pelvic organs and contribute to urinary and fecal continence. Continence is supported by baseline tonic contractions as well as "fast-twitch" muscle fibers, which, when contracted, constrict the lumens of the urethra, vagina, and rectum. Kegel exercises strengthen this muscle group, thereby alleviating or eliminating urinary stress incontinence. (From Wall LL. Incontinence, prolapse, and disorders of the pelvic floor. In: Berek JS, Adashi EY, Hillard PA, eds. Novak's Gynecology, 12th ed. New York: Williams & Wilkins; 1996:621; with permission.)

trusor contractions (31). All incontinent patients should be offered pelvic floor exercise, because they supplement all forms of incontinence treatment and have no adverse side effects.

The ability to localize and contract the pelvic floor muscles can be determined by intentionally interrupting the urinary stream while voiding or by performing contractions around two fingers placed in the vagina. Once the appropriate muscle contractions are identified, performing the exercises during urination is not appropriate. Patients should be advised to perform the exercises as a regular regimen. They should be made aware that because the movement is barely perceptible to others, they may incorporate the exercises into their daily activities (such as a daily commute to work). The number of contractions recommended per day ranges from 20 to 200, with the duration of each contraction ranging from 5 to 10 seconds. With very weak muscles, the initial regimen may start with 10 repetitions of 3 seconds performed once or twice daily. Improvement is generally seen after 2 to 3 weeks, but the full effect is not seen until the exercises are performed daily for 2 to 3 months. For patients who are compliant, pelvic floor exercises can cure 30% to 70% of women with incontinence (34), and surgery can often be avoided.

It should be noted that many women are unable to properly localize the pelvic floor muscles and erroneously contract their abdominal, thigh, and gluteal muscles (35). Biofeedback is then indicated, because it helps the patient identify the proper muscle groups (36,37). A single biofeedback session is often adequate. Pelvic floor exercises may also be performed with the aid of vaginal cones weighing from 20 to 90 g, with progression to heavier cones as strength improves (38).

ELECTRICAL STIMULATION

Another, more complex and less proven, option to help women rehabilitate the pelvic musculature is electrical stimulation. An electrode-containing probe connected to a stimulator unit is placed into the vagina or anus and delivers electrical stimulation to the pelvic floor and urethral musculature, typically twice daily for 15 min, which yields increases in levator ani tone and bladder support (39-41), but with variable overall results. A recent trial found both subjective and objective incontinence outcomes to be inferior to those from simple Kegel exercises (42). Moreover, stimulator units are expensive and not always covered by insurers.

MAGNETIC STIMULATION

Recently a pulsating magnetic chair that stimulates the pelvic floor musculature has been FDA approved. The patient sits fully clothed in the chair for 20-min sessions. An uncontrolled trial suggests possible benefit (43).

BLADDER TRAINING

Another form of behavioral therapy is bladder training. Bladder training (or "bladder drill") manages urinary incontinence with timed voiding (44-46). The patient is instructed to void at frequent predetermined intervals rather than responding to urinary urge, with the schedule determined by review of the voiding diary. The goal is for the patient to regain control of continence by suppressing urinary urges through the maintenance of low but gradually increasing bladder volumes. Mild fluid restriction can therefore be a helpful adjunct. During the course of treatment, the patient records the number of voids and incontinent episodes, which serves as a reinforcement and also helps to gauge the gradual lengthening of the voiding interval. Bladder training is effective for treating detrusor instability and mild cases of genuine stress incontinence. Short-term response rates of 50% (with subjective response rates as high as 85%) have been documented with this method, although with longer follow-up 43% of patients subsequently suffer relapse (47,48).

DIETARY MODIFICATION

Dietary substances that are spicy, acidic. or carbonated can irritate the bladder through unclear mechanisms and contribute to urinary incontinence. Common potential offenders include coffee, tea, carbonated beverages, citrus fruits. and tomatoes, all of which presumably exert an effect on the bladder via their breakdown products in the urine. Decreasing or eliminating the intake of any dietary irritant can sometimes be a useful measure. In such situations, the patient should also be cautioned to not limit fluid intake, because doing so would only concentrate the urine and intensify the irritant effect.

TREATMENT OF NONGENITOURINARY FACTORS

Treatment of incontinence must be based upon an accurate assessment of all the factors contributing to the incontinence after a complete history and physical examination and simple testing. Successful treatment plans must take into account not only the type(s) of incontinence but also any mitigating factors involved. Medical problems and social or environmental factors that may exacerbate incontinence must be addressed, especially as, once identified, nongenitourinary causes of incontinence are often easily treated. For example, incontinence related to restricted mobility may improve with simple interventions such as prescribing a bedside commode. Treatment of stool impaction or chronic constipation allows complete bladder emptying and relieves overflow incontinence. Adjusting the type and dosage of medications can correct pharmaceutical-related incontinence. Treatment of hyperglycemia, hypercalcemia, and psychological disturbances can also alleviate voiding symptoms.

PESSARIES AND OTHER MECHANICAL DEVICES

Intravaginal support prostheses (i.e., "pessaries") and the contraceptive diaphragm are also options for treating urinary incontinence and other symptoms of pelvic organ prolapse (Fig. 10-3) (49,50). With proper fitting, a pessary should reduce prolapse and the patient should be able to void without any urinary retention. The pessary should be removed for intercourse and monthly cleaning and requires office examination (typically every 6 months after initial close follow-up), at which time the pessary is removed, cleaned, then replaced. These follow-up visits determine whether voiding is complete and if vaginal ulceration has occurred. Some physicians routinely recommend concomitant use of vaginal estrogen cream to help prevent mucosal erosions.

Other devices include urethral caps and plugs; these have demonstrated modest benefit (51) but have failed to gain acceptance by women and consequently for the most part are no longer available.

When it has been determined that a woman has overflow incontinence resulting from chronic urinary retention, careful consideration should be given to the possibility of such reversible causes as alpha-adrenergic agonists, anticholinergic agents, large cystocele, fecal impaction, and urethral obstruction. Once these causes are excluded, the patient should have a urethral catheter placed for a few weeks, because bladder decompression for up to one month can relieve the retention, restore bladder tone, and sometimes cure the incontinence. If incontinence recurs or persists after catheter removal, a

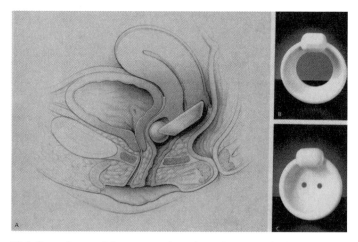

Figure 10-3 Pessaries used for stress urinary incontinence typically elevate the bladder neck and correct the angle between the bladder and the urethra. The incontinence ring and dish pessaries are the most frequently used pessaries for this indication. (From Culligan PJ, Heit M. Urinary incontinence in women: evaluation and management. Am Fam Physician. 2000;62:2441; with permission.)

chronic indwelling catheter should be considered. In such circumstances, a suprapubic catheter is preferred to an indwelling urethral catheter because there is less bacterial colonization on the lower abdominal wall than on the perineum. A temporary urethral catheter may also be useful in the setting of skin breakdown resulting from any form of urinary incontinence, until definitive treatment is undertaken.

PHARMACOLOGIC TREATMENTS

Many patients with pelvic floor relaxation and stress incontinence are perimenopausal or postmenopausal; if their exam reveals signs of hypoestrogenism, their urinary incontinence sometimes responds to estrogen replacement. Estrogen replacement therapy increases blood flow to the submucosal plexus and epithelium of the urethra, increases the number of alpha-receptors in the urethra, and increases skin collagen content. Even women already taking oral replacement sometimes manifest signs of hypoestrogenism and may benefit from the addition of topical estrogen in the form of either vaginal cream or Estring. When the uterus is present and systemic estrogen is used, progesterone is added to decrease the risk of endometrial cancer from unopposed estrogen replacement (see Chapter 16). It should be noted that the evidence to support benefit for urinary incontinence (52,53) is not as strong as that for preventing urinary tract infections. However, topical estrogen remains a cornerstone of treatment for the estrogen-deficient patient, because most experts observe excellent clinical benefit for incontinence and anticipate more supportive evidence from future trials.

In addition to estrogen, other pharmacologic agents may be prescribed either alone or in combination with other nonsurgical therapy (Table 10-6). The alpha-adrenergic agonist pseudoephedrine (usually prescribed in the long-acting form) binds to alpha-receptors in the urethra and increases urethral pressure. It may be a helpful adjunct in treating stress incontinence, particularly when used in conjunction with pelvic floor exercises and topical estrogen.

Anticholinergic agents are typically the first-line medications for treating urge incontinence. They produce bladder relaxation and improve bladder storage. A commonly prescribed anticholinergic agent is oxybutynin 5 mg PO tid (often initiated at 1/2 tablet tid in older patients), increased as necessary to 10 mg PO tid. Recently, a once-daily extended release form of oxybutynin (Ditropan XL) has become available. The recommended starting dose is 5 mg once daily, which can be increased by 5 mg increments at approximately weekly intervals to a maximum of 30 mg daily. The extended release form is associated with a decreased incidence of side effects but is more expensive than the generic formulation. Another new anticholinergic agent is tolterodine (Detrol), which appears to be better tolerated but slightly less efficacious

Table 10-6 Medications Commonly Used To Manage Incontinence

Medication Type	Mechanism of Action
Topical estrogen	Increases blood flow to urethra and increases skin collagen content (for stress incontinence)
Anticholinergics Oxybutynin (Ditropan) Dicyclomine (Bentyl) Imipramine (Tofranil) Flavoxate (Urispas) Tolterodine (Detrol)	Detrusor relaxation (for urge incontinence)
Alpha-adrenergic agonists Ephedrine Pseudoephederine (Sudafed) Imipramine (Tofranil)	Increase bladder outlet resistance and urethral pressure (for stress incontinence)
Alpha-adrenergic antagonists Doxazosin (Cardura) Terazosin (Hytrin) Tamsulosin (Flomax)	Decrease bladder outlet resistance (for overflow incontinence)

than short-acting oxybutynin (54). The recommended starting dose for the long-acting tolterodine formulation (Detrol LA) is 4 mg once daily and that for the twice daily formulation is 2 mg bid. These doses may be halved if needed.

Anticholinergic agents should be avoided in patients with urinary retention and narrow angle glaucoma and should be used with caution in the setting of gastrointestinal hypomotility, severe gastrointestinal reflux disease, or concomitant bisphosphanate use. When anticholinergic agents are prescribed, it is important to alert the patient to the potential side effects, namely dry mouth, constipation, inability to void, blurred vision, and occasionally confusion. A stool-bulking agent is often helpful in treating the constipation. Blurred vision and dry mouth generally require alteration of the dosage or type of medication. Post-void residuals should be checked 1 to 2 weeks after initiation of medical therapy; if residual volumes start to increase, the options are to decrease the dose of medication or begin intermittent clean catheterization along with the medication.

Imipramine, a tricyclic antidepressant, has both anticholinergic and alpha-adrenergic properties, and is useful in treating both urge and stress urinary incontinence by suppressing involuntary bladder contractions and increasing urethral contractility. Because it is sedating, imipramine is usually dosed at bedtime, beginning at 25 mg PO qhs and increasing as necessary to 100 mg. If required, a low dose may be taken in the morning as well.

Sometimes more than one drug may be needed to increase efficacy or minimize side effects, and different drug combinations may be tried. Behavioral treatments, such as pelvic exercises and timed voiding schedules, are useful adjuncts to medical therapy and are often necessary to achieve continence.

It should be noted that certain medications are unhelpful in the treatment of incontinence. For instance, while the alpha-adrenergic antagonists (terazosin, doxazosin, tamsulosin) are commonly prescribed for men to relieve bladder outlet obstruction and urinary retention, such conditions are unusual in women, and use of these medications would aggravate stress incontinence. Note also that while in theory cholinergic agonists improve bladder contractility, in practice their effect is limited, and consequently these medications are generally not prescribed.

PERIURETHRAL INJECTIONS

Another option to incontinence surgery is periurethral injection of bovine collagen, carbon-coated beads, or autologous fat, perfomed under cystoscopic guidance. This is often effective for women with stress incontinence and intrinsic urethral sphincter defect (55,56) and has the advantage of being a minimally invasive office procedure (57). At each given session one or two injections may be placed into the urethral submucosa at the region of the bladder neck. Coaptation of the walls of the proximal urethra and bladder neck should be seen. The procedure can usually be performed with local anesthesia with or without low doses of intravenous sedation. Multiple treatment sessions are typically required to maintain continence or improvement.

A large multicenter study of periurethral collagen injections indicated that 78% of women reported continued improvement after more than 2 years of follow-up (55), with 50% of these patients reporting being completely dry. Complications were rare, and none of the women suffered hypersensitivity to the injected material; however, because 1% to 4% of the population is allergic to bovine collagen, a skin test is required before consideration for treatment with collagen. A separate study of patients treated with autologous fat injection found that at 6-month follow-up 12% were cured of symptoms, 44% were improved, and 44% were deemed failures. Complications were unusual but included urinary tract infections and subcutaneous abdominal wall hematoma (56).

Surgical Treatment

Surgical treatment of incontinence is reserved for those patients who fail or who are not candidates for nonsurgical therapy. Surgery can treat symptomatic pelvic floor defects, intrinsic urethral sphincter deficiency, low bladder compliance, urinary tract fistulae, ectopic ureters, and urethral diverticula. The patient must always be advised of the risks of anti-incontinence surgery, which include subsequent urinary retention with the need for catheterization, new symptoms of frequency and urgency or persistence

Surgical treatment of incontinence is reserved for those patients who fail nonsurgical therapy.

of the original urinary incontinence problem.

Surgical procedures for stress incontinence include retropubic suspensions, needle suspensions, pubovaginal slings, anterior colporrhaphies with suburethral plication, paravaginal repairs, and placement of artificial urinary sphincters. Retropubic suspensions anchor the pubocervical fascia to ligaments located on the bony pelvis (58). They are performed either laparoscopically or via laparotomy. Needle suspensions utilize a suprapubic and transvaginal approach (59). Sutures are placed on both sides of the urethra (incorporating the endopelvic fascia), then secured to the rectus abdominis fascia or ligaments inserting into the pubic bone. Anterior colporrhaphy plicates the pubocervical fascia underneath the bladder neck via a transvaginal approach. The retropubic and needle suspensions and anterior colporrhaphy restore the bladder neck to a high retropubic position.

A newer surgical treatment is the pubovaginal sling procedure, which utilizes a strip of rectus abdominis fascia or fascia harvested from the fascia lata of the thigh and places it between the bladder neck and anterior vaginal wall (60,61). The ends of the strip or "sling" are secured to the remaining rectus abdominis fascia. The pubovaginal sling is effective in treating bladder neck hypermobility with intrinsic sphincter defect, because mobility is restricted and urethral coaptation promoted. More recently, a vaginal wall sling has been used to successfully treat patients with these problems (62). Sling procedures can utilize a transabdominal and/or a transvaginal approach and have become increasingly popular in the surgical treatment of incontinence, especially for patients with previously failed repair.

In any type of incontinence surgery, concomitant repair of pelvic floor defects (including enterocele, rectocele, and uterine prolapse) is performed; this improves total pelvic floor support and minimizes voiding dysfunction postoperatively. If inadequate, the perineal body should be restored as well, because the perineal body is the insertion site for muscular components of the external urethral sphincter and contributes to pelvic support and continence.

Post-operatively, post-void residual volumes are checked to ensure complete bladder emptying. Detrusor instability with urgency and frequency may result from partial outlet obstruction or from denervation of the bladder neck from dissection. These symptoms are usually transient; however, if they do not resolve spontaneously, anticholinergic medication may be required. Lifestyle changes must follow surgical treatment, and prolonged standing, abdominal straining, and heavy lifting should be avoided indefinitely. Pulmonary conditions associated with cough should be treated promptly. Lastly, stool softeners are frequently recommended to decrease the risk of constipation and its attendant effect on urinary continence.

Summary

Urinary incontinence is common and treatable. Successful management rests upon the accurate evaluation of lower urinary tract storage and function. A thorough history must first be elicited. Next, the presence and degree of any pelvic prolapse, estrogen deficiency or neurologic deficits are noted. A urinalysis is performed to rule out pyuria and hematuria, and the post-void residual is measured. Sometimes simple office cystometry is performed to uncover a component of urge incontinence.

Following surgical treatment for urinary incontinence, activities such as heavy lifting must be avoided and conditions such as cough and constipation aggressively treated.

Using this information a differential diagnosis can be formed. For those patients with straightforward cases of urinary incontinence, the primary physician can initiate treatment and follow the patient's progress, often with the help of the voiding diary. For many patients, more than one type of treatment modality is required to maintain improvement or achieve cure, and the side effects of each treatment modality must be monitored. Referral to a specialist is recommended for patients with complex voiding disorders or unsuccessful outcomes.

Urinary incontinence must not be viewed as a normal outcome of childbirth or aging. Furthermore, physicians should actively screen for this problem, just as is done for other major health conditions. Although urinary incontinence may not be life threatening, it can be devastating to a patient's quality of life. Indeed, urinary incontinence is an epidemic health issue begging for our attention.

REFERENCES

1. **Diokno AC, Brock BM, Brown, MB, et al.** Prevalence of urinary incontinence and other urologic symptoms in the non-institutionalized elderly. J Urol. 1986;136:1022.
2. **Johnson MJ, Werner C.** We have no choice: a study of familial guilt feelings surrounding nursing home care. J Geront Nurs. 1982;8:641-5,654.
3. **Ouslander JG, Kane RL, Abrass IB.** Urinary incontinence in elderly nursing home patients. JAMA. 1982;248:1194.
4. **Starer P, Libow LS.** Obscuring urinary incontinence. J Am Geriatr Soc. 1985;33:842.

5. **Wolin LH.** Stress incontinence in young, healthy nulliparous females. J Urol. 1969; 101:545.

6. **Cardozo L.** Urinary incontinence in women: have we anything new to offer? BMJ. 1991;303:1453.

7. **Norton P, MacDonald L, Stanton S.** Distress associated with female urinary complaints and delay in seeking treatment. Neurourol Urodyn. 1987;6:170.

8. **Raz S, Little NA, Juma, S.** Female urology. In: Walsh PC, Retik AB, Stamey TA, Vaughan DE Jr., eds. Campbell's Urology, 6th ed. Philadelphia: WB Saunders; 1992: 2782-2828.

9. **Stamey TA.** Urinary incontinence in the female. In: Walsh PC, Retik AB, Stamey TA, Vaughan DE Jr., eds. Campbell's Urology, 6th ed. Philadelphia: WB Saunders; 1992: 2829-50.

10. **McGuire EJ, Lytton B, Pepe V, et al.** Stress incontinence. Am J Obstet Gynec. 1976;47:255.

11. **McGuire EJ, Savastano JA.** Stress incontinence and detrusor instability/urge incontinence. Neurourol Urodyn. 1985;4:313.

12. **Farrar DJ, Osborne JL, Stephenson TP, et al.** A urodynamic view of bladder outflow obstruction in the female: factors influencing the results of treatment. Br J Urol. 1976;47:815.

13. **Axelrod SL, Blaivas JG.** Bladder neck obstruction in women. J Urol. 1987;137:497.

14. **Stephens FD.** Anatomic vagaries of double ureters. Aust N Z J Surg. 1958;28:27.

15. **Ellerker AG.** The extravesical ectopic ureter. Br J Surg. 1958;45:344.

16. **Hinman F Jr, Cohlan WR.** Gartner's duct carcinoma in a urethral diverticulum. J Urol. 1960;83:414.

17. **Benjamin J, Eliot L, Cooper JF, et al.** Urethral diverticulum in adult females: clinical aspects, operative procedures, and pathology. Urology. 1974;3:1.

18. **Peters WH, Vaughan ED Jr.** Urethral diverticulum in the female. Obstet Gynecol. 1976;47:549.

19. **Leach GE, Bavendam TG.** Female urethral diverticula. Urology. 1987;30:110.

20. **Resnick NM.** Geriatric urinary incontinence. AUA Update Series. 1992;11: 66.

21. **Resnick NM.** Voiding dysfunction in the elderly. In: Yalla SV, McGuire EJ, Elbadawi A, Blaivas JG, eds. Neurourology and Urodynamics: Principles and Practice. New York: Macmillan; 1988: 303-30.

22. **Wein AJ.** Practical uropharmacology. Urol Clin North Am. 1991;18:269.

23. **Hilton P.** Urinary incontinence during sexual intercourse: a common, but rarely volunteered symptom. Br J Obstet Gynecol. 1988;95:377.

24. **Khan Z, Bhola A, Starer P.** Urinary incontinence during orgasm. Urology, 1988;31: 279.

25. **Snooks SJ, Swash M, Henry MM, et al.** Risk factors in childbirth causing damage to pelvic floor innervation. Int J Colorect Dis. 1986;1:20.

26. **Smith ARB, Hosker GL, Warrell DW.** The role of partial denervation of the pelvic floor in the aetiology of genitourinary prolapse and stress incontinence of urine: a neurophysiological study. Br J Obstet Gynecol. 1989;96:24.

27. **Blaivas JG, Zayed AAH, Labib KB.** The bulbocavernous reflex in urology: a prospective study of 299 patients. J Urol. 1981;126:197.

28. **Schmidt RA, Senn E, Tanagho EA.** Functional evaluation of sacral nerve root integrity. Urology. 1990;35:5.

29. **Marshall FC, Uson AC, Melicow MM.** Neoplasms and caruncles of the female urethra. Surg Gynecol Obstet. 1960;110:723.

30. **Fantl JA, Newman DK, Colling J, et al.** Urinary incontinence in adults: acute and chronic management. Rockville, MD: US Department of Health and Human Services, Agency for Health Care Policy and Research, March 1996; AHCPR Publication 96-0682, Clinical Practice Guideline No. 2, 1996 Update.

31. **Burgio KL, Locher JL, Goode PS, et al.** Behavioral vs. drug treatment for urge urinary incontinence in older women. JAMA. 1998;280:1995-2000.

32. **Klarov P, Belving D, Bischiff N, et al.** Pelvic floor exercises versus surgery for female urinary stress incontinence. Urol Int. 1986;41:129.

33. **Mauritsen L.** Pelvic floor exercises for female stress urinary incontinence. Int Urogynecol J. 1994;5:44.

34. **Kegel A.** Progressive resisting exercises in the functional restoration of the perineal muscles. Am J Obstet Gynecol. 1949;56:238.

35. **Bo K, Larger S, David S, et al.** Knowledge about and ability to correct pelvic floor muscle exercises in women with urinary stress incontinence. Neurourol Urodyn. 1988;71:261.

36. **Cardoza LD, Abrams PD, Stanton SL, et al.** Idiopathic bladder instability treated by biofeedback. Br J Urol. 1978;50:521.

37. **Stroebel CF, Glueck BC.** Biofeedback treatment in medicine and psychiatry: an ultimate placebo? Sem Psychiatr. 1973;5:379.

38. **Plevnik S.** New method for testing and strengthening of pelvic floor muscles. In: Proceedings of the 15th Annual General Meeting, International Incontinence Society, 1985.

39. **Erickson BC, Bergman S, Eiknes SH.** Maximal electrostimulation of the pelvic floor in female idiopathic detrusor instability and urge incontinence. Neurourol Urodyn. 1989;8:219.

40. **Tanagho E.** Electrical stimulation. J Am Geriatr Soc. 1990;38:353.

41. **Bazeed MA, Thuroff JW, Schmidt RA, et al.** Effect of chronic electrostimulation of the sacral roots on the striated urethral sphincter. J Urol. 1982;128:1357.

42. **Bo K, Talseth T, Holme I, et al.** Single blind, randomised controlled trial of pelvic floor exercises, electrical stimulation, vaginal cones, and no treatment in management of genuine stress incontinence in women. BMJ. 1999;318:487-93.

43. **Galloway NT, El-Galley RE, Sand PK, et al.** Exracorporeal magnetic innervation therapy for stress urinary incontinence. Urology. 1999;53:1108-11.

44. **Frewen WK.** Role of bladder training in the treatment of the unstable bladder in the female. Urol Clin North Am. 1979;6:273.

45. **Holmes DM, Stone AR, Berry PR.** Bladder training: three years on. Br J Urol. 1983;55:660.

46. **Frewen WK.** An objective assessment of the unstable bladder of psychosomatic origin. Br J Urol. 1978;50:246.

47. **Abrams PH, Torrens M.** Urine flow studies. Symposium on Clinical Urodynamics. Urol Clin North Am. 1979;6:63.

48. **Farrar DJ, Whiteside CG, Osborne JL, et al.** A urodynamic analysis of micturition symptoms in the female. Surg Gyn Obstet. 1975;141:875.

49. **Nygaard I.** Prevention of exercise incontinence with mechanical devices. J Reprod Med. 1995;40:89.

50. **Suarez GM, Baum NH, Jacobs J.** Use of contraceptive diaphragm in management of stress urinary incontinence. Urology. 1991;37:119.

51. **Miller JL, Bavendam T.** Treatment with the Reliance urinary control insert: one-year experience. J Endourol. 1996;10:287.

52. **Fantl JA, Cardozo L, McClish DK.** Estrogen therapy in the management of urinary incontinence in post-menopausal women: a meta-analysis. First Report of the Hormones and Urogenital Therapy Committee. Obstet Gynecol. 1994;83:12-8.

53. **Fantl JA, Bump RC, Elser DM, et al.** Efficacy of estrogen supplementation in the treatment of urinary incontinence. Obstet Gynecol. 1996;88:745-9.

54. **Appell RA.** Clinical efficacy and safety of tolterodine in the treatment of overactive bladder: a pooled analysis. Urology. 1997;50(Suppl):90-6.

55. **Burch JC.** Urethrovaginal fixation to Cooper's ligament for correction of stress incontinence, cystocele, and prolapse. Am J Obstet Gynecol. 1961;81:281.

56. **Gittes RF, Loughlin KR.** No-incision pubovaginal suspension for stress incontinence. J Urol. 1987;138:568.

57. **Culligan PJ, Heit M.** Urinary incontinence in women: evaluation and management. Am Fam Physican. 2000;62:2433-44,2447,2452.

58. **Stamey TA.** Endoscopic suspension of the vesical neck for urinary incontinence. Surg Gynecol Obstet. 1973;136:547.

59. **Marshall VF, Marchetti AA, Krantz, KE.** The correction of stress incontinence by simple vesico-urethral suspension. Surg Gynecol Obstet. 1988;88:509.

60. **Raz S.** Modified bladder neck suspension for female stress incontinence. Urology. 1981;7:82.

61. **Parker RT, Addison WA, Wilson, CJ.** Fascia lata urethrovesical suspension for recurrent stress urinary incontinence. Am J Obstet Gynecol. 1979;135:843.

62. **McGuire EJ, Lytton, B.** Pubovaginal sling procedure for stress incontinence. J Urol. 1979;119:82.

CHAPTER 11

Endometriosis

JOHN C. PETROZZA, MD
ALAN H. DeCHERNEY, MD

ndometriosis is the presence of functional endometrial tissue (glands and stroma) outside the uterine cavity. Although first described in 1860 by von Rokitansky, many aspects of this disease, including its etiology, remain obscure. It is well established, however, that endometriosis is a common cause of pelvic pain and infertility.

In many ways, endometriosis behaves similar to a cancer. It has the ability to "metastasize" to different areas of the body either directly via the lymphatics or through the bloodstream. It can behave aggressively and cause extensive damage to affected organs. In addition, like many cancers, the treatment of endometriosis is often primarily palliative rather than curative.

The most common sites of endometriosis are the ovaries, uterine ligaments, posterior cul-de-sac, fallopian tubes, pelvic parietal peritoneum, large bowel, and rectovaginal septum (Table 11-1) (1). Less commonly, endometriosis may be found on the small bowel, ureter, appendix, vagina, umbilicus, inguinal areas, diaphragm, vulva, skin, pleura, episiotomy wounds, and abdominal incision scars. When endometriosis occurs at distant sites such as the lung, unusual presentations such as monthly hemoptysis can result.

At times, making the diagnosis of endometriosis can be difficult. In the past, the diagnosis was based on symptomatology and the exclusion of other common diseases that caused pelvic pain. Today the diagnosis is still fre-

Table 11-1 Common Sites of Endometriosis

Site	Percentage
Uterosacral ligaments	63.0
Ovaries	
Superficial	56.0
Deep (endometrioma)	19.5
Ovarian fossae	32.5
Anterior vesicle pouch	21.5
Posterior cul-de-sac	18.5
Broad ligament	7.5
Intestines	5.0
Fallopian tube	
Mesosalpinx	4.5
Salpingitis isthmica nodosa	3.0
Uterus	4.5
Gastrointestinal tract	5.0
Urinary tract	10.0

quently made on clinical grounds; however, the availability of laparoscopy often allows for definitive diagnosis. Some physicians have advocated administering a trial of medication that induces a hypoestrogenic state as an adjunct to making the diagnosis. Although potentially cost-effective in the short run, this approach limits the ability to make a definite diagnosis, remove adhesions, and perhaps is inferior when considering long-term prognosis, particularly infertility. In part because the average time from symptom onset to the diagnosis of endometriosis is typically prolonged (frequently 7 years) (2), recent debate has focused on the potential therapeutic value of early laparoscopic diagnosis and intervention.

Epidemiology

Because the definitive diagnosis of endometriosis is surgical, estimates of its prevalence are based on data from surgical series, which are limited in number and are biased according to the indication for the procedure. Among patients undergoing tubal ligation the prevalence is 1.8%, whereas that of teenagers undergoing operative procedures who reported pelvic pain is 53% (3). Recent studies evaluating the general population estimate the prevalence to be 2.5% to 3.3 % of women of reproductive age (4). Approximately one third of women who present with pelvic pain are eventually diagnosed with

Approximately one third of women with chronic pelvic pain have endometriosis. The incidence may be higher in women who also have infertility.

endometriosis (3); the incidence may be higher if the woman also has infertility. The disease is found primarily in women of reproductive age and is rarely seen in women younger than 15 years or older than 65 years, supporting the idea that estrogen is needed for endometriosis to grow (5). Endometriosis can occur in any social stratum but has been more frequently diagnosed in Asians and Caucasians than in Blacks.

Risk Factors

Many factors are associated with increased or decreased likelihood of endometriosis (Table 11-2) (6). Many of the protective factors are those that either render a relatively low estrogen state or decrease the amount or duration of menstrual flow. Congenital obstructive anomalies of the müllerian system, such as a transverse vaginal septum or imperforate hymen, have the potential to allow a large amount of retrograde flow into the pelvic cavity, placing the patient at risk for endometriosis (7). Note, however, that tampon use has not been similarly implicated.

Table 11-2 Risk Factors for Endometriosis

Factor	Odds Ratio	Confidence Interval
Protective		
Current oral contraceptive use	0.4	0.2–0.7
Cigarettes >1 ppd	0.5	0.3–0.9
Regular exercise (>2 h/wk of conditioning/sports)	0.6	0.4–0.8
Definite risk		
Length of menstrual cycle <27 days	2.1	1.4–2.7
Duration of menstrual flow ≥8 days	2.4	1.5–2.9
Unrelated		
Age at menarche		
<11 years	1.2	0.9–1.7
>16 years	0.8	0.4–1.7
Tampon use	0.9	0.7–1.3
Douching	0.9	0.6–1.4

Adapted from Cramer DW, Wilson E, Stillman RJ, et al. The relation of endometriosis to menstrual characteristics, smoking, and exercise. JAMA. 1986;255:1904-8.

Genetics appears to play a role, because having a first-degree relative with documented endometriosis increases a patient's risk to about 7%, approximately double that of the general reproductive-aged population (8). Usually, familial cases present at a younger age and are more severe in nature (9).

Etiology

As stated earlier, the exact etiology of endometriosis is unknown. Several theories have been postulated; however, none adequately explains all of the characteristics of the disease or all the extrapelvic sites described. There are currently six theories that attempt to describe the cause of endometriosis: transplantation, transformation, immunologic, genetic, cell adhesion factors, and environmental.

Transplantation Theory

The transplantation theory holds that fragments of endometrium spread to areas of the body through retrograde flow, lymphatic or hematogenous spread, or iatrogenic dispersion. The endometrial effluent has definitely been shown to contain viable endometrial cells that are capable of transplantation (10). Retrograde flow through the fallopian tubes permits endometrial fragments access to areas conducive to implantation and growth (11). Areas such as the peritoneum are thin and well vascularized, allowing a rich estrogenized environment in which to bathe the endometrial implants and support their growth, while, conversely, areas that are keratinized, such as the skin or vaginal mucosa, are rarely involved with endometriosis. The dependent nature of endometriosis in the lower pelvis supports this retrograde flow theory. Further evidence for this theory is that increased retrograde flow due to a congenital anomaly, such as a transverse septum or hemivagina, increases the susceptibility to endometriosis (12). Also, women with frequent and long menses are at increased risk for endometriosis. However, intraperitoneal menstrual fluid and debris is almost a universal finding when peritoneal dialysis or laparoscopy is performed during the perimenstrual period, which suggests that other factors must also be involved (13,14).

The spread of endometrial tissue to sites beyond the pelvis occurs via lymphatic and venous channels, especially during the perimenstrual phase of the menstrual cycle (15). However, that such minuscule amounts of endometrial tissue could be the nidus for an endometrial implant suggests once again that other, unknown, factors must be involved. The finding of endometriosis in surgical skin wounds after pelvic surgery, especially uterine surgery, clearly implicates an iatrogenic transplantation model.

Transformation Theory

During embryonic development the endometrium and parietal and visceral peritoneum all arise from the same peritoneal pluripotent cells; thus it is conceivable that these cells could differentiate into endometrial cells (16). This may be a spontaneous event or secondary to irritants, growth factors, hormones, inflammation, cytokines, or trauma. These factors must be female specific, because men rarely get endometriosis, except those on high-dose tamoxifen therapy for prostate cancer, who can develop endometriosis in müllerian remnants.

Immunologic Theory

Dysfunction of the immune system has been implicated as contributing to endometriosis. Some have proposed that a defect in cell-mediated immunity is responsible, leading to decreased surveillance, recognition, and destruction of transplanted endometrium. The data are at first glance misleading, because studies demonstrate that the numbers of macrophages, T-helper cells, natural killer cells, and interleukin-1 are all actually *increased* in both serum and peritoneal fluid in women with endometriosis. However, as the severity of endometriosis increases, these numbers decrease and approach the levels of the normal population (17). Moreover, even when present in high concentration, these immune cells demonstrate decreased activity in experimental studies.

The humoral arm also appears to be affected. Alterations in the B-cell response, complement levels, and immunoglobulin production, as well as the development of autoantibodies to endometrial cells, have all been reported in women with endometriosis (18). As well documented as these various findings are, however, they fail to explain whether the immune dysfunction is the cause or a consequence of the endometriosis.

Genetic Theory

The familial occurrence of endometriosis raises the possibility of a genetic predisposition. As stated earlier, the risk of disease doubles to approximately 7% if a first-degree relative is affected (8), and endometriosis has also been reported in monozygotic twins (19). The genetic theory is attractive for its ability to explain the shortcomings of the other theories and for its potential utility in identifying susceptible women before they develop symptoms or sequelae. Ongoing research is currently evaluating several candidate genes.

Cell Adhesion Factors Theory

Alterations in the structural and cellular biochemical makeup of the endometrium may predispose a woman to endometriosis. Integrins are cell adhesion molecules that undergo dynamic changes at the cellular level during a woman's menstrual cycle. A lack of the beta-3 subunit has been shown to be closely associated with the diagnosis of endometriosis (20). Other cell adhesion molecules are being investigated.

Environmental Theory

Dioxin is a potent chemical toxin that belongs to a large class of halogenated aromatic hydrocarbons created in industrial processes. Investigations in rhesus monkeys have demonstrated a clear association between dioxins and endometriosis (21). Epidemiologic studies of humans from areas exposed to dioxin or polychlorinated biphenyls (PCBs) have shown a higher incidence of endometriosis in women with higher levels of these compounds in their blood (22). Because dioxin appears to behave like an antiestrogen rather than an estrogen (23), it is speculated that its effects of immunosuppression and hormonal dysregulation are the factors leading to endometriosis. Further studies are needed to help determine whether the relationship between dioxin exposure and endometriosis is causal or only associated.

Endometriosis and Infertility

Infertility occurs in 30% to 40% of women with the diagnosis of endometriosis. The pathogenesis of infertility in patients with endometriosis is not definite and may be multifactorial. Proposed mechanisms include tubal damage from adhesions that occlude the fimbriae or constrict the fallopian tubes, and interference with ovulation by endometriomas. Hostile factors in the peritoneal fluid, such as activated macrophages (which may phagocytize sperm) and excess prostaglandins (which may impair ovulation or fallopian tube motility), have also been suggested (17).

Until recently, most experts agreed that mild or minimal endometriosis did not play a role in infertility (24). However, recent pooled data (25) suggest that laparoscopic surgery led to a higher incidence of subsequent pregnancy (odds ratio, 2.7; 95% confidence interval, 2.1 to 3.5) than danazol or no treatment. More recently, a prospective, randomized trial of 341 infertile women with minimal or mild endometriosis, demonstrated fertility benefit of laparoscopic resection or ablation compared with diagnostic laparascopy alone. The 36-week cumulative incidence of subsequent pregnancy was 30.7% in the treated group compared with 17.7% in the diagnostic laparoscopy group (26).

It has long been apparent that conservative surgical treatment of more severe disease is associated with enhanced pregnancy rates, probably due in part to the correction of mechanical factors that were preventing pregnancy. Follow-up studies suggest that if spontaneous conception does not occur within 3 years after removal of endometriosis, a successful, spontaneous pregnancy is rare. Pregnancy is nonetheless sometimes possible with assisted reproductive technologies (see Chapter 20).

Diagnosis

Definitive diagnosis of endometriosis requires direct visualization and biopsy of suspected lesions. For pelvic endometriosis, this is usually accomplished laparoscopically by a gynecologist familiar with its various appearances. However, a thorough history and physical examination can usually yield a presumptive diagnosis.

History

The typical patient with endometriosis presents with a history of chronic pelvic pain or infertility or both (Table 11-3). The pelvic pain can be quite variable, but the classic symptom is secondary dysmenorrhea (i.e., painful menses beginning years after menarche) (see Chapter 12). The dysmenorrhea of endometriosis often begins 1 to 2 days before the onset of menses and continues throughout the duration of bleeding. The pain most likely stems from prostaglandin secretion by the ectopic endometrial tissue and, while typically

Table 11-3 Frequency of Symptoms in Patients with Endometriosis

Symptom	Frequency, %
Dysmenorrhea	60–80
Pelvic pain	30–50
Infertility	30–40
Dyspareunia	25–40
Menstrual irregularities	10–20
Cyclical dysuria/hematuria	1–2
Dyschezia	1–2
Rectal bleeding (cyclic)	<1

intermittent and cyclic, in some women the pain may be continuous. When endometriosis involves the deeper aspects of the posterior cul-de-sac, recto-vaginal septum, and uterosacral ligaments, patients may also complain of dysuria, dyschezia, backache, and dyspareunia, especially with deep penetration. Many symptoms of pelvic endometriosis therefore overlap with those associated with disorders of the genitourinary tract or gastrointestinal system (Table 11-4).

Patients may also report cyclic premenstrual spotting beginning within a few days before the onset of normal menstrual flow. One should therefore elicit a menstrual history as well as a careful description of the pain and its precise relationship to menses. Although the onset of the secondary dysmenorrhea may be abrupt, an insidious onset with gradual worsening of pelvic pain over successive menses is more typical of endometriosis. A presentation of acute onset of pain requires that such processes as pelvic inflammatory disease (PID), adnexal torsion, hemorrhagic luteal cysts, urinary tract infections, renal stones, and diverticulitis be excluded (see Chapter 9). A menstrual diary is often useful to record the timing of the pain and any premenstrual spotting.

One should also inquire whether there is a family history of endometriosis and elucidate any potential risk factors such as short menstrual cycle intervals or longer duration of menses. However, not all patients with endometriosis have risk factors. One should also carefully question the patient regarding

Table 11-4 Symptoms of Endometriosis in Relation to Site of Lesions*

Anatomical Site	Symptoms
Female reproductive tract	Dysmenorrhea Lower abdominal and pelvic pain Dyspareunia Infertility Menstrual irregularity Rupture/torsion of endometrioma Low-back pain
Gastrointestinal tract	Cyclical tenesmus/rectal bleeding Diarrhea Colonic obstruction
Urinary tract	Cyclical hematuria or pain Ureteral obstruction
Surgical scars, umbilicus	Cyclical pain and bleeding
Lung	Cyclical hemoptysis

*Surgical studies have demonstrated that the location and depth of endometrial implants may produce distinctive symptom patterns. Note, however, that pain severity often correlates poorly with the extent of the disease (1,27,28).

symptoms related to the urinary and gastrointestinal tracts to help exclude these potential sources of the pelvic pain.

Because patients with endometriosis are commonly misdiagnosed with cystitis or pelvic inflammatory disease, endometriosis should be considered in women for whom supportive laboratory evidence for these diagnoses is repeatedly lacking.

It is not uncommon for the patient with endometriosis to describe prior visits to physician offices or emergency rooms where her symptoms were attributed to such diagnoses as cystitis or PID. One should not be misled by this history, however, and one should recognize that many patients with endometriosis are stigmatized (sometimes repeatedly) by a presumptive diagnosis of PID. These patients often benefit from additional time in the office visit to validate the emotional responses to both the chronic pelvic pain and incorrect diagnoses and to educate the patient regarding the challenge of diagnosing endometriosis.

Physical Examination

A general physical examination, including careful attention to the abdomen, should precede the pelvic exam. The pelvic exam often yields the most findings when performed just before or during menstruation, when lesions are most active and symptoms most severe. Although endometriosis is uncommon in the vagina, it can occasionally be seen in the vaginal fornices or cervical canal as small, bluish, grape-like nodules. Any lesions should be biopsied and a histologic diagnosis obtained. To exclude infections as the source of the chronic pelvic pain, any abnormal vaginal discharge or evidence of cervical inflammation requires further investigation; even in the absence of exam findings, cervical specimens for chlamydia and gonorrhea are usually sent.

Bimanual exam may reveal tenderness in the vaginal fornices or cervical motion tenderness. Adnexal fullness and tenderness may represent an endometrioma of the ovary. A retroverted, fixed uterus is suggestive of adhesions due to endometriosis in the posterior cul-de-sac. The rectovaginal exam is essential, because it may demonstrate thickening or nodularity of the uterosacral ligaments and cul-de-sac peritoneum. Isolated tenderness in the anterior vaginal wall is more likely due to a primary urological process such as bladder disease, urethritis, or an urethral diverticulum.

If the patient is not menstruating, a stool guaic should be performed. A positive test may be due to endometriosis, but it should be assumed to result from a primary gastrointestinal lesion until such pathology is appropriately excluded. The patient who is menstruating is given three guaic cards to complete at home and return.

Laboratory Evaluation and Imaging Techniques

The CA-125 is a high-molecular-weight glycoprotein expressed on the cell surface of derivatives of embryonic coelomic epithelium. While commonly elevated in women with epithelial ovarian cancers, pelvic infections, uterine fibroids, pancreatitis, chronic liver disease, and during pregnancy or menstruation, it is also a marker for endometriosis (29). One study reported that 80% of women with pain and endometriosis had a serum CA-125 concentration greater than 16 U/mL (29). However, the CA-125 may be in the normal range in women that have only mild or minimal disease, and in general this marker lacks adequate sensitivity and specificity for general use as a diagnostic tool (30). However, for patients with elevated levels who subsequently undergo surgical treatment for their endometriosis, serial monitoring may help signal disease recurrence, and for those patients with infertility, a low postoperative CA-125 concentration predicts greater likelihood of spontaneous pregnancy (31).

A pelvic transvaginal ultrasound is often useful in confirming ovarian endometriomas detected on pelvic exam. These ovarian cysts may be unilocular or septated and typically have a sonographic "ground glass" appearance. They tend to persist and often become quite large. When a "chocolate" cyst (named such for its content of brown blood debris) is diagnosed, often plans are made for its surgical drainage and resection. Such a cyst is at risk for rupture, which causes acute pelvic pain from irritation of the peritoneum by the "chocolate" material contained inside. The subsequent inflammatory response can result in dense adhesions that may be particularly difficult to dissect.

Laparoscopy

Laparoscopy is an outpatient surgical procedure often used to confirm the diagnosis of endometriosis and allow for surgical treatment. The procedure involves placement of a laparoscope 2 to10 mm in diameter through a puncture site in the umbilicus. One to three more puncture sites, usually 5 to 12 mm in diameter, are placed in the lower abdomen. The peritoneal cavity is then insufflated with carbon dioxide to elevate the anterior abdominal wall and permit visualization of the lower pelvis. General anesthesia is most often used; however, the patient usually goes home within a few hours after the procedure and is back to work or normal home activities within 24 to 48 hr. Side effects following the procedure include mild pelvic discomfort, occasional shoulder pain due to diaphragmatic irritation from the carbon dioxide, and anesthetic sequelae. Newer techniques to visualize the pelvis include gasless laparoscopy, which can be performed without general anesthesia, and office laparoscopy using a smaller (2 mm) diameter laparoscope, small amounts of intraperitoneal gas insufflation, and intravenous sedation.

The "classic" laparoscopic appearance of endometriosis is a blue or black lesion with a "powder burn" appearance. Other presentations include white, "scarred" lesions resembling old operative scars or fibrotic remnants from previous pelvic infections, and reddish, hemorrhagic lesions, which are the most active (32). Clear, vesicular lesions are usually seen in younger women and probably represent early disease (32). These lesions are also difficult to visualize during laparoscopy unless it is performed by an experienced laparoscopist. Biopsies should be taken from lesions to help confirm the diagnosis. Lesions may invade as deeply as 5 mm into the peritoneum or remain as superficial as 1 to 2 mm (32), and it is often difficult to appreciate the depth of an endometriotic implant. Lesions commonly mistaken for endometriosis include hemangiomas, old sutures, necrotic areas from old ectopic pregnancies, cancer cells, epithelial inclusion cysts, residual carbon from previous laser surgery or coagulation devices, hysterosalpingogram dye reaction, and inflammatory cysts (32).

Adhesions are another common finding in patients with endometriosis. These typically result from the inflammatory process of endometriosis or from the rupture of endometriomas. Adhesions may completely obliterate the cul-de-sac or adnexae and involve the bowel (33). Though adhesions represent an important cause of infertility, they generally do not cause pelvic pain. In some cases, the extent of adhesions may prohibit laparoscopy, forcing the surgeon to resort to a laparotomy at a later date following adequate bowel preparation.

The American Society for Reproductive Medicine (formerly the American Fertility Society) has classified endometriosis based on surgical findings (Table 11-5) (34). In this classification, endometriosis is divided into stages of severity based on extent and size of peritoneal disease, ovarian involvement, and severity of adhesions involving the ovaries and fallopian tubes; thus the system attempts to quantitate the effect on fertility. A major shortcoming is that it makes little attempt to designate the expected degree of pelvic pain. Nonetheless, the classification system provides a framework for the surgeon to document the location and size of lesions as well as the extent of adhesions, and allows for objectivity and standardization, and therefore is included in the operative report.

Table 11-5 American Society for Reproductive Medicine Revised Endometriosis Classification

Endometriosis		<1 cm	1–3 cm	>3 cm
Peritoneum	Superficial	1	2	4
	Deep	2	4	6
Ovary	R Superficial	1	2	4
	Deep	4	16	20
	L Superficial	1	2	4
	Deep	4	16	20

		Partial	Complete
Cul-de-sac	Posterior cul-de-sac obliteration	4	40

Adhesions		<$^1/_3$ Enclosre	$^1/_3$–$^2/_3$ Enclosure	>$^2/_3$ Enclosure
Ovary	R Filmy	1	2	4
	Dense	4	8	16
	L Filmy	1	2	4
	Dense	4	8	16
Tube	R Filmy	1	2	4
	Dense	4	8	16
	L Filmy	1	2	4
	Dense	4	8	16

Classification	Stage	Total Score
Minimal	I	1–5
Mild	II	6–15
Moderate	III	16–40
Severe	IV	>40

Data from American Fertility Society. Revised American Fertility Society classification of endometriosis. Fertil Steril. 1985;43:351. (The American Fertility Society is now the American Society for Reproductive Medicine.)

Treatment

In discussing any treatment modality, it is important to understand that there is no cure for endometriosis. Treatment is directed solely towards improving fertility, reducing symptoms, and preventing disease progression. Surgical treatment is invasive and carries the risk of complications; however, it is the only treatment demonstrated to improve fertility outcomes. Medical therapy avoids operative risks but is fraught with side effects and is only beneficial in relieving symptoms.

The choice of treatment is influenced by the severity of the patient's symptoms, age, fertility desires, willingness for surgery, and ability to tolerate side effects, and therefore must be individualized. For example, a young patient with unwanted infertility might choose surgical treatment, even if her symptoms are only mild. On the other hand, a woman with severe symptoms but for whom fertility is not an issue may opt for either surgical or medical therapy. Medical therapy may be more appropriate for women nearing menopause and for those who have already undergone surgical treatment without significant success. Not infrequently, patients who have suffered years of severe pelvic pain despite numerous and various treatment trials may opt to undergo definitive surgery (hysterectomy and oophorectomy)—even young, nulliparous patients.

Expectant Management

Though endometriosis is usually a progressive disease, it may vary widely from one individual to another, and sometimes spontaneous improvement occurs. Expectant management avoids the risks of surgery and the side effects of medications; however, its disadvantage is the lost opportunity to intervene and potentially prevent disease progression. For those who opt for expectant management—in fact, for all patients with endometriosis—the nonsteroidal anti-inflammatory medications (NSAIDs) offer some symptom relief.

Conservative Surgery

With the advent of laparoscopy and recent advances in instrumentation, endometriosis is almost always treated surgically at the time of diagnostic laparoscopy. Doing so prevents implants from infiltrating more deeply or diffusely and may improve fertility rates as well as eliminate pelvic pain. Most mild and moderate cases can be handled well through laparoscopy. Severe cases, especially those where dissection is difficult, or those involving large endometriomas, are more commonly managed with laparotomy. In such cases, preoperative ovarian suppression may be useful in decreasing the amount of vascularity and inflammation.

Laparoscopy may be used for mild or moderate endometriosis, and may improve fertility as well as eliminate pain.

Elimination of endometriosis is achieved by excision, fulguration using bipolar coagulation, or laser vaporization. The peritoneal defects created during surgery will spontaneously reperitonealize but if extremely large are reapproximated with fine sutures. Lysis of adhesions can be performed with the laser, bipolar cautery, hydrodissection, or sharply with scissors. Adhesion reformation is found at 37% to 72% of surgical sites. New adhesion formation is less common during laparoscopy than with surgery at laparotomy. Often, adhesion barriers or gels may be placed over adnexae, the uterus, or "raw" sites to prevent formation of further adhesions. Many surgeons will remove the appendix, because up to 13% of patients will have histologic evidence of endometriosis; however, appendectomy is contraindicated in infertility patients due to the remote chance of infection from stump leakage and subsequent adhesion formation. The rate of recurrence of endometriosis following conservative surgery is reported to range from 2% to 50%, and a repeat surgical procedure is required in at least 15% of patients.

Endometriosis of the ovary usually starts as a small lesion, then develops into a cyst filled with brownish fluid, the so-called "chocolate" cyst. These cysts cannot be simply drained, since the recurrence rate is at least 50% (1). The cyst must be opened, drained, and the cyst wall dissected and removed in order to eradicate any functioning endometriotic tissue.

For those patients with significant pelvic pain, several adjuvant procedures can be employed. In patients with primarily midline pelvic pain, a presacral neurectomy has been shown to be quite effective. The procedure involves excising a small portion of the hypogastric plexus as it passes over the sacral promontory. Constipation, vaginal dryness, and bladder dysfunction are potential complications but usually disappear in a few months. Sixty to seventy percent of these patients may have complete resolution of their pain for many years (35,36). A uterine suspension may be utilized in those women with endometriosis and a retroflexed uterus. Its purpose is to prevent the formation of dense adhesions in the posterior cul-de-sac as well as re-adhesion of the tubes and ovaries to a site that has been extensively denuded. Laparoscopic uterine nerve ablation (LUNA) can treat the dysmenorrhea associated with endometriosis. Using the laser or electrocautery technique, the uterosacral ligaments are divided at the point of attachment to the cervix, thereby interrupting most of the sensory innervation of the cervix and uterine corpus. Up to 80% of patients experience some relief, although the duration of benefit is unknown (37).

There are some women with severe pelvic pain, who are either young or desire the potential for future fertility, who are unresponsive to medical and surgical therapy. For some of these women, a multi-disciplinary approach that includes a chronic pain clinic may be useful. For others, a hysterectomy with ovarian preservation may offer pain relief. However, following hysterectomy pain will sometimes recur, and approximately 3% to 10% of patients will require a second operation to remove the ovaries. Medical hypoestrogenic therapy after surgical intervention may be useful in helping avoid a second procedure if endometriotic implants remain.

Definitive Surgery

Definitive surgery consists of hysterectomy and bilateral oophorectomy and in effect, is surgical castration. In addition, the appendix and areas of the pelvic parietal peritoneum that are covered with endometriosis are removed. This approach is primarily for women with long-standing disease and uncontrollable pain who no longer desire fertility. The patient will develop menopausal symptoms shortly after surgery due to the rapid fall in her estrogen level. Many surgeons will opt to delay placing the patient on estrogen replacement therapy for 3 to 6 months, especially if a large amount of residual endometriosis is left behind.

Medical Therapy

There are four commonly used medical strategies in the treatment of endometriosis: oral contraceptives, progestins, gonadotropin-releasing hormone antagonists, and danazol (Table 11-6). Each has been shown to reduce both the amount of endometriosis and the severity of pelvic pain. However, unlike surgery, none has been shown to improve fertility compared to expectant management.

Medical therapy is useful in reducing the amount of endometriosis and avoids operative risks, but it does not improve fertility.

Oral Contraceptives

Combined oral contraceptives have long been used to treat endometriosis. Rationale for their use was based on the observation that pregnancy provided pain relief and diminished the number and extent of endometrial implants. Endometriotic tissue decidualizes, undergoes necrosis, and involutes with this therapy. Although most data are from studies using the older, high-dose estrogen pills, the usual low-dose combination pills are now standard. Importantly, only monophasic regimens can be used.

The first tablet is taken by day 3 of the patient's menses, then taken continuously (without using the placebo pills) until breakthrough bleeding occurs, at which time the dose is doubled to eliminate the breakthrough bleeding. If breakthrough bleeding persists, the dose is increased to one tablet three times daily until the bleeding stops. After 5 days of the increased dose, the patient is then weaned back to 1 to 2 pills a day in order to maintain the amenorrheic state. It is essential to emphasize to the patient that this is a continuous, rather than a cyclic, regimen. Most patients can maintain this protocol for 6 to 9 months. The same contraindications that apply to contra-

Table 11-6 Endometriosis Treatment Regimens

Drug	Dose	Success Rate, %
Danazol ($)	100–400 mg PO q day for 3–9 months	90
GnRHa ($)		
Intramuscular (leuprolide acetate [Lupron])	3.75 mg/month for 6 months	90
Intranasal (nafarelin [Synarel])	200 mg/spray bid for 6 months	90
Subcutaneous (goserelin acetate implant [Zoladex])	3.6 mg every month for 6 months	90
Progestins		
Medroxyprogesterone	30-40 mg PO q day for 6 months	80
Depot progesterone (Depo-Provera)	100–200 mg/month for 6 months	80
Megestrol	40 mg/day for up to 24 months	86
Norethindrone	5 mg/day up to 15 mg/day for 6 months	80
Oral contraceptives	1 tablet/day and increase dose to control breakthrough bleeding for 6–9 months	50–80

ceptive use of birth control pills also apply to these patients. Approximately 50% to 80% of patients experience pain relief (38). Side effects are characteristic of oral contraceptive use and include weight gain, nausea, breast tenderness, increased appetite, depression, irritability, depression, and increased vaginal discharge. Approximately one-third of women will discontinue treatment due to these side effects (38).

Progestin Regimens

Progestin-only regimens have gained popularity due to the multiple side effects of the continuous combined oral contraceptive regimen. Progestins work by suppressing ovarian steroidogenesis, promoting decidualization of endometrial tissue, opposing the growth-promoting effects of estrogen, decreasing the density of the nuclear estrogen receptor at the cellular level, and helping convert the potent estradiol to the weaker estrone. By eliminating cyclic bleeding, progestins also prevent menstrual reflux.

Medroxyprogesterone acetate is usually given in an oral daily dose of 30 to 40 mg per day for at least 6 months, with relief of pain noted in up to 80% of women (39,40). Megestrol acetate in a daily oral dose of 40 mg per day for up to 24 months offers relief in up to 86% of patients (41). Norethindrone acetate is another option, begun at 5 mg per day and increased by 2.5 mg per day every 2 weeks up to a maintenance dose of 15 mg per day. Depot medroxyprogesterone acetate (Depo-Provera) has been found effective when dosed more frequently than that required for contraception; it is usually pre-scribed as a dose of 100 to 200 mg IM monthly. The progestins are usually continued for 6 to 9 months. Side effects include depression, irritability, breakthrough bleeding, minor weight gain, and edema. In addition, depot medroxyprogesterone acetate may be complicated by a delayed (up to 1 or 2 years) return of ovulatory function and fertility.

Gonadotropin-Releasing Hormone Agonists

Gonadotropin-releasing hormone agonists (GnRHa) are structurally altered forms of endogenous gonadotropin-releasing hormone which, when given in continuous fashion beyond one week, paradoxically inhibit LH and FSH re-lease from the pituitary, resulting in decreased ovarian steroid production (42,43). Estrogen levels reach near-menopausal levels and amenorrhea re-sults. GnRHa is usually administered for up to 6 months. Longer periods of therapy are associated with significant bone loss, albeit with uncertain clini-cal importance (44–46).

There are three GnRHa formulations available: a depot form given monthly (depot leuprolide acetate [Lupron] 3.75 mg IM), a nasal spray (na-farelin [Synarel] 200 mcg/spray bid), and a long-acting subcutaneous implant (goserelin acetate implant [Zoladex] 3.6 mg implanted SC monthly). All forms are equally effective. Side effects relate to the induction of the hypoestrogenic state and, in addition to the bone loss, include hot flashes, vaginal dryness, in-somnia, emotional lability, chronic fatigue, headaches, and depression.

Recently "add-back" hormone replacement therapy (HRT) has been added to the GnRHa regimens to ameliorate these side effects. This strategy has been shown to be effective while not attenuating the endometriosis benefit. One study demonstrated that either usual-dose HRT (conjugated estrogen 0.625 mg/day plus medroxyprogesterone acetate 5 mg/day) and low-dose HRT (conjugated estrogen 0.3 mg/day plus medroxyprogesterone acetate 5 mg/day) are equally effective (47).

Danazol

Danazol is a 2,3-isoxazole derivative of the synthetic steroid ethisterone (17-alpha-ethinyltestosterone) that has multiple mechanisms of action—many of them androgenic, and all of which lead to atrophy of endometriotic implants. The dose ranges from 200 to 800 mg orally per day divided into two to four doses; however, doses greater than 400 mg per day have been shown to be no more effective than lower doses (48). At least 6 months of therapy is needed to achieve good results in the face of extensive disease, and often ovarian en-dometriomas do not respond. Side effects include weight gain, muscle cramps, decreased breast size, mood changes, oily skin, depression, sweating, edema, appetite changes, acne, hirsutism, and deepening of the voice. Regular menses usually continue, but irregular bleeding is not uncommon, especially with lower doses of danazol (48). Due to its androgenic effects, bone loss is not significant (49); however, danazol does temporarily decrease high-density lipoprotein (HDL) and increase low-density lipoprotein (LDL) cholesterol (50). Because of these multiple adverse side effects and the availability of other agents, danazol is now used infrequently as a first-line medical therapy.

Recurrence

Recurrent endometriosis is heralded by the reappearance of symptoms and/or signs that led to the initial diagnosis. Recurrence rates ranging from 2% to 20% have been reported. The reoperation rate for recurrent disease is approximately 15%; most second operations occur within 1 to 5 years of the first (51). Many studies show a decreased recurrence rate following a second procedure; however, these studies have limited follow-up.

Conclusion

Despite its discovery over a century ago endometriosis remains an enigmatic disease without definite etiology or cure. Current treatment, whether medical or surgical, is often only temporarily beneficial. Many women have had their reproductive years shortened due to this devastating disease. In extreme cases patients suffer with severe symptoms of chronic pain until definitive surgery. Earlier detection by the primary care physician may allow for more timely intervention and, perhaps, better outcomes.

REFERENCES

1. **Shaw RW.** Atlas of Endometriosis. New York: Parthenon Publishing Group; 1993:25.
2. **Thomas EJ.** Questioning the approaches. Intl J Gynecol Obstet. 1999;64(Suppl 1), S23.
3. **Guzick DS.** Clinical epidemiology of endometriosis and infertility. Obstet Gynecol Clin North Am. 1989;16:43.
4. **Houston DE, Noller KL, Melton LJ, et al.** Incidence of pelvic endometriosis in Rochester, Minnesota, 1970-1979. Am J Epidemiol. 1987;125:959-69.
5. **Barbieri RL.** Etiology and epidemiology of endometriosis. Am J Obstset Gynecol. 1990;162:565.
6. **Cramer DW, Wilson E, Stillman RJ, et al.** The relation of endometriosis to menstrual characteristics, smoking and exercise. JAMA. 1986;225:1904-8.
7. **Olive DL, Henderson DY.** Endometriosis and müllerian anomalies. Obstet Gynecol. 1987;69:412.

8.   Simpson JL, Elias S, Malinak LR, Buttram VC. Heritable aspects of endometriosis. I—Genetic studies. Am J Obstet Gynecol. 1980;137:327.

9.   Malinak LR, Buttram VC, Elias S, Simpson JL. Heritable aspects of endometriosis. II—Clinical characteristics of familial endometriosis. Am J Obstet Gynecol. 1980;137: 332.

10.   Kruitwagen RF, Poels LG, Willemsen WN, et al. Endometrial epithelial cells in peritoneal fluid during the early follicular phase. Fertil Steril. 1991;55:297.

11.   Sampson JA. Peritoneal endometriosis due to menstrual dissemination of endometrial tissue into peritoneal cavity. Am J Obstet Gynecol. 1927;14:422.

12.   Hanton EM, Malkasian GD, Dockerty MB, Pratt JH. Endometriosis associated with complete or partial obstruction of menstrual egress. Obstet Gynecol. 1966;28:626.

13.   Halme J, Hammond MG, Hulka JF. Retrograde menstruation in healthy women and in patients with endometriosis. Obstet Gynecol. 1984;64:151.

14.   Blumenkrantz MJ, Gallagher N, Bashore RA. Retrograde menstruation in women undergoing chronic peritoneal dialysis. Obstet Gynecol. 1981;57:667.

15.   Javert CT. Pathogenesis of endometriosis based on endometrial hyperplasia, direct extension exfoliation and implantation, lymphatic and hematogenous metastasis. Cancer. 1949;2:399.

16.   Gruenwald P. Origin of endometriosis from the mesenchyme of the coelomic walls. Am J Obstet Gynecol. 1942;44:470.

17.   Hill JA, Faris HMP, Schiff I. Characterization of leukocyte subpopulations in the peritoneal fluid of women with endometriosis. Fertil Steril. 1988;50:216.

18.   Meek SC, Hodge DD, Musich JR. Autoimmunity in infertile patients with endometriosis. Am J Obstet Gynecol. 1988;158:1365.

19.   Moen MH. Endometriosis in monozygotic twins. Acta Obstet Gynecol Scand. 1994; 73:59.

20.   Lessey BA, Castelbaum AJ, Sawin SW, et al. Aberrant integrin expession in the endometrium of women with endometriosis. J Clin Endocrinol Metab. 1994;79:643.

21.   Rier SE, Martin DC, Bowman RE, et al. Endometriosis in rhesus monkeys (*Macaca mulatta*) following chronic exposure to 2,3,7,8-tetrachlorodibenzo-*p*-dioxin. Fundam Appl Toxicol. 1983;21:433.

22.   Bois FY, Eskenazi B. Possible risk of endometriosis for Seveso, Italy residents: an asessment of exposure to dioxin. Environ Health Perspect. 1994;102:476.

23.   Safe S, Astroff B, Harris M, et al. 2,3,7,8-Tetrachlorodibenzo-*p*-dioxin (TCDD) and related compounds as antiestrogens: characterization and mechanism of action. Pharmacol Toxicol. 1991;69:400.

24.   Schenken RS, Malinak LR. Conservative surgery versus expectant management for the infertile patient with mild endometriosis. Fertil Steril. 1982;37:183.

25.   Hughes EG, Fedorkow DM, Collins JA. A quantitative overview of controlled trials in endometriosis-associated infertility. Fertil Steril. 1993;59:963-70.

26.   Marcoux S, Maheux R, Berube S, and the Canadian Collaborative Group on Endometriosis. Laparoscopic surgery in infertile women with minimal or mild endometriosis. N Engl J Med. 1997;337:217-22.

27.   Redwine DB. The distribution of endometriosis in the pelvis by age group and fertility. Fertil Steril. 1987;47:173.

28. **Fedele L, Parazzini F, Bianchi S, et al.** Stage and localization of pelvic endometriosis and pain. Fertil Steril. 1990;53:155.

29. **Mashashi T, Matsuzawa K, Onsawa M.** Serum CA-125 levels in patients with endometriosis: changes in CA-125 levels during menstruation. Fertil Steril. 1988;72:328.

30. **Pittaway DE.** CA-125 in women with endometriosis. Obstet Gynecol Clin N Am. 1989;16:237.

31. **Pittaway DE, Rondinone D, Miller KA, Barnes K.** Clinical evaluation of CA-125 concentrations as a prognostic factor for pregnancy in infertile women with surgically treated endometriosis. Fertil Steril. 1995;64:321-4.

32. **Martin DC, Hubert GD, Vander Zwaag R, El-Zeky FA.** Laparoscopic appearances of peritoneal endometriosis. Fertil Steril. 1989;51:63.

33. **Weed JC, Ray JE.** Endometriosis of the bowel. Obstet Gynecol. 1987;69:727.

34. **American Fertility Society.** Revised American Fertility Society classification of endometriosis. Fertil Steril. 1985;43:351.

35. **Tjaden B, Schlaff WD, Kimball A.** The efficacy of presacral neurectomy for the relief of midline dysmenorrhea. Obstet Gynecol. 1990;76:89.

36. **Polan ML, DeCherney A.** Presacral neurectomy for pelvic pain in infertility. Fertil Steril. 1980;34:557.

37. **Lichten EM, Bombard J.** Surgical treatment of primary dysmenorrhea with laparoscopic uterine nerve ablation. J Reprod Med. 1987;32:37.

38. **Noble AD, Lechtworth AT.** Medical treatment of endometriosis: a comparative trial. Postgrad Med J. 1979;55(Suppl 5):37.

39. **Luciano AA, Turksoy RN, Carleo J.** Evaluation of oral medroxyprogesterone acetate in the treatment of endometriosis. Obstet Gynecol. 1988;72:323.

40. **Moghissi KS, Boyce CRK.** Management of endometriosis with oral medroxyprogesterone acetate. Obstet Gynecol. 1976;47:265.

41. **Schlaff WD, Dugoff L, Damewood MD.** Megestrol acetate for treatment of endometriosis. Obstet Gynecol. 1990;75:646.

42. **Vickery BH, Nestor JJ.** Luteinizing hormone-releasing analogues: development and mechanism of action. Semin Reprod Endocrinol. 1987;5:353.

43. **Henzl MR.** Gonadotropin-releasing hormone (GnRH) agonists in the management of endometriosis: a review. Clin Obstet Gynecol. 1988;31:840.

44. **Jacobsen JB.** Effects of nafarelin on bone density. Am J Obstet Gynecol. 1990;162:591.

45. **Schenken RS.** Gonadotropin-releasing hormone analogs in the treatment of endometriosis. Am J Obstet Gynecol. 1990;162:579.

46. **Henzl MR.** Administration of nasal nafarelin as compared with oral danazol for endometriosis: a multicenter double-blind comparative clinical trial. N Engl J Med. 1988;318:485.

47. **Moghissi KS, Schlaff WD, Olive DL, et al.** Goserelin acetate (Zoladex) with or without hormone replacement therapy for the treatment of endometriosis. Fertil Steril. 1998;69:1056-62.

48. **Barbieri RL.** Comparison of the pharmacology of nafarelin and danazol. Am J Obstet Gynecol. 1990;162:581.

49. **Dawood MY, Lewis V, Ramos J.** Cortical and trabecular bone content in women with endometriosis: effect of gonadotropin-releasing hormone agonist and danazol. Fertil Steril. 1984;42:709.

50. **Allen JK, Fraser IS.** Cholesterol, high density lipoprotein and danazol. J Clin Endocrinol Metabol. 1981;53:149.

51. **Wheeler JM, Malinak LR.** Recurrent endometriosis. Contemp Gynecol Obstet. 1987; 41:14-9.

CHAPTER 12

Chronic Pelvic Pain

JODI L. FRIEDMAN, MD

ANDREA J. RAPKIN, MD

Chronic pelvic pain (CPP) is generally defined as pelvic pain that persists for at least 6 months. It is one of the more common gynecologic complaints encountered, yet both the diagnosis and management of this disorder remain challenging and often unsatisfying. Unfortunately, even after thorough evaluation the etiology of the pain often remains obscure; indeed, even when certain types of pathology are discovered at laparoscopy (e.g., endometriosis, adhesions, venous congestion), there is not always a clear or consistent relationship to the patient's pain symptomatology (1). Furthermore, over one third of patients with CPP have no identifiable somatic pathology after a thorough evaluation.

Patients with CPP are frequently anxious and depressed and usually have experienced significant disruption of their social, marital, and occupational lives. Protracted disability, inappropriate health care utilization, and high rates of undiagnosed psychological morbidity have all been observed in cross-sectional studies (2).

Epidemiology and Demographics

While the exact prevalence of CPP is not known, one survey of 651 women revealed a current prevalence of 12% and a lifetime occurrence rate of 33% (3). The mean age of presentation of CPP is between 25 and 30 years old; there does not appear to be any difference between races or educational status. Women with CPP often have a longstanding pattern of somatic symptomatology, and there is a high rate of history of sexual and physical abuse (48% vs. 7% in controls according to one large study) (2,4). Approximately 10% of referrals to gynecologists are for CPP, and 12% of hysterectomies performed in the United States are for CPP. Interestingly, 12% to 30% of patients who present to pain clinics for CPP have already undergone a hysterectomy, clearly underscoring the point that hysterectomy is not always definitive treatment for CPP.

Differential Diagnoses

The differential diagnosis of CPP is extensive and includes both gynecologic and nongynecologic conditions (Box 12-1). Gynecologic causes of CPP are classically divided into cyclic versus noncyclic patterns of pain, with the inference being that cyclic pain is caused by conditions directly related to menstruation. However, several conditions may cause both cyclic and noncyclic patterns of pain. Additionally, there are nongynecologic conditions, such as irritable bowel syndrome, that may be exacerbated by the menstrual cycle and therefore present with a cyclic pain pattern. Nevertheless, this dichotomous schema remains a useful diagnostic construct, provided the clinician is aware of these potential confounding factors.

Because some nongynecologic conditions may be exacerbated by the menstrual cycle and therefore present with a cyclic pain pattern, the pain may be mistakenly interpreted as gynecologic.

The laparoscopic findings of women with and without CPP are shown in Table 12-1. As stated previously, over one third of patients have no identifiable somatic pathology after undergoing a complete work-up including laparoscopy. Among the women with CPP and no identifiable pathology at the time of laparoscopy, the most common diagnoses are irritable bowel syndrome and myofascial pain (5).

Even after a full work-up that includes laparoscopy, more than one third of patients have no identifiable cause of pelvic pain.

Cyclic Pelvic Pain

Cyclic pelvic pain refers to pain occurring at the time of, or beginning up to 2 weeks before, menses that is due to primary or secondary dysmenorrhea. Pain

---

Box 12-1 Causes of Chronic Pelvic Pain

Gynecologic
Noncyclic
  Adhesions
  Endometriosis
  Salpingo-oophoritis
  Ovarian remnant syndrome
  Pelvic congestion syndrome (varicosities)
  Pelvic neoplasms
  Pelvic relaxation
Cyclic
  Primary dysmenorrhea
  Secondary dysmenorrhea
    Imperforate hymen
    Transverse vaginal septum
    Cervical stenosis
    Uterine anomalies (congenital malformation, bicornuate uterus, blind uterine horn)
    Intrauterine synechiae (Asherman's syndrome)
    Endometrial polyps
    Uterine leiomyoma
    Adenomyosis
    Pelvic congestion syndrome (varicosities)
    Endometriosis
Atypical cyclic
  Endometriosis
  Adenomyosis
  Ovarian remnant syndrome
  Chronic functional cyst formation
Gastrointestinal
  Irritable bowel syndrome
  Inflammatory bowel disease
  Carcinoma
  Infectious diarrhea
  Recurrent partial small bowel obstruction
  Diverticulitis
  Hernia (inguinal or femoral)
  Abdominal angina
Genitourinary
  Recurrent or relapsing cystourethritis
  Painful bladder syndrome
  Urethral syndrome
  Interstitial cystitis
  Ureteral diverticuli or polyps
  Carcinoma of the bladder
  Ureteral obstruction
  Pelvic kidney
Neurologic
  Nerve entrapment syndrome
  Neuroma
Musculoskeletal
  Low back pain syndrome
    Congenital anomalies
    Scoliosis and kyphosis
    Spondylarthropathies
    Spinal injuries
    Tumors
    Osteoporosis
    Degenerative changes
    Coccydynia
  Myofascial syndrome
  Fibromyalgia
Systemic
  Acute intermittent porphyria
  Abdominal migraine
  Systemic lupus erythematosus
  Lymphoma
  Neurofibromatosis

Table 12-1 Laparoscopic Findings in Women with and without CPP*

	No. of Patients	No Visible Pathology	Endo-metriosis	Adhesions	Myomas	Ovarian Cysts	Chronic PID	Pelvic Vari-cosities	Other
						(%) ──────→			
With CPP	1318	39	28	25	<1	3	6	<1	4
Without CPP	1103	72	5	17	2	—	1	—	2

*Combined data from 15 published studies. Adapted from Howard FM. The role of laparoscopy in chronic pelvic pain: promise and pitfalls. Obstet Gynecol Survey. 1993;48:357.

that occurs cyclically but not just before menses is called *atypical cyclic pelvic pain* and may be due to endometriosis, adenomyosis, ovarian remnant syndrome, or chronic functional cyst formation.

Dysmenorrhea

Dysmenorrhea affects up to 50% of menstruating women. *Primary dysmenorrhea* is menstrual pain without pelvic pathology, whereas *secondary dysmenorrhea* refers to painful menses with underlying pathology. Primary dysmenorrhea usually appears within 1 to 2 years of menarche, once ovulatory cycles are established. Younger women are more commonly affected, but it may persist throughout a woman's ovulatory years. The etiology of dysmenorrhea is related to increased endometrial prostaglandin production and elevated uterine tone. The pain of dysmenorrhea usually begins within hours of the onset of a menstrual period and can last up to 72 hr. The pain is colicky in nature with suprapubic cramping that often is accompanied by lumbosacral back pain and pain radiating down the anterior thighs. Like other visceral pain, it is deep, often poorly localized, and may be accompanied by nausea, vomiting, diarrhea, and, rarely, syncope.

Secondary dysmenorrhea commonly begins many years after menarche. Compared with primary dysmenorrhea, the duration of the cyclic painful episodes tends to be significantly longer, with pain sometimes beginning about 1 to 2 weeks before menses and persisting as long as a few days beyond cessation of bleeding. The nature of the pain is similar to that described for primary dysmenorrhea. Endometriosis is the most common cause of secondary dysmenorrhea, followed by adenomyosis. However, the differential diagnosis is long (see Box 12-1).

Endometriosis

The incidence of endometriosis is unknown but is estimated to be anywhere from 3% to 43% in the general female population; endometriosis is detected in 20% to 90% of patients undergoing a laparoscopy for CPP (6). However, there does not appear to be a consistent correlation between the extent of the endometriosis and the pain symptoms experienced by the patient (7). Endometriosis usually presents in women in their 30's or 40's but may be seen in younger women and adolescents as well. As can be seen in Box 12-1, endometriosis can present as classic cyclic pain, atypical cyclic pain, or as noncyclic pain. Endometriosis is discussed in detail in Chapter 10.

Adenomyosis

Adenomyosis refers to endometrial glands and stroma that have penetrated into the myometrium and is found in 8% to 20% of hysterectomy specimens. The peak incidence is in women aged 40 to 50 years. Dysmenorrhea due to adenomyosis often begins up to 1 week before menses and may persist throughout menstruation. Associated dyspareunia and dyschezia are common, and menorrhagia may also be present. On examination the uterus is diffusely enlarged, though usually less than 14 cm, and it is often soft and tender during menses.

Ovarian Remnant Syndrome

The ovarian remnant syndrome may occur following bilateral salpingo-oophorectomy. This syndrome results from residual ovarian tissue that is left *in situ,* usually due to difficult visceral dissection. The tissue can become functional and cystic and occasionally cause other complications such as ureteral obstruction. The patient usually complains of pain beginning about 2 to 5 years after the surgery. The pain may or may not be cyclic. The diagnosis can usually be confirmed by ultrasonography (especially if aided by clomiphene stimulation) and with an estradiol and FSH level that reveals a premenopausal picture, which can be determined after the patient has withheld hormone replacement therapy for at least 1 month.

Pelvic Congestion

It is controversial whether pelvic congestion is truly a cause of pelvic pain. Transuterine venography studies have revealed larger mean ovarian and uterine vein diameters, delayed disappearance of contrast medium, and ovarian congestion in a significantly greater percentage of women with CPP without obvious pathology than in those with identifiable pathology or control patients (1). Because of these findings, it has been postulated that perhaps autonomic dysfunction leading to pelvic congestion plays a primary role in pelvic pain in these patients. However, because vascular congestion may also be seen in pregnant and postpartum women who are completely asymptomatic, the true relationship between pelvic congestion and pelvic pain is uncertain. Symptoms of pelvic congestion consist of secondary dysmenorrhea, low back pain, dyspareunia, menorrhagia, and a high incidence of irritable bowel syndrome and chronic fatigue syndrome (6). Additionally, the ovaries are often enlarged with multiple functional cysts.

Noncyclic Pelvic Pain

Unlike cyclic and atypical cyclic pelvic pain, noncyclic pelvic pain is unaffected by the menstrual cycle. The causes of noncyclic pelvic pain are both gynecologic and nongynecologic.

Gynecologic Sources

ADHESIONS

Pelvic adhesions are thought to result from pelvic inflammatory disease (PID), endometriosis, prior surgery, perforated viscus (e.g., appendix, diverticulum), and inflammatory bowel disease, though only about 50% of women found to have pelvic adhesions have a known history of one of these conditions. Despite being a relatively common finding at laparoscopy, the role of adhesions in CPP remains uncertain. As can be seen in Table 12-1, the prevalence of adhesions is greater in patients with CPP than in patients without pain (25% vs. 17%); however, this difference is somewhat modest and it certainly does not establish a causal relationship. It has not been possible to demonstrate a relationship between the duration and severity of pain and the extent or location of adhesions (8). Studies have shown mixed results with regard to improvement in CPP after adhesiolysis. Women with dense bowel adhesions appear to have the best outcomes, whereas women with significant anxiety, depression, and somatic symptomatology pre-operatively appear to have the poorest outcomes (9,10).

SALPINGO-OOPHORITIS

Salpingo-oophoritis usually presents as an acute infection; however, atypical or partially treated infections may present as CPP without associated fever or peritoneal signs. Symptoms of subclinical disease may include noncyclic pelvic pain, menstrual irregularities, dyspareunia, increased vaginal discharge, and occasionally dysuria and suprapubic pain (11). Subacute, or atypical, salpingo-oophoritis is often a sequela of *Chlamydia* or *Mycoplasma* infection, or it may be due to active recurrent infection (6). Examination reveals abdominal tenderness, cervical motion tenderness, and bilateral adnexal tenderness. A purulent cervical discharge may be present. Diagnosis is established with positive cervical cultures; however, if physical examination is suggestive and/or the erythrocyte sedimentation rate is elevated, the patient should be treated empirically for salpingo-oophoritis.

PELVIC MASSES

When symptomatic, pelvic neoplasms and cysts most commonly cause acute pelvic pain (due to torsion, rupture, or degeneration) but may cause chronic symptoms, especially if large enough to encroach on adjacent pelvic structures. Uterine leiomyomata are the most common pelvic neoplasm; approximately 20% of women of reproductive age have fibroids that are clinically apparent. About 30% of women with fibroids will experience some pain or discomfort produced by direct pressure on supporting ligaments or other somatic structures such as bladder or bowel. Pelvic pressure, urinary frequency or urgency, and constipation may all be associated symptoms due to fibroids. Menorrhagia may also be present if the tumors are intramural or submucosal.

Ovarian cysts or neoplasms are less commonly the cause of CPP. Laparoscopic studies have revealed ovarian cysts in only 3% of patients undergoing laparoscopy for CPP (8). The majority of symptomatic cysts present as acute pelvic pain because of rupture, hemorrhage, or torsion, with chronic pain being distinctly less common, except in the case of an endometrioma. Ovarian neoplasms are even less common, occurring in less than 1% of women presenting with CPP. Ovarian cancer, about which the patient often has an underlying fear, is generally asymptomatic until peritoneal disease is present; even then, vague discomfort, abdominal distention, and nonspecific gastrointestinal symptoms predominate, not pain.

Nongynecologic Sources
GASTROENTEROLOGIC CONDITIONS
Gastroenterologic conditions are a common cause of pelvic (lower abdominal) pain. Because the cervix, uterus, and adnexa share the same visceral innervation with the lower ileum, sigmoid colon, and rectum, it is often difficult to differentiate pelvic pain of gynecologic from enterocoelic origin (12). Painful stimuli from the left hemicolon usually produce pain in the midline and suprapubic area, similar to where pain of uterine origin is perceived.

Approximately 60% of patients referred to gynecologists for chronic pelvic pain actually have irritable bowel syndrome.

It is estimated that irritable bowel syndrome (IBS) accounts for up to 60% of referrals to gynecologists for CPP. Because IBS symptoms are often exacerbated by the menstrual cycle, the pain may be erroneously interpreted as gynecologic in nature. In general, pelvic pain originating from the gastrointestinal tract shows some relationship to bowel movements, food intake, or other digestive functions. Pain that improves following a bowel movement and that worsens after eating is certainly suggestive of IBS. Likewise, the presence of bloating, belching, anorexia, nausea, excessive flatulence, diarrhea, or constipation raises the suspicion for IBS. Pelvic pain associated with dyspareunia is usually more likely to be gynecologic; however, dyspareunia does occur in a high percentage of patients with IBS. Coexistent psychopathology (e.g., somatization disorder, stress, anxiety disorders, depression) are also seen in a high percentage of patients with IBS.

Other gastroenterologic causes of CPP occur at a much lower incidence but include inflammatory bowel disease, diverticular disease, intestinal neoplasm, hernias, and ischemic bowel disease.

UROLOGIC CONDITIONS

As with enterocoelic pain, pain of urologic origin may also be difficult to distinguish from gynecologic pain. The more common urologic disorders associated with CPP are recurrent urinary tract infection, urethral syndrome, painful bladder syndrome, and interstitial cystitis. Any patient with CPP who complains of irritative urinary symptoms should undergo a thorough urologic work-up (13).

MUSCULOSKELETAL CONDITIONS

Musculoskeletal abnormalities commonly contribute to the symptoms of CPP. Musculoskeletal dysfunction from the lumbar spine, pelvis, and hips may cause pain that has a similar character and location as gynecologic pain, often making it difficult to identify the true site of pathology. Additionally, there is often a cyclic pattern of exacerbation to musculoskeletal pain of the pelvis and low back that further confuses the picture. Most musculoskeletal abnormalities associated with CPP result from long-standing postural changes that lead to a variety of muscular dysfunctions (14). A lordotic, anterior pelvic tilt posture is most common and may lead to muscle imbalance involving the abdominal muscles, thoracolumbar fascia, lumbar extensors, hip muscles, and pelvic floor musculature.

In addition to these structural abnormalities, myofascial pain syndrome has been found to be a primary etiology of pain in approximately 15% of patients with CPP (5). This disorder is characterized by the presence of trigger points along the abdominal wall that, when compressed (which can be done externally or by muscle contraction), are tender and generate referred pain in a dermatomal distribution. Trigger points are often present in women with CPP irrespective of the presence or type of underlying pathology. Indeed, in Slocomb's series of 122 women with CPP, he found abdominal wall trigger points in 89%, vaginal trigger points in 71%, and sacral trigger points in 25% of patients. Fifty-two percent of these patients were pain-free after treatment for their myofascial pain (15).

The symptoms of myofascial pelvic pain are often exacerbated by the premenstrual period and stimulation to the dermatome of a trigger point (e.g., full bladder or bowel or other stimuli to organs that share the dermatome of the involved nerve(s)). As with nerve entrapment, local anesthetic infiltration to areas of tenderness can be an extremely useful diagnostic maneuver, because often the patient will experience immediate improvement in pain.

NERVE ENTRAPMENT

Abdominal cutaneous nerve entrapment or injury may occur spontaneously or within weeks to years after transverse suprapubic skin or laparoscopy incisions. The syndrome of spontaneous abdominal nerve entrapment most commonly involves the ilioinguinal and iliohypogastric nerves becoming trapped between the transverse and internal oblique muscles. Symptoms of nerve entrapment include a burning, stabbing, or aching pain in the dermatomal distribution of the involved nerve, though the pain is usually perceived to be coming from within the abdomen, not from the skin. The pain may also be described as stabbing and colicky that is exacerbated by hip flexion and exercise and is relieved by bed rest. Occasionally pain is described as radiating to the labia and inner aspect of the thigh or hip. On examination, tenderness is often localized along the line of the lateral edge of the rectus muscle, medial and inferior to the anterior iliac spine. Diagnosis may be confirmed by nerve block; patients usually report immediate relief after local infiltration with 0.25% bupivicaine.

PSYCHOSOCIAL FACTORS

Women who have chronic pelvic pain without obvious pathology have traditionally been considered to have psychogenic pain. This would imply that all pain must be either *somatic* (physical, "organic") or *psychogenic* (mental, "functional"), and that these are discreet, mutually exclusive entities. This is an inadequate model of pain. It is now understood that not only are painful stimuli modulated by many peripheral factors other than the original painful stimulus but there are also a variety of central modulators of pain including motivational and affective states mediated by neuropeptides, endorphins, and a variety of other neurotransmitters. Thus the distinction between *mental* and *physical* causes of pain becomes somewhat blurred and often not very useful.

It is certainly true that women with CPP have high rates of psychological morbidity, though this does not appear to be unique to chronic pain of the pelvis as compared to other types of chronic pain syndromes (16). From a psychological perspective, various factors may promote the chronicity of pain, including the meaning attached to the pain, anxiety, the ability to redirect attention, personality, mood state, experience, and reinforcement contingencies that may amplify or attenuate pain (1).

Conversely, chronic pain itself may certainly promote the development of significant psychopathology. The Minnesota Multiphasic Personality Inventory (MMPI) studies of women with CPP have shown a high prevalence of a particular personality profile characterized by high scores on the hypochondriasis, hysteria, and depression scales. In studies comparing women with CPP who have no identifiable somatic pathology to women who have CPP due to endometriosis, MMPI profiles were unable to distinguish between the two groups. That is, these two groups were psychologically indistinguishable from each other, and both were clearly abnormal compared with the control group (6).

Another common condition among women with CPP is depression (17). Depression and pain are very closely related and often coexist, one exacerbating the other. Both can lead to behavioral and social withdrawal and decreased activity. The low levels of norepinephrine, serotonin, and GABA postulated to be associated with depression also facilitate pain transmission.

Several studies have looked at the role of sexual abuse as a specific risk factor for CPP. A history of both physical and sexual abuse has been shown to be more prevalent in women with CPP than those with other types of chronic pain (52% vs. 12%) and control groups (6). Abuse clearly seems to play a significant role in promoting the chronicity of painful conditions in the pelvis.

Clinical Evaluation

A complete evaluation of the patient with CPP requires an extensive and meticulous history be obtained, a thorough physical examination with obvious emphasis on certain areas, and some simple blood and urine tests at the very least. The goals of this evaluation are to rule out life-threatening conditions (e.g., cancer, major depression with significant risk of suicide), to diagnose treatable sources of pain, and to identify those patients whose source of pain is not identifiable or who have not responded to conventional therapies. It is this last group of patients who clearly benefit from a multidisciplinary pain-management approach. It should be noted that the entire evaluation may require several visits, particularly with regard to some of the more sensitive aspects of the history that the patient may not feel comfortable enough discussing on the initial visit (Figure 12-1, page 334).

History

The evaluation of CPP should begin with a thorough history of the nature of the pain including severity, location, radiation patterns, and aggravating or alleviating factors. Major goals of the history include differentiating between visceral and somatic sources of pain (though referred pain may complicate this distinction) and determining whether the pain has a cyclic pattern. The patient should be questioned regarding the effect of menstruation, stress, work, exercise, intercourse, and orgasm. If a history of dyspareunia is elicited, further questioning should distinguish between *entrance dyspareunia* (suggesting vulvar or urethral pathology), *vaginal dyspareunia* (suggesting vaginal changes or pelvic floor spasm), and *deep-thrust dyspareunia* (suggesting possible pelvic source of pathology such as endometriosis). The context in which the pain arose (e.g., post-partum, post-rape) and the social and occupational toll of pain should also be ascertained, because this has a significant impact on therapy and its effectiveness.

A pain diary is very helpful in detecting cyclic patterns, and the patient should be instructed on its use at her first office visit. The diary should be used for at least 2 months, noting the onset, intensity, and duration of pain, relationship to the menstrual cycle, and any aggravating or alleviating factors. The pain intensity is graded on a 1–10 scale, allowing for easy comparison of painful episodes.

A past medical and surgical history should be elicited. A detailed review of systems is essential and should be focused around the disorders listed in Box 12-1. Abnormal vaginal bleeding, discharge, dysmenorrhea, dyspareunia, and history of infertility all suggest a gynecologic process. Constipation, diarrhea, flatulence, abdominal bloating, tenesmus, hematochezia, and relationship of pain to bowel movements or eating should prompt further investigation into gastroenterologic causes. Pain that is exacerbated with exercise or postural changes may suggest a musculoskeletal process. Urologic disorders are associated with irritative symptoms such as frequency, urgency, dysuria, nocturia, or incontinence.

Given the relationship between CPP and psychosocial dysfunction, a thorough psychosocial and psychological history is essential for proper evaluation and management of these patients. This history should include past or current physical, sexual, or emotional abuse, history of psychiatric disorders and hospitalizations, suicide attempts, and chemical dependency.

Physical Examination

A complete physical examination should be performed, but particular attention should be paid to the abdomen, lumbosacral area, external genitalia, and bimanual and rectovaginal exams. The patient should be examined for hernias while standing. Then, before performing a pelvic exam, the abdominal wall should be evaluated thoroughly for trigger points. This examination should include evaluation of the abdomen with muscles tensed (by having the patient raise her head and shoulders off the table or with straight leg raising) to differentiate abdominal wall pain from visceral sources of pain. Abdominal wall pain is exacerbated and visceral pain is usually diminished with this maneuver. If trigger points are identified, it is worthwhile to inject them before

proceeding with the pelvic exam, because this will enable a thorough bimanual exam not influenced by abdominal wall pain. If administered in the correct locations, 3 mL of 0.25% bupivicaine or 2% lidocaine will provide almost
immediate relief of trigger point or nerve entrapment pain.

Diagnostic Testing

Initial laboratory tests should include a pregnancy test, complete blood
count, erythrocyte sedimentation rate, urine analysis and urine culture, cervical specimens for gonorrhea and chlamydia, Pap smear, and stool guaiac. A
pelvic ultrasound should be reserved for those women with an abnormal
pelvic exam that suggests adnexal pathology or a possible endometrioma, or if
the pelvic exam is hampered by the patient's body habitus or by pain. Other
investigations (e.g., endoscopy, cystoscopy, other imaging studies) are
prompted by findings of the in-depth review of systems and physical exam.

Laparoscopy

Laparoscopy has played a prominent role in the medical evaluation of CPP;
indeed, many gynecologists have viewed it as a necessary diagnostic study in
the "comprehensive evaluation of the patient with pelvic pain". In Howard's
extensive review of the literature (8), laparoscopically diagnosable abnormalities were found in 61% of the patients who had CPP compared with abnormalities found in 28% of women without CPP. Women with disabling cyclic
pain that does not respond to nonsteroidal anti-inflammatory agents and oral
contraceptives should be referred for possible laparoscopic evaluation.
Women with either cyclic or noncyclic pain who are found to have an abnormal pelvic exam or have signs or symptoms of significant endometriosis
should be considered for possible laparoscopy. Finally, laparoscopy is often indicated for women with chronic noncyclic pelvic pain for whom nongynecologic
somatic and visceral causes have been excluded and initial multidisciplinary pain
management has failed (see below).

Management

After completing a thorough evaluation as outlined above, the first task of
the clinician is to ensure that the patient does not have an acute condition.
Recall that, by definition, chronic pelvic pain has been present for at least 6
months. Symptoms such as fevers, anorexia, nausea, vomiting, or uterine
bleeding should raise suspicion of a superimposed acute process. Likewise,
orthostasis, peritoneal signs, or leukocytosis each warrants immediate atten-

tion. A history of a recent pregnancy or abortion should also alert the clinician to the possibility of an acute gynecologic cause of pain. If cervical cultures are positive for chlamydia or gonorrhea, or if the patient has cervical motion tenderness plus a purulent discharge or an elevated sedimentation rate, she should be treated for salpingo-oophoritis before proceeding with any further evaluation.

Nongynecologic Pain

If a nongynecologic cause of CPP is suggested by the initial work-up (e.g., IBS, urogenital disease, major depression), the next steps in management will of course be directed at that particular condition. If myofascial pain syndrome is suspected (on the basis of either a suggestive physical exam or a positive response to trigger point injections), the patient should be more fully evaluated for this condition. Although pain relief from trigger point injections usually outlasts the duration of anesthetic action, the relief is usually only partial and requires repeated injections. One should expect long-lasting relief after approximately four to five biweekly injections (6). TENS (transcutaneous electric nerve stimulator) units and acupuncture have also been shown to be useful adjuncts in the treatment of chronic myofascial pain. Exercise and other modifying factors such as stress may need to be addressed. Medical therapy with tricyclic antidepressants or GABA agonists (e.g., carbamazepine, gabapentin, baclofen) can often be a useful adjunct as well.

Cyclic Gynecologic Pain

Cyclic gynecologic pain, as stated before, is due to primary or secondary dysmenorrhea. The initial treatment of these entities consists of nonsteroidal anti-inflammatory drugs (NSAIDs), which are effective in approximately 80% of cases. The medication should be taken for the first few days of menses just before or at the onset of pain and continued regularly to prevent re-formation of prostaglandin by-products (6). Therapy should be a 4 to 6 month trial, with trials of different types of NSAIDs and higher doses if necessary, before declaring such treatment a failure. If the patient does not respond to NSAIDs or if she desires contraception, she should be treated with oral contraceptives. Oral contraceptives decrease prostaglandin production by decreasing endometrial proliferation, and more than 90% of patients with primary dysmenorrhea will enjoy relief with this therapy (6). If the patient does not respond to this regimen, or if she is not a candidate for oral contraceptives, a codeine preparation can be added for 2 to 3 days per month. Secondary dysmenorrhea is more likely to be refractory to all of these measures. Patients with unresponsive cyclic pain should be referred to a gynecologist for more intensive menstrual suppression and consideration of laparoscopy (Fig. 12-1).

Noncyclic Gynecologic Pain

Treatment of noncyclic CPP is less straightforward (see Fig. 12-1). As discussed above, diagnostic and operative laparoscopy has traditionally been considered standard procedure to evaluate women with noncyclic CPP. More recently, however, several studies have suggested that initial nonsurgical multidisciplinary treatment focusing on the pain management model provides the best long-term prognosis for these patients (18-20).

Multidisciplinary Pain Management

The multidisciplinary approach to the patient with CPP is similar to that of other chronic pain conditions, where a therapeutic, supportive, and sympathetic physician-patient relationship must be established. Follow-up appointments should be scheduled on a regular basis to avoid reinforcing pain behavior as a means to elicit sympathy and medical attention.

The management team should include the primary care physician or gynecologist, a mental health professional, and, if possible, an anesthesiologist or acupuncturist. The mental health professional may provide cognitive or behavioral training such as stress management, relaxation techniques, biofeedback, assertiveness training, or other adaptive coping mechanisms. Some patients may also benefit from additional psychological therapy, marital counseling, or sexual counseling. Given the high prevalence of depression in this population it is imperative that patients be formally screened for this disorder and, if present, appropriately treated with therapeutic doses of antidepressant medication and psychotherapy. The high incidence of a history of both physical and sexual abuse in these patients also requires considerable attention and counseling skills on the part of the mental health professional.

Medical therapy of CPP should be maintained in conjunction with behavioral and psychological counseling. Tricyclic antidepressants (TCAs) have been effective in the treatment of many pain syndromes by improving pain tolerance, restoring normal sleep patterns, and reducing depressive symptoms (19). Although there are no randomized controlled data on the efficacy of TCAs on CPP, several published observational studies suggest that antidepressants may be useful as part of a biopsychosocial treatment plan (21). When used to treat pain, TCA therapy is initiated with very low doses, such as 10 to 25 mg of nortriptyline or amitriptyline at bedtime. This is titrated up to 50 to 75 mg as needed. Full therapeutic effects may not be reached until approximately 4 weeks. GABA agonists may also be useful in the medical management of chronic pain. Only one randomized controlled trial has evaluated a selective serotonin reuptake inhibitor on pelvic pain (22). This was a very small study of 23 women that compared 6 weeks of sertraline versus placebo; the investigators found no significant difference in measures of pain or functional disability. Clearly further investigation with larger numbers of patients is needed.

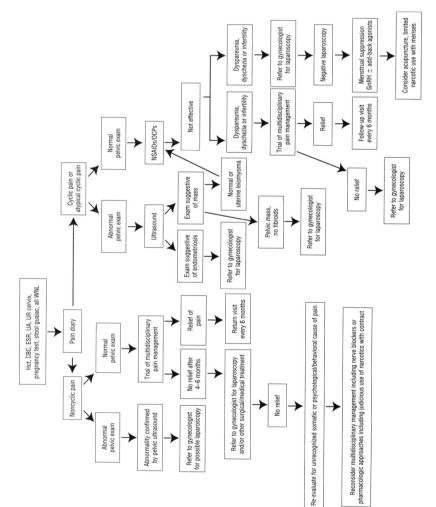

Figure 12-1 Algorithm for chronic pelvic pain treatment.

Acupuncture and various nerve blocks (e.g., caudal, epidural) have been used with varying success in the treatment of CPP. Such treatment may be worthwhile pursuing if a specialist with the appropriate expertise is available. Trigger-point injections (as discussed earlier in the section on Musculoskeletal Conditions) have proven to be extremely effective in treating myofascial pain (or even the myofascial components of pain).

Surgery
Clinical improvement after operative laparoscopy has been reported in 65% to 80% of patients who were found to have pathology at the time of the laparoscopy. Overall, however, a woman undergoing diagnostic and operative laparoscopy for CPP has (at best) a less than 50% chance that the procedure will result in an improvement in her pain (8,18).

Presacral neurectomy (PSN) or sympathectomy is a procedure that may be effective for a subset of patients with refractory primary or secondary dysmenorrhea who do not respond to multidisciplinary pain management. The response rate to PSN for secondary dysmenorrhea is 50% to 77% (6), and the procedure will only relieve pain originating from the cervix, uterus, and proximal fallopian tubes. Temporary resolution of pain after a fluoroscopically guided hypogastric nerve block predicts a favorable response to this operation.

Finally, hysterectomy may be considered in severe cases of pain that are determined likely to be of uterine origin. Generally this pain is cyclic or associated with irregular bleeding. One author noted a 75% success rate for treatment of "uterine pain", but the criteria for diagnosis of uterine pain were not noted (23). Clearly a hysterectomy is not a panacea for CPP; indeed, up to 30% of patients seeking treatment at pelvic pain clinics have already undergone a hysterectomy (24). Hysterectomy appears to be particularly useful for women who have completed childbearing and who have secondary dysmenorrhea or chronic pain due to endometriosis, adenomyosis, or pelvic congestion. It is imperative that the patient be well informed that this procedure provides no guarantee that her pain will resolve, because many women are not aware of the possibility of persistent pelvic pain after hysterectomy.

Conclusion

Chronic pelvic pain can pose a diagnostic challenge, because the range of possible causes is vast and includes nongynecologic conditions. Evaluation of this problem requires a thorough history and physical examination and is often best accomplished over more than one office visit. Pain diaries are often helpful. Standard laboratory studies sometimes reveal the cause; however, radiologic studies are not usually necessary in the absence of worrisome history or abnormal exam findings. Careful attention to the patient's psychological health is often beneficial. The treatment of cyclic chronic pelvic pain is fairly straightforward, whereas that for noncyclic pain is more challenging and is often best approached in a multidisciplinary fashion.

REFERENCES

1. **Rapkin AJ, Reading AE.** Chronic pelvic pain. Curr Probl Obstet Gynecol Fertil. 1991; 14:105.

2. **Reiter RC, Gambone JC.** Demographic and historical variables in women with idiopathic chronic pelvic pain. Obstet Gynecol. 1990;75:428.

3. **Walker EA, Katon WJ, et al.** The prevalence of chronic pain and irritable bowel syndrome in two university clinics. J Psychosom Obstet Gynaecol. 1991;12(Suppl):65.

4. **Rapkin AJ, Kames LD, Darke LL, et al.** History of physical and sexual abuse in women with chronic pelvic pain. Obstet Gynecol. 1990;76:92.

5. **Reiter RC, Gambone JC.** Nongynecologic somatic pathology in women with chronic pelvic pain and negative laparoscopy. J Reprod Med. 1991;36:253.

6. **Berek JS, Rapkin A.** Pelvic pain and dysmenorrhea. In: Novak ER, ed. Gynecology, 12th ed. Philadelphia: Williams and Wilkins; 1996:329-428.

7. **Fedele L, Parazzini F, Bianchi S, et al.** Stage and localization of pelvic endometriosis and pain. Fertil and Steril. 1990;53:155.

8. **Howard FM.** The role of laparoscopy in chronic pelvic pain: promise and pitfalls. Obstet Gynecol Survey. 1993;48:357.

9. **Steege JF, South AL.** Resolution of chronic pelvic pain after laparoscopic lysis of adhesions. Am J Obstet Gynecol. 1991;165:278.

10. **Peters AAW, Trimbos-Kemper GCM, et al.** A randomized clinical trail on the benefit of adhesiolysis in patients with intraperitoneal adhesions and chronic pelvic pain. Br J Obstet Gynaecol. 1992;99:59-62.

11. **Centers for Disease Control and Prevention.** 1993 sexually transmitted disease treatment guidelines. MMWR. 1993;42(RR-14):1.

12. **Rapkin AJ, Mayer EA.** Gastroenterologic causes of chronic pelvic pain. Obstet Gynecol Clin North Am. 1993;20:663.

13. **Lewis L, Wall MD, Norton PA, et al.** Practical Urogynecology. Philadelphia: Lippincott, Williams & Wilkins; 1993:264-73.

14. **Baker PL.** Musculoskeletal origins of chronic pelvic pain. Obstet Gynecol Clin North Am. 1993;20:719.

15. **Slocumb JC.** Neurological factors in chronic pelvic pain: trigger points and the abdominal pelvic pain syndrome. Am J Obstet Gynecol. 1984;149:536.

16. **Rosenthal RH.** Psychology of chronic pelvic pain. Obstet Gynecol Clin North Am. 1993;20:627.

17. **Walker EA, Katon WJ, Harrop-Griffiths J, et al.** Relationship of chronic pelvic pain to psychiatric diagnosis and childhood sexual abuse. Am J Psychiatry. 1988;145:75.

18. **Peters AAW, Von Dorst E, Jellis B, et al.** A randomized clinical trial to compare two different approaches in women with chronic pelvic pain. Obstet Gynecol. 1991;77:740.

19. **Milburn A, Reiter RC, Rhomberg AT.** Multidisciplinary approach to chronic pelvic pain. Obstet Gynecol Clin North Am. 1993;20:643.

20. **Kames LD, Rapkin AJ, Naliboff BD, et al.** Effectiveness of an interdisciplinary pain management program for the treatment of chronic pelvic pain. Pain. 1990;41:41.

21. **Walker EA, Sullivan MD, Stencherer MA.** Use of antidepressants in the management of women with chronic pelvic pain. Obstet Gynecol Clin North Am. 1993;20:743.

22. **Engel CC, Walker EA, Engel AL, et al.** A randomized, double-blind crossover trial of sertaline in women with chronic pelvic pain. J Psychosom Res. 1998;44:203-7.

23. **Stoval TG, Laing FW, Crawford DA.** Hysterectomy for chronic pelvic pain of pressured uterine etiology. Obstet Gynecol. 1990;75:676.

24. **Reiter RC.** A profile of women with chronic pelvic pain. Clin Obstet Gynecol. 1990; 33:130.

CHAPTER 13

Evaluation of the Pelvic Mass

ANITA L. NELSON, MD
ROBERT M. SINOW, MD

The pelvic mass is a clinical problem commonly faced by primary care physicians. The differential diagnosis of a pelvic mass may depend upon a woman's age, hormonal state, symptomatology, and exam findings. However, the initial evaluation often requires an imaging study, and ultimately determining the diagnosis may depend upon surgical exploration.

Uterine masses, masses arising from the fallopian tubes, ovarian masses, and nongynecologic pelvic masses are discussed in this chapter. A general management protocol is outlined to aid primary care physicians in their assessment of pelvic masses, to assist them in deciding when to refer to specialists, and to enable them to counsel patients as to the expected course of action. Lastly, ovarian cancer screening is discussed for both usual and high-risk populations.

Acutely symptomatic pelvic masses that result from infection, torsion, or rupture are discussed in Chapters 8 and 9. Pelvic pain of greater than 6 months' duration without any abnormalities on examination is discussed in Chapter 12.

History

Often the patient with a pelvic mass is completely asymptomatic and the mass is detected on routine pelvic examination. However, depending on the origin, extent, and possible hormone production of the mass, a patient may present with any of a myriad of symptoms.

Pain emanating from pelvic viscera is generally vague and poorly localized; thus the patient's description may not be helpful in identifying the source. In eliciting the history from a patient who notes pain, the presence of a cyclical component sometimes helps narrow the differential diagnosis. Enquiry should also include whether intercourse exacerbates the pain, because deep dyspareunia generally suggests possible uterine or adnexal involvement. Pelvic pain may also stem from gastrointestinal or urologic sources, and the patient should be questioned regarding the presence of symptoms related to these organ systems.

However, significant overlap may occur. For example, an ovarian malignancy in the early stages, if not completely asymptomatic, may cause symptoms such as dyspepsia and early satiety. After ovarian tumor enlargement, tumor spread and/or ascites have occurred, the tumor may continue to manifest itself in other nonlocalizing symptoms such as urinary frequency, abdominal fullness and constipation. The presentation of acute-on-chronic pain can result from acute torsion of an ovary containing a previously asymptomatic neoplasm, or bleeding into or rupture of an ovarian mass.

Although a history of abnormal menstrual bleeding commonly results from endometrial abnormalities, it can also be the presenting symptom of various pelvic masses such as uterine fibroids or sarcomas, cervical polyps, and cervical carcinomas. Rarely, abnormal vaginal bleeding may result from the stimulation of the endometrium by estrogen-producing ovarian masses. Certain ovarian tumors may alternatively secrete androgens, resulting in a presentation of virilization (hirsutism and clitoromegaly).

An abnormal vaginal discharge is most frequently an indication of infection, but other causes such as postmenopausal atrophy are also common. In rare instances, an abnormal discharge may herald a cervical carcinoma or fallopian tube malignancy, the latter generally being associated with a profuse watery discharge, sometimes blood-tinged.

Despite the various symptoms described above, pelvic masses are frequently asymptomatic, and therefore lack of symptoms should not diminish the potential clinical import of an abnormal mass found on examination.

Physical Examination

Pelvic masses are not uncommonly encountered on routine exam. When performed carefully, each element of the pelvic exam can yield different information (see also Chapter 1). The abdominal examination can reveal peritoneal signs, ascites, and large abdominopelvic masses. Speculum examination can demonstrate pelvic relaxation and masses protruding into the vagina. Maneuvers performed in the bimanual exam may reveal other important findings.

Evaluation for cervical motion tenderness can identify and localize tubal pathology, such as ectopic pregnancy and salpingitis. Cervical motion tenderness is assessed by grasping the cervix between the two vaginal examining fingers, then gently pivoting the cervix from side to side to stretch each of the fallopian tubes in turn while avoiding contact with the peritoneal surfaces. Next, the uterus is carefully examined to identify and characterize possible uterine masses. The examining vaginal fingers should be placed behind the uterine corpus to gently lift the entire uterus toward the abdominal wall to stabilize it and to permit a careful examination of its size, shape, tenderness, mobility, and consistency by the abdominal examining fingers. Adnexal structures are detected on bimanual examination if the examining vaginal fingers are first swept deep and laterally in the posterior pelvis, then elevated to present the adnexa to the abdominal wall for examination by the external examining fingers. In contrast to the technique used to palpate the uterus, the adnexa are best felt as they slip between the internal and external examining fingers, at which time their size, consistency, tenderness, shape, and mobility can be determined.

An important component of the pelvic exam is the rectal examination, which often can better define a pelvic mass than can the digital vaginal examination alone. During the rectovaginal exam, the posterior aspect of the uterus should be explored for irregularities on its surface and the rectovaginal septum and the cul-de-sac are examined for tenderness, pelvic masses, or implants along the uterosacral ligaments. Adnexae deep in the pelvis are more completely characterized by elevating them with the rectal finger and sliding them between the rectal and abdominal fingers. In an obese woman, the rectal exam may be the only way to evaluate her pelvic structures.

Nongynecologic Causes of Pelvic Masses

Any differential diagnosis for pelvic masses must include nongynecologic causes (Box 13-1). For instance, a distended bladder can be mistaken for a cystic pelvic mass, and hard stool in the bowel can mimic a firm adnexal mass. Other gastrointestinal processes such as diverticulosis, appendiceal abscess, Chrohn's disease, and colon cancer or other gastrointestinal tumors need to be included in the differential diagnosis. Pelvic masses may also be due to anatomic variations such as an ectopic (pelvic) kidney, urachal cyst, or sacral meningocele. Neoplasms of the urinary tract as well as peritoneal, mesenteric and omental cysts can present as pelvic masses. Retroperitoneal sarcomas, lymphomas, and teratomas in the sacrococcygeal areas can be palpated during the rectovaginal examination and mistaken for reproductive tract pelvic pathology.

Box 13-1 Differential Diagnosis of Pelvic Mass in Women of Reproductive Age

Confounding processes	**Uterine masses**
Distended bladder	Müllerian anomalies
Stool or gas in the bowel	Adenomyosis
Pelvic kidney	Multiparity
Appendiceal abscess	Neoplasms
Diverticulosis	
Colon cancer	**Ovarian masses**
Urinary tract neoplasms	Functional cysts
	Hyperplastic changes
Pregnancy-related masses	Neoplasms
Ectopic pregnancy	
Molar pregnancy	
Luteoma of pregnancy	
Fallopian tube masses	
Salpingitis	
Tubo-ovarian abscess	
Hydrosalpinx	
Paratubal cysts	
Neoplasms	

A complete history and careful and methodic abdominal, pelvic, and rectal examinations (which should include testing for occult blood in the stool) may help distinguish a gynecologic from a nongynecologic source. However, imaging studies are often necessary to identify the origin of the mass and define its characteristics.

Uterine Masses

On bimanual examination, uterine masses are often midline, firm, and moveable. Interaction between the vaginal and abdominal examining fingers can generally determine if a mass is uterine. Specifically, if movement of the cervix results in motion of the mass and if downward pressure on the mass causes the cervix to move, the mass is likely to be uterine. Exceptions to this rule can occur with pedunculated fibroids (which do not necessarily move with cervical manipulation) and adnexal masses adherent to the uterus (which do move with the uterus).

Failure of fusion of the müllerian ducts results in a wide range of possible congenital uterine abnormalities such as a didelphic uterus (complete duplication of the vagina, cervix, and uterus), bicornuate uterus, or septate uterus. The first two defects may be palpated on physical exam; the last often evades detection unless more invasive tests are performed for evaluation of infertility or recurrent spontaneous abortion. In early adolescence, an imperforate hymen or complete transverse vaginal septum can result in hematocolpos (accumulation of blood in the vagina) and hematometra (accumulation of blood in the uterus), which can present as a pelvic mass and/or as primary amenorrhea. Prompt surgical intervention is important to relieve symptoms and to reduce the risk of future endometriosis.

Any uterine mass that is rapidly growing requires evaluation even in the absence of symptoms. An exception to this rule may be growth of a known leiomyoma (uterine fibroid) in postmenopausal women initiating hormone replacement therapy. However, even in this instance, characterization of the mass would be prudent and close monitoring is mandatory.

Several imaging tests may be helpful in evaluating uterine masses. Transabdominal and transvaginal sonography aid in defining leiomyomata (Fig. 13-1) and by excluding any endometrial deformities. Furthermore, ultrasonography can image the adnexae and identify other pelvic pathology

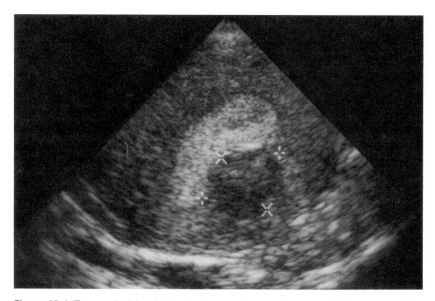

Figure 13-1 Transvaginal longitudinal ultrasound image of uterus with leiomyoma. The hypoechoic solid fibroid (outlined by calipers) can be seen distorting the endometrium (*thick bright white stripe*). This particular fibroid is both intramural (located within the wall of the uterus) and submucosal (protruding into the endometrial cavity).

that may otherwise be masked by the uterine enlargement. However, ultrasonography has recognized limitations. It may not be able to detect small (< 1.5 cm) myomata. Occasionally, sonography is unable to distinguish between a leiomyoma and adenomyosis (endometriosis within the myometrium), especially if the fibroid lacks a definitive pseudo-capsule. Fibroids that are degenerating may have both solid and cystic components, making their diagnosis less secure based on ultrasonography alone. Magnetic resonance imaging (MRI) is expensive but more sensitive in detecting myomata and in quantifying their sizes. Therefore, in some cases, MRI may have a role in monitoring the effect of medical therapy, predicting the feasibility of myomectomy, and distinguishing leiomyoma from adenomyosis.

Other tests have more limited applications. Office hysteroscopy is used to visualize polyps and submucosal fibroids. By revealing filling defects, sonohysterography (Fig. 13-2) or hysterosalpingography can demonstrate the presence of endometrial pathology. Diagnostic laparoscopy may occasionally be necessary to exclude other significant pathology when imaging studies are not helpful.

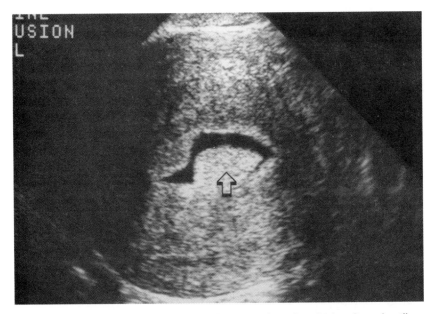

Figure 13-2 Sonohysterogram. Saline infusion opens the endometrial cavity and outlines the large endometrial polyp (*open arrow*) for better visualization by transvaginal ultrasound. This procedure is particularly useful when there is thickening of the endometrial stripe.

Fibroids

Leiomyomata of the uterus are the most common type of solid pelvic tumors. They occur in at least 20% of women aged 35 and older (1) and are more frequent in African-American women. They are usually multiple and slow growing. Fortunately, their malignant potential is low; less than 1% of women with fibroids develop leiomyosarcoma.

The clinical significance of fibroids depends primarily upon their location and size. All leiomyomata start as intramural lesions. They can continue to grow within the uterine walls or extend either into the uterine cavity (submucosal fibroids) or to the peritoneal surface (subserosal fibroids). Occasionally, a fibroid will continue its evolution and emerge entirely from the uterine wall on a stalk, which can extend either into the peritoneal cavity (as a pedunculated fibroid) or into the uterine cavity (where it might present with hemorrhage as an aborting fibroid). Rarely, fibroids lose their connection with the uterus altogether and parasitize to other organs.

Symptoms and Findings

The specific features and locations of fibroids are associated with characteristic symptoms and physical findings. Patients with small fibroids may be asymptomatic. Submucosal and intramural fibroids are associated with the greatest frequency of symptoms, most commonly menorrhagia, infertility, or both. Large fibroids can produce pelvic and abdominal compression problems (e.g., urinary frequency, constipation) and, in extreme cases, can create problems with lower extremity edema and respiratory compromise (Fig. 13-3). Leiomyomata can overlie the adnexae or displace them from the pelvis, preventing satisfactory bimanual examination of the tubes and ovaries. A rapidly expanding leiomyoma, as can be found in pregnancy, may outgrow its blood supply, necrose, and cause considerable pain.

Management

An incidental finding of small fibroids in an asymptomatic woman seldom requires an extensive workup. It is usually sufficient to perform another bimanual exam in 6 to 12 months to document that the uterus is not rapidly enlarging (which would raise concern for a uterine sarcoma or other malignancy). However, leiomyomata large enough to prevent adequate examination of the adnexae warrant ultrasound study both to confirm the diagnosis and to exclude adnexal pathology. This step is important because ovarian masses adherent to the uterus can be too easily mistaken for fibroids.

For symptomatic reproductive-age women with small or moderately sized fibroids, first-line treatment is medical therapy. Low-dose birth control pills significantly reduce menstrual blood loss and help correct anemia yet do not

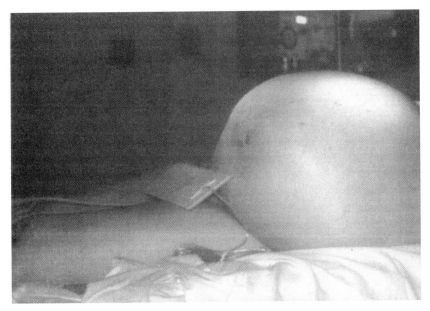

Figure 13-3 Preoperative photo of a woman with a 18,800 g (41 lb) leiomyoma. This massive fibroid caused obstruction of the patient's venous and lymphatic return and consequent edema and skin breakdown in her lower extremities. In addition, the patient complained of significant dyspnea due to pulmonary compression.

stimulate growth of myomata (2). Continuous use (i.e., skipping the placebo pills) of monophasic oral contraceptives can completely eliminate menses in some women. Other estrogen-containing contraceptives such as the patch, the once-monthly injection, and the vaginal ring can also decrease blood loss. Progestin-only methods may be similarly helpful. Depot medroxyprogesterone acetate (DMPA or Depo-Provera) induces amenorrhea in 50% of women by 12 months. The levonorgestrel-releasing IUD (Mirena) reduces menstrual blood loss by 70% to 90% in 6 to 9 months and can be used to treat menorrhagia due to fibroids or adenomyosis. All of these methods simultaneously provide effective contraception.

Long-acting gonadotropin releasing hormone (GnRH) agonists induce amenorrhea. By suppressing ovarian function they also remove endogenous estrogen support of the leiomyoma and result in some shrinkage of the size of the lesions. Unfortunately, this benefit is only temporary, and because the hypoestrogenic effects of GnRH agonists include a decline in bone density, their use is not recommended for longer than 6 to 9 months unless estrogen/progestin add-back therapy is given. For further discussion of the management of fibroids, see Chapter 14.

A uterine mass associated with symptoms of pain or abnormal bleeding deserves additional attention. The temptation to attribute all abnormal bleeding to leiomyoma must be resisted. Evaluation of such bleeding includes endometrial sampling and sometimes biopsies of the endocervical canal to exclude hyperplasia, cancer, or polyps (see Chapter 3). In postmenopausal women, transvaginal ultrasonography evaluation of the endometrium is emerging as an acceptable noninvasive alternative, particularly in women with cervical stenosis. The thickest portion of the endometrium should measure less than 5 mm in the anterior-posterior dimension on a sagittal view and the contour of the endometrial lining must be smooth for the test to be completely reassuring. A thickness in excess of 11 mm is worrisome and mandates endometrial biopsy. The presence of fluid in the endometrial cavity may raise concerns for local pathology but should be considered in the context of the appearance and thickness of the endometrial lining, because such fluid may result from nothing more than cervical stenosis.

The presence of fibroids does not necessarily mean the source of abnormal vaginal bleeding has been identified; a thorough evaluation should be made to exclude other causes.

Other Uterine Masses

A rapidly growing or unusually firm uterus is most typically associated with uterine sarcomas, but such findings may on rare occasions be a presentation of endometrial cancer. The more typical presentation of endometrial hyperplasia or carcinoma is simply irregular bleeding without any abnormal findings on pelvic exam. Similarly, one may rarely encounter an especially firm or unusually shaped ("barrel shaped") uterine cervix, which raises suspicion for cervical malignancy. The more classic presentation of cervical cancer is, of course, a complaint of postcoital bleeding or unusual vaginal discharge, usually associated with a visible lesion on the cervix. In both of these situations, endocervical and endometrial biopsies should both be performed to provide a tissue diagnosis.

In addition to uterine fibroids, other benign uterine conditions such as adenomyosis can present as pelvic masses. *Adenomyosis* is defined as the presence of endometrial glands and stroma in the myometrium. The majority of women who have symptomatic adenomyosis are parous and in the latter half of their reproductive years. Common complaints associated with adenomyosis include dysmenorrhea, menorrhagia, and deep-thrust dyspareunia. On exam the uterus is boggy and diffusely enlarged (sometimes two to three times normal size) and usually tender, particularly just before and during menses. There are no specific tests to diagnose adenomyosis, although ultrasonography and, more recently, MRI may be helpful. The diagnosis can be formally made only by histologic exam following hysterectomy, but therapy can be initiated on the basis of clinical findings. Management with nonsteroidal anti-inflammatory drugs and hormonal contraceptives has been tried with limited success; hysterectomy is often required. Appropriately timed pelvic examinations (every 6 to 12 months) are used to rule out a rapidly growing uterine mass.

Fallopian Tube Masses

Healthy fallopian tubes are not palpable on bimanual examination. Acute salpingitis, pelvic abscess, hydrosalpinx, paratubal cyst, torsed adnexa, and neoplasms can cause palpable tubal masses. Torsion and infectious tubal diseases are discussed in Chapter 9.

Chronic adnexal masses (e.g., hydrosalpinx) and neoplasms may be cystic or firm, mobile or fixed. Large paratubal and paraovarian cysts can be palpated on bimanual exam, but smaller ones are more frequently found incidentally at the time of a surgical procedure. These thin-walled, fluid-filled cysts attached to the fallopian tube are now recognized to be accessory lumina. If detected on bimanual examination, they are difficult to distinguish from ovarian masses. Ultrasonography typically reveals one or multiple simple cystic structures, which may vary widely in size and measure 20 cm or more. Although these cysts are generally benign, surgical removal of larger cysts is recommended to exclude the possibility of malignancy and to eliminate the risk of torsion. The role of nonsurgical aspiration of these masses is being researched.

Other types of fallopian pathology are more difficult to accurately diagnose by exam or with ultrasonography. On bimanual exam firm, fixed masses may be consistent with extensive endometriosis, carcinoma, or adhesions resulting from previous pelvic surgery or infection. History of previous tubal infection can suggest chronic hydrosalpinx, which may be a permanent sequela. Carcinoma of the fallopian tube is rare and accounts for less than 1% of all female genital tract malignancies. The classic triad of fallopian carcinoma includes a profuse watery vaginal discharge, pelvic pain, and a pelvic mass. However, the full triad is rare, and the majority of patients are asymptomatic when the pelvic mass is detected on routine exam. Whenever a persistent watery or bloody discharge (not explained by endometrial pathology) is present in a postmenopausal woman, the practitioner should be alerted to a possible fallopian-type cancer. Surgical evaluation is mandatory whenever a patient is symptomatic or there is a question of malignancy. Diagnostic laparoscopy may be sufficient in some instances, but the patient should be prepared for exploratory laparotomy and possible extirpative procedures.

Tuberculosis of the pelvis is more common in developing countries. Tuberculosis of the uterus or fallopian tube can present as a pelvic mass even without evidence of prior pulmonary involvement. A reactive PPD may indicate this possibility, but endometrial sampling for direct staining and culture and hysterosalpingography to image the contours of the tube are more definitive in establishing a diagnosis of pelvic tuberculosis.

Ovarian Masses

During the reproductive years, the ovary undergoes predictable changes related to the menstrual cycle. Each cycle, dozens of follicles are stimulated. A dominant follicle emerges, extrudes an oocyte, and forms a corpus luteum. Distinguishing between these and other cysts on the basis of clinical examination alone is difficult. Contraceptive methods can influence physical findings and their interpretation. For instance, users of birth control pills or DMPA may form small follicles, but these women should not ovulate or form corpora lutea.

In a woman with an ovarian mass, the recommended approach is to first determine if the mass is functional or neoplastic, because management of these two entities differs. The commonest diagnoses, functional cysts, include follicular cysts, corpus luteum cysts, and theca lutein cysts. The other important etiologies of ovarian enlargement are polycystic ovary syndrome, ovarian neoplasms (both benign and malignant), and tumors metastatic to the ovary. The likelihood of each lesion is related to the woman's hormonal status and her use of hormonal contraception. Characteristics of the mass on physical exam and ultrasonography over time can also help distinguish among functional cysts, benign neoplasms, and malignancy, although surgical and histological evaluation may sometimes be necessary.

Management

Overall, only 10% of all ovarian tumors are malignant (3), but any mass that causes enlargement of the ovary to more than 8 cm in the reproductive years or any palpable ovary at any other time of life must be considered potentially malignant until proven otherwise. Upon detection of an ovarian mass, one generally proceeds to ultrasonography for further characterization. Typically, transvaginal probe ultrasonography is requested in addition to transabdominal ultrasonography because the former is often able to better image adnexal structures. Patient receptivity to this testing may be optimized with education at the time of the office visit.

Ultrasonography findings that are supportive of the benign nature of a cyst (Fig. 13-4) include size less than 8 cm (less than 5 cm in premenarchal girls and postmenopausal women), unilaterality, negligible free peritoneal fluid, and simple cystic appearance. Sonographically, a simple cyst is one that appears unilocular, anechoic, and devoid of septa, papillae, or solid areas. If a patient with such ultrasonography findings is of reproductive age and asymptomatic, one can usually avoid surgery and instead manage her by reevaluating the ovarian mass with a second ultrasound study in 4 to 6 weeks to confirm that it is decreasing in size. This is because an adnexal mass in this setting is most often due to a functional cyst (4). Subsequent follow-up may only require serial ultrasounds to document complete resolution of the mass over the ensuing 2 to 3 months. It should be emphasized that this practice is acceptable only if the mass is less than 8 cm, cystic and smooth, unilateral, and not associated with any symptoms or ascites.

It must be noted, however, that ultrasonography cannot definitively distinguish benign from malignant processes. The negative predictive value for excluding a malignancy has been reported to be approximately 95%, with the positive predictive value for diagnosing malignancy to be approximately 70%

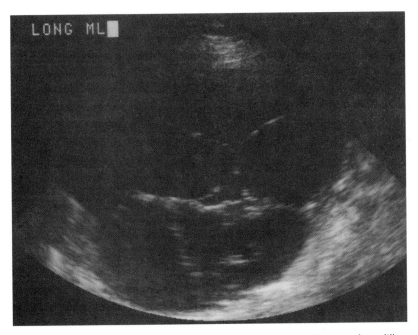

Figure 13-4 Ultrasound image of serous cystadenoma. This particular mass is multiloculated. The thin walls of the septations help to distinguish this benign lesion from its malignant counterpart shown in Figure 13-5. However, because serous cysts may assume a variety of appearances, surgical excision is often necessary to exclude malignancy.

to 75% (5). In some studies, ultrasonography has been found to be frankly misleading in 15% of cases (6).

Ultrasound findings that suggest the need for surgical exploration include masses greater than 8 cm (greater than 5 cm for premenarchal girls and postmenopausal women), masses that grow or persist over a 2 to 3 month period of observation, and masses that are solid, irregular in contour, or fixed (Fig. 13-5). The finding of bilateral ovarian masses warrants surgical exploration because it increases concern for malignancy. The presence of pain or other symptoms of an acute process or ascites also represents an indication for surgery, except in women who are experiencing ovarian hyperstimulation or who have evidence of infection.

The finding of bilateral ovarian masses increases the concern for malignancy.

The menopausal patient is managed somewhat differently, using separate criteria. At menopause, the ovary undergoes atresia and, within a year, is generally not palpable. Occasionally, however, benign cysts can develop within the postmenopausal ovary and enlarge it into the palpable range. The proportion of malignant tumors in women over 50 with palpable ovaries is about 30%. However, with the more widespread use of ultrasound, as many as 10% to 15% of postmenopausal women have the incidental finding of small cysts in their ovaries (7). If the cyst is less than 5 cm, simple in character, unilateral, and thin walled, and the CA-125 is normal (<35), and if she is asymptomatic and without ascites, the patient should be a candidate for conservative management (8). The American College of Obstetricians and Gynecologists guidelines recommend that such women be offered tests (CA-125 and transvaginal ultrasonography) at 1 month and every 3 months for the first year and every 4 to 6 months thereafter (9), especially if she is a poor surgical risk. If there is any change in the size or morphology of the ovary or the mass, or if the CA-125 level rises for otherwise unexplained reasons, the patient should be referred to a gynecologist for surgical resection because with these findings she has a 70% to 80% chance of ovarian malignancy.

The ovaries atrophy at the time of menopause and within 1 year generally become nonpalpable. The incidence of malignant tumors in women over 50 with palpable ovaries is about 30%.

The approach and extent of surgery and the specialization of the staff needed at operation depend upon the probability of carcinoma. If the physical examination or adjunctive testing suggests carcinoma, it is important to

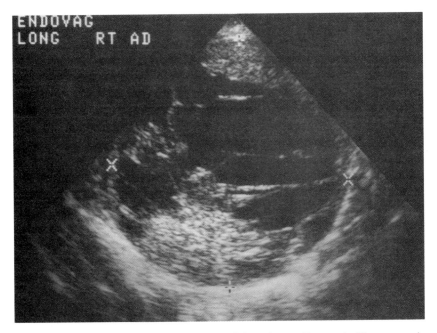

Figure 13-5 Ultrasound image of ovarian epithelial carcinoma. Transvaginal image reveals a multiseptated, complex mass with thick septa and a substantial solid component. Such findings indicate malignancy is likely.

thoroughly stage the extent of the cancer at the time of surgery and optimally debulk the tumor. In women under age 30 with solid components in their masses, preoperative serum alpha-fetoprotein (AFP) and human chorionic gonadotropin (hCG) levels should be drawn to identify germ cell tumors. Postoperatively, older women suspected of having ovarian cancer may benefit from baseline CA-125 levels to monitor their response to treatment.

Ovarian masses thought to be benign are best approached laparoscopically; referral to gynecologists experienced in those procedures can reduce overall costs and shorten recovery time. A prospective randomized trial compared laparotomy with laparoscopy for treatment of premenopausal women with benign-appearing adnexal masses measuring <10 cm (10). No differences were found in operating time or in the risk of inadvertent rupture of the ovarian mass, but laparoscopy was associated with less operative morbidity, fewer hospital days, and less postoperative pain (10). Postmenopausal women with persistent masses at low suspicion for cancer (e.g., simple cystic masses measuring <4 cm with normal CA-125 levels), for whom the decision has been made to operate, may also benefit from laparoscopic approach (10).

Some investigators have advocated transvaginal aspiration of ovarian simple cysts in premenopausal women, especially those cysts that are small and thin walled where cure rates exceed 50% (11). However, fine-needle aspiration is currently not recommended as the management of choice, because the recurrence rate after 1 year is 25% to 40% and the sensitivity of cytologic examination of aspirated fluids is variable (40% to 95%) (12). Some have also voiced concern for the possibility of seeding the abdomen with malignant cells (13).

Functional Ovarian Cysts

Functional cysts differ from their normal counterparts (ovarian follicle, corpus luteum) solely on the basis of excessive size. Functional cysts are normal according to the phase of the menstrual cycle during which they develop (i.e., there are follicular and corpus luteum cysts). Theca lutein cysts are a third, less common, type of function cyst that are associated with pregnancy or use of reproductive technologies. Functional cysts are common; an estimated 65% of women undergoing surgery for ovarian enlargement are found to have functional cysts.

Follicular Cysts
Follicular cysts are common in young menstruating women and form during the preovulatory (i.e., follicular) phase of the menstrual cycle. As with a normal ovarian follicle, a follicular cyst initially develops from cyclical gonadotropin stimulation; however, it then persists abnormally either as a result of a failure of the dominant follicle to rupture or from failure of an immature follicle to undergo atresia. While the upper limit of diameter of a normal ovarian follicle is 2.5 cm, follicular cysts range from 2.5 to 15 cm in diameter. (Therefore it is by definition inaccurate to inform a woman with a 1.5 cm follicle that she has an ovarian "cyst".) Structurally, follicular cysts are fluid-filled, thin-walled structures located in the ovarian cortex. Most are asymptomatic and incidental findings on routine exam, although larger follicular cysts may cause a sensation of pelvic fullness or dull aching. Occasionally, these cysts are ruptured during the bimanual exam and may cause transient tenderness. Such large cysts may also predispose the patient to ovarian or adnexal torsion, which typically presents as an acute abdomen (see Chapter 9).

As stated above, management of follicular cysts depends upon the patient's age and symptoms as well as the size of the mass and sonographic appearance. In reproductive-age women, masses greater than 8 to 10 cm are surgically explored, the only possible exception being a rapidly resolving simple cyst in an asymptomatic woman. Smaller follicular cysts (5 to 8 cm) may be managed conservatively with a repeat pelvic examination in 2 months, because most of these cysts should spontaneously resolve in 8 to 9 weeks. In such instances, sonographic studies are not mandatory but may be helpful to document the character of the mass and trends in size of the cyst over the observation period. Neither combined oral contraceptive pills nor DMPA (Depo-Provera) will hasten the rate of spontaneous regression of a follicular cyst (14), but these are often prescribed as they reduce the likelihood that a second follicle may arise to confuse the clinical picture (15). Furthermore, these contraceptives will help prevent pregnancy from complicating management. Follicular cysts that persist for 8 to 12 weeks in reproductive-age women require surgical intervention, because it is not possible to exclude carcinoma on clinical grounds alone. Simple cystectomy, commonly performed laparoscopically, is the preferred procedure unless other pathology is detected intraoperatively.

Postmenopausal women occasionally develop cysts that clinically appear to be "follicular cysts". Because these postmenopausal women are not ordinarily expected to have responsive follicles, these cysts should be viewed with suspicion. However, estimates of the prevalence of these cysts are increasing as more menopausal women undergo ultrasound studies.

Corpus Luteum Cysts

Corpus luteum cysts differ from follicular cysts in that the former develop during the postovulatory (i.e., luteal) phase of the cycle, usually as a consequence of the follicle immediately re-sealing following ovulation. Retention and then further accumulation of cystic fluid occurs, thereby preventing the normal degeneration and fibrosis of the follicle. Sometimes progesterone production is prolonged as well. A corpus luteum cyst (CLC) must be at least 3 cm in diameter to distinguish it from a normal corpus luteum; the average diameter of a CLC is 4 cm. Corpus luteum cysts are therefore generally smaller and less common than follicular cysts but because of the generation of progesterone are clinically more significant.

A CLC may be an incidental finding on routine exam but may cause the woman dull unilateral lower abdominal or pelvic pain. Because a CLC is often associated with prolonged progesterone production, the clinical presentation of a symptomatic woman with a CLC often resembles that of a woman with an early ectopic pregnancy: she may have delayed menses, pelvic pain, and a tender adnexal mass. Sensitive pregnancy tests are necessary to distinguish between these diagnoses (see Chapter 9). Ultrasonography is not always diagnostic. The sonographic appearance of a CLC in nonpregnant women can be quite similar to that of a cystadenoma or an endometrioma.

Unruptured CLCs in asymptomatic women may be managed with a follow-up pelvic examination in 4 to 6 weeks. If resolution does not occur spontaneously, surgical evaluation and a cystectomy are performed to confirm the diagnosis. The objective of surgery should be to remove the pathology while preserving ovarian function.

Postmenopausal women and women using hormonal methods that reliably suppress ovulation (oral contraceptives, DMPA) are highly unlikely to develop such cysts.

Theca Lutein Cysts

Theca lutein cysts are the third and least common of the functional cysts. They result from excess hCG stimulation and consequently usually occur in pregnancy, the so-called "luteoma of pregnancy" (discussed later in this chapter). However, exogenous gonadotropins prescribed to infertility patients to induce ovulation also can also cause theca lutein cysts; rarely, paraneoplastic processes in which hCG is elaborated may also create theca lutein cysts. Both ovaries are usually affected, and they can become moderately or massively enlarged (up to 20 to 30 cm in diameter) as a result of this excess stimulation and contain hundreds of cysts. Medication history and pregnancy testing often suggest the diagnosis, which can be confirmed by ultrasonography. Management consists of close observation with serial pelvic exams and ultrasound studies, because these cysts will generally spontaneously regress within 2 to 3 months after the source of excessive stimulation is removed. Occasionally supportive care becomes necessary when massive ascites develops and compromises respiration.

Polycystic Ovary Syndrome

Polycystic ovary (PCO) syndrome is a complex and heterogeneous state. As it was originally defined in 1935 by Stein and Leventhal (13), PCO was diagnosed in women who had oligomenorrhea, hirsutism, obesity, and infertility and who were found to have enlarged, polycystic ovaries. Today, most experts agree that PCO is a problem of chronic anovulation that may present with a wide range of clinical manifestations, no single one of which is diagnostic, and in fact does not necessarily include the finding of polycystic ovaries. The majority of women with PCO do have enlarged ovaries with at least ten follicles on an ultrasound plane and an increased volume of stroma (Fig. 13-6). However, ap-

Polycystic ovary syndrome is a problem of chronic anovulation. Most women with PCO have enlarged and cystic ovaries; however, approximately 30% of affected women have normal-appearing ovaries on ultrasonography.

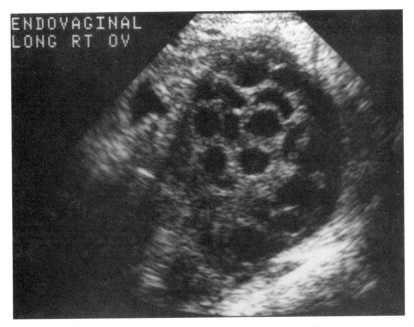

Figure 13-6 Ultrasound image of polycystic ovary. Multiple small cystic structures of similar size within an enlarged ovary are consistent with, but not diagnostic of, polycystic ovary syndrome. Conversely, this morphologic finding is not necessarily present in this disorder of chronic anovulation.

proximately 30% of women with clinically diagnosed PCO have normal-appearing ovaries on ultrasonography. Conversely, ultrasound findings of polycystic ovaries may be found in approximately 25% of normal cycling women and even 14% of women on oral contraceptives. Several etiologies have been suggested for this poorly understood and complex syndrome (see Chapter 3).

The finding of bilaterally enlarged, cystic ovaries on pelvic exam in a woman with irregular menses necessitates further evaluation. After the possibility of pregnancy has been eliminated, an ultrasound study is ordered to exclude other pelvic pathology. Once the diagnosis of PCO is made on clinical grounds, treatment should focus on normalizing androgen levels, preventing unopposed estrogen stimulation of the endometrium, and treating insulin resistance. Typically contraceptives, DMPA, or cyclic oral medroxyprogesterone are prescribed. Oral contraceptives decrease circulating free testosterone levels and prevent endometrial hyperplasia. DMPA suppresses endometrial growth and cyclic oral medroxyprogesterone can induce regular withdrawal bleeding. Each of these methods prevents the unopposed endometrial stimulation. When weight loss in not achieved, treatment with metformin or a thiazolidinedione is often indicated. For women desiring pregnancy, ovulation induction will likely be necessary and such patients should be appropriately referred.

Ovarian Neoplasms

Each year nearly 26,000 women in the United States are diagnosed with ovarian cancer and over half that number die of the disease (16). Ovarian cancer is now the fourth leading cause of cancer deaths in women (after lung, breast, and colon cancer) (17), and a woman's lifetime risk of ovarian carcinoma is 1.4%. Women of all ages are affected, but for a young woman (age 20 to 35 years) with an ovarian mass there is only a 1% chance that the mass is malignant, whereas the likelihood is much higher for a mass detected in a peri- or post-menopausal woman. The peak incidence of ovarian cancer occurs at age 62.

> *Ovarian cancer is now the fourth leading cause of cancer deaths in women. The peak incidence occurs at age 62, but women of all ages are affected.*

Ovarian neoplasms are classified according to the predominant cell type involved (e.g., epithelial, germ cell) and histologic appearance—benign, borderline ("low malignant potential"), or invasive. Therefore each of the cell types discussed below may be benign, borderline, or malignant in its behavior (Table 13-1).

Epithelial Ovarian Neoplasms
BENIGN
The coelomic epithelium covering the ovary gives rise to 75% of all primary ovarian neoplasms, the overwhelming majority of which are benign. The major cell types in this category include serous, mucinous, endometrioid, clear cell, transitional, and undifferentiated. The benign tumors are lined by a single layer of cells without nuclear stratification or atypia.

Serous cysts may assume a variety of appearances and may be difficult to differentiate from malignant tumors, making frozen sections at the time of surgery important. *Mucinous cystadenomas* are distinguished by their ability to gradually grow to massive dimensions (albeit slowly). This distinguishes them from rapidly growing malignant masses; some mucinous tumors weigh more than 100 kg and literally fill the peritoneal cavity. These benign tumors may also be complicated by pseudomyxoma peritonei, in which a massive amount of mucinous material collects in the peritoneal cavity, leading to the formation of adhesions. *Endometrioid tumors* of the ovary include endometrioid adenoma and adenofibroma. Many also classify ovarian endometrioma

Table 13-1 Ovarian Neoplasms

Benign	Malignant	Comments
Epithelial neoplasms		
Serous cystadenoma	Serous cystadenocarcinoma	*Need tissue specimen to distinguish*
Most common; benign		*between benign and malignant*
epithelial neoplasm		*tumors*
Mucinous cystadenoma	Mucinous cystadenocarcinoma	
May be very large; spill of	*CA-125 levels not elevated*	
contents may result in		
pseudomyxoma peritonei		
Endometrioid	Endometrioid adenocarcinoma	
"Chocolate cysts" often		
associated with other		
pelvic endometriosis;		
benign endometrial tumor		
(adenofibroma)		
Mesonephroid (clear cell)		*Small, rare, solid tumors,*
tumors		*unilateral Meig's syndrome*
Brenner tumor		*associated with ovarian fibroma (as-*
Fibroma		*cites and hydrothorax)*
Solid tumor usually 6 cm		
but may weigh up to to		
50 lb		
Germ cell neoplasms		
Benign cystic teratoma	Immature teratoma	*Benign version most common tumor in*
("Dermoid cyst" or "mature	*Presence of immature*	*adolescents and women in their 20's;*
teratoma") contains teeth,	*neural tissue; usually*	*malignancy types differ by age: im-*
hair, sebum; rupture may	*unilateral*	*mature types more likely in young;*
cause chemical peritonitis	Malignant degeneration of mature cys-	*malignant degeneration more likely in*
Struma ovarii	tic teratoma	*postmenopausal women*
Thyroid glands overgrow	*Rare, usually squamous*	
other elements in	Dysgerminoma	*Male counterpart: seminoma; can occur*
dermoid; may cause		*at any age but mostly in young*
hyperthyroidism		*adults; one of most*
		common neoplasms found in preg-
		nancy
	Endodermal sinus tumor	*Bilateral 10%–15%; AFP levels*
	("yolk sac" tumor)	*often elevated; median age 19*
	Embryonal carcinoma	*Extremely fast growing; one of the most*
		malignant ovarian cancers; resembles
		same tumor in testes.
	Choriocarcinoma	*AFP and HCG levels elevated; HCG lev-*
		els elevated; may follow pregnancy or
		start spontaneously
	Gonadoblastoma	*Often appears in women with primary*
		amenorrhea, virilization, abnormal
		sexual maturation
Stroma cell neoplasms		
(sex cord tumors)		
Granulosa-theca cell thecoma	Granulosa-theca	*Call-Exner bodies found on histology;*
Rarely malignant;		*produce estrogen that can cause pre-*
usually unilateral;		*cocious puberty, endometrial cancer,*
postmenopausal women		*postmenopausal bleeding; usually*
		low malignant potential
Sertoli-Leydig	Sertoli-Leydig	*Results in masculinization; also called*
		androblastoma or arrhenoblastoma;
		moderately well or poorly differenti-
		ated malignancy
Metastatic tumors	Krukenberg	*Primary in GI tract, breast, or other mu-*
		cous gland; signet ring cells
	Metastatic adenocarcinoma from	*More common than Krukenberg*
	Large intestine	
	Breast	
	Endometrium	*Most common metastases*
	Lymphoma	

("chocolate cysts") in this category. An endometrioma forms when cystic hemorrhagic spaces develop within the ovary as a result of monthly shedding from the endometrial implants below the cortex. Medical therapy for endometriosis is often quite successful; however, endometriomas larger than a few centimeters do not respond to hormonal suppression and require surgical removal.

Other benign epithelial cell neoplasms of the ovary are less common. *Clear cell* tumors are relatively rare but are the most common type of ovarian neoplasm associated with hypercalcemia or hyperpyrexia.

MALIGNANT

Approximately 90% of all ovarian carcinoma derive from the ovarian epithelium. Most women who develop ovarian cancer are older and, unfortunately, remain asymptomatic until their disease is advanced. If early symptoms do occur, they are usually vague, nonspecific and refer to the upper GI tract (e.g., early satiety, dyspepsia). As a result, these women often undergo a thorough GI evaluation but not a pelvic examination. Later in the disease process, ascites and metastases to the bowel and omentum can cause abdominal distention, dyspnea, nausea, vomiting, and anorexia. Mechanical effects of tumor impingement may also result in complaints of urinary frequency or constipation. Menstrual changes may occur in premenopausal women and vaginal bleeding in postmenopausal ones.

Most women with early-stage ovarian cancer are asymptomatic. Some note vague, nonspecific symptoms referable to the upper GI tract, such as early satiety and dyspepsia.

The most common sign of ovarian cancer is a pelvic mass, usually solid, irregular, and fixed. If an abdominal mass (usually an omental cake) or ascites is also found, advanced ovarian cancer is highly likely. Whenever suspicion of an ovarian carcinoma is raised on pelvic examination, sonographic studies, particularly transvaginal ultrasound, should be obtained because these often provide useful information about the character of the lesion (solid or cystic, simple or complex) and its spread. CT scanning is performed next as it is better able to evaluate lymph node involvement. The elevated levels of the tumor marker CA-125 may increase the suspicion of a malignant process, but low levels are not reassuring. CA-125 is normal in more than 50% of stage 1 serous cystadenocarcinomas and is not able to de-

The tumor marker CA-125 may increase the suspicion of a malignant process if it is elevated but is not reassuring if it is low.

tect mucinous cystadenocarcinoma. When elevated, this tumor marker is valuable in assessing the effectiveness of therapy in women being treated for many types of ovarian carcinoma and, following surgery, is helpful in detecting early recurrences. The definitive diagnosis of epithelial ovarian carcinoma and its formal staging are obtained at surgery. Prognosis is dependent on tumor type and stage of disease.

Germ Cell Tumors

BENIGN

Germ cell tumors tend to present earlier in life than do epithelial cell neoplasms. The range of tumor types that arise in this category reflects the full potential of the primordial germ cells.

Benign cystic teratomas (commonly called *dermoid cysts*) are among the most common ovarian neoplasms, comprising 20% to 25% of ovarian neoplasms in reproductive years. They are slow-growing tumors that can present as early as infancy but generally are detected in the early reproductive years. Cystic teratomas can range in size from millimeters to 25 cm in diameter; 80% are less than 10 cm. A cystic teratoma usually gives rise to no symptoms and is discovered on pelvic examination or ultrasonography performed for some other indication.

Classically, cystic teratomas are found anteriorly and are quite mobile on bimanual exam, often migrating to the upper quadrants during manipulation. Occasionally, the weight of the mass will trap it behind the uterus in the posterior cul-de-sac. Cystic teratomas are bilateral in 10% to 15% of cases.

Cystic teratomas are derived from totipotential stem cells and include elements of ectodermal, mesodermal, and, rarely, endodermal tissue. As a result, they are often filled with viscous sebaceous fluid, hair, cartilage, and teeth. Most of the solid material is contained in a protrusion of the cyst wall (tubercle of Rokitansky) that forms the calcifications that can be seen on pelvic X-ray film. Ultrasonography can image an adnexal mass with solid and cystic components, often with a fluid line or Rokitansky's protuberance as a confirmatory finding. Although the sonographic image is very characteristic, malignancy can only be ruled out histologically. Therefore, except for the very small lesions, surgical extirpation (usually by cystectomy) of cystic teratomas is required to verify the benign nature of the mass and to avoid potential complications such as torsion, rupture, and malignant degeneration. In some series, torsion occurred in over 10% of dermoids, usually in younger women. Although uncommon, rupture of the cyst contents can occur at any time but is more likely in pregnancy and presents as a chemical peritonitis caused by the leak of sebaceous material into the peritoneal cavity. Malignant degeneration of benign cystic teratomas occurs in less than 2% of cases; its most common presentation is squamous cell carcinoma in older women.

MALIGNANT

Malignant germ cell tumors grow rapidly and often cause pelvic pain as a result of hemorrhage, necrosis, or distention of the capsule. Most appear in younger women, even prepubescent girls, and can be detected as a mass on pelvic exam. Many of these tumors have quantitative tumor markers such as alpha-fetoprotein (AFP) and hCG, which assist in making the diagnosis and in monitoring the effectiveness of treatment.

Dysgerminoma is the most common type of malignant germ cell tumor; it is analogous to seminoma of the male testis. *Immature teratomas* contain immature extra-embryonal or embryonal elements. *Endodermal sinus tumors* (formerly called *yolk sac tumors*) are always unilateral, are detectable by monitoring serum AFP, and are best treated by unilateral oophorectomy. *Choriocarcinoma* can be diagnosed by the presence of hCG in nonpregnant women but can be first suggested by pregnancy symptoms.

Sex Cord/Stromal Tumors

Sex cord/stromal tumors are capable of producing sex steroids and are generally characterized by the impacts of their "female" or "male" hormone production. *Granulosa* cell tumors secrete estrogen and are seen in women of all ages, although more often in postmenopausal women. Because of its estrogen production, this tumor is frequently associated with endometrial hyperplasia (25% to 50% of cases) and even endometrial carcinoma (5% of affected women). *Sertoli-Leydig* tumors, on the other hand, produce androgens that can cause clinical virilization in 70% to 85% of women. *Thecomas,* particularly luteinized thecomas, are usually unilateral and almost always benign; 50% of thecomas produce estrogen.

Tumors Metastatic to the Ovary

The ovary is a common site for hematogenously disseminated carcinomas due to the richness of its blood supply. Krukenberg tumors are metastatic lesions to the ovary that arise most frequently from gastric carcinoma, but other abdominal neoplasms may also be the source. Nearly one-fourth of women who die from breast cancer have evidence of metastatic disease to the ovaries. Lymphomas and leukemias can also metastasize to the ovary. Women with personal histories of these malignancies need careful monitoring of the size, consistency, and tenderness of their ovaries over time.

Pelvic Masses Related to Pregnancy

Three specific problems unique to the state of pregnancy need to be considered when a pelvic mass is encountered in a gravid woman: ectopic pregnancy, molar pregnancy, and luteoma of pregnancy.

Ectopic Pregnancy

When faced with a positive pregnancy test and a pelvic mass, a provider must have a high index of suspicion for ectopic pregnancy, even in an asymptomatic woman. Many ectopic pregnancies occur in the absence of any identifiable risk factors. Physical exam findings may be misleading, because the uterus typically enlarges due to hormonal stimulation. It should also be mentioned that in the majority of cases the ecoptic pregnancy is not palpable. Women with suspected ectopic pregnancy should be managed by those experienced with this diagnosis (see Chapter 9).

Molar Pregnancy

Hydatidiform mole (molar pregnancy) is an abnormal pregnancy characterized by the absence of a fetus, embryo, cord, and amnion, and the presence of swelling of the placental villi. Molar pregnancies are uncommon but may be suspected when a woman suffers excessive hormonally related symptoms such as hyperemesis gravidarum and early pregnancy-induced hypertension. The physical findings of absent fetal heart tones and greater than expected uterine enlargement can also suggest the diagnosis. Levels of β-hCG are often abnormally high. Ultrasonography may reveal classic "grape clusters" or "snow storm" appearances or may demonstrate an abnormality consistent with a missed abortion. Treatment is uterine evacuation, and final diagnosis is made upon histologic evaluation of the uterine contents. Molar pregnancies carry an increased risk for development of subsequent trophoblastic disease, including choriocarcinoma; frequent postoperative testing of β-hCG levels is therefore necessary. Follow-up care should be provided by specialists.

Luteoma of Pregnancy

A luteoma of pregnancy results from a benign, hyperplastic reaction of the theca lutein cells and is similar to a theca lutein cyst. However, in contrast to theca lutein cysts, luteoma of pregnancy may significantly elevate serum androgen levels, which is sometimes manifest by signs and symptoms of masculinization. The fetus is less frequently affected, because the placenta rapidly aromatizes androgens into estrogen. Conservative management using serial examinations and ultrasound studies is appropriate once other etiologies have been eliminated. It should be noted that the ovarian masses might persist for months after the β-hCG levels have returned to nonpregnant levels (18).

Pelvic Relaxation

Although not usually thought of as a pelvic mass, pelvic relaxation can cause a woman to complain of a sense of fullness or a mass pressing on her introitus or protruding from her vagina. The examiner generally has little difficulty distinguishing these findings of pelvic relaxation from a true mass (see Chapter 14 for a discussion of evaluation and management).

Ovarian Cancer Screening

Screening in Usual-Risk Women

When ovarian cancer is diagnosed at an early stage, 5-year cure rates approach 100% (19). Because over two-thirds of ovarian cancer is diagnosed at an advanced stage when prognosis is poor, considerable effort has been expended to develop more effective screening programs to detect early, more curable disease. One of the greatest challenges to establishing an ovarian cancer screening program is the sporadic nature of the disease. While there are identified risk factors for ovarian cancer, no subset of women is exclusively at increased risk for the disease. Even women who have undergone oophorectomy are still at some, albeit smaller, risk for developing ovarian carcinoma. Also, because rare as ovarian cancer is so rare, the screening tests must be highly sensitive and specific. Even if a screening test for ovarian cancer had 98% specificity and 80% sensitivity, its positive predictive value would still be low, and for every real case of ovarian cancer identified, 50 women would need to undergo diagnostic surgical procedures (20).

A thorough pelvic examination, emphasizing the bimanual and rectal elements, has been the traditional screening test for ovarian carcinoma. However, the pelvic exam is not very sensitive; pelvic examination may miss as many as 10% of pelvic masses of less than 10 cm.

Investigators have studied many devices to screen women, including transabdominal ultrasound, transvaginal ultrasonography, and tumor markers (e.g., CA-125)—alone and in combination. The results of these trials, as summarized by the Cancer Genetics Studies Consortium (21), the NIH Consensus Conference (20), and others (23), have been discouraging. While transabdominal ultrasound has clearly demonstrated an ability to detect an increase in ovarian volume, it is not able to distinguish accurately between benign and malignant lesions. The sensitivity of transabdominal ultrasound is therefore superior to pelvic examination, but its specificity is low. Transvaginal ultrasound represents an improvement over transabdominal ultrasound, demonstrating both superior sensitivity (>95%) and specificity for detecting ovarian cancer, but in clinical trials 90% of lesions detected by transvaginal ultrasound were still benign. Consequently, because of the rarity of the ovarian carcinoma, transvaginal ultrasound screening would result in 10 laparotomies for every case of ovarian cancer detected in postmenopausal women.

CA-125 is generally held to be the most specific serum marker for ovarian cancer; however, as a screening test, CA-125 lacks both sensitivity and specificity. CA-125 has only a sensitivity of 50% in clinically detected stage I disease, and it is even lower in sonographically detected stage I tumors. Its specificity is similarly poor, stemming from the fact that CA-125 levels can be elevated in a wide range of unrelated processes including pregnancy, menstruation, endometriosis, pelvic inflammatory disease (PID), and pancreatic cancer.

Some researchers have coupled CA-125 with ultrasonography to increase the sensitivity of screening programs (24-26). However, estimates project that if every woman in America over age 45 were screened on an annual basis with transvaginal ultrasound and serum CA-125 levels, the cost would approach $45 billion each year without evidence that any lives would be saved. Given these cost issues and the poor sensitivity of both CA-125 and transvaginal ultrasound, the 1994 NCI Consensus Conference (20) reached the following conclusion:

> There is no evidence available yet that current screening modalities of CA-125 and transvaginal ultrasound can be effectively used for widespread screening to reduce mortality from ovarian cancer nor that their use will result in decreased rather than increased morbidity and mortality.

A prospective, randomized trial of ovarian cancer screening of 74,000 postmenopausal women was initiated in 1993 by the National Cancer Institute (NIH) and may provide better guidance in upcoming years.

Currently, the annual pelvic examination is the preferred screening test for the low-risk woman. In the future, better screening tests may become available such as new ovarian cancer antigens and new imaging techniques such as implanted telemetry systems with high-resolution pixel cameras and three-dimensional ultrasound imaging (27).

Screening in High-Risk Women

Family history has long been recognized as a risk factor for epithelial ovarian cancer. If a woman has one affected first-degree relative, she has a two- to four-fold increased risk of developing epithelial ovarian carcinoma. If a woman has one first-degree relative and a second-degree relative with ovarian carcinoma, she faces a three- to ten-fold increased risk (up to 15% lifetime risk) of developing ovarian cancer. With two first-degree relatives affected, genetic inheritance may be of an autosomal dominant mode and the patient's lifetime risk of ovarian cancer may be as high as 50%. Women with these hereditary risk factors tend to develop ovarian cancer a decade earlier than women with nonhereditary disease.

High-risk women fall into one of three groups: specific family history of ovarian carcinoma (site-specific), hereditary breast/ovarian familial cancer syndrome, and the Lynch II syndrome. It is now thought that 90% of familial ovarian cancer falls into the second category (i.e., the woman's risk is due to mutations in the *BRCA1* breast/ovarian cancer susceptibility gene).

Women with hereditary breast/ovarian familial cancer syndrome (including those with *BRCA1* gene mutations) may face up to an 85% risk of developing breast cancer by age 70 and a lifetime risk for ovarian cancer of 10% to 25% (21). Usually the family pedigree reveals affected first- and second-degree relatives from the maternal and/or paternal side, with transmission in an autosomal dominant pattern. *BRCA2* mutations have less impact on a woman's risk for ovarian cancer; the cumulative risk is estimated to be 10% by age 70. Lynch II syndrome reflects a combination of Lynch I syndrome (familial colon cancer) and a high rate of ovarian, endometrial, and breast cancers in addition to other colon and genitourinary cancers.

Management of women in these high-risk groups depends upon their age, fertility desires, and the magnitude of their individual risk. With appropriate counseling, *BRCA1* testing may be offered to women with a family history of two or more family members with ovarian/breast cancer. Those found free of mutations may be less intensively monitored, while those with the mutation could benefit from more intensive preventive strategies.

Prophylactic oophorectomy will reduce, but not eliminate, the risk of ovarian carcinoma. It should be offered to high-risk women (especially those with two or more first-degree relatives with ovarian cancer) by age 35 or earlier if they complete their families at a younger age. Such surgery can be performed laparoscopically on an outpatient basis.

For women at high risk for ovarian cancer, prophylactic oophorectomy can reduce (but not eliminate) the risk of ovarian carcinoma. It can be offered by age 35, or earlier if the woman has completed her family.

For those high-risk women who do not undergo prophylactic oophorectomy, the ACOG Committee on Gynecologic Practice (9) advocates CA-125 and transvaginal ultrasound studies every 6 months.

The Cancer Genetics Studies Consortium consensus statement recommends that *BRCA1* mutation carriers undergo annual or semiannual screening with serum CA-125 levels and transvaginal ultrasound starting at age 25 to 35 (21). Ideally the transvaginal ultrasounds should be coupled with color-flow Doppler and morphologic index determination. In younger women, such studies need to be carefully timed to avoid false positive results arising from ovulation (which could confound ultrasound findings) and menstruation (which can falsely elevate the CA-125). In addition, patients should be advised to use measures to reduce the risk of ovarian cancer (see below).

It should be noted that over 5% postmenopausal women and over 35% of premenopausal women who are being treated for breast cancer with tamoxifen will develop reversible ovarian cysts. Because some of these women may be at high risk for ovarian carcinoma due to *BRCA1* mutations they deserve prompt but measured evaluation. The cysts will resolve if the tamoxifen is discontinued (28).

Ovarian Cancer Prevention

Only about 5% of the women who develop ovarian carcinoma have an identifiable genetic risk factor. Incessant ovulation is the other variable that has been identified as an important risk factor for development of epithelial ovarian carcinoma, for a woman's risk is related to the number of ovarian cycles she experiences. Injectable and combination oral contraceptives effectively suppress ovulation. In epidemiologic studies, oral contraceptives have been shown to significantly reduce the risk of epithelial ovarian cancer. Use of oral contraceptives for only 12 months reduces the risk by 40%, and women who have used birth control pills for 10 years have a relative risk of 0.2 for epithelial ovarian carcinoma. In a manner analogous to childbearing, it is likely that this use would have greatest impact in the early reproductive years—before age 30 or 35.

Contraception that suppresses ovulation, higher parity, and tubal ligation all appear to protect against future development of ovarian cancer.

Injectable contraceptives probably provide a similar protection effect, although data currently available from international studies have shown only a slight protective effect, likely because the studies preferentially enrolled multiparous women already at significantly lower risk for ovarian cancer. It is predicted that as young women in the United States use injectable methods in greater numbers, the magnitude of protection against ovarian cancer afforded by injectable methods will become more evident.

Recent studies have also shown that bilateral tubal ligation lowers a woman's risk of ovarian cancer (29). The reason for this protection has not been fully elucidated but may in part be related to subsequent decrease in the vascular perfusion of the ovaries. Consequently, there may possibly be inhibition of ovulation, or perhaps lower estrogen levels, or a disturbance in the utero-ovarian circulation that results in a reduction in the uterine growth factors delivered to the ovaries. An alternative explanation is that tubal ligation may afford protection by blocking carcinogens (e.g., perineal asbestos and possibly other substances such as talc) from reaching the ovaries (29). Some studies (30-32), including two large meta-analyses (33,34), have demonstrated an association between the development of ovarian cancer and the use of talcum powder and possibly also deodorant spray (30) in the perineal area. More recent studies fail to support such a link (35-37), however, suggesting that perhaps in the past the known problem of asbestos contaminating talc may have been responsible (37). Nonetheless, some clinicians advise their patients to avoid such hygiene practices until evidence is conclusive.

Summary

A pelvic mass can represent any of several possibilities, ranging from hard stool in the colon to ovarian carcinoma. Through careful elicitation of the history, thorough physical examination, and appropriate use of ultrasound study, the experienced physician can usually determine the initial course of action before the involvement of the gynecologist. Clinical competence at the level of the primary care physician can contribute to efficient management, leading to prompt intervention of pelvic malignancies and timely reassurance when all is benign.

REFERENCES

1. Uterine leiomyomata. ACOG Technical Bulletin. 1994;192:1-9.
2. **Friedman AJ, Thomas PP.** Does low-dose combination oral contraceptive use affect uterine size or menstrual flow in premenopausal women with leiomyomas? Obstet Gynecol. 1995;85:631-5.
3. **Tanos V, Schenker JG.** Ovarian cysts: a clinical dilemma. Gynecol Endocrinol. 1994;8: 59-67.
4. **Osmers RGW, Osmers M, von Maydell B, et al.** Preoperative evaluation of ovarian tumors in the premenopause by transvaginosonography. Am J Obstet Gynecol. 1996; 175:428-34.
5. **Herrmann UJ, Locher GW, Goldhirsch A.** Sonographic patterns of ovarian tumors: prediction of malignancy. Obstet Gynecol. 1987;69:777-81.

6. **Benacerraf BR, Finkler NJ, Wojciechowski C, Knapp RC.** Sonographic accuracy in the diagnosis of ovarian masses. J Reprod Med. 1990;35:491-5.

7. **Wolf SI, Gosink BB, Feldesman MR, et al.** Prevalence of simple adnexal cysts in postmenopausal women. Radiology. 1991;180:65-71.

8. **Goldstein SR.** Postmenopausal adnexal cysts: how clinical management has evolved. Am J Obstet Gynecol. 1996;175:1498-501.

9. **ACOG Committee on Gynecologic Practice.** Routine cancer screening. Committee Opinion 128. American College of Obstetricians and Gynecologists; 1993.

10. **Parker WH, Berek JS.** Laparoscopic management of the adnexal mass. Obstet Gynecol Clin N Am. 1994;21:79-92.

11. **Weinraub Z, Avrech O, Fuchs C, et al.** Transvaginal aspiration of ovarian cysts: prognosis based on outcome over a 12-month period. J Ultrasound Med. 1994;13:275-9.

12. **Ganjei P.** Fine-needle aspiration cytology of the ovary. Clin Lab Med. 1995;15:705-26.

13. **Stein IF, Leventhal ML.** Amenorrheic association with bilateral polycystic ovaries. Am J Obstet Gynecol. 1935;29:181-91.

14. **Steinkampf MP, Hammond, KR, Blackwell RE.** Hormonal treatment of functional ovarian cysts: a randomized, prospective study. Fertil Steril. 1990;54:775-7.

15. **Lanes SF, Birmann B, Walker AM, Singer S.** Oral contraceptive type and functional ovarian cysts. Am J Obstet Gynecol. 1992;166:956-61.

16. **Wingo PA, Tong T, Bolden S.** Cancer statistics, 1995. CA Cancer J Clin. 1995;45:8-30.

17. **DiSaia PJ.** Ovarian neoplasms. In: Scott JR, DiSaia PJ, Hammond CB, Spellacy WN, eds. Danforth's Obstetrics and Gynecology, 7th ed. Philadelphia: Lippincott-Raven; 1997.

18. **Fossum GT, Davajan V, Kletzky OA.** Early detection of pregnancy with transvaginal ultrasound. Fertil Steril. 1988;41:788-91.

19. **Young RC, Walton LA, Wllenberg SS, et al.** Adjuvant therapy in stage I and stage II epithelial ovarian cancer: results of two prospective randomized trials. N Engl J Med. 1990;322:1021-7.

20. **NIH Consensus Development Panel on Ovarian Cancer.** Ovarian cancer: screening, treatment and follow-up. JAMA. 1995;273:491-7.

21. **Burke W, Daly M, Garber J, et al, for the Cancer Genetics Studies Consortium.** Recommendations for follow-up care of individuals with an inherited predisposition to cancer: II—*BRCA1* and *BRCA2*. JAMA. 1997;277:997-1003.

22. Reference deleted in proof.

23. **Teneriello MG, Park RC.** Early detection of ovarian cancer. CA Cancer J Clin. 1995;45:71-87.

24. **Schwartz PE, Chambers JT, Taylor KJ.** Early detection and screening for ovarian cancer. J Cell Biochem Suppl. 1995;23:233-7.

25. **Fiorica JV, Roberts WS.** Screening for ovarian cancer. Cancer Control. 1996;3:120-9.

26. **Jacobs IJ, Skates SJ, MacDonald N, et al.** Screening for ovarian cancer: a pilot randomised controlled trial. Lancet. 1999;353:1207-10.

27. **Karlan BY, Platt LD.** Ovarian cancer screening: the role of ultrasound in early detection. Cancer. 1995;76:2011-5.

28. **Shushan A, Peretz T, Uziely B, et al.** Ovarian cysts in premenopausal and postmenopausal tamoxifen-treated women with breast cancer. Am J Obstet Gynecol. 1996; 174:141-4.

29. **Miracle-McMahill HL, Calle EE, Kosinski AS, et al.** Tubal ligation and fatal ovarian cancer in a large prospective cohort study. Am J Epidemiol. 1997;145:349-57.

30. **Cook LS, Kamb ML, Weiss NS.** Perineal powder exposure and the risk of ovarian cancer. Am J Epidemiol. 1997;145:459-65.

31. **Chang S, Risch H.** Perineal talc exposure and risk of ovarian carcinoma. Cancer. 1997;79:2396-401.

32. **Cramer DW, Liberman RF, Titus-Ernstoff L, et al.** Genital talc exposure and risk of ovarian cancer. Int J Cancer. 1991;81:351-6.

33. **Gross, AJ, Berg PH.** A meta-analytical approach examining the potential relationship between talc exposure and ovarian cancer. J Expo Anal Environ Epidemiol. 1995;5:181-95.

34. **Harlow BL, Cramer DW, Bell DA, Welch WR.** Perineal exposure to talc and ovarian cancer risk. Obstet Gynecol. 1992;80:19-26.

35. **Wong C, Hempling RE, Piver MS, et al.** Perineal talc exposure and subsequent epithelial ovarian cancer: a case-control study. Obstet Gynecol. 1999;93:372-6.

36. **Tzonou A, Polychronopoulou A, Hsieh CC, et al.** Hair dyes, analgesics, tranquilizers, and perineal talc applications as risk factors for ovarian cancer. Int J Cancer. 1993;55:408-10.

37. **Whysner J, Mohan M.** Perineal application of talc and cornstarch powders: evaluation of ovarian cancer risk. Am J Obstet Gynecol. 2000;182:720-4.

CHAPTER 14

Hysterectomy and Alternatives

SAMANTHA M. PFEIFER, MD

PAMELA CHARNEY, MD

NICOLE PILEVSKY, MD

STEVEN J. SONDHEIMER, MD

Hysterectomy is defined as the removal of the uterus including the uterine body (corpus) and cervix (1). The terms *total hysterectomy* or *complete hysterectomy* are synonymous with hysterectomy; however, these terms are commonly misused by the lay population to denote simultaneous removal of the adnexae (ovaries and fallopian tubes). To avoid this confusion, it is probably best to avoid these terms and to always indicate removal of the ovaries and tubes separately by stating "hysterectomy with or without bilateral/unilateral salpingo-oophorectomy."

Specific variants of hysterectomy include supracervical and radical. A supracervical hysterectomy refers to the removal of only the corpus leaving the cervix in place. Radical hysterectomy involves removal of most of the parametrial and upper vaginal tissue. Because of the wider dissection it is associated with greater surgical risk but also with a higher cure rate for limited invasive cervical cancer (stages I and II). Removal of the ovaries is not necessarily simultaneously performed with a radical hysterectomy.

The first vaginal hysterectomy in the United States was performed in 1829 by John Collins Warren of Harvard University. Abdominal hysterectomies followed later, in the mid-19th century; however, patients frequently died of hemorrhage, infection, and other post-operative complications. In the early 20th century, mortality was reduced to less than 1%, largely by employing reliable techniques to secure individual ligation of the uterine and ovarian vessels. By 1965, hysterectomy was the most common major surgery in the United States and it remained so until replaced by cesarean section in 1982 (2).

The rates for hysterectomy in the population vary substantially depending on patient characteristics and location (3,4). Relevant patient characteristics include age group, parity, and level of education, with highest hysterectomy rates occurring among women 40 to 54 years old (4). Multiple live births or miscarriages are associated with higher hysterectomy rates (3). In several studies, the level of education has been found to be inversely related to hysterectomy rates, including a recent study of women under age 45 (5). However, the Wisconsin Longitudinal Study found a woman's occupation to be more important than level of education on multivariate analysis (6). Whether this association is related to limited access to alternative treatments and/or delays in obtaining medical care is unclear. Geographic location has also been associated with wide variations in hysterectomy rates, with the United States (4) and Finland (7) having substantially higher rates than comparable developed countries. Overall, about one third of American women undergo hysterectomy by age 50, with higher rates noted in the South and the West (4). In some studies, hysterectomy rates also varied by race (8). In a study of women under 45 years of age, the most important risk factors for hysterectomy were self-reported uterine fibroids, endometriosis, severe dysmenorrhea, cancer, or previous ovarian surgery (5).

This chapter reviews hysterectomy, its common indications, and alternative treatments for many of these conditions. The natural history and management of fibroids and genital prolapse are discussed in detail. (Endometriosis, chronic pelvic pain, and urinary incontinence are reviewed in Chapters 11, 12, and 10, respectively.) Pre-operative and post-operative considerations are addressed. Additionally, the potential benefits and risks of hysterectomy are described.

Indications

Hysterectomy is performed to alleviate the discomfort, suffering, and morbidity caused by benign conditions of the uterus, and to treat malignant or pre-malignant conditions of the cervix, uterus, or ovaries. Most hysterectomies are performed for nonmalignant conditions such as abnormal vaginal bleeding, uterine fibroids, genital prolapse, or pelvic pain.

The most common indication for hysterectomy is difficult to assess because often more than one indication is reported on discharge summaries and in clinical summations. Several studies have reported analysis of hospital discharge coding using only the first indication listed on the discharge summary

(3,7,8). Recognizing this limitation, uterine fibroids are the most common indication followed by endometriosis (Table 14-1). Other common reasons for hysterectomy are cancer, prolapse, and menstrual or menopausal symptoms. Where it has been analyzed (7), the indications have remained stable over time. Hysterectomy is indicated for nonmalignant conditions when the symptoms are affecting the woman's quality of life and medical interventions are not successful, tolerated, or desired. The most common presenting symptoms that eventually lead to hysterectomy are abnormal vaginal bleeding and pelvic pain.

Abnormal Vaginal Bleeding

Abnormal vaginal bleeding is any vaginal bleeding pattern that varies from a woman's usual pattern (i.e., amenorrhea, menorrhagia, intermenstrual bleeding) and can stem from a variety of causes, including fibroids, endometrial hyperplasia, endometrial cancer, anovulation, bleeding disorders, pregnancy, or hypothyroidism. However, even after thorough evaluation, sometimes no pathologic explanation may be found (see Chapter 3 for a detailed discussion of the evaluation and treatment of abnormal bleeding patterns). Bleeding longer than 7 days or exceeding 80 mL blood loss in a cycle is considered excessive (menorrhagia), and treatment is necessary if the patient is anemic or the symptoms are affecting her quality of life. Medical therapy should always be attempted first, but when medical therapy is contraindicated, not tolerated, or fails, surgical treatment is often necessary.

Table 14-1 Estimated Percentage of Hysterectomies by Diagnosis and Age, 1988–1990.

Diagnosis	25–34 Years	45–54 Years	All Ages
	←	(%)	→
Fibroids	14.0	53.0	33.5
Endometriosis	29.0	13.3	18.2
Prolapse	14.5	11.7	16.2
Cancer	9.7	6.8	11.2
Endometrial hyperplasia	3.0	8.4	6.0
Menstrual/menopausal symptoms	8.3	2.6	4.5
Cervical dysplasia	3.4	—	1.4
Pain	1.9	—	0.6
Other	15.5	3.8	8.5

Adapted from Wilcox LS, Koonin LM, Pokras R, et al. Hysterectomy in the United States, 1988–1990. Obstet Gynecol. 1994;83:549-55.

Leiomyomata

Uterine fibroids (leiomyomata) are benign tumors consisting of proliferations of uterine smooth muscle and connective tissue. They may be located in the uterine wall (intramural), beneath the serosal surface of the uterus (sub-serosal), or beneath the endometrial lining (submucosal). The last are most likely to cause bleeding abnormalities. Fibroids are the most common neoplasm of the female pelvis, occurring in up to 20% to 25% of women of reproductive age (9), and are reported to be more common in black women than in other groups (8). The etiology of fibroids is not known, but because fibroids enlarge with pregnancy and decrease after menopause, estrogen is assumed to be a stimulant to growth. The natural history of untreated fibroids has not been well elucidated, but when fibroids are large enough, symptoms can be precipitated. Malignant degeneration is fortunately rare, especially because there are no risk factors to reliably predict the patient with sarcoma. Uterine sarcoma, including leiomyosarcoma, is found at the time of surgery in only 0.2% of patients with myomata (10).

Symptoms associated with fibroids include excessive bleeding, pelvic pressure or pain, bladder or rectal pressure, and infertility. Some women may experience more than one symptom, whereas others with even large fibroids remain asymptomatic. When leiomyomata are asymptomatic, most physicians concur that nothing need be done. For small to moderately sized fibroids, first-line treatment is medical therapy. If the uterine mass measures the size of 3 months' gestation or greater, however, intervention with surgical and nonsurgical procedures should be strongly considered. Once the uterus reaches this size it becomes virtually impossible to reliably palpate the ovaries, thus precluding the possibility of detecting an adnexal mass. The type of procedure performed (myomectomy, hysterectomy, uterine artery embolization) and the timing depend on the patient's symptoms and her preferences regarding preservation of the uterus and future fertility.

Genital Prolapse

Genital prolapse refers to protrusion of the uterus, cervix, and vagina into the barrel of the vagina or, in severe cases, through the vaginal introitus. Conditions of genital prolapse include uterine prolapse, cystocele, enterocele, and vaginal prolapse. These conditions are due to relaxation of the pelvic support muscles and fascia caused by childbirth, trauma, stress, and aging. The largest general population survey of genital prolapse found the overall prevalence of the condition to be 31% (11). In this study, all types of prolapse increased in frequency with increasing age (Fig. 14-1); however, among Swedish women aged 20 to 59, 44% of prolapse occurred in parous women

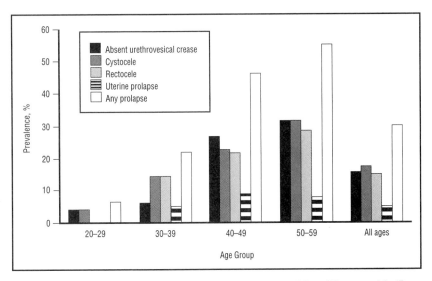

Figure 14-1 Prevalence of genital prolapse among women 20 to 59 years old. (From Samuelsson EC, Victor FTA, Tibblin G, Svardsudd KF. Signs of genital prolapse in a Swedish population of women 20 to 59 years of age and possible related factors. Am J Obstet Gynecol. 1999;180:299-305; with permission.)

and only 6% occurred in women who had never carried a child to term. In this relatively younger age group, no prolapse extended beyond the introitus, and only 8 of 150 women were noted to have prolapse that reached the introitus with straining.

Prolapse of the uterus is also referred to as *decensus* or *procidentia* and is described in three degrees. *First-degree prolapse* is defined as descent of the cervix to the upper portion of the vagina, *second-degree prolapse* is descent of the cervix to the introitus, and *third-degree prolapse* is protrusion of the cervix/uterus through the introitus (Fig. 14-2). Common causes of uterine prolapse include multiple births (especially of large infants), large uterine fibroids, and morbid obesity. Prolapse of the cervical stump or vaginal cuff after hysterectomy may be a complication of the procedure (e.g., a short vaginal canal) or the subsequent development of morbid obesity or menopause. In general, the degree of prolapse may remain unchanged or increase when the pelvic examination is performed with the patient upright rather than in the dorsal lithotomy position (12).

Rectocele is the protrusion of the rectum into the vagina, signifying relaxation of rectal support. Symptoms may include constipation and a sensation that the vagina is "falling out". Some patients must manually (using their fingers or an aid such as a spoon placed against the posterior vaginal wall) reduce a rectocele before being able to defecate successfully. *Enterocele* refers

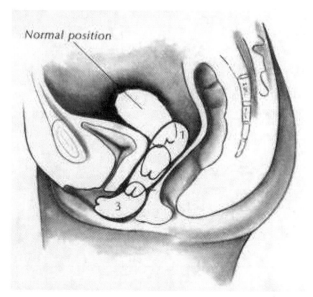

Figure 14-2 Stages of uterine (or "uterovaginal") prolapse. *First-degree prolapse* refers to descent of the uterus wherein the cervix still lies in the upper portion of the vagina. With *second-degree prolapse*, the cervix is at the vaginal introitus. *Third-degree prolapse*, defined as descent of the uterus such that the cervix lies outside of the introitus, includes complete procidentia, wherein the entire uterus is located outside the vagina. Because of connective tissue attachments, uterine prolapse is necessarily accompanied by vaginal prolapse and, when advanced, cystocele and enterocele as well. (From Bickley LS, Hoekelman RA. Bates' Guide to Physical Examination and History Taking, 7th ed. Philadelphia: Lippincott Williams & Wilkins; 1999:428; with permission.)

to herniation of the pouch of Douglas into the rectovaginal septum, creating a bulge in the upper vagina. It usually contains small bowel. (Bladder prolapse (*cystocoele*) is discussed in Chapter 10.)

The definitive treatment of advanced prolapse is surgery. The surgical approach for hysterectomy in a patient with uterine prolapse is usually vaginal. However, in the setting of uterovaginal prolapse, additional procedures (e.g., repair of a cystocele, rectocele, or enterocele, or suspension of the vaginal vault to the sacrospinous ligament) should be performed to attempt cure (13). It should be noted that when bladder suspension procedures are planned to correct stress urinary incontinence, available evidence does not support the removal of a normal, well-supported uterus; hysterectomy generally should be reserved for gynecologic indications alone (14).

For milder forms of prolapse, surgery is often unnecessary. If intervention is indicated, patients can often be managed with a pessary, of which there are multiple types available (15). Weight loss, although difficult to achieve, may also improve many chronic symptoms of genital prolapse.

Endometriosis

Endometriosis is the presence of endometrial glands and stroma in a location other than the uterine lining. It is usually located in the pelvis and only rarely in more remote locations such as the lung. The etiology is unclear, and various theories abound. For many women, endometriosis is a progressive disease that leads to infertility and chronic pelvic pain. Hormonal therapies often relieve the discomfort, and laparoscopic removal or destruction of endometriotic lesions can improve both pain and fertility outcomes. For some patients, hysterectomy with ovarian preservation offers pain relief; however, pain will recur in approximately 3% to 10% of such patients. Definitive therapy therefore includes removal of the uterus, ovaries, and all foci of endometriosis. (For a more extensive discussion, see Chapter 11.)

Adenomyosis

Adenomyosis is defined as the presence of endometrial glands and stroma in the uterine wall (myometrium) at a depth approximately 2.5 mm beneath the endometrium (16). The condition can be diagnosed definitively only by histologic examination of surgical specimens, although MRI has been shown to have approximately 90% accuracy (16a,16b). Interestingly, the incidence of simultaneous endometriosis is low. Patients with adenomyosis are usually parous, suggesting that the condition is possibly related to a postpartum event. Patients with adenomyosis are frequently asymptomatic; symptomatic patients are usually between 35 and 50 years old and typically present with menorrhagia and cyclic pelvic pain that progressively worsens. On examination the uterus is diffusely enlarged and may be boggy and tender. Although adenomyosis is often treated with nonsteroidal anti-inflammatory agents or hormonal contraception, there is currently no medical therapy that is reliably effective and hysterectomy is the definitive treatment.

Pelvic Pain

Pelvic pain is defined as either *acute* or, when it persists for more than 6 months, *chronic*. Acute pelvic pain rarely necessitates a hysterectomy except in the setting of tubo-ovarian abscess or an ectopic pregnancy located in the cervix or uterine cornua. Chronic pelvic pain is by far a more common reason for hysterectomy.

Chronic pelvic pain can be divided into cyclic and noncyclic patterns of pain. *Cyclic pain* is caused by dysmenorrhea, either primary or secondary, whereas *noncyclic pain* is independent of the menstrual cycle. *Primary dysmenorrhea* has its onset at or shortly after menarche, whereas *secondary dysmenorrhea* arises later and is more commonly associated with pelvic pathology such as endometriosis, adenomyosis, or fibroids. Other etiologies of persistent pelvic pain include adhesive or malignant disease, incompletely treated or recurrent pelvic infections, and diseases of the urinary or gastrointestinal tract. Evaluation for chronic pelvic pain commonly involves a diagnostic laparoscopy. However, in up to 30% of cases no disease is found (17).

Hysterectomy may not necessarily benefit a patient with chronic pelvic pain. Even for those patients with surgically correctable conditions, both the physician and the patient must understand the possibility (if not the probability) that the pain may be unchanged or even worsened (related to scarring occurring during the healing process) by the surgical procedure. If necessary, nonsurgical therapies may be employed after hysterectomy (18). The use of hysterectomy for the treatment of severe dysmenorrhea without documented pathology is controversial. (For additional information, see Chapter 12.)

Malignancies

Cervical, ovarian, endometrial, and uterine malignancies may be treated with a hysterectomy. These malignancies are reviewed in other chapters. For cervical carcinoma *in situ,* minimally invasive cervical carcinoma, and endometrial carcinoma, simple hysterectomy without salpingo-oophorectomy is indicated because malignant spread to the ovaries is exceedingly rare with these cancers. However, surgical treatment of ovarian cancer typically involves removal of the uterus with the ovaries even when there is no apparent extension of cancer to the uterus. In the uncommon presentation of the younger patient who desires future childbearing potential and who appears to have a curable ovarian cancer, it may be appropriate to preserve the uterus and contralateral ovary if wedge biopsy of this ovary confirms the absence of disease (19). Even when both ovaries must be removed from these young women, consideration should be given to preservation of the uterus to allow for possible future pregnancy using donor egg.

Alternatives

In recent years, there has been exponential growth in the number of medical and surgical alternatives to hysterectomy. The specific therapeutic options depend on the diagnosis and include medical management, pessary use, alternative surgical techniques, and interventional radiology.

Medical Alternatives

Medical therapy should not be initiated in a middle-aged woman with heavy vaginal bleeding until the possibilities of pregnancy and malignancy have been addressed. Initial assessment usually includes a careful bleeding history and a pregnancy test for women at risk. In addition, a pelvic ultrasound to assess the endometrial stripe is often warranted as well as sampling of the endometrium by endometrial aspiration (endometrial biopsy). Abnormal findings may necessitate further evaluation with dilatation and curettage (D&C). If no pregnancy or malignancy is demonstrated and no bleeding disorder is suspected, one of several types of hormonal therapy may be used to control bleeding until menopause occurs. Use of such agents can often help avoid hysterectomy.

Hormonal therapies commonly used include combination oral contraceptive pills, medroxyprogesterone acetate (Provera or Depo-Provera), and gonadotropin-releasing hormone (GnRH) agonists. Combination oral contraceptive pills (COCs) are progestin dominant and, when taken in the usual fashion used for contraceptive purposes, reduce endometrial proliferation and menstrual blood loss. This effect is useful for women with fibroids, adenomyosis, or unexplained menorrhagia. Chronic pain from endometriosis may also be improved with the use of COCs, particularly when taken in a continuous (noncyclic) fashion. If the woman is a nonsmoker without other relative contraindications, oral contraceptive pills may be used into menopause. (For further discussion of COC use in perimenopause, see Chapter 5.)

Medroxyprogesterone acetate is another alternative for the woman with significant bleeding problems and pain caused by endometriosis. It can be given orally as Provera 10 to 30 mg daily for 10 to 14 consecutive days of each month, or in a long-acting formulation (Depo-Provera) administered as an intramuscular injection 150 mg every 3 months or as frequently as monthly if necessary. The high dose of progesterone suppresses ovarian function and leads to atrophy of the endometrium. With continued use, complete amenorrhea is achieved by 50% of users within 1 year (20).

All patients with heavy vaginal bleeding and anemia should be treated with iron replacement therapy. Although the constipation often associated with oral iron therapy may limit compliance with thrice-daily regimens, any iron supplementation is beneficial. Aggressive treatment of the associated constipation may improve compliance. Often, iron therapy alone can successfully treat the iron deficiency anemia caused by vaginal bleeding.

When used beyond a few weeks, GnRH agonists paradoxically down-regulate the pituitary, leading to suppression of ovarian estrogen production. Thus these agents induce a pharmacological, reversible menopause. GnRH agonists have been successfully employed to treat endometriosis and have also been approved for treatment of small to moderately sized uterine fibroids because they inhibit bleeding and correct anemia. In addition, these agents have been shown to shrink the size of the fibroids, although the regression varies widely, from a slight decrease in size to as much as an 85% reduction in volume (21-25).

Unfortunately, however, once the GnRH agonist is discontinued the fibroids return to their original size within 3 months, so to achieve long-term benefit the GnRH agonists must be continued indefinitely. However, long-term use of GnRH agonists places the patient at risk for consequences associated with the menopausal state, namely hot flashes, vaginal dryness, and, most importantly, osteoporosis. Because of these risks and the expense of GnRH agonists, they are typically used for 6 months or less and have been implemented primarily in the pre-operative setting.

When used for 3 to 6 months pre-operatively, GnRH agonists may substantially decrease the size of the uterine fibroid and allow for a vaginal rather than abdominal hysterectomy, reducing morbidity and length of hospital stay. Also, the amenorrhea induced by GnRH agonists can help correct anemia, thereby allowing for storage of autologous blood or preventing the need for blood transfusion either pre-operatively or post-operatively. Pre-operative GnRH use can also decrease the size of submucous fibroids to facilitate hysteroscopic resection and therefore help avoid a hysterectomy. However, when used before myomectomy, GnRH use may result in a higher frequency of myoma recurrence when compared with those who had not received GnRH agonists pre-operatively (26). Therefore routine use of GnRH agonists before myomectomy remains controversial.

GnRH agonists should not be used before myomectomy due to an associated increased risk of myoma recurrence.

GnRH agonists have also been used in patients with moderate-to-severe endometriosis to control symptoms and delay hysterectomy. The hypoestrogenic state induced by GnRH agonists suppresses the endometriosis. With the GnRH agonist leuprolide acetate, a decrease in endometriosis-associated dysmenorrhea, pelvic pain, pelvic tenderness, and induration has been confirmed in placebo-controlled studies (27). As previously stated, however, long-term use of these medications is fraught with concern for osteoporosis and other "menopausal" sequelae. However, add-back therapy using postmenopausal doses of estrogen alone or in combination with progesterone has successfully ameliorated some of the side effects of the GnRH agonist, with no apparent compromise in efficacy (28). (For more detailed discussion, see Chapter 11.)

Pessary

The pessary is a device made of silicone (or sometimes latex) that is worn in the vagina for the nonsurgical management of uterine prolapse, vaginal prolapse following hysterectomy, or stress urinary incontinence (Fig. 14-3). Pessaries are available in many shapes; the ring shape is most often utilized when urinary symptoms are significant (29). Pessaries require an office fitting with different shapes and sizes, testing for comfort and stability while the patient stands, sits, squats, and performs the Valsalva maneuver. The patient should have a voiding trial with the pessary in place before leaving the office. The device is worn continuously but removed for intercourse and intermittent cleaning (e.g., monthly, but as per manufacturer's instructions), and periodic pelvic examinations are required (often biannually after initial close follow-up) to exclude such complications as vaginal ulceration. The physician placing the pessary is responsible for providing follow-up care for the duration of its use. Adjuncts include exercises to strengthen pelvic floor musculature (Kegel excercises) and vaginal estrogen therapy for postmenopausal women. Some patients may avoid surgery for years by choosing to use a pessary. Indications for surgery include the desire for definitive cor-

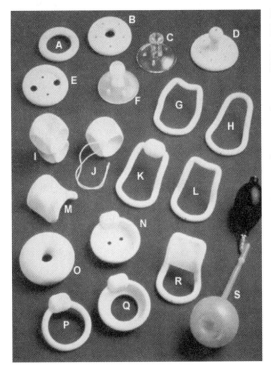

Figure 14-3 Various types of pessaries. *A*, Ring; *B*, Shaatz; *C*, *D*, Gellhorn; *E*, Ring with support; *F*, Gellhorn; *G*, Risser; *H*, Smith; *I*, Tandem cube; *J*, Cube; *K*, Hodge with knob; *L*, Hodge; *M*, Gehrung; *N*, Incontinence dish with support; *O*, Donut; *P*, Incontinence ring; *Q*, Incontinence dish; *R*, Hodge with support; *S*, Inflatoball (latex). (From Viera AJ, Larkins-Pettigrew M. Practical use of the pessary. Am Fam Physician. 2000;61:2719; with permission.)

rection, recurrent vaginal ulcerations with pessary use, and stress urinary incontinence that the patient finds unacceptable (14).

Surgical Alternatives

With the development of new surgical instruments and techniques, an increasing number of surgical alternatives to total hysterectomy have evolved over the last several years. These include abdominal myomectomy, hysteroscopy for the diagnosis and management of submucosal myomas and endometrial polyps, and endometrial ablation. Finally, laparoscopy has also allowed for the introduction of new procedures.

Abdominal Myomectomy

Abdominal myomectomy involves removing fibroids from the uterus through an abdominal incision, leaving the uterus and cervix in place. The American College of Obstetricians and Gynecologists has detailed the criteria for myomectomy and hysterectomy in women with a fibroid uterus (9). In general, myomectomy is indicated for women who have symptomatic fibroids but desire future childbearing or for women who are determined to retain their reproductive organs. The procedure is usually considered less appropriate for women who have reached an age of decreasing fertility. The surgical approach for fibroid removal and the likelihood of complications depend on the number, location, and size of the myomata, as well as the age and fertility desires of the patient.

Two issues surrounding myomectomy are the possibility of malignant degeneration and the risk of fibroid recurrence. It should be noted that though rapidly enlarging myomata often raise the concern for malignancy, studies have shown that the incidence of malignancy is not higher in this group of women (10), so myomectomy is a feasible alternative. The other, more common sequela of myomectomy is fibroid recurrence. Studies using pelvic ultrasound show a 50% incidence of fibroid recurrence within 5 years of the surgery (30), and 10% to 35% of myomectomy patients require subsequent surgery for this reason (31-33). As discussed previously, the use of GnRH agonists should be avoided in patients for whom myomectomy is planned because its use is associated with a higher frequency of myoma recurrence compared with those who had not received GnRH agonists (26).

Hysteroscopy

Hysteroscopy involves placing a hysteroscope through the cervical canal and into the uterine cavity to allow visualization of the entire uterine cavity. Once an abnormality is diagnosed by this technique, treatment can usually be accomplished via the same approach. Hysteroscopy is particularly useful in the diagnosis and management of submucosal myomata or endometrial polyps.

For technical reasons, hysteroscopic resection of myomata should be limited to myomata measuring less than 3 to 5 cm diameter, with at least 50% of the myoma projecting into the uterine cavity. Pretreatment with GnRH agonists has been used to facilitate the surgery by decreasing the size of the fibroid to be resected; however, this agent increases the likelihood of recurrence. Although complications of hysteroscopic resection of myomata are rare, perforation of the uterus can occur. For the removal of larger myomata, simultaneous laparoscopy allows for observation of the outside of the uterus and may help decrease the risk of perforation. Other complications are related to the use of specific uterine distending fluids. Dextran has been associated with acute hypervolemia, pulmonary edema, and severe coagulopathy (34). Glycine solution is therefore preferred, but this agent is associated with the risk of post-operative hyponatremia (35).

Hysteroscopy can also be used to perform endometrial ablation, which involves destroying the endometrial lining of the uterus in order to cause amenorrhea. The procedure is indicated for women who have a normal uterine cavity and lack fibroids and who are without coagulation defects. Endometrial ablation may be selected for patients who are considered poor surgical risks for hysterectomy. The technique is 60% effective in causing amenorrhea. In a follow-up study of 1000 consecutive procedures (36), of the women who did not have a subsequent hysterectomy and for whom follow-up information was available, 38% had amenorrhea and, of those still menstruating, 86% reported lighter bleeding. The projected hysterectomy rate over 6.5 years after the procedure was 21% and was lower on multivariate analysis if intrauterine pathology was defined. Patients should be properly counseled that endometrial ablation should not be considered for those who wish to maintain fertility. Complications of the procedure are similar to those of hysteroscopic resection.

Endometrial ablation is contraindicated for those women interested in maintaining their fertility.

Newer techniques of endometrial ablation include thermal balloon endometrial ablation (37). This technique involves inserting a fluid-filled balloon into the endometrial cavity, then heating the balloon to 70 to 92°C for 6 to 9 min. Amenorrhea occurs in approximately 40% of patients, and oligomenorrhea-hypomenorrhea occurs in 40% to 50% of patients (38,39). Data from the British National Health Service from 1989 to 1996 show that the rate of endometrial ablation has been gradually increasing, whereas the number of hysterectomies has remained stable.

Laparoscopy

Laparoscopy is a valuable technique for evaluating and treating pathologic conditions in the pelvis and may offer alternatives to hysterectomy in the management of endometriosis, uterine fibroids, pelvic adhesions, and pain. A laparoscope is placed through an incision in the abdominal wall into the abdominal cavity to allow visualization of the pelvic and abdominal organs after insufflation with carbon dioxide for abdominal expansion. Laparoscopy is usually performed under general anesthesia but may be performed under epidural or spinal anesthesia and, more recently, when used for tubal sterilization or diagnostic purposes, with local anesthesia/sedation alone.

The management of endometriosis, pelvic adhesions, uterine fibroids, and pain is often facilitated by laparoscopy. With technical improvements in laparoscopic equipment, aggressive resection of endometriosis and pelvic adhesions can be performed. In addition, small pedunculated uterine fibroids can be removed. Larger fibroids are more difficult to remove laparoscopically because of the risk of significant bleeding. In addition, morcellation is often needed to remove the myoma through the operative laparoscopy portals, unless a culdotomy incision is used through the pouch of Douglas.

A newer technique is laparoscopic myolysis for the treatment of symptomatic myomata (40). Laparoscopic myolysis involves the application of the Nd:Yag laser or the bipolar needle for coagulation of the blood supply of the myoma. The intent is to cause atrophy and necrosis of the myoma by destroying its immediate blood supply. Pyomyoma is a possible consequence. Also, necrosing leiomyoma can produce pain, fever, and other symptoms.

Interventional Radiology

Radiologists and gynecologists have studied the use of transcatheter embolization of the uterine artery for the control of fibroids and abnormal bleeding (41). Also, catheterization of the branches of the uterine artery has been utilized to embolize the major blood supply to the myomata, resulting in the regression of the myomata (42). In studies of patients with fibroids and menorrhagia treated with bilateral uterine artery embolization, approximately 80% experienced moderate to marked improvement in bleeding and pelvic pressure and pain symptoms (42a,42b). This technique does not appear to be successful in the treatment of adenomyosis, however (42c). Also, it should be noted that transient severe pelvic pain has been reported with this technique, and further experience will define its appropriate uses and success.

Specific Pre-Operative Considerations

Ultrasonography and magnetic resonance imaging (MRI) are the best radiographic studies for the evaluation of the pelvis. Pelvic ultrasound is the best method for screening the pelvis for abnormalities such as uterine myomata or adnexal pathology. MRI is reserved for specific and focused evaluation of pelvic organs (e.g., distinguishing between ovarian and tubal pathology or better characterizing adnexal pathology). With good resolution, MRI may not only offer the advantage of distinguishing between myoma and adenomyosis but also alert the surgeon to a sarcomatous appearance of a fibroid (43).

In general, the primary care physician is responsible for identification and management of medical problems existing before surgery. A careful pre-operative evaluation can screen for limitations in exercise tolerance and identify cardiac, pulmonary, and endocrine problems not previously diagnosed. This can allow for optimal management both pre-operatively and in the perioperative period.

Although hysterectomy is often indicated for treatment of conditions leading to chronic anemia, the procedure itself causes blood loss. Most patients respond well to aggressive iron replacement therapy before surgery, but for those who do not, pre-operative use of combined oral contraceptive pills, Depo-Provera, or GnRH agonists may help correct the anemia. If the anemia is not severe, many surgeons recommend the patient donate two units of blood for autologous use during surgery. However, it should be recognized that transfusion of even autologous blood is not entirely innocuous because it can lead to cardiac overload and other complications (44).

Patients requiring allogeneic transfusions should be reassured that in the United States the risk of acquiring HIV is believed to have been lowered to 1 in 26 million per unit of blood as a result of improvements in the donor screening process and the use of more sensitive assays (45,46). Transmission of hepatitis C virus is also a concern with transfusion of blood products. Blood from a directed donor such as a relative or friend may put the patient at ease, but this blood is typically less safe than the supply procured from regular donors.

Types of Hysterectomy

Once the decision has been made to perform a hysterectomy, the surgeon must determine the most appropriate approach. Important considerations are uterine size, history of previous surgery, previous surgical findings, suspected pathology (i.e., malignancy), the surgeon's level of expertise with a given approach, and the patient's preference.

Total Abdominal Hysterectomy and Total Vaginal Hysterectomy

When the uterus is enlarged enough to make the vaginal approach excessively difficult, an abdominal hysterectomy (TAH) is typically performed. An abdominal hysterectomy is also appropriate when other pelvic pathology is present, such as a malignancy, severe endometriosis or pelvic adhesions. Otherwise, vaginal hysterectomy (TVH) is preferred, particularly in cases of genital prolapse and obese patients. In addition, vaginal hysterectomy is adequate for pre-invasive cervical neoplasia or minimally invasive cervical cancer.

Laparoscopic Hysterectomy

Laparoscopic hysterectomy includes a broad range of procedures by which laparoscopic technique is used in completing hysterectomy. The laparoscope may be employed in a diagnostic fashion to determine the feasibility of a vaginal approach or to assess a pelvic mass. Varying amounts of surgical dissection can be performed, including ligation of the ovarian vessels to help with vaginal removal of the ovaries. Laparoscopy utilized to facilitate a vaginal hysterectomy in a patient who otherwise may not have been a candidate is called *laparoscopy-assisted vaginal hysterectomy* (LAVH). A true laparoscopic hysterectomy (LH), which is a relatively new procedure, involves liberating the entire uterus endoscopically using the vagina as a portal for removal. When performing a laparoscopic supracervical hysterectomy (see below), the uterus can be removed either by morcellation, through an extended abdominal incision, or via a culdotomy. The disadvantage of morcellation is that it may complicate the diagnosis of unexpected pathology such as endometrial cancer. With both LAVH and LH, there is a learning curve, and operative time is particularly dependent on experience.

Supracervical Hysterectomy

In the woman with normal Papanicolaou smears, preservation of the cervix by a supracervical hysterectomy is an option. Supracervical hysterectomy offers reductions in both operative time and risk compared with either multiple myomectomy or total hysterectomy. It also avoids shortening and scarring of the vaginal apex, which can occur with a TAH. Supracervical or subtotal hysterectomy was common until the mid-20th century, until concern for cervical cancer in the remaining stump and decreased morbidity associated with total

Women who have undergone a supracervical hysterectomy require continued cervical cancer screening.

hysterectomy led to shifts in thinking. However, interest in supracervical hysterectomy has been renewed in the United States, in part because of the perception that the cervix may play a role in the female sexual response (47). It has also been proposed that supracervical hysterectomy is associated with a lower incidence of vault prolapse, infection, adjacent organ injury, and hemorrhage; however, this is not clearly supported in the literature (48,49). Patients should be carefully selected for supracervical hysterectomy. However, previous or current cervical dysplasia is now only a relative contraindication, because colposcopy may allow conservative management of cervical dysplasia. Because the cervix remains *in situ* after a supracervical hysterectomy, regular Pap smear screening must be continued.

Prophylactic Oophorectomy

Prophylactic removal of the ovaries at the time of hysterectomy for benign disease is still a controversial subject. The major reason to remove the ovaries is to prevent ovarian cancer, a disease not readily diagnosed at an early or curable stage. Studies have shown that 4.5% to 14.1% of women develop ovarian cancer after hysterectomy for benign nonovarian indications (50). Also, in patients for whom ovaries are conserved during hysterectomy, 0.9% to 5.1% will eventually require surgery for adnexal pathology (50-52). Prophylactic oophorectomy should be considered for women with a family history of ovarian cancer and those approaching menopause (i.e., over the age of 40 to 45).

On the other hand, prophylactic removal of the ovaries results in surgical menopause, with its attendant risks. Osteoporosis may result, and sexuality, libido, and self-image may be affected (53). Issues surrounding the use of postmenopausal hormone replacement therapy are becoming increasingly complex. Also, gestational surrogacy has enabled women who have had hysterectomies to have a biological child by donating an egg, whereas this is obviously not possible after removal of the ovaries. Thus the decision of whether to perform prophylactic oophorectomy must be based on the careful weighing of the advantages and disadvantages for each individual woman (53).

Benefits and Risks

The benefits of hysterectomy are primarily derived from an improvement in the patient's quality of life (4,54,55). In particular, those patients with genital prolapse, bleeding abnormalities, pelvic pain, or a significantly enlarged uterus report improved health status after recuperation from a hysterectomy. In a prospective cohort study of 300 patients in Great Britain, 80% of patients reported that they felt a lot better or somewhat better 3 months post-operatively, 16% noted no change, and only 4% felt somewhat worse, with one patient (0.3%) feeling a lot worse (55). The benefit is clear in those diseases where hysterectomy serves as definitive therapy, such as for early-stage endometrial or cervical cancer, adenomyosis, and fibroids. Also, patients who have severe symptoms before hysterectomy usually experience a more significant improvement in their quality of life post-operatively. However, those patients who undergo a hysterectomy for pelvic pain may have persistent or worse pain post-operatively and should be counseled appropriately.

Many women are reluctant to proceed with hysterectomy because of concerns about quality-of-life issues after the surgery. Carlson's survey of women in Maine found that women undergoing hysterectomy with and without bilateral salpingo-oophorectomy experienced a significant improvement in symptoms that had been present before surgery such as back pain, dyspareunia, urinary frequency, and fatigue (54). Physical symptoms that develop after hysterectomy include urinary problems in 4% to 20% of patients and depression or anxiety in 6% to 8% of patients (54). Hot flashes develop more frequently in women who have their ovaries removed compared with those who do not undergo oophorectomy (14% versus 3%, respectively) (54). There has been limited research on the impact of hysterectomy on family members and the woman's sexual partner (4).

Sexuality is an important concern for most women. Although diminished sexual function has been reported in 7% to 21% of patients after hysterectomy (54,56,57), other studies have revealed improved sexual function. The studies revealing diminished sexual functioning are complicated by the observation that the patients were mixed in regard to diagnosis and surgical technique, so that patients who had abdominal or vaginal hysterectomy with or without bilateral oophorectomy were analyzed together. Helstrom et al reported that approximately 50% of patients had an improved sense of sexuality after hysterectomy (56), and pre-operative sexual activity appears to be the best predictor of post-operative sexuality. Women who undergo supracervical hysterectomy report better subsequent libido and more frequent sexual activity compared with those who underwent total hysterectomy (47). Dennerstein reported 89 women undergoing hysterectomy with bilateral salpingo-oophorectomy and found that 33 experienced a deterioration in sexual function, which suggests that loss of endogenous hormones may adversely affect sexual well-being (57a).

Complications of hysterectomy can occur intraoperatively or during the post-operative period. Intraoperative complications include excessive blood loss, unanticipated removal of an organ such as an ovary, and damage to adjacent organs such as the bladder, bowel, or ureters. The amount of blood loss depends on the size of the uterus and the difficulty of removal. Blood loss is typically considered excessive if a transfusion is required. Damage to the bladder or gastrointestinal tract is more likely in cases where the dissection of the uterus is difficult such as in patients with endometriosis or with extensive pelvic adhesive disease. The incidence of ureteral injury is between 0.5% and 1.5% of major gynecologic surgeries and occurs more commonly during an abdominal procedure than during a vaginal approach (58,59).

Post-operative complications may be recognized in the hospital or have a delayed presentation. Febrile illness (secondary to infection or atelectasis), ileus, and voiding dysfunction are examples of early problems that are not infrequent. Wound complications are less common but include abdominal incision or vaginal cuff infections or bleeding, and superficial or deep wound separation. Thromboembolic phenomenon, in particular deep vein thrombosis, is also of concern after pelvic surgery. Thromboembolic complications occur early in the post-operative course: 50% within the first 24 hr, 75% within the first 72 hr, and only 15% occurring after the seventh post-operative day (60).

Delayed complications include both vesicovaginal or rectovaginal fistula formation, bowel obstruction from post-operative adhesions, and fascial wound dehiscence. The incidence of major complications (bowel trauma, bladder trauma, fistula, ureter trauma, transfusion, sepsis, and pulmonary embolism) varies significantly with the surgical approach and different case series, but in general complication rates are higher for abdominal hysterectomy.

Length of Stay, Convalescence, and Cost

Post-operative length of hospital stay varies with the type of hysterectomy. In a study from Ohio, during the period 1988 to 1994, the median hospital stay was 4 days for an abdominal hysterectomy and 3 days for a vaginal hysterectomy or LAVH (61). In another review of the literature, the average lengths of stay were 2 days for LAVH and 3 days for TAH (62). Average convalescent periods from a randomized prospective trial from Sweden were 16 days for LAVH and 35 days for TAH (55). Data from other studies show the time to return to work ranges from 2 to 6 weeks for LAVH and 5 to 9 weeks for TAH (63-66).

The cost of a hysterectomy depends on the approach and on any additional procedures that may need to be performed. Physician fees may vary widely. In one institution, the average total charges (including professional and facility fees) for patients undergoing a hysterectomy without any secondary procedures were $5804 ± $1581 for LAVH, $4548 ± $763 for TAH, and $3522 ± $737 for TVH (67). Although patients undergoing LAVH typically have a shorter length of stay by 1 day compared with TAH or TVH patients, the cost of this procedure tends to be highest because of the equipment required, especially when disposable instruments are used. In other reports, the charges for LAVH ranged from $3772 to $11,931 and for TAH from $4368 to $7031 (66,68,69).

Summary

Hysterectomy is indicated for the management of cancer and pre-cancerous conditions of the cervix, uterus, and ovaries, as well as nonmalignant conditions when symptoms are adversely affecting a woman's quality of life. Nonsurgical measures appropriate to the specific etiology should be the first approach for nonmalignant conditions. For example, when genital prolapse is symptomatic but not advanced, a trial of a pessary may delay or obviate the need for surgery. Hormonal therapy can be used to treat a variety of conditions associated with pelvic pain and abnormal bleeding, such as fibroids, endometriosis, and dysfunctional uterine bleeding. When surgery is required, new conservative techniques that preserve fertility or control symptoms, such as myomectomy, endometrial ablation, or new techniques involving laparoscopic surgery, may be used instead of hysterectomy. Such approaches are ideal for women who want to preserve their reproductive organs and understand the limitations of these alternative treatments and procedures.

In recent years, the number of different surgical techniques for hysterectomy have increased, whereas the length of stay and recuperation time have decreased. Follow-up studies demonstrate that after hysterectomy, women often report fewer symptoms and an improved quality of life, including sexual functioning.

REFERENCES

1. Stedman's Medical Dictionary. Baltimore: Williams and Wilkins; 1979.
2. **Pokras R, Hufnagel VG.** Hysterectomy in the United States, 1965-1984. Am J Public Health. 1988;78:852-3.
3. **Brett K, Marsh JVR, Madans JH.** Epidemiology of hysterectomy in the United States: demographic and redproductive factors in a nationally representative sample. J Womens Health. 1997;6:309-16.
4. **Lewis CE, Groff JY, Herman CJ, et al.** Overview of women's decision making regarding elective hysterectomy, oophorectomy, and hormone replacement therapy. Review. J Womens Health Gend Based Med. 2000;9(Suppl)2:S5-14.
5. **Harlow BL, Barbieri RL.** Influence of education on risk of hysterectomy before age 45 years. Am J Epidemiol. 1999;150:843-7.
6. **Marks NF, Shinberg DS.** Socioeconomic differences in hysterectomy: the Wisconsin Longitudinal Study. Am J Public Health. 1997;87:1507-14.
7. **Vuorma S, Teperi J, Hurshainen R, et al.** Hysterectomy trends in Finland, 1987-1995: a register-based analysis. Acta Obstet Gynecol. 1998;77:770-6.
8. **Wilcox LS, Koonin LM, Pokras R, et al.** Hysterectomy in the United States, 1988-1990. Obstet Gynecol. 1994;83:549-55.
9. Uterine leiomyomata. ACOG Technical Bulletin. 1994;192:1-9.
10. **Parker WH, Fu YS, Berek JS.** Uterine sarcoma in patients operated on for presumed leiomyoma and rapidly growing leiomyoma. Obstet Gynecol. 1994;83:414-8.

11. **Samuelsson EC, Victor FTA, Tibblin G, Svardsudd KF.** Signs of genital prolapse in a Swedish population of women 20 to 59 years of age and possible related factors. Am J Obstet Gyncol. 1999;180:299-305.

12. **Barber M, Lambers A, Visco AG, Bump RC.** Effect of patient position on clinical evaluation of pelvic organ prolapse. Obstet Gynecol. 2000;96:18-22.

13. Pelvic organ prolapse. ACOG Technical Bulletin. 1995;214:686-93.

14. Urinary incontinence. ACOG Technical Bulletin. 1995;123:1-11.

15. **Viera AJ, Larkins-Pettigrew M.** Practical use of the pessary. Am Fam Physician. 2000;61:2719-29.

16. **Blaustein A, Kurman RJ, eds.** Blaustein's Pathology of the Female Genital Tract, 4th ed. New York: Springer-Verlag; 1994.

16a. **Reinhold C, McCarthy S, Bret PM, et al.** Diffuse adenomyosis: a comparison of endovaginal US and MR imaging with histopathologic correlation. Radiology. 1996; 1999:151-8.

16b. **Togashi K, Ozasa H, Konishi I, et al.** Enlarged uterus: differentiation between adenomyosis and leiomyoma with MR imaging. Radiology. 1989;171:531-4.

17. **Cunanan RG, Courey NG, Lippes J.** Laparoscopic findings in patients with pelvic pain. Am J Obstet Gynecol. 1983;146:589.

18. Chronic pelvic pain. ACOG Technical Bulletin. 1996;223:1-9.

19. **Hoskins WJ, Perez CA, Young RC, eds.** Principles and Practice of Gynecologic Oncology, 2nd ed. Philadelphia: Lippincott-Raven; 1997.

20. **Kaunitz AM, Mishell DR.** Progestin-only contraceptives: current perspectives and future directions. Dialogues in Contraception. 1994;4.

21. **Friedman AJ, Hoffman DI, Comite F, et al.** Treatment of leiomyomata uteri with leuprolide acetate depot: a double-blind placebo-controlled, multicentered study. The Leuprolide Study Group. Obstet Gynecol. 1991;77:720-5.

22. **Andreyko JL, Jaffe RB, et al.** Use of an agonist analog of gonadotropin-releasing hormone (naferelin) to treat leiomyomas: assessment by magnetic resonance imaging. Am J Obstet Gynecol. 1988;158:903-10.

23. **Letterie GS, Coddington CC, Winkel CA, et al.** Efficacy of a gonadotropin releasing hormone agonist in the treatment of uterine myomata: long-term follow-up. Fertil Steril. 1989;51:951.

24. **Matta WH, Shaw RW, Nye M, et al.** Long-term follow-up of patients with uterine fibroids after treatment with LHRH agonist buseralin. Br J Obstet Gynecol. 1989; 96:200-6.

25. **Schlaff WD, Zerhouni EA, Huth JA, et al.** A placebo-controlled trial of a depot gonadotropin-releasing hormone analogue(leuprolide) in the treatment of uterine leiomyomata. Obstet Gynecol. 1989;74:856-62.

26. **Fedele L, Bianchi S, Baglioni A, et al.** Intranasal buserelin versus surgery in the treatment of uterine leiomyomata: long-term follow-up. Eur J Obstet Gynecol Reprod Biol. 1991;38:53-7.

27. **Dlugi AM, Miller JD, Knittle J.** Lupron depot (leuprolide acetate for depot suspension) in the treatment of endometriosis: a randomized, placebo controlled, double-blind study. The Lupron Study Group. Fertil Steril. 1990;54:419-27.

28. **Friedman AJ, Hornstein MD.** Gonadotropin-releasing hormone agonist plus estrogen-progestin "add-back" therapy for endometriosis-related pelvic pain. Fertil Steril. 1993; 60:236-41.

29. **Cundiff GW, Weidner AC, Visco AG, et al.** A survey of pessary use by members of the urogynecologic society. Obstet Gynecol. 2000;95:931-5.

30. **Fedele L, Parazzini F, Luchini L, et al.** Recurrence of fibroids after myomectomy: a transvaginal ultrasonographic study. Human Reprod. 1995;10:1795-6.

31. **Malone LJ, Ingersoll FM.** Myomectomy in infertility. In: Behrman SJ, Kistner RW, eds. Progress in Infertility. Boston: Little, Brown; 1975.

32. **Babaknia A, Rock JA, Jones JW Jr.** Pregnancy success following abdominal myomectomy for infertility. Fertil Steril. 1978;30:644.

33. **Buttram VC Jr, Reiter RC.** Uterine leiomyomata: etiology, symptomatology and management. Fertil Steril. 1981;36:433.

34. **Vercellini P, Rossi R, Pagnoni B, Fedele L.** Hypervolemic pulmonary edema and severe coagulopathy after intrauterine dextran instillation. Obstet Gynecol. 1992;79: 838-9.

35. **Gonzales R, Brensilver JM, Rovinski JJ.** Posthysteroscopic hyponatremia. Am J Kidney Dis. 1994;23:735-8.

36. **Phillips G, Chien PFW, Garry R.** Risk of hysterectomy after 1000 consecutive endometrial laser ablations. Br J Obstet Gynecol. 1998;105:897-903.

37. **Neuwirth RS, Duran AA, Singer A, et al.** The endometrial ablator: a new instrument. Obstet Gynecol. 1994;83:792-4.

38. **Singer A, Almanza R, Gutierrez A, et al.** Preliminary clinical experience with a thermal balloon endometrial ablation method to treat menorrhagia. Obstet Gynecol. 1994;83:732-4.

39. **Soderstrom RM, Brooks PG, Corson SL, et al.** Endometrial ablation using a distensible multielectrode balloon. J Am Assoc Gynecol Laparosc. 1996;3:403-7.

40. **Goldfarb HA.** Laparoscopic coagulation of myoma (myolysis). Obstet Gynecol Clin North Am. 1995;22:807-19.

41. **Yamashita Y, Harada M, Yamamoto H, et al.** Transcatheter arterial embolization of obstetrical and gynecological bleeding: efficacy and clinical outcome. Br J Radiol. 1994;67:530-4.

42. **Ravina JH, Aymard A, Ciraru-Vigneron N, et al.** Arterial embolization to treat uterine myomata. Lancet. 1995;346:671-2.

43. **Mayer DP, Shipilov V.** Ultrasonography and magnetic resonance imaging. Obstet Gynecol Clin North Am. 1995;22:667-721.

44. **Penner M Sibrowski W.** Benefits and risks of autologous blood donation. Infusion Ther Transfusion Med. 1994;21:64-8.

45. **Lackritz EM, Satten GA, Arberle-Grasse J, et al.** Estimated risk of transmission of the human immunodeficiency virus by screened blood in the United States. N Engl J Med. 1995;333:1721-5.

46. **Sloand EM, Pitt E, Klein HG.** Safety of the blood supply. JAMA. 1995;274:1368-73.

47. **Kilkku P.** Supravaginal uterine amputation vs. hysterectomy: effects on coital frequency and dyspareunia. Acta Obstet Gynecol Scand. 1983;62:153-8.

48. **Scott JR, Sharp HT, Dodson MK, et al.** Subtotal hysterectomy in modern gynecology: a decision analysis. Am J Obstet Gynecol. 1997;176:1186-92.

49. **Jones DDE, Shackelford P, Brame RG.** Supracervical hysterectomy: back to the future? Am J Obstet Gynecol. 1999;180:512-5.

50. **Piver MS, Wong C.** Prophylactic oophorectomy: a century-long dilemma. Hum Reprod. 1997;12:205-6.

51. **Grogan RH, Duncan CJ.** Ovarian salvage in routine abdominal hysterectomy. Am J Obstet Gynecol. 1955;70:1277-83.

52. **Ranney B, Abu-Ghazaleh S.** The future function of ovarian tissue which is retained in vivo during hysterectomy. Am J Obstet Gynecol. 1977;70:626-34.

53. Prophylactic oophorectomy. ACOG Technical Bulletin. 1987;111:1-5.

54. **Carlson KJ, Miller BA, Fowler FJ.** The Maine Women's Health Study: I—-Outcomes of hysterectomy. Obstet Gynecol. 1994;83:556-65.

55. **Olsson J-H, Ellstrom M, Hahlin M.** A randomised prospective trial comparing laparoscopic and abdominal hysterectomy. Br J Obstet Gynaecol. 1996;103:345-50.

56. **Helstrom L, Lundberg PO, Sorbom D, Backstrom T.** Sexuality after hysterectomy: a factor analysis of women's sexual lives before and after subtotal hysterectomy. Obstet Gynecol. 1993;81:357-62.

57. **Gath D.** Hysterectomy and psychiatric disorder: levels of psychiatric morbidity before and after hysterectomy. Br J Psychiatr. 1982;140:335-50.

57a. **Dennerstein L.** Sexual response following hysterectomy and oophorectomy. Obstet Gynecol. 1977;49:92-6.

58. **Mann WJ, Arato M, Patsner B, Stone ML.** Ureteral injuries in an obstetrics and gynecology training program: etiology and management. Obstet Gynecol. 1988;72:82-5.

59. **Daly JW, Higgins KA.** Injury to the ureter during gynecologic surgical procedures. Surg Gynecol Obstet. 1988;167;19-22.

60. **Herbst AL, Mishell DR, Stencherer MA, Droegemueller W, eds.** Comprehensive Gynecology, 2nd ed. St. Louis: Mosby-Year Book; 1992.

61. **Weber AM, Lee JC.** Use of alternative techniques of hysterectomy in Ohio, 1988-1994. N Engl J Med. 1996;335:483-9.

62. **Meickle SF, Nugent EW, Orleans M.** Complications and recovery from laparoscopy-assisted vaginal hysterectomy compared with abdominal and vaginal hysterectomy. Obstet Gynecol. 1997;89:304-11.

63. **Raju KS, Auld BJ.** A randomized prospective study of laparoscopic vaginal hysterectomy vs. abdominal hysterectomy, each with bilateral salpingo-oophorectomy. Br J Gynaecol. 1994;101:1068-71.

64. **Bronitsky C, Payne RJ, Stuckey S, Wilkins D.** A comparison of laparoscopically assisted vaginal hysterectomy vs. traditional total abdominal and vaginal hysterectomies. J Gynecol Surg. 1993;9:219-24.

65. **Railton P, Kurylko L, Shah CM.** Laparoscopic-assisted vaginal hysterectomy. Can Oper Room Nurs J. 1994;12:19-29.

66. **Messina MJ, Garavaglia MM, Walsh RT, et al.** Laparoscopy-assisted vaginal hysterectomy cost analysis and review of initial experience in a community hospital. J Am Osteopath Assoc. 1995;95:31-6.

67. **Dorsey JH, Holtz PM, Griffiths RI, et al.** Costs and charges associated with three alternative techniques of hysterectomy. N Engl J Med. 1996;335:476-82.

68. **Liu CY.** Laparoscopic hysterectomy: a review of 72 cases. J Reprod Med 1992;37:351-4.

69. **Harris MB, Olive DL.** Changing hysterectomy patterns after introduction of laparoscopically assisted vaginal hysterectomy. Aust J Obstet Gynaecol. 1994;171:340-4.

CHAPTER 15

Menopause

ANNE W. MOULTON, MD
CAROL LANDAU, PHD
MICHELE G. CYR, MD

Epidemiology

More than 13 million women in the United States are now in or past menopause, and another 6 million women will enter menopause during the next decade (1). The average age of menopause is 51, with a range of 45 to 55. Cigarette smoking, some chemotherapeutic agents, and radiation exposure have been associated with earlier onset of menopause. Later onset of menopause is seen in multiparous women. Age of maternal menopause is a strong predictor of age of daughters at menopause. Because the current average female life expectancy is 78 years, a woman can expect to spend more than one-third of her life in the postmenopausal period.

Definitions

Menopause is defined as a cessation of ovarian function that results in permanent amenorrhea. Because 12 months of amenorrhea ensures a cessation of ovarian function in older women, definitive diagnosis is usually made retrospectively. *Perimenopause* refers to the time before actual menopause when the menstrual cycle first becomes irregular. In the United States, this usually occurs at approximately age 47 (2). *Climacteric,* a rarely used broad term, characterizes the entire transition from the reproductive to the postreproductive phase of a woman's life and thus includes both the perimenopause and postmenopause periods.

Physiology

Each woman is born with approximately 400,000 primordial follicles in her ovaries but will ovulate less than 500 times. As menopause approaches, a smaller number of the follicles remain, which are increasingly unresponsive to gonadotropin stimulation.

Hormonal changes reflecting this decrease in ovarian function begin to occur in the decade before the development of irregular cycles. The earliest evidence of these endocrine changes is a mild increase in follicle-stimulating hormone (FSH) levels toward the upper limit of normal. There is a concomitant fall in estrogen levels but only a slight decline in progesterone secretion. During the course of the perimenopausal transition, the menstrual cycle interval often shortens (because of a shorter follicular phase), and gradually these cycles become interspersed with abnormally long intermenstrual intervals (secondary to anovulatory cycles).

When menstrual cycles cease, the secretion of steroid hormones and gonadotropins changes dramatically. The FSH level rises sharply, and estradiol levels fall. After menopause most of the circulating estrogen is no longer produced by the ovaries but is derived from the peripheral conversion of androstenedione to estrone by adipose tissue. Androstenedione, the principal ovarian androgen, is also reduced by about 50% (2); however, because of the reduction in estrogen, there is relative androgen excess. After menopause, the ovaries continue to atrophy until they ultimately are replaced by fibrotic tissue.

Cultural Variations

Although 75% of menopausal women in the United States experience hot flashes, only 10% to 15% of women seek care from a physician for them. Research suggests that there are cultural variations in the development and perception of menopausal symptoms. Symptom reporting in Japan among a population sample of women experiencing natural menopause was significantly lower than in North America. Only 12% of Japanese women report hot flashes; in fact, there is no equivalent term in Japanese. One survey of Nigerian women revealed that only 30% experienced hot flashes (3). These differences need to be viewed in light of cultural variations in diet, exercise, and

Because patients who are experiencing perimenopause are often reluctant to report their concerns or symptoms, it is important that the primary care physician initiate discussion about menopause.

medical illnesses (4). Also, in cultures with more positive attitudes toward mid-life, women's menopausal symptoms are reported less frequently.

There are limited data on the experience of menopause for non-whites in the United States. The health care professional should be aware that the average menopausal African-American woman has a decreased risk of developing osteoporosis and an increased risk of coronary heart disease. In addition, African-American women are more likely to experience prolonged dysfunctional bleeding in the perimenopausal transition. One recent study suggests that African-American women view menopause more positively than white women (5).

Short-Term Symptoms

Irregular Bleeding

Unpredictable vaginal bleeding is perhaps the most common clinical occurrence during the perimenopausal transition. Most women experience between 2 and 8 years of irregular menses before the onset of menopause. This change in cycle length occurs most commonly from anovulation. Although changes in cycle length and frequency of bleeding are common at this time, it is still essential to determine whether this is caused by menopause or some underlying pathology. If an episode of bleeding occurs more often than every 21 days, is profuse for longer than 7 to 10 days, or occurs after a 6-month interval of amenorrhea or in a very irregular pattern, then additional

Although menstrual cycle changes are common during perimenopause, secondary causes should be excluded if bleeding occurs more often than 21 days, is profuse for longer than 7 to 10 days, or occurs after a 6-month period of amenorrhea.

evaluation is indicated (Box 15-1). Work-up might include a pregnancy test, pelvic exam, Pap smear, pelvic ultrasonography, endometrial biopsy, and endocervical curettage. Referral to a gynecologist is often indicated for biopsy or D&C. After evaluation, treatment options often include low-dose combined oral contraceptives or cyclic progestins, depending on whether the patient smokes, has need for contraception, and other factors (see Chapter 3).

Box 15-1 Irregular Bleeding in a Perimenopausal Woman

When to refer for further evaluation:
- Episodes of bleeding occur more frequently than every 21 days
- Bleeding is profuse for more than 7 to 10 days
- Bleeding occurs after a 6-month interval of amenorrhea
- Bleeding occurs in a very irregular pattern

Additional evaluation could include:
- Pregnancy test as indicated
- Bimanual examination and PAP test
- Endometrial biopsy
- Transvaginal ultrasonography

Hot Flashes

The most widely acknowledged symptom of menopause is the *hot flash,* occurring in about 70% to 80% of all women and often beginning several years before menses cease (6). Flashes are sometimes triggered by stress, hot weather, confining spaces or by the ingestion of caffeine, alcohol, or spicy foods. The etiology of the hot flash remains unclear but it probably originates from neurotransmitter activity and is influenced by a combination of hormonal, metabolic, and psychological factors. A vasomotor flash has two stages. It begins with a hot flash, which is a sudden transient sensation ranging from warmth to intense heat that spreads over the body, particularly on the upper chest, face, scalp, and head. This is followed by the physiologically measurable hot flash, with visible erythema and perspiration in the same distribution. Hot flashes can be objectively measured as changes in skin temperature, diminished skin resistance, and decreased core temperature. Some women also experience palpitations and feelings of anxiety. The duration of hot flashes ranges from 30 seconds to several minutes, but the frequency and severity are often quite variable. Symptoms are more likely to occur at night.

Most women remain symptomatic for more than a year. The percentage of women who experience hot flashes for longer than 5 years ranges from 29% to 50%. There is wide variability in the distress associated with hot flashes (7). Only 10% to 15% of women who report any hot flashes describe them as being severe or very frequent (1). For these women, hot flashes may significantly disrupt sleep and adversely affect their lives. Treatment is discussed later in this chapter.

Genitourinary Symptoms

The vagina, vulva, urethra, and trigone of the bladder have a large number of estrogen receptors and thus undergo atrophy as estrogen levels start to decline, even before the onset of menopause. The vulva loses most of its collagen adipose tissue and water-retaining ability and becomes flattened and thin. Sebaceous glands remain, but secretions decrease. Vaginal shortening and narrowing occur as the vaginal walls become thin, lose elasticity, and become pale in color. Postmenopausally, the vagina produces fewer secretions and loses most of its lubricating ability in response to sexual stimulation. There is a decrease in cellular glycogen production leading to a less acidic pH, which can then predispose to the replacement of the usual lactobacilli with fecal flora. All of these postmenopausal changes predispose the patient to atrophic vaginitis with an increased potential for bleeding, infection, and discomfort, as well as, in some cases, decreased sexual interest. Patients with atrophic vaginitis usually complain of dryness, vaginal burning, external dysuria, or dyspareunia. If necessary, a saline wet mount of the vaginal secretions can help confirm the diagnosis with the finding of a less uniform appearance of the epithelial cell population, including smaller, more oval-shaped cells. Similarly, a Pap smear may demonstrate atrophic cells. In addition, estrogen deficiency is also sometimes the cause of ASCUS (atypical squamous cells of uncertain significance) in postmenopausal women. See Chapter 7 for discussion of the management of Pap smear abnormalities.

Atrophy of the connective tissues and blood vessels surrounding the urethra causes a decrease in the normal pressure generated by the urethra and surrounding tissues, a major determinant of continence. A lower threshold for the urge to void has also been reported in postmenopausal women. Loss of pelvic tone also contributes to diminished functional integrity of the lower urinary tract. As a result of decreased pelvic support, prolapse of the urethrovesicular junction occurs, and some measure of bladder control is lost. The *senile urethra syndrome* is characterized by the following symptoms in the absence of either infection or detrusor instability: dysuria, frequency, urgency, suprapubic discomfort, stress incontinence, and urge incontinence.

Between 15% and 35% of women over the age of 60 have urinary incontinence. *Stress incontinence,* the involuntary loss of small amounts of urine with maneuvers that increase abdominal pressure such as coughing, is probably the most common form of chronic urinary incontinence in older women. *Urge incontinence* is the loss of large volumes of urine because of inability to delay voiding once bladder fullness is sensed. Diagnosis and treatment of these disorders is discussed in more detail in Chapter 10.

Depression

Results of studies on the relationship between psychological symptoms and menopausal transition conflict. However, a biological mechanism is supported by two findings. First, neurons in several areas of the brain bear specific nuclear receptors for estrogen. Secondly, estrogen alters the concentration and availability of certain neurotransmitters, including serotonin (8). In addition to these effects, hot flashes can cause nighttime awakening and predispose some perimenopausal and postmenopausal women to fatigue, cognitive impairment, irritability, and depressed mood. It should also be recognized that sociocultural factors, individual characteristics, and the environment all contribute to the menopause experience.

Despite the documented neurologic findings, there is no evidence that natural menopause is a time of increased risk for depression (9). In a large longitudinal study, no correlation was found between depression and hormonal status (10). Identified risk factors for depression during menopause include a history of previous depression, a long duration of vasomotor symptoms, and multiple worries about family members. There is some evidence that new, paid employment may have a positive effect on mood in menopausal-age women (11). Treatment is discussed later in this chapter.

Miscellaneous Symptoms

Many symptoms are listed as potentially related to menopause, but research has not established a definite causation for most of them. The long list of symptoms reported during the period extending from perimenopause through menopause includes palpitations, chest pain, headache, fatigue, change in bowel habits, lack of interest in sex, dry skin, and formication (the sensation of bugs crawling on the skin).

Long-Term Issues

Osteoporosis

Osteoporosis is a diffuse skeletal disease characterized by low bone mass and micro-architectural deterioration of bone tissue with a consequent increase in bone fragility and risk of fracture (12). It is a major medical problem for women, causing increased morbidity and mortality, loss of function, long-term physical and emotional disability, and suffering. Twenty-five million people in the United States have osteoporosis; 1.3 million fractures are attributable to osteoporosis each year, and the annual cost of caring for patients with osteoporosis-related fractures is 10 billion dollars.

Peak bone mass for women is achieved in the early thirties. After a period of equilibrium, bone mass starts to decline and several years later further accelerates, particularly in the first 20 years after menopause. The hip, vertebrae, and distal portion of the forearm are the most common sites of osteoporotic fractures, although fractures at other sites can occur. Of the estimated 1.3 million osteoporotic fractures annually, more than 500,000 are of the vertebrae, and 250,000 are of the hip. At age 50 the average white woman has a lifetime risk of 17.5% for hip fracture and a lifetime risk for any fracture of 40%.

There are several known risk factors for bone loss. Age-related osteoporosis accounts for 80% to 90% of all osteoporosis in women. White or Asian race predisposes to osteoporosis. Africans and people of African descent have a bone mass that, adjusted for body size, is generally 5% to 10% higher than that of whites, as well as a slower rate of bone loss after menopause. There is also evidence that peak bone mass attained is predictive of the subsequent development of osteoporosis and fractures. Nutrition and lifestyle factors also affect the development of osteoporosis. Adequate calcium intake is especially important; conversely, diets high in protein, phosphorus, fat, fiber, sodium, and caffeine may be harmful. Immobilization, even for short periods of time, can cause significant bone loss, whereas regular weight-bearing exercise has been associated with maintenance of bone density.

Finally, many hormones are important in bone development. These include estrogens, androgens, parathyroid hormone, and vitamin D and its metabolites. Secondary causes sometimes need to be considered and include endocrine disorders such as thyrotoxicosis, primary hyperparathyroidism, and glucocorticoid excess, as well as certain malignancies, immobilization, alcohol abuse, nutritional deficiencies, and chronic corticosteroid or heparin use. Screening, prevention, and treatment are discussed later in this chapter.

Cardiovascular Disease

Cardiovascular disease is a major cause of mortality for women in the United States, accounting for 250,000 deaths each year, with 100,000 of these deaths occurring prematurely. It is the leading cause of death in women over the age of 40. One in three women will die of heart disease. Although coronary disease develops approximately 10 to 15 years later in women than in men, by the age of 70 the male/female ratio incidence of coronary artery disease starts to approach one (13). African-American women have higher rates of coronary artery disease, with higher subsequent morbidity and mortality rates as well. Rates of coronary artery disease in Hispanic and Asian women are somewhat lower. Data from the Framingham Study suggest that traditional cardiac risk factors (diabetes, hypertension, elevated cholesterol, smoking, positive family history) play a role in women as they do in men. The magnitude of the effect of these factors may be different for women, however, and there are also unique coronary artery disease risk factors and thus different preventive strategies for women.

The delay in the development of coronary disease in women has been attributed to the beneficial effects of circulating estrogen before the development of menopause. After menopause the risk of developing coronary artery disease increases gradually. Further evidence that estrogen is protective comes from the strong association between early menopause, especially surgical menopause, and increased risk of heart disease.

There have been more than 30 epidemiologic studies on the use of postmenopausal hormones (in most cases unopposed estrogen replacement therapy); the majority found a reduction in the risk of developing coronary artery disease, on average 50%. It is known that estrogen has beneficial effects on plasma lipids, at least in the short term (14). Studies suggest that only 33% to 50% of estrogen's beneficial effect is actually mediated through improvement in serum lipids, however (15). Estrogen also has direct effects on the coronary vasculature by way of estrogen receptors in the arterial endothelial and smooth muscle cells. Estrogen lowers blood pressure, and *in vitro* studies (16) suggest that estrogen has other beneficial effects on the vasculature, including antioxidant effects.

However, in contrast to the foregoing data derived from observational studies, one recent randomized prospective double-blind placebo-controlled study of women with existing coronary artery disease (HERS Study) found that treatment with hormone replacement therapy (HRT) for an average of 4 years did not offer any overall reduction in cardiac events. Particularly worrisome was an apparent initial increase in cardiovascular events in women on HRT (17). By the fourth year, however, there were fewer cardiovascular events in the treated group than in the placebo group. The authors concluded that they

... do not recommend starting this treatment for the purpose of secondary prevention of coronary artery disease. However, given the favorable pattern of coronary artery disease events after several years of therapy, it could be appropriate for women already receiving hormone treatment to continue.

Of course, the results of the HERS Study cannot be extrapolated to primary prevention of coronary artery disease in healthy postmenopausal women. However, information released early from the ongoing Women's Health Initiative, a controlled trial of healthy postmenopausal women, reveals a similar pattern of "early harm, late benefit." For the first 2 years, more cardiovascular events were noted in the HRT group. However, the trend of subsequent years suggests that further follow-up may possibly demonstrate cardioprotection from HRT. Thus, although the observational data strongly support the use of HRT to prevent coronary artery disease, prospective trials reveal a more complex interaction. More data from this large prospective study are eagerly awaited. For a more detailed discussion, see Chapter 16. Screening and treatment of coronary artery disease is discussed later in this chapter.

Evaluation of the Patient

In recent years there has been a great deal of public attention to menopause. The negative tone of much of this information as well as many of the prevailing stereotypes of mid-life women have fostered unfounded fears (18). Patients experiencing perimenopause are often reluctant to express their concerns. Thus it is important for the physician to inform patients that menopause is a positive developmental phase for most women. Many women enjoy their sexuality more because they no longer have a fear of unwanted pregnancy. For some women, midlife allows them more time to pursue individual rather than family goals.

Negative expectations can also cause poor tolerance of symptoms. Thus it is essential for the primary care physician to be able to educate and reassure patients about what to expect at menopause, and such counseling should ideally be part of routine primary care visits for women in their forties (Box 15-2). The perimenopausal transition is also an appropriate time to review health maintenance and routine preventive measures.

The diagnosis of menopause usually requires merely an adequate menstrual history along with a brief review of systems. For women who have symptoms suggestive of menopause yet continue to experience fairly regular menses, or for women who have undergone hysterectomy, an elevated serum follicle-stimulating hormone (FSH) may be useful in verifying the diagnosis.

A rapidly changing knowledge base necessitates the use of resources that provide updated information on menopause. Scheduling extra time during office visits is necessary in order to share this information, answer complex questions, and assess the patient's risk of breast cancer, heart disease, and osteoporosis. One should also generally discuss the pros and cons of hormone replacement (see Chapter 16) and the use of alternative therapies.

Screening for osteoporosis should be offered to asymptomatic menopausal patients who have additional risk factors for osteoporosis or for whom the results are likely to affect treatment decisions or lifestyle changes. Although screening identifies women who have or are at risk for the development of osteoporosis, it is unable to accurately predict the risk of fracture. This together with the high cost of bone density testing prohibits mass screening of all postmenopausal women.

Box 15-2   Role of the Primary Provider in the Care of the Menopausal Woman

---

Counseling on the average woman's experience with menopause:
- Mean age of 51
- Considerable individual variation in the experience of menopause
- Most women do not have severe symptoms
- Most women do not become depressed

Assessment and treatment, as needed, for symptoms:
- Assess menstrual history
- Screen for hot flashes, vaginal dryness, changes in mood

Review of health maintenance and routine preventive measures:
- Cancer screening
- Exercise, diet

Establish risk factors for heart disease and osteoporosis:
- Assess patient's past medical history, exercise, diet, alcohol intake
- Assess patient's family history

Screening for heart disease and osteoporosis if warranted by risk factors, symptoms, or HRT decision:
- Glucose, total and HDL cholesterol (fasting panel if indicated)
- Stress testing, coronary angiography
- Bone densitometry

Provide resource information:
- Educational materials
- Local support groups
- Community resources
- Books, periodicals, Internet

There are currently five techniques for assessing bone density: radiographic absorptiometry, single-photon absorptiometry, dual-photon absorptiometry, dual-energy x-ray absorptiometry, and quantitative computed tomography. Although these techniques vary in cost, accuracy, and amount of radiation exposure, the choice of procedure is typically determined by what is available locally. Ordinary radiographs are not helpful in screening for osteoporosis because they lack sensitivity to detect early bone loss.

The results of bone density testing are expressed in standard deviations, with the more negative number implying lower bone density. The T-score compares the individual patient's bone density with the mean peak value of young healthy persons of the same sex. When this score is lower than –2.5 on a DXA scan, the patient has osteoporosis, and some form of pharmacologic treatment is indicated. A T-score between –1 and –2.5 indicates osteopenia, which may be addressed with similar medications or with more conservative intervention and close follow-up, depending on the patient's risk factors and overall clinical picture. When a patient's Z-score (which compares the patient's bone density with the gender-matched *and* age-matched mean) is lower than –2, accelerated bone loss has occurred, and secondary causes of osteoporosis (e.g., endocrinopathies, multiple myeloma) must be excluded (19). Initial evaluation includes measuring serum levels of calcium, alkaline phosphatase, and 25-hydroxy vitamin D. Such testing may uncover a vitamin D deficiency or suggest hyperparathyroidism, which can be confirmed with measurement of the intact parathyroid hormone level. Further investigation is guided by the clinical presentation.

Assessment of risk for cardiovascular disease in an asymptomatic perimenopausal or postmenopausal woman includes a detailed history and physical examination. Routine bloodwork should include a random total and high-density lipoprotein cholesterol and a fasting glucose. Although a baseline electrocardiogram is occasionally helpful in some circumstances, no data support routine use. Similarly, there is no proven benefit to performing screening stress tests on asymptomatic women, even those who have risk factors for CAD.

Prevention and Treatment of Symptoms

Hot Flashes

Medications
Severe hot flashes are treated most effectively with estrogen (with concurrent progesterone if the patient has a uterus (see Chapter 16 for further discussion). Recent studies suggest that the addition of androgens may be helpful if estrogen alone does not relieve symptoms (6). However, many women may choose not to take estrogen, and there are alternative treatments available to them (Table 15-1) (1). Medroxyprogesterone acetate (MPA) 20 mg daily has been shown in two double-blind crossover studies to decrease hot flashes by 70% to 90%. Vitamin E, propranolol, and oral clonidine 0.1 mg daily have also been effective in small studies. Recent pilot studies suggest reduction of hot flashes with antidepressants such as fluoxetine (Prozac), paroxetine

Table 15-1 Alternative Treatments for Menopausal Symptoms

Symptom	Treatment Modality
Hot flashes	Paced respirations
	Medications
	Environmental planning
	Increase plant estrogens in diet
	Decrease caffeine and spicy foods
Sexual dysfunction	Kegel exercises
	Regular sexual activity
	Vaginal lubricants
Overall health	Exercise
	Stress management and relaxation techniques
	Well-balanced diet

(Paxil) 20 mg daily, and venlafaxine (Effexor) 75 mg daily (20). Also, a recent report describes beneficial effect with gabapentin (Neurontin), presumably via its direct action on the thermoregulatory center (21). All of these agents await large placebo-controlled trials for confirmation of benefit. Interestingly, some studies have observed a 40% decrease in hot flash symptoms with placebo.

Behavioral Techniques

Behavioral and environmental planning techniques can be beneficial and have few side effects. Most patients benefit from sleeping in a cool room, keeping a cold glass of water nearby, wearing layered clothing in lighter colors and weave, using sheets and linens that breathe, avoiding foods that trigger hot flashes (e.g., caffeine, heavy spices), and carrying a small fan. Woodward and colleagues found that ventilation increased significantly during the beginning of a hot flash (22), and that hot flashes can be reduced by training the patient to perform slow, deep abdominal breathing (23).

Nutrition and Nutritional Supplements

In addition to the dietary changes mentioned above, both vitamin E (400 IU) and phytoestrogens (plant estrogens) appear to help hot flashes. Many believe that the average Asian diet of about 3 to 4 oz of certain soy foods (e.g., tofu, soy cheese, but not soy sauce) is responsible for the lower frequency of hot flashes reported by Japanese women compared with Americans. However, double-blind, placebo-controlled trials of soy products have failed to show a significant reduction in hot flashes over placebo. Although some have postulated that phytoestrogens act more like selective estrogen receptor modulators, with estrogen effect on some tissues yet anti-estrogenic effect on others, their action on breast tissue is not known. Because many women, such as breast cancer patients, turn to nutritional supplements because they have been advised not to use estrogen, they should be cautioned about the lack of information regarding the risks and benefits of phytoestrogens.

Health food stores in the United States also sell a variety of herbs for treating menopausal symptoms. Black cohosh, red clover, mandrake, dong quai, gotu kola, sarsaparilla, and tea made from dried garden sage have been touted as successful remedies for hot flashes or other menopausal symptoms. However, a clinical trial of dong quai found it to be no more helpful than placebo (24). Moreover, for the majority of herbs no scientific studies have been conducted to test either efficacy or toxicity. Also, because these nutritional supplements are unregulated, there is wide variation in quality and dosage. Thus at present it is difficult to endorse the use of these products.

Acupuncture

A study by Wyon et al found that two forms of acupuncture were effective in reducing hot flashes by 50% compared with baseline, but that electro-acupuncture was a more long-lasting treatment (25). However, further research is necessary because this study followed subjects for only 3 months post-treatment.

Exercise

Although it has not been studied systematically, many women report a reduction in hot flashes with regular exercise. Additionally, the benefits of weight bearing and aerobic exercise in the prevention of osteoporosis and coronary artery disease are well documented.

Summary

Overall, alternative therapies offer promise as adjuncts to or replacements for hormone therapy. More long-term controlled studies are necessary before definite conclusions and treatment recommendations can be made, however (26).

Genitourinary Atrophy

Initial therapies for stress and urge incontinence include Kegel exercises (27), scheduled voiding, and prompt treatment of urinary tract infections. For those women who fail to respond to these measures, referral to a urologist, urogynecologist, or specialized nurse for further evaluation or biofeedback training may sometimes be indicated (see Chapter 10). Assessment and treatment of potential vaginal infections are important as well as educating the patient to avoid feminine hygiene products that might further increase infection or inflammation.

Estrogen vaginal cream is highly effective and sometimes necessary even in women already taking systemic HRT. Alternative therapies for atrophic vaginitis, in addition to Kegel exercises, include regular use of vaginal acidifier/lubricants (e.g., Replens, Aci-Jel) to relieve vaginal dryness and restore the normal vaginal pH, and the use of lubricants such as K-Y jelly during sexual intercourse (see Chapter 8).

Depression

The best approach to depression during menopause is to carefully assess the patient in standard fashion with respect to DSM-IV criteria and to treat the patient accordingly (28). As in all cases of depression, the physician needs to rule out medication effects and medical illnesses associated with depression. In a woman of menopausal age, likely culprits include antihypertensive medication and endocrine disorders. When treating a major depressive episode, antidepressant medication can be extremely beneficial and cost-effective. Short-term cognitive or behavioral psychotherapy is also beneficial and, in contrast to medication, is without side effects. It is extremely important to attend to any marital and family problems as well.

Women who have experienced a long period of untreated menopausal symptoms that result in a sleep disturbance are at increased risk for depression. This has been referred to as the "domino effect" of menopausal symptoms. When sleep disturbance is implicated in precipitating depression, HRT or another treatment of hot flashes is indicated. The direct effect of HRT on depression is highly variable, reducing symptoms in some women and exacerbating the condition in others.

Because the effect of HRT on depression is highly variable, adjusting such therapy is often warranted before beginning psychopharmacologic therapy.

Therefore HRT is not currently a recommended first-line treatment for depression, and the HRT regimen, if used to treat physiologic symptoms, should be adjusted before prescribing adjunctive psychopharmacologic treatment.

Possibly due to the known effects of estrogen on the serotonin system, some postmenopausal women appear to benefit from the facilitative effects of estrogen taken with a selective serotonin reuptake inhibitor (SSRI). Conversely, postmenopausal women not taking estrogen sometimes respond better to tricyclic antidepressants than to SSRIs.

Osteoporosis

Preventing bone loss is essential because there are no safe and proven means for strengthening the skeleton and restoring skeletal integrity once osteoporosis and fractures have occurred. However, this goal is tempered by the finding that some women with low bone density never suffer fractures or other clinical effects.

Estrogen replacement has been shown to be effective for prevention of osteoporosis and is commonly used for the treatment of established disease as well (see Chapter 16). Raloxifene (Evista) 60 mg daily is a selective estrogen receptor modulator approved for both prevention and treatment of osteoporosis. Compared with estrogen, raloxifene appears to have more favorable effects on breast and endometrial tissue; however, a large study failed to demonstrate a reduction in nonvertebral fractures (29), and overall raloxifene's effect on increasing bone mineral density is less than that of estrogen or alendronate.

The bisphosphonate alendronate (Fosamax) is approved for both prevention (5 mg) and treatment (10 mg) of osteoporosis. Because of alendronate's poor absorption and its risk of causing esophageal ulceration, this medication must be taken on an empty stomach with a large glass of water. Food must then be avoided for 30 min, and the patient should not assume the recumbent position until after having eaten. Because of these restrictions, the alternative dosing regimen of 70 mg taken once weekly likely improves compliance. Women with active upper gastrointestinal tract disease, including significant gastroesophageal reflux, should avoid alendronate. The newer bisphosphonate, risedronate (Actonel 5 mg daily), is associated with less upper gastrointestinal effects than alendronate, but the suggestion of slightly inferior efficacy (30,31) begs for a trial directly comparing the two drugs. Both bisphosphanates should be avoided in patients with renal impairment.

Calcitonin decreases bone breakdown by inhibiting osteoclast activity and is approved for the treatment of established osteoporosis. Calcitonin has been shown to reduce bone loss when used for up to 2 years. It is available in a nasal spray (Miacalcin) and is dosed as one spray daily, using alternate nostrils. Although calcitonin is the least efficacious medication affecting bone density, its beneficial effects on pain transmission make it particularly useful for the first several months after a fracture.

With any of the aforementioned preventive or treatment regimens, it is important to include calcium and vitamin D supplementation. In addition, it has been shown that the combination of calcium and vitamin D supplementation by itself increases total body bone mineral density and reduces the incidence of fracture in postmenopausal women. Thus all postmenopausal women should be advised to ingest 1500 mg of calcium daily as well as vitamin D 400 I/U per day. Calcium can be obtained from any combination of dairy products, calcium-rich vegetables (e.g., bok choi), and calcium-fortified juices. If sufficient calcium cannot be obtained from food sources (which may be related to lactose intolerance and low fat diets), then calcium supplementation is necessary. To help ensure absorption, calcium supplementation should be taken

For the purpose of preventing osteoporosis and fractures, all postmenopausal women should be advised to ingest 1500 mg of calcium and 400 I/U of vitamin D daily. Supplements should be recommended when dietary sources are inadequate.

with meals, often as 500 mg tid. Vitamin D deficiency is common in elderly persons, especially those who are chronically ill, poorly nourished, or housebound and therefore receiving inadequate sunlight exposure. Standard multivitamins contain 400 I/U of vitamin D.

There is also growing evidence that exercise is beneficial to bone. In addition to maintaining bone density, exercise may also reduce fracture risk by strengthening back muscles, improving agility and mobility, and maintaining a sense of well-being. Once a patient has developed osteoporosis or experienced a fracture, referral to a physical therapist is often helpful to institute an appropriate exercise program.

Coronary Artery Disease

Menopause is a particularly good time to assess cardiac risk factors such as diabetes, hypertension, and hyperlipidemia. Counseling about appropriate diet and exercise is indicated as well as addressing any psychosocial factors that may affect the development of heart disease in women, including depression and anxiety. There is no clear evidence that antioxidants prevent the development of heart disease in women. It should also be noted that the recommendation for moderate drinking (1 to 3 drinks per day) in order to increase HDL is not based on evidence of benefit for women. In fact, women may experience toxicity, increased risk of breast cancer, and even cirrhosis with as few as 1 to 1½ drinks per day. Although there is no consensus regarding the use of aspirin for primary prevention of myocardial infarction in women, many physicians recommend low-dose (81 mg per day) aspirin for their older female patients. Observational studies provide good evidence that physically active women have a reduced risk for the development of heart disease (32). Current recommendations call for regular exercise for all women, gradually increased to consist of moderate activity of 30-min duration for most days of the week (33).

Resources

Results from a study in a large HMO suggest that approximately one-third of patients surveyed felt that their menopause care was fair to poor, with one-half of the women agreeing that a menopause support group would be useful

(34). These findings highlight the need to expand the resources available to menopause patients.

There are many resources available to perimenopausal and post-menopausal patients, including books, pamphlets, and newsletters. Information given to the patient at the appropriate time will help to clarify the normal experience of menopause. Many Web sites on the Internet provide educational material. The North American Menopause Society (NAMS) offers a series of consumer brochures on various aspects of menopause (http://www.menopause.org). Other Web sites of interest include those of the American Heart Association (http://www.americanheart.org) and the National Osteoporosis Foundation (http://www.nof.org). Two federal agencies also provide research update sites: http://www.healthfinder.gov and the National Center for Complementary and Alternative Medicine (http://nccam.nih.gov).

Summary

Menopause is a unique period in a woman's life that is accompanied by many physiologic changes, some of which may manifest as troublesome symptoms. In addition, the menopause transition heralds the onset of increasing incidence of chronic problems such as osteoporosis and coronary artery disease. Thus, for the astute and well-informed primary care physician, the menopausal patient offers a wealth of opportunity for intervention in the form of basic patient education, symptom management, risk factor reduction, and primary prevention. By meeting these challenges, the physician can help optimize the last one-third of the woman's life.

REFERENCES

1. **Hammond CB.** Menopause and hormone replacement therapy: an overview. Obstet Gynecol. 1996;87S:2-15.
2. **Santoro NF.** Endocrinology of the climacteric. In: Seifer DB, Kennard EA, eds. Menopause: Endocrinology and Management. Totowa, NJ: Humana Press; 1999:21-34.
3. **Okonofua FE, Lawal A, Bamgbose JK.** Features of menopause and menopausal age in Nigerian women. Int J Gynecol Obstet. 1990;31:341-5.
4. **Lock M.** Menopause in cultural context. Exp Gerontol. 1994;29:307-17.
5. **Pham K-TC, Grisso JA, Freeman EW.** Ovarian aging and hormone replacement therapy. J Gen Intern Med. 1997;12:230-6.
6. **Bachmann GA.** Vasomotor flashes in menopausal women. Am J Obstet Gynecol. 1999;180:S312-6.
7. **Kronenberg F.** Hot flashes: epidemiology and physiology. In: Flint M, Kronenberg F, Utian W, eds. Multidisciplinary Perspectives on Menopause. Ann N Y Acad Sci. 1990; 592:52-86.

8. **Sherwin BB.** Hormones, mood, and cognitive functioning in postmenopausal women. Obstet Gynecol. 1996;87S:20-7.

9. **Matthews KA, Wing RR, Kuller LH, et al.** Influences of natural menopause on psychological characteristics and symptoms of middle-aged healthy women. J Consul Clin Psychol. 1990;58:345-51.

10. **McKinlay JB, McKinlay SM, Brambilla D.** The relative contributions of endocrine changes and social circumstances to depression in mid-aged women. J Health Social Behav. 1987;28:345-63.

11. **Bromberger JT, Matthews KA.** Employment status and depressive symptoms in middle aged women: a longitudinal investigation. Am J Public Health. 1994;84:202-6.

12. **Lindsay R.** The menopause and osteoporosis. Obstet Gynecol. 1996;87S:16-9.

13. **Moulton AW.** Coronary artery disease. In: Carlson KJ, Eisenstat SA, Fregoletto FD, Schiff I, eds. Primary Care of Women. St. Louis: Mosby; 1995:8-15.

14. **Writing Group for the PEPI Trial.** Effects of estrogen or estrogen/progestin regimens on heart disease risk factors in post-menopausal women. JAMA. 1995;273:199-208.

15. **Sullivan JM, Fowlkes LP.** The clinical aspects of estrogen and the cardiovascular system. Obstet Gynecol. 1996;87S:36-43.

16. **Wild RA.** Estrogen: effects on the cardiovascular tree. Obstet Gynecol. 1996;87S: 27-35.

17. **Hulley S, Grady D, Bush T, et al.** Randomized trial of estrogen plus progestin for secondary prevention of coronary heart disease in postmenopausal women. JAMA. 1998; 280:605-13.

18. **Martin KA.** Menopause and estrogen replacement therapy. In: Carlson KJ, Eisenstat SA, Fregoletto FD, Schiff I, eds. Primary Care of Women. St. Louis: Mosby; 1995: 251-6.

19. **McGarry KA, Kiel DP.** Postmenopausal osteoporosis. strategies for preventing bone loss, avoiding fracture. Postgrad Med. 2000;108:79-82, 85-88, 91.

20. **Gottlieb N.** Nonhormonal agents show promise against hot flashes. J Nat Cancer Inst. 2000;92:1118-20.

21. **Guttuso TJ.** Gabapentin's effects on hot flashes and hypothermia. Neurology. 2000; 54:2161-3.

22. **Woodward S, Greville HW, Freedman RR.** Ventilatory response during menopausal hot flashes. Menopause. 1995;2:81-8.

23. **Freedman RR, Woodward SW.** Behavioral treatment of menopausal hot flashes: evaluation by ambulatory monitoring. Am J Obstet Gynecol. 1992;167:436-9.

24. **Hirsata JD, Swiersz LM, Zell B, et al.** Does dong quai have estrogenic effects in postmenopausal women? A double-blind, placebo-controlled trial. Fertil Steril. 1997;68: 6981-6.

25. **Wyon Y, Lindgren R, Lundeberg T, Hammar M.** Effects of acupuncture on climacteric vasomotor symptoms, quality of life, and urinary excretion of neuropeptides among postmenopausal women. Menopause. 1995;2:3-12.

26. **Kronenberg F.** Alternative therapies: new opportunities for menopause research. Menopause. 1995;1:1-2.

27. **Kegel AM.** Physiologic therapy for urinary stress incontinence. JAMA. 1951;146:915-17.

28. **Landau C, Milan F.** Assessment and treatment of depression during menopause: a preliminary report. Menopause. 1996;3:201-7.

29. **Ettinger B, Black DM, Mitlak BH, et al.** Reduction of vertebral fracture risk in postmenopausal women with osteoporosis treated with raloxifene: results from a 3-year randomized clinical trial. Multiple Outcomes of Raloxifene Evaluation (MORE) Investigators. JAMA. 1999;282;7:637-45.

30. **Harris ST, Watts NB, Genant HK, et al.** Effects of risedronate treatment on vertebral and nonvertebral fractures in women with postmenopausal osteoporosis: a randomized controlled trial. JAMA. 1999;282:1344-52.

31. **Leder BZ, Kronenberg HM.** Gastroenterologists and choosing the right bisphosphonate. Gastroenterology. 2000;119:866-71.

32. **Kushi LH, Fee RM, Folsom AR, et al.** Physical activity and mortality in postmenopausal women. JAMA. 1997;277:1287-92.

33. **Burress J, Christiani D, Berwick DM.** Counseling to promote physical activity. In: U.S. Preventive Services Task Force Guide to Clinical Preventive Services, 2nd ed. Baltimore: Williams & Wilkins; 1996:611-24.

34. **Livingston WW, Healy JM, Jordan HS, et al.** Assessing the needs of women and clinicians for the management of menopause in an HMO. J Gen Intern Med. 1994;9:385-9.

CHAPTER 16

Hormone Replacement Therapy

REBEKAH WANG-CHENG, MD
ANN BUTLER NATTINGER, MD, MPH

Hormone replacement therapy (HRT) is appropriate for many post-menopausal women because of the associated bone-sparing and possible long-term cardiovascular benefits that have a direct effect on mortality. In addition, HRT provides more immediate improvement in vasomotor and urogenital symptoms (Box 16-1). Some studies have suggested that estrogen may improve cognitive function and delay or decrease the risk of Alzheimer's dementia (1), and that it may help protect against colon cancer (2); however, other evidence (2a,27) does not support such claims. Similarly, recent trials such as the Women's Health Initiative raise questions as to the degree of benefit for preventing cardiac disease, and other studies suggest that HRT may contribute to an increased risk of breast cancer (3,4). Thus, while for some women the decision regarding HRT is straightforward, for many patients the decision involves a careful analysis of the relative risks for osteoporosis, breast cancer, and heart disease.

In addition to these issues, women often have concerns regarding endometrial cancer risk, the inconvenience of monthly bleeding and other potential side effects, and the prospect of taking life-long medication. While women can receive HRT information from sources such as women's magazines, books, friends, and television, most women still benefit from a discussion with their physician. The primary care physician must remain up-to-date and knowledgeable about HRT so that he or she can help patients make informed decisions regarding their health and well-being in this unique time of life.

Box 16-1 Risks and Benefits of Hormone Replacement Therapy

Short-term benefits
Improvement in vasomotor symptoms
Improvement in urogenital symptoms
Increased libido
Decrease in mood swings
Decrease in weight gain

Long-term beneficial effects
Total mortality: 35%–45% decrease in overall mortality
Cardiovascular: 30%–50% decrease in risk of MI
Osteoporosis: 25%–50% decrease in hip, wrist, and nonspinal fractures
Alzheimer's disease: ~30% decrease in risk

Risks
Endometrial cancer: four- to five-fold increased risk with *unopposed* estrogen; progestin eliminates this increased risk
Breast cancer: 25%–35% increased risk with 5 or more years of HRT

Throughout this chapter case studies of sample patients illustrate different aspects of clinical decision-making. The risks and benefits of HRT are reviewed and applied to these very practical clinical situations. Also to be discussed are the contraindications to HRT and the importance of monitoring for complications. In addition, an overview of the various available regimens and their advantages, disadvantages, and side effects is given. Finally, compliance issues, which impact greatly on long-term treatment, are addressed.

Beneficial Effects of Hormone Replacement Therapy

Cardiovascular Disease

CASE 16-1

Connie B is a 52 year-old corporate attorney for a large insurance company. Her job is stressful, and she admits to eating fast food and not exercising much. She was considering taking estrogen until she read an article in the Wall Street Journal about estrogen and heart disease, and she is now very confused. Her father died of a myocardial infarction at age 47, and her older sister underwent coronary artery bypass grafting this year at age 59. Her mother is alive and well at age 75 and has no osteoporosis. On exam she is moderately obese and has border-line hypertension.

Coronary artery disease (CAD) remains the largest single cause of death in the United States, accounting for almost a million deaths per year. In every year since 1984, heart disease has killed more women than men, and the gap continues to widen. CAD claimed the lives of 505,930 women and 435,297 men in 1996 (5). More women (44%) than men (27%) die within one year of a myocardial infarction (MI), which in part may be due to the fact that women are older than men when cardiac disease becomes clinically apparent. CAD develops about 10 years later in women than in men, with the risk increasing rapidly after menopause.

More than 30 observational studies have examined the effects of HRT on cardiovascular morbidity and mortality, and meta-analyses of these studies are consistent with a 50% reduction in heart disease risk (6). In most of these studies, unopposed estrogen was used. A recent follow-up study of the very large Nurses' Health Study (7) suggests that this cardioprotective effect is also present with the combination estrogen-progestin regimen (relative risk [RR], 0.39; 95% confidence interval [CI], 0.19 to 0.78) as well as with estrogen alone (RR, 0.60; 95% CI, 0.43 to 0.83) compared with nonusers. Thus the addition of progestin does not appear to attenuate the cardioprotective effects of estrogen alone, which had been a previous concern.

In contrast to the findings from these observational studies, however, a Northern California study rather surprisingly failed to detect any cardioprotective effect of estrogen (8). This retrospective case-control study of 438 women hospitalized for MI compared with 438 controls did not show a statistically significant decrease in the odds ratio (0.96; 95% CI, 0.66 to 1.4) for MI for current users of estrogen or estrogen-progestogen. These data suggest that estrogen's beneficial effects on the heart may not be as great as previously thought.

The recent Heart and Estrogen/Progestin Replacement Study (HERS) also raises doubt as to the cardioprotective effect of estrogen. This randomized, placebo-controlled trial examined the efficacy of combined estrogen and progestin (0.625 mg of conjugated estrogen and 2.5 mg of medroxyprogesterone) in preventing coronary events in 2763 U.S. women with established CAD (9). A greater number of recurrent coronary events were noted in the

HRT group in year one of the study, but there was a trend towards benefit in years four and five (Fig. 16-1). However, at the end of the five years, there was still no significant difference in MI or death (172 HRT and 172 placebo) between the two groups (although gallbladder disease was increased and throm-

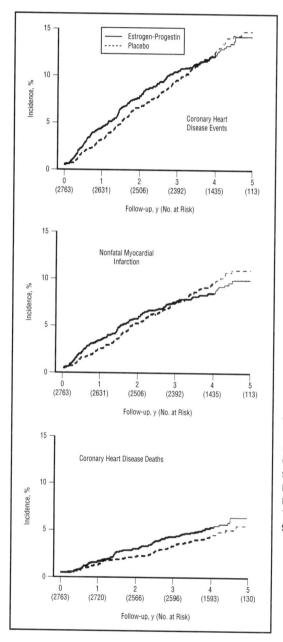

Figure 16-1 Kaplan-Meier estimates of the cumulative incidence of primary coronary heart disease (CHD) events (*top*) and to its constituents: nonfatal myocardial infarction (MI) (*middle*) and CHD death (*bottom*). The number of women observed at each year of follow-up and still free of an event are provided in parentheses, and the curves become fainter when this number drops below half of the cohort. Log rank *P* values are 0.91 for primary CHD events, 0.46 for nonfatal MI, and 0.23 for CHD death. This randomized prospective study of women with established coronary disease failed to demonstrate the cardioprotection from HRT that had been noted in observational studies. In fact, for the first year, the estrogen-progestin arm had a greater number of coronary events than the placebo group. Further follow-up detected a trend toward benefit in later years. (From Hulley SH, Grady D, Bush T, et al. Randomized trial of estrogen plus progestin for secondary prevention of coronary heart disease in postmenopausal women. JAMA. 1998;280;609; with permission.)

boembolic disease was almost triple in the HRT group). Some have postulated that HRT is associated with an initial higher risk of MI by possibly contributing to a procoagulable state in susceptible hosts, thus explaining the decreasing number of cardiac events as the course of HRT continued. As a result, many authors have recommended against *initiating* HRT in women with known coronary disease, yet endorse continuing therapy in those who have already tolerated it for a few years. It should be emphasized that little can be inferred from the HERS study regarding the effects of HRT on women without coronary disease.

> *Because HRT is associated with an initial higher risk of MI, many authors have recommended against initiating HRT in women with known coronary disease but endorse continuing therapy in those who have already tolerated it.*

The surprising findings of the Northern California and HERS studies raise the possibility that the benefit of HRT in observational studies could actually be a reflection of confounders such as the "healthy user effect". These more recent studies underscore the importance of completing randomized prospective trials before drawing definitive conclusions.

The Women's Health Initiative Study, sponsored by the National Institutes of Health, is a randomized prospective controlled trial following more than 27,000 women to assess the efficacy and safety of HRT on cardiovascular disease, breast cancer, fractures, colon cancer, and dementia. Full results of this 15-year project will not be available until 2006 (10), but preliminary data from the first two years of the study were released in April 2000 because of the unexpected finding of a trend toward increased risk of cardiovascular events in the hormone using group. Fewer than 1% of women in either the estrogen/progestin group or the unopposed estrogen group suffered a complication, but it was still a higher rate than that of the control group, so the investigators notified all participants for ethical reasons. Close scrutiny of these data reveals a trend toward decreasing disparity between the two groups, and perhaps with longer follow-up will demonstrate eventual cardioprotection from HRT, as the HERS trial suggested. In Europe a prospective study similar in design to the Women's Health Initiative is underway, the Women's International Study of Long Duration Oestrogen after Menopause (WISDOM) trial.

Another prospective randomized trial, the Estrogen Replacement and Atherosclerosis (ERA) trial, compared the effects of estrogen, estrogen plus medroxyprogesterone, or placebo on atherosclerotic lesions in women with known CAD (11). After three years of therapy, repeat coronary angiograms revealed no difference in the progression of atherosclerosis between the three groups. However, it may be difficult to interpret the significance of this study's results, given the questionable relevance of angiographic findings, the brief duration of the trial, and the timing of the initiation of HRT (average 23 years following the onset of menopause).

Estrogen certainly does have established beneficial effects on the cardiovascular system, mediated through several mechanisms such as changes in lipid metabolism, blood pressure, coagulation factors, antioxidant properties, and direct vascular effects. Estrogen's improvement of the lipid profile probably accounts for less than half of its cardioprotective effect. Given the prevalence of heart disease in this country (one-half of postmenopausal women develop cardiovascular disease) and the large reduction in cardiovascular and other mortality noted with HRT use in several observational studies, one could project that universal postmenopausal HRT use would improve life expectancy overall from a population standpoint. However, the unexpected difficulty in demonstrating cardioprotection in prospective trials calls this into question. Given that HRT can also contribute to adverse events such as an increased risk of breast cancer, efforts have been directed toward helping to predict the relative potential risks and benefits on an individual basis.

Using data from the many trials that showed cardiovascular benefit, a decision analysis was developed to examine the effect of HRT on mortality in hypothetical women with varying risk factors for CAD, breast cancer, hip fracture, and endometrial cancer (12). According to this model a woman with at least one cardiac risk factor would enjoy mortality benefit from HRT use—even if such a woman had first-degree relatives with breast cancer. Gains in life expectancy would also occur from preventing hip fractures. Calculations using this model predict that the only women for whom HRT would not extend life expectancy would be those at lowest risk for heart disease yet at increased risk for breast cancer. However, this model was designed before publication of the aforementioned prospective trials, and its premise of cardioprotection from estrogen is now in question.

Recognizing that bias alone may possible be responsible for the apparent beneficial effect of HRT on CAD in observational trials, and that prospective trials of HRT use have demonstrated a complex association with cardiovascular events, the American Heart Association (AHA) has offered updated clinical recommendations. The AHA stated that "There are insufficient data to suggest that HRT should be initiated for the sole purpose of primary prevention of coronary vascular disease" (12a). Instead, decisions regarding starting and continuing HRT should be baseed on "established noncoronary benefits and risks, and patient preference." Regarding HRT use in women with established CAD, the AHA assumed a more flexible position than the authors of the HERS study, stating that HRT could be initiated in women with existing CAD—but not for the purpose of secondary prevention, as it considers available data inconclusive. Another AHA recommendation recognizes the recent association of thromboembolic events with HRT use. When women taking HRT develop an acute coronary event or become immobilized, one should consider either temporarily discontinuing the HRT or using DVT prophylaxis. The decision to subsequently resume HRT should, again, "be based on noncoronary benefits and risks, as well as patient preference" (12a).

Many now feel that women considering HRT use should be advised that during the first few years they may possibly be at slightly increased risk for cardiovascular events. Also, new emphasis is being placed on encouraging women at risk for heart disease to address modifiable lifestyle factors, such as diet, exercise, and smoking, as well as raising physician awareness to prescribe women lipid-lowering and blood pressure agents when needed.

Future directions in the study of HRT and coronary disease may involve screening for and excluding women with genetic susceptibility to thrombosis, using lower doses of ERT, comparing different preparations and routes of delivery of estrogen and progesterone, and initiating HRT use sooner after the menopause (12a).

DISCUSSION OF CASE 16-1

This case has no easy answer. Even though Connie B has no menopausal symptoms and is not at great risk for osteoporosis because of her obesity, she may be a candidate for HRT. Additional history reveals she lacks significant increased risk for breast cancer, and she has at least one risk factor for CAD (her strongly positive family history). In helping her make an informed decision, it would be important to explain the conflicting data regarding cardioprotection and the possibility of an increased chance of breast cancer after 5 to 10 years of HRT use. Of course, one would also advise her that for prevention of CAD she should make major lifestyle changes in nutritional habits, stress, and exercise.

If she agrees to HRT, a trial of continuous HRT would be recommended for this 52 year old, with the understanding that unpredictable spotting may be expected in the first few months of therapy and should not be a cause for alarm. As with most postmenopausal women, it is highly unlikely that Connie B would appreciate the resumption of cyclic bleeding. Her blood pressure will be monitored, but the literature suggests that it is not raised by HRT (see PEPI Trial findings in Box 16-2). In addition, any symptoms or signs of thromboembolism would be addressed quickly.

Box 16-2 Findings from the Postmenopausal Estrogen/Progestin Interventions (PEPI) Trial

- Estrogen alone resulted in the greatest increase in HDL.
- Estrogen combined with progestin in a cyclic fashion still resulted in HDL increase.
- LDL levels were reduced by about 20% regardless of which regimen was used.
- HRT reduced fibrinogen levels in all treatment groups over placebo.
- There were no adverse effects on insulin levels or blood pressure in any group.
- Adenomatous endometrial hyperplasia was significantly increased in the unopposed estrogen group (34% vs. 1%) compared with other regimens.

Data from Writing Group for the PEPI trial. Effects of estrogen/progestin regimens on heart disease risk factors in postmenopausal women. JAMA. 1995;273:199-208.

Lipids

CASE 16-2

Norma G is a 54-year-old nurse who has hyperlipidemia. Although she has no family or personal history of coronary artery disease, her total and LDL-cholesterol levels have remained elevated in spite of aggressive dietary modification, and her HDL remains in the mid-30s despite regular exercise and HRT for one year. She has been taking combination estrogen-progestin and is interested in continuing HRT, but she is concerned about whether the progestin is blunting the favorable effects of the estrogen.

Conjugated estrogen is associated with increased high-density lipoprotein cholesterol (HDL) and apolipoprotein A-I levels, both of which favorably affect cardiovascular risk. Concerns were raised previously by studies suggesting progestins had an adverse effect on estrogen's beneficial lipid alterations. The Postmenopausal Estrogen/Progestin Interventions (PEPI) Trial (13) was the first multicenter, randomized, double-blind trial addressing very issue. It determined that HDL levels increased the most in women receiving estrogen alone, but that HDL levels also rose in women receiving combination estrogen/progestin. Conjugated estrogen plus medroxyprogesterone acetate (MPA) administered cyclically had a more favorable effect on HDL than did a continuous regimen, and micronized progesterone led to the most increase in HDL. More findings from this major trial are listed in Box 16-2.

Since these beneficial lipid effects occur with oral estrogen preparations because of the hepatic metabolism and are not as pronounced with transdermal estrogen, oral estrogens are the preferred route in women with hyperlipidemia.

DISCUSSION OF CASE 16-2

Based on the PEPI trial, it would be reasonable to either try estrogen alone or switch from MPA to a micronized progesterone and monitor her lipid response. The effects on lipids appear to be dependent on current use, so Norma G must understand that ideally HRT should be life-long. If she elects to take unopposed estrogen, she will require annual endometrial surveillance.

Osteoporosis

CASE 16-3

Karen L is a thin, fair-skinned flight attendant. Karen had a long history of smoking before quitting last year at the age of 50. Her mother had severe osteoporosis and sustained a hip fracture at the age of 72, and her father and older sister both had gallstones. Her menses stopped about 3 years ago, and she says her vasomotor symptoms and dyspareunia are now mild. Though she agrees to undergo bone densitometry, she is unsure about HRT.

Osteoporosis is an important cause of morbidity and mortality in elderly women. An estimated 25 million people in the United States are at risk for bone loss, and 80% of them are women. Some 1.5 million fractures occur per year: 500,000 vertebral fractures, 300,000 hip fractures, and 200,000 wrist fractures. It is estimated that 17.5% of white women who are 50 years of age will have a hip fracture during their remaining lifetime (14). Declining estrogen levels are the major risk factor for postmenopausal osteoporosis, which mainly affects trabecular bone.

The Osteoporotic Fractures Study Group (15) studied 9516 women 65 years of age or older to identify risk factors for hip fracture (Box 16-3). A history of hip fracture in the mother, especially before the age of 80, doubled the risk of hip fracture for the woman, even after adjustment for bone density. The incidence of hip fracture varied greatly from 1.1 per 100 woman-years among women with no more than two risk factors and normal calcaneal bone density for their age, to 27 per 1000 woman-years for women with five or more risk factors and bone density in the lowest third for their age. Gaining weight after the age of 25 reduced the risk of fracture. Current smokers had almost twice the risk of hip fracture as nonsmokers, but the association was not significant after adjusting for factors such as weight, health, and exercise.

This same study group (16) found that current estrogen use was associated with a decrease in the risk for wrist fractures (RR, 0.39; CI, 0.24-0.64) and for all nonspinal fractures (RR, 0.66; CI, 0.54-0.80) when compared with nonuse. These results were similar for women using unopposed estrogen or combination estrogen/progestin, for women older or younger than 75 years of age, and for smokers or nonsmokers.

Duration of use appears to play a role in fracture reduction (Table 16-1) (16). Hormone use of 10 years or greater reduced the risk of wrist fractures by 75%; short-term use resulted in only a 25% reduction. This study also found the time of initiation of HRT to be important. Women who began HRT early

---

Box 16-3   Risk Factors for Hip Fracture: Findings from the Osteoporotic Fractures Study Group

- Maternal history of hip fracture
- Previous fracture after the age of 50
- Tall height at the age of 25
- Self-rating of health as fair or poor
- Previous hyperthyroidism
- Treatment with long-acting benzodiazepines
- Treatment with anticonvulsants
- High caffeine intake
- Less than 4 h/day on feet
- Little or no weight gain after the age of 25

Data from Cauley JA, Seeley DG, Ensrud K, et al. The Osteoporotic Fractures Study Group. Estrogen replacement therapy and fractures in older women. Ann Intern Med. 1995; 122: 9-16.

In reducing the risk of osteoporosis, the time of initiation of HRT plays an important role. Women who begin HRT early in menopause have been found to have a significantly reduced risk of wrist and nonspinal fractures.

in menopause had a significantly reduced risk for wrist and all nonspinal fractures. The relative risk for all nonspinal fractures among current long-term users who initiated estrogen within 5 years of menopause was 0.53 (CI, 0.37 to 0.74), but the risk was 0.97 (CI, 0.56 to 1.68) in current long-term users who began estrogen more than 5 years after menopause.

A recent case-control study of more than 4500 Swedish women conflicts with this finding, however, because differences in hip fracture protection were not related to timing of initiation of therapy but only to duration of use (17). This study also showed that this protection afforded by HRT was lost soon after it was stopped, such that 5 years following cessation of HRT the risk reduction had fallen to 25%. Although some studies have shown that low-dose esterified estrogen (0.3 mg) increases bone mineral density (18), in this Swedish study low-dose estrogen was found to be ineffective in preventing hip fractures.

Although there are now other treatment options available for osteoporosis (e.g., alendronate, risedronate, intranasal calcitonin), estrogen remains the treatment of choice for both prevention and treatment of osteoporosis because of its superior efficacy as well as its cost-effectiveness. A daily dosage of 0.625 mg of conjugated estrogens helps preserve bone mass and prevent fractures. Transdermal estrogen also appears to work well, with one study demonstrating a 5.3% increase in lumbar spine bone mineral density and a 50% reduction in vertebral fracture rate (19).

Raloxifene, a selective estrogen receptor modulator (SERM) similar to tamoxifen that was released in 1998, is another alternative to HRT. Approved by the FDA for the prevention of osteoporosis, raloxifene has an estrogen agonist

Table 16-1   Effect of Estrogen on Fractures: Findings from the Osteoporotic Fractures Study Group

	Relative Risks for Current Users (95% CI)	
	Use <10 years	Use >10 years
Hip fractures (*n* = 134)	0.81 (0.40–1.65)	0.27 (0.08–0.85)
Wrist fractures (*n* = 200)	0.75 (0.42–1.36)	0.25 (0.10–0.61)
All nonspinal (*n* = 824)	0.67 (0.49–0.92)	0.60 (0.45–0.83)

Modified from the Osteoporotic Fractures Study Group. Estrogen replacement therapy and fractures in older women. Ann Intern Med. 1995;122:9-16.

effect on bone but an antagonist effect on both breast and uterine tissue. Consequently, concurrent progesterone is not required to protect the endometrium.

In a double-blind two-year trial in 601 postmenopausal women, Delmas et al (20) reported that a daily dose of 60 mg of raloxifene increased bone mineral density about 2% more than placebo in the lumbar spine, hip, and total body ($P < 0.0001$ for all comparisons). Endometrial thickness was similar in the raloxifene and placebo groups throughout the study, and both total cholesterol and low-density lipoprotein cholesterol serum levels were decreased significantly in the raloxifene group.

The Multiple Outcomes of Raloxifene Evaluation (MORE) study (21) involved 7705 women in 25 countries who had been postmenopausal at least 2 years and who met World Health Organization criteria for having osteoporosis. The women were randomized to either 60 mg/d or 120 mg/d of raloxifene or to placebo and followed for 3 years. Raloxifene increased bone mineral density in the femoral neck and spine and reduced vertebral but not hip fractures in both dosage groups (RR 0.7 for 60 mg group and RR 0.5 for 120 mg group). The failure to prevent hip fracture is of concern, because mortality benefit from treating osteoporosis is correlated with this endpoint.

Raloxifene effects on serum lipids and coagulation factors were compared with placebo and HRT in 390 healthy postmenopausal women in a double-blind, randomized trial (22). Dosages of 60 mg/d and 120 mg/d of raloxifene significantly lowered LDL-cholesterol by 12% (similar to the 14% reduction with HRT), but did not significantly change HDL-cholesterol, triglycerides, or plasminogen activator inhibitor-1. Further trials are necessary to see if these biochemical effects offer protection against cardiac disease.

Long-term studies of raloxifene, such as the Raloxifene Use for the Heart (RUTH) trial, are still in progress, but available data suggest the drug is inferior to HRT for treating osteoporosis and lipid abnormalities. However, raloxifene appears to decrease rather than increase the risk of breast and endometrial cancer and thus may be the preferred medication for osteoporosis in women at high risk for breast cancer.

DISCUSSION OF CASE 16-3

Karen L is at high risk for osteoporosis and fracture for several reasons: a long smoking history, thin body habitus, Caucasian race, and, most importantly, having a mother with severe disease. Because her mother had a hip fracture at a relatively young age, Karen's own risk of hip fracture is doubled regard-

less of her own bone density. Data from the Osteoporotic Fractures Study Group suggest that initiation of HRT should begin within 5 years of menopause to have optimal effect, so Karen needs to make a decision fairly soon. Baseline bone densitometry may help persuade her of the importance of early intervention. She should be advised that long-term therapy is necessary for reducing fracture risk, because bone loss will ensue once HRT is stopped. Because she travels so much in her work, she might find the transdermal estrogen to be more convenient, but she needs to be informed that, aside from the decreased risk of hypertriglyceridemia, she will lose some of the beneficial effect on lipids with this route. A second and better reason for transdermal rather than oral estrogen is the decreased risk of gallstone formation, which was present in other family members.

Cognitive Functioning

Studies in experimental animal models show a role for estrogen in the regeneration and preservation of neuronal elements within the central nervous system. Degeneration resulting from estrogen deficiency is postulated to be one of the factors leading to Alzheimer's disease (AD). Estrogen also affects several neurotransmitter systems such as the cholinergic system, which is linked to learning and memory. Estrogen has also been shown to improve cerebral blood flow and to increase cerebral glucose utilization. In addition, recent *in vitro* studies demonstrated that estradiol can influence the production of amyloid proteins by brain cells (23).

By the third decade after menopause, 50% of women manifest the histopathologic changes of AD, but half of these women do not have clinical evidence of disease (24). Still, a staggering 30% to 50% of women over the age of 85 suffer from dementia, resulting in a tremendous toll on families, caregivers, and society.

A recent meta-analysis (1) of the ten observational studies of the effect of postmenopausal estrogen on dementia suggests a 29% decreased risk of dementia among estrogen users. Thirteen studies on cognitive function in nondemented postmenopausal women show no clear benefit of estrogen in those who are asymptomatic, although cognitive improvement was at times linked to estrogen use due to general improvement in depression and other menopausal symptoms.

Table 16-2   Risk for Alzheimer's Disease by Route of Estrogen Administration

Route	No. of Cases	Odds Ratio (95% CI)
Oral only	60	0.70 (0.50–0.98)
Oral + injection and/or vaginal cream	21	0.59 (0.35–0.98)
Injection and/or vaginal cream only	11	0.48 (0.24–0.94)

Modified from Paganini-Hill A, Henderson VW. Estrogen replacement therapy and risk of Alzheimer disease. Arch Intern Med. 1996;156:2213-7.

A case control study (25) of a cohort of 8877 women residents of the Leisure World retirement community in Southern California, one of the largest studies to date, revealed that HRT may be useful for preventing or delaying onset of AD. The risk of AD and other dementia was significantly reduced in estrogen users (odds ratio [OR], 0.65; CI, 0.49 to 0.88) compared with nonusers. This reduced risk was present for both oral and other routes of administration, although it was most reduced in the nonoral group (Table 16-2). Another interesting finding from this study was that risk decreased significantly with both higher dosages (1.25 mg oral conjugated estrogen) and increasing duration of therapy of 15 years or more (test for trend, $p = 0.01$ for both variables). Caution must be used in interpreting these findings, however, because the sample size was not large.

Small numbers of women with existing AD have also been treated with estrogen in clinical trials (26), and cognitive improvement has been demonstrated in memory, orientation, and calculation. Women with mild or moderate dementia show greater improvement than those severely affected. These beneficial effects are lost, however, after treatment is discontinued. Of interest, the addition of progestin may have a detrimental effect.

However, a recent randomized controlled trial (27) that included 32 sites in the United States studied 120 women with mild-to-moderate AD (Mini-Mental Status Exam score, 12 to 28) failed to demonstrate any beneficial effect of estrogen. These women, whose average age was 75, were given 0.625 mg/day, 1.25 mg/d, or placebo for one year. No differences in global, cognitive, or activities of daily living were found between the groups, with some suggestion of worsening in the Clinical Dementia Rating Scale for estrogen takers ($P = 0.01$).

The Women's Health Initiative, a large prospective randomized placebo-controlled trial, should help clarify the effect of HRT on cognitive function and the risk of developing dementia.

Risks of Hormone Replacement Therapy

Endometrial Cancer

CASE 16-4

Michelle B is a 50-year-old woman who has significant symptoms and signs of urogenital atrophy but has been reluctant to take HRT because of a sister and aunt with endometrial cancer. She has no risk factors for coronary artery disease and is in otherwise excellent health that she maintains through exercise and a prudent diet.

The risk of endometrial cancer is clearly elevated in women who take estrogen without adequate doses of progestin (28). The risk is related to both dosage and duration of use. For women taking 0.625 mg of unopposed conjugated estrogen daily for at least 5 years, the relative risk of endometrial cancer is increased four- to five-fold (29,30). To put this in perspective, however, this rare cancer has a baseline incidence of only 1 per 1000 women. Moreover, the risk of dying from endometrial cancer is even lower than the risk of developing endometrial cancer, because women taking estrogen tend to have earlier stage disease and better prognosis. Nonetheless, invasive, potentially fatal endometrial tumors can arise. Taking unopposed estrogen on a cyclic schedule does *not* decrease these risks.

Progestins taken with estrogen therapy are effective in preventing the development of endometrial hyperplasia (31) and lowering the increased risk of development of endometrial carcinoma (32). Progestins are effective whether prescribed in a cyclic fashion for 10 to 14 days per month or in a continuous fashion. The addition of the progestin may cause unwanted bleeding, emotional lability, and other symptoms. Therefore, some have proposed using progestin administered in a cyclic fashion every 3 months (termed *long-cycle*) instead of every month. Though two studies have found no increase in endometrial hyperplasia or carcinoma in women on long-cycle regimens (33,34), a recent study sounds a note of caution.

The Scandinavian Long-Cycle Study was an open, randomized, multicenter trial of 240 women taking estrogen comparing cyclic progestin taken every 3 months to that taken every month (35). This study was recently terminated prematurely when it was found that the long-cycle patients had a 6%

incidence of endometrial hyperplasia or carcinoma compared with a 0.8% incidence for the control patients receiving progestin monthly. A promising alternative is the postmenopausal use of a progestin-releasing IUD (Mirena), which provides local endometrial protection while avoiding the adverse systemic effect of progestin.

Monitoring for endometrial hyperplasia and cancer are important in women on HRT. Criteria are listed in Box 16-4 for the various regimens of HRT. Withdrawal bleeding occurs in 30% to 80% of women taking estrogen plus a monthly cyclic progestin (28). The usual time for withdrawal bleeding to begin is from the fourth day of progestin until the fourth day after the progestin cycle for that month has been concluded. Bleeding that begins outside of the usual time range is a possible marker of endometrial pathology and should prompt endometrial evaluation. Many women taking estrogen plus progestin in a continuous fashion bleed irregularly for the first 6 to 12 months of therapy, but beyond that time the endometrium becomes atrophic and bleeding should cease.

Women on continuous regimens require endometrial evaluation if bleeding persists for more than 10 days at a time, is particularly heavy, or persists for more than 12 months. Women who have a uterus yet still opt to take unopposed estrogen probably should have endometrial evaluation before initiation of therapy, and at least annually. Endometrial evaluation should also be done if such women experience bleeding.

Box 16-4   Criteria for Endometrial Evaluation for Women on Hormone Replacement Therapy

Unopposed estrogen
Before initiation of therapy
Annual evaluation
Any bleeding (if evaluation not done recently)

Cyclic estrogen/progestin
Early bleeding before 4th day of progestin or >4 days after progestin ends

Continuous estrogen/progestin
Heavy bleeding
Bleeding more than once a month
Bleeding >10 days at a time
Persistent bleeding after 12 months of therapy

Currently available methods of endometrial evaluation include transvaginal ultrasonography, office-based endometrial biopsy, and surgical dilatation and curettage. Office-based endometrial biopsy is generally well tolerated without sedation or anesthesia, and is quite accurate (36). Transvaginal ultrasonography also appears to be quite accurate when a cutoff of 4 mm endometrial thickness is used (37,38), but most authorities still recommend the use of a direct sampling technique. Dilatation and curettage may also be used for surveillance when office-based endometrial biopsy is not technically possible.

DISCUSSION OF CASE 16-4

Because of her significant urogenital symptomatology, we would encourage a trial of HRT for Michelle B with the assurance that she would undergo regular, careful surveillance because of her very positive family history for uterine cancer. We would definitely recommend combination estrogen-progestin for endometrial protection. A baseline sampling would be considered for her personal reassurance, and the endometrium would be evaluated if any unexpected vaginal bleeding occurred (see Box 16-4). If her symptoms fail to respond adequately to systemic therapy, topical vaginal estrogen cream may be added. Although raloxifene would help lower her risk of endometrial cancer, this SERM is indicated only for the prevention and treatment of osteoporosis and would not be expected to treat urogenital atrophy.

Breast Cancer

CASE 16-5

Susan T is a 52-year-old woman who has been experiencing hot flashes for several years, even before the cessation of her menses a year ago. They have progressed to the point where they are now interfering with her daily functioning. She has also been suffering mood swings (most notably depression) and finally presents for evaluation. Because a sister died of breast cancer that was diagnosed at a late stage, she is very fearful of taking estrogen.

Breast cancer is the most common cancer among women in the United States, with over 180,000 new cases each year. There is understandably a great deal of concern about this disease on the part of women contemplating HRT. Over 40 studies, including several meta-analyses (3,39-43), have addressed the question of whether HRT use increases the risk of breast cancer. Most of these meta-analyses have found no association of breast cancer with short-term (less than 5 years) use of estrogen, but a 25% to 30% increase in the risk of breast cancer associated with longer use. While one study found the risk of HRT was most strongly associated with tumors of favorable histology (44), this information awaits confirmation.

A well-designed study reanalyzed 90% of the worldwide epidemiologic evidence of breast cancer and HRT (3). For the 53,865 postmenopausal women in this study, the relative risk of developing breast cancer increased significantly by 1.023 for each year of HRT use (Table 16-3). This risk was similar in magnitude to the risk conveyed by undergoing menopause one year later. Women who had used HRT for at least 5 years (mean use, 11 years) had a 35% increase in risk of breast cancer. The relative risk returned to baseline within 5 years after stopping HRT use (see Table 16-3). Although there has been concern that HRT use could reduce mammographic sensitivity (45), this study found that the excess of breast cancers were of local stage rather than more advanced stage.

How can we explain these risks to patients? When a hypothetical cohort of 1000 women who do not use HRT ages from 50 to 70 years, 45 women would be expected to develop breast cancer (3). If these 1000 women all used HRT

Table 16-3   Relative Risk of Breast Cancer Associated with Hormone Replacement Therapy: Meta-Analysis of 53,865 Postmenopausal Women

Risk Factor	RR (95% CI)
One year of HRT use	1.023 (1.011–1.036)
Menopause one year later	1.028 (1.021–1.034)
Five or more years of HRT (mean use of 11 years)	1.35 (1.21–1.49)
Time Since Last Use	**RR**
Current use	1.21
Cessation 1–4 years ago	1.10
Cessation 5–9 years ago	1.01

Adapted from Sillero-Arenas M, Delgade-Rodriquez M, Rodiques-Canteras R, et al. Menopausal hormone replacement therapy and breast cancer: a meta-analysis. Obstet Gynecol. 1992;79:286-94.

for 5, 10, or 15 years, the excess breast cancers expected would be 2, 6, and 12 cases respectively.

Two cohort studies have suggested that the breast cancer risk of estrogen combined with cyclic progestin is greater than the risk of unopposed estrogen (4,46). Further data regarding this possibility would be helpful, as would data comparing the risk of estrogen combined with continuous versus cyclic progestin.

The Nurses' Health Study analyzed competing mortality risks (47,48). Current HRT users were found to have a lower overall risk of mortality than never-users (RR, 0.63; 95% CI, 0.56-0.70). However, after HRT use of 10 or more years, the improvement in mortality was lessened (RR, 0.80; 95% CI, 0.67-0.96), due mainly to an increase in breast cancer mortality. In general, the survival benefit from HRT use is greater among women with more CAD risk factors and lesser for women at low risk for CAD (48).

One group recently developed a decision model to help compare the mortality benefits of HRT, alendronate, raloxifene, and conservative care for hypothetical women with varying risk factors for CAD, breast cancer, and hip fracture (48a). For women at high risk for developing CAD, HRT was preferred. (It should be noted that this model assumed that the beneficial effect of HRT in preventing cardiac events will be supported by the prospective trials that are in progress.) For women at high risk for breast cancer but not CAD, raloxifene would be the optimal treatment. For those women at low risk for CAD, breast cancer, and hip fracture, the calculations in this model supported conservative care.

While women with a family history of breast cancer have a greater risk of developing breast cancer than those with no such family history, the relative risk associated with HRT use appears to be no higher among women with a family history compared with women without (3,43,49). In the Nurses' Health Study an overall mortality benefit among women who took HRT was seen even for women whose mother or sister had breast cancer (48). In another prospective cohort study limited to women with a family history of breast cancer (50), the overall mortality was also lower among women who had ever used HRT (RR, 0.67; 95% CI, 0.51-0.89). Overall the available evidence suggests that the magnitude of risk conveyed by HRT use in women with a family history of breast cancer is similar to that of women without such a family history. However, the baseline risk of women with a family history is higher, and groups such as the ACP-ASIM have in the past recommended against prescribing HRT to such patients (see also Chapter 18).

What about the woman with a personal history of breast cancer? Due to concern about the hormone responsiveness of some breast cancers, both doctors and breast cancer survivors have been reluctant to use estrogen, even many years beyond the treatment of a breast cancer. However, because there are few data to support or refute this position, this practice has recently been questioned (51). The National Cancer Institute is currently conducting trials of estrogen use in breast cancer survivors; data should be forthcoming in a few years. In the meantime, standard practice would generally be to avoid HRT in such women outside the realm of clinical trials (52). See Box 16-5 for other contraindications to HRT.

DISCUSSION OF CASE 16-5

Because of the family history of breast cancer, Susan T should be religious about yearly mammograms and continuing her monthly breast self-exams. She has already had a screening mammogram, which should always be obtained before initiation of HRT (preferably within 6 months). This is true for all women, regardless of age. The increased risk of breast cancer is associated with HRT use of 5 years or longer duration; therefore it is not an important consideration when HRT is prescribed for short-term treatment of vasomotor symptoms.

Although the available data do not support a greater risk of estrogen use among women with a family history of breast cancer, her level of concern may preclude this option. Raloxifene, while possibly decreasing her risk of developing breast cancer, would not help Susan's hot flashes and in fact would be expected to worsen them. If she is reluctant to use HRT, the use of either progestin alone (i.e., without estrogen) or other medications such as clonidine (see Chapter 15) could be considered for treating her vasomotor symptoms. Further evaluation and treatment of her depression is also a good idea.

Box 16-5   Contraindications to Estrogen Replacement Therapy

- Known or suspected breast cancer
- Known or suspected endometrial cancer
- Active thromboembolic disease
- Past history of thromboembolic disease associated with estrogen use
- Hypertriglyceridemia (>600 mg/dL) or pancreatitis associated with estrogen use

Hormone Replacement Therapy Regimens

Unopposed Estrogen

Jane S is a 49-year-old health-conscious teacher who has been experiencing severe hot flashes but who initially did not want hormone replacement because she does not believe in taking medicines. Eventually, after obtaining no relief with her "natural" estrogens from the health food store, she agrees to continuous combination therapy. However, after a few months of combined HRT she becomes frustrated with the unpredictable bleeding, bloating, and weight gain, and requests to take estrogen alone.

For the woman without a uterus, estrogen alone is clearly the regimen of choice. Estrogen is available in a variety of preparations (Table 16-4), along with recommended dosages and cost. Although progestin may have some synergistic effect on preservation of bone density, its contribution appears to be low—less than 5% of the total benefit. Moreover, progesterone has been implicated in many of the untoward side effects of HRT, and a recent study suggests that it contributes additional risk of breast cancer over estrogen replacement therapy alone (43).

Monitoring for endometrial hyperplasia and cancer in women receiving HRT is important, particularly in women who elect to take unopposed estrogen.

There may be a few women with an intact uterus who elect to take unopposed estrogen, typically because they do not want to deal with cyclic or unpredictable bleeding. If they do so, they must be fully informed of the markedly increased risk of endometrial hyperplasia and cancer, and the need for regular surveillance (53). Unopposed estrogen can still be considered a viable option, however, because benefits of estrogen probably outweigh the risk of endometrial cancer (53).

Jane S is a woman who is well-read and keeps informed on women's health issues but steers away from traditional medicine.

Table 16-4   Hormone Replacement Drugs

Drug	Available Strengths
Oral estrogen	
Conjugated estrogen	
Premarin	0.3, 0.625, 0.9, 1.25, 2.5 mg
Esterified estrogen	
Estratab	0.3, 0.625, 1.25, 2.5 mg
Menest	0.3, 0.625, 1.25, 2.5 mg
Estropipate	
Ogen	0.625, 1.25 mg
Ortho-Est	0.625, 1.25 mg
Estropipate tablets	0.75, 1.5, 3.0 mg
Estradiol	
Estrace	0.5, 1.0, 2.0 mg
Estradiol tablets	0.5, 1.0, 2.0 mg
Gynodiol	0.5, 1.0, 1.5 mg
Oral estrogen combinations	
Conjugated estrogen + progestin	
Premphase	0.625 mg Premarin × 14 days + 0.625 mg Premarin + 5.0 mg medroxy-progesterone-acetate (MPA) × 14 days
Prempro	0.625 mg Premarin + 2.5 mg MPA
	0.625 mg Premarin + 5.0 mg MPA
Estradiol + norgestimate	
Ortho-Prefest	1.0 mg estradiol for 3 days followed by estradiol + 0.09 mg norgestimate for 3 days, repeated continuously
Estradiol + norethindrone	
Activella	1 mg estradiol + 0.5 mg norethindrone
Ethinyl estradiol + norethindrone acetate	
Femhrt	5 mg ethinyl estradiol + 1 mg NETA
Esterified estrogen + androgen	
Estratest	1.25 mg Estratab + 2.5 mg methyltestosterone
Estratest H.S.	0.625 mg Estratab + 1.25 mg methyltestosterone
Transdermal estrogen	
Estradiol	
Alora	0.05, 0.075, 0.1 mg/day
Climara	0.025, 0.05, 0.1 mg/day
Vivelle	0.375, 0.05, 0.075, 0.1 mg/day
Fem Patch	0.025 mg/day
Estraderm	0.05, 0.1 mg/day
Transdermal estrogen combinations	
Estradiol + norethindrone aceatate (NETA)	
CombiPatch	0.05 mg/day estradiol + 0.14 mg/day NETA, 0.05 mg/day estradiol + 0.25 mg/day NETA
Vaginal estrogen	
Conjugated estrogen	
Premarin	0.625 mg estrogen/g cream
Estradiol	
Estrace	0.1 mg estradiol/g cream
Estring Vaginal Ring	2.0 mg/90 days (7.5 μg/day)
Oral progestin	
Medroxyprogesterone acetate	
Provera	2.5, 5.0, 10 mg
Amen	10 mg
Cycrin	2.5, 5.0 10 mg
Norethindrone	
Micronor	0.35 mg
Nor-QD	0.35 mg
Norethindrone acetate	
Aygestin	5.0 mg
Micronized progesterone	
Prometrium	100 mg

Because of her "intolerance" for combined therapy and her personal comfort with risk-taking, she is willing to take unopposed estrogen and agrees to comply with baseline and yearly endometrial sampling. Another alternative is for her to try long-cycle combination estrogen-progestin but, given the recent data, consideration should still be given to periodic endometrial sampling.

Combination Estrogen/Progestin: Short-Cycle Administration

In earlier regimens estrogen was given for about 25 days of the month with one week off because it was felt that the break from estrogen stimulation would reduce endometrial hyperplasia and cancer. This has proven not to be true, so now estrogen is administered daily and a progestin is added for 10 to 14 days of the month. When 5 to 15 mg of medroxyprogesterone (MPA) is taken for the first 2 weeks of the month, the vaginal bleeding occurs in the middle of the month (usually days 14 to 20). Many women find this to be more convenient, because holidays often occur near the end of the month. From the 15th to the end of the month they take estrogen alone. A combination pill, Premphase, is available in a dial pack similar to birth control pills. Fourteen pills of conjugated estrogen 0.625 mg are followed by 14 pills containing both estrogen 0.625 mg combined and MPA 5.0 mg. The packaging is very convenient and the directions easy to follow (see Table 16-4).

Short-cycle administration has the major disadvantage of a monthly period, but this may be more protective of the endometrium because of the monthly shedding (see next section). Also, some women who do not tolerate progestins well find the cyclic regimen to have fewer side effects than daily progestin.

Combination Estrogen/Progestin: Long-Cycle Administration

In recent years long-cycle administration was developed as a middle ground to avoid the problems of monthly bleeding with the short-cycle pattern and also the breakthrough bleeding with continuous administration of estrogen and progestin. Medroxyprogesterone at a dose of 10 mg/day is given for 14 days on a quarterly basis. With this every 3-month period, women experience longer menses of about 8 days' duration, heavier bleeding, and increased unscheduled bleeding as compared with monthly MPA (32). Despite this, women still preferred the quarterly regimen by almost four to one. As mentioned above, there are discrepant results in the literature regarding the adequacy of endometrial protection with long-cycle regimens (32-34). Until more data are available, consideration should be given to annual endometrial sampling for patients on long-cycle regimens.

Combination Estrogen/Progestin: Continuous Administration

In the continuous HRT regimen, 2.5 or 5.0 mg of daily medroxyprogesterone is taken along with daily estrogen. The continuous regimen has the advantage of eliminating monthly bleeding, although it may take 8 to 12 months (or even longer) of unpredictable spotting before most women achieve amenorrhea. Because many women find unpredictable spotting unacceptable, it may be wise to start with cyclic administration for a year or so and then switch to the continuous regimen. With this strategy the woman undergoes regular withdrawal bleeds on the cycled regimen, then experiences a presumably brief period of unpredictable spotting before becoming amenorrheic on the continuous regimen. This sequenced approach also allows the woman to compare both regimens. A single pill is available that combines estrogen 0.625 mg with MPA in a dosage of 2.5 or 5 mg (Prempro 0.625/2.5 mg or 0.625/5 mg), packaged in a dial pack.

Combination Estrogen/Progestin: Pulsed Administration

Because of breakthrough bleeding and other side effects associated with continuous estrogen and progestin use, a pulsed regimen was recently developed. This new preparation (Ortho-Prefest) is packaged in a dose pack similar to oral contraceptives and contains repeating cycles of 3 days of micronized 17-beta estradiol 1 mg alone alternating with 3 days of estradiol plus norgestimate 0.9 mg (a progestin). A 12-month, multi-center study (54) of 1253 postmenopausal women found the regimen to be well tolerated and detected no cases of endometrial hyperplasia with the commercially available dose.

Transdermal Hormones

Transdermal estrogen can substitute for oral estrogen with any of the regimens. Patches, which come in many dosage strengths, are worn on the abdomen or buttock and are changed once or twice weekly, depending on the formulation. Those that can be changed once per week may be ideal for enhancing compliance in the busy woman.

Skin irritation, which may occur in up to one-fourth of women, is the main side effect. The patches are more costly than oral estrogen, approximately double the price. Another disadvantage of transdermal estrogen is a decrease in the beneficial effects on lipid metabolism, presumably due to loss of first-pass liver metabolism that occurs with oral estrogen. Positive effects on HDL and LDL are evident, however, after 2 years of treatment at higher doses (55). On the other hand, because of the lack of liver involvement, transdermal estrogen is ideal for the woman who develops hypertriglyceridemia from oral estrogen (56). Other advantages and disadvantages of transdermal delivery of estrogen are listed in Box 16-6. It should be noted that transdermal estrogen is just as likely to cause endometrial cancer as the oral form, so the same considerations apply regarding use of a progestin and the importance of endometrial surveillance.

In January 1999 the first combination estrogen-plus-progestin transdermal system (CombiPatch) was introduced. Combining estradiol with norethindrone acetate, this system requires twice-weekly application but appears to effectively relieve vasomotor symptoms while providing endometrial protection.

Vaginal, Intranasal, and Injectable Forms of Estrogen

Urogenital atrophy is one of the most persistent signs of menopause and one that may even worsen with age. Vaginal application of estrogen avoids the first pass through the liver, does not provoke the vaginal bleeding associated with systemic therapy, and entails fewer risks than systemic therapy. However, the beneficial effects of systemic estrogen are absent and thus vaginal cream provides only local treatment. Cream forms of estrogen have been available for over 30 years, and though dosing is flexible it is commonly pre-

---

Box 16-6   Advantages and Disadvantages of Transdermal Estrogen Compared with Estrogen

Advantages
Minimal nausea
Lower dose
Decreased risk for gallstones/cholestasis
Continuous delivery
Ease of administration
Minimal hepatic protein induction
Does not raise triglyceride levels (preferable for diabetic patients?)

Disadvantages
Blunted increase in HDL and decrease in LDL
Skin irritation
Cost

scribed as $^1/_2$-1 applicatorful intravaginally at bedtime for 2 weeks followed by a reduction in frequency to approximately three times weekly.

In a large study of 196 postmenopausal women, Nachtigall (57) compared conjugated estrogen cream with the estradiol ring regarding efficacy for urogenital atrophy and frequency of endometrial overstimulation. The ring and cream treatments produced equivalent effects on the vaginal mucosa and improved vaginal pH toward levels seen in fertile women. With regard to endometrial stimulation, significantly more patients bled with a progestin challenge test after 3 months of treatment with cream than with the ring, which suggests that the ring has a more favorable safety profile.

It should be noted that there are no published cases of endometrial cancer attributed to unopposed vaginal estrogen use. One study looking for possible endometrial changes examined 337 biopsies from 12 pooled studies of 214 subjects but found atrophic endometrium in all specimens (58). The most recent population-based, case-control study in Sweden of 789 women with endometrial cancer and 3368 controls (59) also did not show an increased relative risk of endometrial cancer with unopposed vaginal estrogens. Nevertheless, patients and physicians must keep in mind that vaginal estrogen without progestin protection may possibly increase the risk for endometrial cancer, and, of course, any unexplained bleeding occurring with the use of Estring or conjugated estrogen vaginal cream necessitates endometrial biopsy.

In the early 1990s an estradiol vaginal ring that releases higher doses of estrogen over 3 months became available in Europe; this ring represents a new alternative delivery system. In a small study of 21 postmenopausal women (60), three different doses of the estradiol ring (100, 150, and 200 μg/24 hr) were found to markedly increase the maturation of vaginal cells, suppress FSH, and decrease total and LDL cholesterol significantly. Furthermore, all women reported relief of climacteric symptoms. Although twelve of the women noted some vaginal discomfort during the first three days of use, overall satisfaction was high. Ideally the intravaginal ring will eventually also be available in a second formulation that incorporates progestin as well as estradiol. Estring, a 2-mg vaginal ring containing estradiol, continuously releases estradiol (7.5 μg/24 hr for 90 days). Because only 8% of the total daily dose is systemically absorbed, this device treats local, urogenital symptoms only. For the same reason, concomitant progesterone to protect the endometrium is not required.

Recently, in England, an intranasal form of 17 beta-oestradiol was developed and studied in a double-blind fashion in 420 postmenopausal women (61). Patients were randomized to receive the nasal spray in 4 different dosages (100, 220, 300, or 400 μg) or placebo spray or 1 or 2 mg of oral estradiol. Serum estradiol concentrations were similar with using either the nasal spray or oral estradiol, and the nasal spray was significantly better than placebo at reducing menopausal symptoms such as hot flashes. Patients on the nasal spray experienced some prickling at the site, nosebleeding, and excessive sneezing, but 84% expressed willingness to continue this route at the end of the study.

Depot estrogen is available for injection about every 3 to 4 weeks. Subcutaneous pellets and intramuscular implants are also available but rarely used. Although women may experience relief from hot flashes or urogenital atrophy, no good data exist to support any of these routes for long-term benefits.

Estrogen/Testosterone Combinations

Increasing evidence suggests that androgens play a role in the normal physiology and well-being of women. Androstenedione and testosterone are the two major circulating androgens in women. Testosterone, in particular, may have beneficial effects on sexuality (62), bone (63), and even cognitive functioning (64). As with any androgenic therapy, side effects of hirsutism, male-pattern baldness, deepening of the voice, and acne are of concern. In one ongoing study, these effects were minimal with methyltestosterone dosages of 1.25 or 2.5 mg (65). A few combination estrogen/androgen preparations are commercially available (see Table 16-4). Adverse effects of androgens on lipids (lowering of HDL) and liver function tests should be monitored, and long-term cardiovascular risks remain to be determined.

Compliance Issues

Patient compliance with any therapy is a challenge, but this is especially true with preventive, long-term treatment where the benefits are not readily apparent. Most women understand that HRT will enhance quality of life in the long run, but quality of life in the short-term is a variable that also must be considered when discussing the various options of HRT with a patient.

Hammond (66) has estimated that up to 70% of patients fail to comply with the HRT regimen prescribed. Fear of breast cancer is the leading cause of noncompliance, followed by concerns about endometrial cancer and side effects, particularly vaginal bleeding.

General Side Effects

With estrogen replacement, women may develop breast tenderness and enlargement, nausea, migraine headaches, and edema. When progestins are added to the regimen, particularly in doses higher than MPA 5 mg, patients tend to experience more side effects, such as emotional lability, depression, lethargy, and headache. Progestins may either aggravate or relieve the breast tenderness. Natural micronized progesterone is probably better tolerated and is now commercially available in the United States as Prometrium 100 mg. Both estrogen and progestin may cause premenstrual-like symptoms of irritability and abdominal bloating.

Many of these side effects are somewhat time- and dose-related. For example, breast tenderness may resolve within a few months, so patients should be encouraged to stay with the regimen for a few cycles. Migraine headaches precipitated by HRT may improve with the use of combination androgen-estrogen therapy. Other persistent side effects may be alleviated with lower dosages, different regimens, or routes.

Vaginal Bleeding

The resumption of periodic uterine bleeding represents a major deterrent to compliance with HRT. In one study, 90% of women using combination therapy discontinued its use after 18 months (67). Unpredictable spotting is even more problematic for women than cyclic bleeding. While most women achieve amenorrhea after 6 to 12 months of continuous combination HRT, irregular bleeding in the first 12 months typically results in early discontinuation rates of 9% to 35% (68). Clisham et al (69) found a similarly high discontinuation rate in women using unopposed transdermal estrogen because of the unpredictability of the bleeding, despite a relatively low frequency of bleeding episodes.

No regimen or preparation for a woman with intact uterus has been found to be superior for compliance (58). Also, none of the common regimens has been able to eliminate breakthrough bleeding, which remains a common side effect, occurring in about 15% of cycles of women on unopposed estrogen, 8% of cycles of women on combined sequential therapy, and 13% to 22% of cycles of women on continuous combined therapy (70).

Is There a Role for Short-Term Hormone Replacement Therapy?

The only role for short-term therapy is in relief of vasomotor symptoms surrounding the menopause. Certainly short-term therapy is more appropriate for women at high risk for breast cancer. All of the benefits for osteoporosis and potential benefits for cardiovascular disease and Alzheimer's dementia are associated with long-term therapy greater than 10 to 15 years and probably life-long. These effects are lost after HRT is discontinued, usually not immediately but over time.

Summary

Hormone replacement therapy has many benefits for postmenopausal women: short-term relief from hot flashes and urogenital atrophy and long-term reduction of morbidity and mortality from osteoporosis, and, possibly, from ischemic heart disease. A decrease in risk for Alzheimer's disease may possibly be another potential benefit.

As with any therapy, HRT is not without side effects and risks. Progestin eliminates the risk of estrogen-induced endometrial cancer but may further increase the modestly increased risk of breast cancer noted with estrogen therapy alone. Each individual's relative risks for breast cancer, osteoporosis, and cardiovascular disease should be assessed, and the appropriateness of intervention with either HRT or other agents such as raloxifene or nonhormonal medications should be determined. Life-style modification should also be encouraged for women at risk for heart disease, regardless of whether or not they choose to take HRT.

Women should be informed of the benefits and risks of HRT. In light of the new information regarding increased risk of cardiovascular and thromboembolic events shortly after initiation of HRT, this discussion may require significant time and more than one office visit. Careful communication of the anticipated effects for her as an individual is also often a useful and practical approach in helping the patient weigh the relative importance of the various actions of HRT.

For those that choose to take HRT, a regimen should be individually tailored to suit the patient's risk profiles and preferences. Unopposed estrogen is clearly the choice for women without a uterus. For women with a uterus a progestin is prescribed in either a continuous fashion or cycled regimen. Unfortunately, unwanted bleeding commonly occurs in these women and leads to early discontinuation of HRT. Taking advantage of the different estrogen preparations and the variety of estrogen-progestin regimens that are now available may help decrease this bleeding and other side effects, enhance compliance, and allow the patient to continue long-term treatment. Overall, the majority of women will find that their years from menopause and beyond will be improved with HRT.

ACKNOWLEDGEMENTS
The authors wish to thank Marilyn Schapira, MD, for her helpful comments and critique of this chapter.

REFERENCES

1. **Yaffe K, Sawaya G, Lieberburg I, Grady D.** Estrogen therapy in postmenopausal women: effects on cognitive function and dementia. JAMA.1998;279:688-95.

2. **Calle EE, Miracle-Mcmahill HL, Thun MJ, et al.** Estrogen replacement therapy and risk of fatal colon cancer in a prospective cohort of postmenopausal women. J Natl Cancer Inst. 1995:87:517-22.

2a. **MacLennan SC, MacLennan AH, Ryan P.** Colorectal cancer and oestrogen replacement therapy: a meta-analysis of epidemiological studies. Med J Aust. 1995:162:491-3.

3. **Collaborative Group on Hormonal Factors in Breast Cancer.** Breast cancer and hormone replacement therapy: collaborative reanalysis of data from 51 epidemiological studies of 52,705 women with breast cancer and 108,411 women without breast cancer. Lancet. 1997;350:1047-59.

4. **Schairer C, Lubin J, Troisi R, et al.** Menopausal estrogen and estrogen-progestin replacement therapy and breast cancer risk. JAMA. 2000;283:485-91.

5. Heart and Stroke Facts: 1999 Statistical Supplement. American Heart Association; 1996:1-29.

6. **Grodstein F, Stampfer M.** The epidemiology of coronary heart disease and estrogen replacement in postmenopausal women. Prog Cardiovasc Dis. 1995;38:199-210.

7. **Grodstein F, Stampfer MJ, Manson JE, et al.** Postmenopausal estrogen and progestin use and the risk of cardiovascular disease. N Engl J Med. 1996:335:453-61.

8. **Sidney S, Petitti DB, Quesenberry P.** Myocardial infarction and the use of estrogen and estrogen-progestogen in postmenopausal women. Ann Intern Med. 1997;127: 501-8.

9. **Hulley S, Grady D, Bush T, et al.** Randomized trial of estrogen plus progestin for secondary prevention of coronary heart disease in postmenopausal women. JAMA. 1998;280:605-13.

10. **Rossouw J, Finnegan L, Harlan WR, et al.** The evolution of the Women's Health Initiative: perspectives from the NIH. JAMA. 1995;50:50-6.

11. **Herrington DM, Reboussin DM, Brosnihan KB, et al.** Effects of estrogen replacement on the progression of coronary-artery atherosclerosis. N Engl J Med. 2000;343:522-9.

12. **Col NF, Eckman MH, Karas RH, et al.** Patient-specific decisions about hormone replacement therapy in postmenopausal women. JAMA. 1997;277:1140-7.

13. **Writing Group for the PEPI Trial.** Effects of estrogen or estrogen/progestin regimens on heart disease risk factors in postmenopausal women. JAMA. 1995:273:199-208.

14. **Melton LJ III, Chrischilles EA, Cooper C, et al.** How many women have osteoporosis? J Bone Miner Res. 1992;7:1005-10.

15. **Cummings SR, Nevitt MC, Browner WS, et al, for the Osteoporotic Fractures Study Group.** Risk factors for hip fracture in white women. N Engl J Med. 1995;332:767-73.

16. **Cauley JA, Seeley DG, Ensrud K, et al, for the Osteoporotic Fractures Study Group.** Estrogen replacement therapy and fractures in older women. Ann Intern Med. 1995; 122:9-16.

17. **Michaelsson K, Baron JA, Farahmand BY, et al.** Hormone replacement therapy and risk of hip fracture: population based case-control study. The Swedish Hip Fracture Study Group. BMJ. 1998;316:1858-63.

18. **Recker RR, Davies KM, Dowd RM, Heaney RP.** The effect of low-dose continous estrogen and progesterone therapy with calcium and vitamin D on bone in elderly women. Ann Intern Med. 1999;130:897-904.

19. **Lufkin EG, Wahner HW, O'Fallon WM, et al.** Treatment of postmenopausal osteoporosis with transdermal estrogen. Ann Intern Med. 1992;117:1-9.

20. **Delmas PD, Bjarnason NH, Mitlak BH, et al.** Effects of raloxifene on bone mineral density, serum cholesterol concentrations, and uterine endometrium in postmenopausal women. N Engl J Med. 1997:337:1641-7.

21. **Ettinger B, Black DM, Mitlak BH, et al.** Reduction of vertebral fracture risk in postmenopausal women with osteoporosis treated with raloxifene. JAMA.1999;282:637-45.

22. **Walsh BW, Kuller LH, Wild RA, et al.** Effects of raloxifene on serum lipids and coagulation factors in healthy postmenopausal women. JAMA. 1998:2790:1445-51.

23. **Xu H, Gouras GK, Greenfield JP, et al.** Estrogen reduces neuronal generation of Alzheimer beta-amyloid peptides. Nature Med. 1998;4;4:447-51.

24. **Morris JC, Storandt M, McKeel DW, et al.** Cerebral amyloid deposition and diffuse plaques in "normal" aging: evidence for presymptomatic and very mild Alzheimer's disease. Neurology. 1996;46:702-19.

25. **Paganini-Hill A, Henderson VW.** Estrogen replacement therapy and risk of Alzheimer disease. Arch Intern Med. 1996;156:2213-7.

26. **Paganini-Hill A.** Oestrogen replacement therapy and Alzheimer's disease. Br J Obstet Gynecol, 1996;103:80-6.

27. **Mulnard RA, Cotman CW, Kawas C, et al.** Estrogen replacement therapy for treatment of mild to moderate Alzheimer disease. JAMA. 2000;283:1007-15.

28. **Grady D, Rubin SM, Petitti DB, et al.** Hormone therapy to prevent disease and prolong life in postmenopausal women. Ann Intern Med. 1992;117:1016-37.

29. **Mach TM, Pike MC, Henderson BE, et al.** Estrogens and endometrial cancer in a retirement community. N Engl J Med. 1976;294:1262-7.

30. **Buring JE, Bain CJ, Ehrmann RL.** Conjugated estrogen use and risk of endometrial cancer. Am J Epidemiol. 1986;124:434-41.

31. **Whitehead MI, Fraser D.** The effect of estrogen and progestogens on the endometrium. Obstet Gynecol Clin North Am. 1987;14:299-320.

32. **Voigt LF, Weiss NS, Chu JR, et al.** Progestogen supplementation of exogenous oestrogens and risk of endometrial cancer. Lancet. 1991;338:274-7.

33. **Ettinger B, Selby J, Citron JT, et al.** Cyclic hormone replacement therapy using quarterly progestin. Obst Gynecol. 1994;83:693-700.

34. **Hirvonen E, Salmi T, Puolokk J, et al.** Can progestin be limited to every third month only in postmenopausal women taking estrogen? Maturitas. 1995;21:39-44.

35. **Cerin A, Heldaas K, Moeller B.** Adverse endometrial effects of long-cycle estrogen and progestogen replacement therapy [Letter]. N Engl J Med. 1996;334:668-9.

36. **Koss LG, Shreiber K, Oberlander SG, et al.** Detection of endometrial carcinoma and hyperplasia in asymptomatic women. Obstet Gynecol. 1984;64:1-11.

37. **Osmers R, Volksen M, Sohauer A.** Vaginosonography for early detection of endometrial carcinoma? Lancet. 1990;335:1569-71.

38. **Granberg S, Wikland M, Karlsson B, et al.** Endometrial thickness as measured by endovaginal ultrasonography for identifying endometrial abnormality. Am J Obstet Gynecol. 1991;164:47-52.

39. **Armstrong B.** Oestrogen therapy after the menopause: boon or bane? Med J Aust. 1988;148:213-4.

40. **Dupont W, Page D.** Menopausal estrogen replacement therapy and breast cancer. Arch Intern Med. 1991;151:67-72.

41. **Steinberg K, Thacker S, Smith S, et al.** A meta-analysis of the effect of estrogen replacement therapy on the risk of breast cancer. JAMA. 1991;265:1985-90.

42. **Sillero-Arenas M, Delgade-Rodriquez M, Rodiques-Canteras R, et al.** Menopausal hormone replacement therapy and breast cancer: a meta-analysis. Obstet Gynecol. 1992;79:286-94.

43. **Colditz GA, Egan KM, Stampfer MJ.** Hormone replacement therapy and risk of breast cancer: results from epidemiologic studies. Am J Obstet Gynecol. 1993;168:1473-80.

44. **Gapstur SM, Morrow M, Sellers TA.** Hormone replacement therapy and risk of breast cancer with a favorable histology. Results of the Iowa Women's Health Study. JAMA. 1999;281:2091-7.

45. **Persson I, Thurfjell E, Holmberg L.** Effect of estrogen-progestin replacement regimens on mammographic breast parenchymal density. J Clin Oncol. 1997;15:3201-7.

46. **Colditz GA, Rosner B, for the Nurses' Health Study Research Group.** Use of estrogen plus progestin is associated with greater increase in breast cancer risk than estrogen alone. Am J Epdemiol. 1998;47(Suppl):645.

47. **Colditz GA, Hankinson SE, Hunter DJ, et al.** The use of estrogens and progestins and the risk of breast cancer in postmenopausal women. N Engl J Med. 1995;332:1589-93.

48. **Grodstein F, Stampfer MJ, Colditz GA, et al.** Postmenopausal hormone therapy and mortality. N Engl J Med. 1997;336:1769-75.

48a. **Col NF, Pauker SG, Goldberg RJ, et al.** Individualizing therapy to prevent long-term consequences of estrogen deficiency in postmenopausal women. Arch Intern Med. 1999;159:1458-66.

49. **Stanford JL, Weiss NS, Voigt LF, et al.** Combined estrogen and progestin hormone replacement therapy in relation to risk of breast cancer in middle-aged women. JAMA. 1995;274:137-42.

50. **Sellers TA, Mink PJ, Cerhan JR, et al.** The role of hormone replacement therapy in the risk for breast cancer and total mortality in women with a family history of breast cancer. Ann Intern Med. 1997;127:973-80.

51. **Cobleigh MA, Berris RF, Bush T, et al.** Estrogen replacement therapy in breast cancer survivors. JAMA. 1994;272:540-5.

52. **Vassilopoulou-Sellin R.** Estrogen replacement therapy in women at increased risk for breast cancer. Breast Cancer Res Treat. 1995;28:167-77.

53. **Wood H, Wang-Cheng R, Nattinger AB.** Postmenopausal hormone replacement: are two hormones better than one? J Gen Intern Med. 1993;8:451-8.

54. **Corson SL, Richart RM, Caubel P, Lim P.** Effects of a unique constant-estrogen, pulsed-progestin hormone replacement therapy containing 17-beta-estradiol and norgestimate on endometrial histology. Int J Fertil. 1999;44:279-85.

55. **Ory SJ, Field CS, Herrmann RR, et al.** Effects of long-term transdermal administration of estradiol on serum lipids. Mayo Clin Proc. 1998;73:735-8.

56. **Nachtigall LE.** Emerging delivery systems for estrogen replacment: aspects of transdermal and oral delivery. Am J Obstet Gynecol. 1995;173:993-7.

57. **Nachtigall LE.** Clinical trial of the estradiol vaginal ring in the US. Maturitas. 1995;22(Suppl):S43-7.

58. **Vooijs GP, Geurts TBP.** Review of the endometrial safety during intravaginal treatment with estriol. Eur J Obstet Gynecol Reprod Biol. 1995;62:101-6.

59. **Weiderpass E, Baron JA, Adami HO, et al.** Low-potency oestrogen and risk of endometrial cancer: a case-control study. Lancet. 1999;353:1824-8.

60. **Nash HA, Brache V, Alvarez-Sanchez F, et al.** Estradiol delivery by vaginal rings: potential for hormone replacement therapy. Maturitas. 1997;226:27-33.

61. **Studd J, Pornel B, Marton, I, et al, for the Aerodiol Study Group.** Efficacy and acceptability of intranasal 17B-oestradiol for menopausal symptoms: randomized dose-response study. Lancet. 1999;353:1574-8.

62. **Burger H, Hailes J, Nelson J, et al.** Effect of combined implants of oestradiol and testosterone on libido in postmenopausal women . BMJ. 1987; 294:936-7.

63. **Colvard DS, Eriksen EF, Keeting PE, et al.** Identification of androgen receptors in normal human osteoblast-like cells. Proc Natl Acad Sci. 1989;86:854-7.

64. **Sherwin BB.** Oestrogen and/or androgen replacement therapy and cognitive functioning in surgically menopausal women. Psychoneuroendocrinology. 1988;13:345-57.

65. **Timmons MC, Barrett-Connor E, Young R, et al.** Interim safety analysis of a two-year study comparing oral estrogen-androgen and conjugated estrogens in surgically menopausal women. Poster at Annual Meeting of North American Menopause Society, San Francisco; Sept. 1995.

66. **Hammond CB.** Women's concerns with hormone replacement therapy: compliance issues. Fertil Steril. 1994;62:157-60S.

67. **Hahn RG.** Compliance considerations with estrogen replacement: withdrawal bleeding and other factors. Am J Obstet Gynecol. 1989;161:1854-8.

68. **Doren M, Schneider HP.** The impact of different HRT regimens on compliance. Int J Fertil Menopausal Stud. 1996;41:29-39.

69. **Clisham PR, Cedars MI, Greendale G, et al.** Long-term transdermal estradiol therapy: effects on endometrial histology and bleeding patterns. Obstet Gynecol. 1992;79:196-201.

70. **Archer DF, Pickar JH, Bottiglioni F, for the Menopause Study Group.** Bleeding patterns in postmenopausal women taking continuous combined or sequential regimens of conjugated estrogens with medroxyprogesterone acetate. Obstet Gynecol. 1994;83: 686-92.

CHAPTER 17

Diseases of the Vulva

MARIA L. CHANCO TURNER, MD

JANICE RYDEN, MD

U nless a patient has symptoms referable to the vulva, this area is often overlooked in the physical examination. Except for the labia majora, most of its structures are out of view during routine gynecologic examination because they fall behind the speculum. However, if one is to detect asymptomatic lesions early, every pelvic exam should include careful inspection of the vulva.

Vulvar symptoms commonly result from a discharge emanating from processes occurring higher in the reproductive tract, such as vaginitis and cervicitis, but primary vulvar processes can occur, such as vulvar dystrophies (e.g., lichen sclerosis), vestibular gland inflammation, and benign and malignant vulvar neoplasms. The vulva is also subject to involvement in diffuse skin processes such as psoriasis and vitiligo. Moreover, systemic illnesses such as Crohn's disease and Behcet's syndrome may have vulvar manifestations. Although vulvar candidiasis and certain sexually transmitted infections (e.g., syphilitic chancres, condyloma acuminata) may have skin findings localized to the vulva, the reader should note that such infections are discussed in Chapter 8. In addition to dermatologic abnormalities, vulvar disorders include vulvodynia and pudendal neuralgia.

Anatomy

The vulva is literally hidden between the thighs. It is bounded anteriorly by the mons pubis, laterally by the inguinal folds, and posteriorly by the perineal body. The vulva consists of the labia majora, labia minora, clitoris, hymen, and vulvar vestibule. The openings of the urethra, vagina, Skene's glands, Bartholin's glands, and minor vestibular glands are located within the vestibule (Fig. 17-1). Excessive and/or abnormal secretions from the cervix, vagina, and vestibular glands, as well as urinary and fecal incontinence, can lead to vulvar irritation (vulvitis). The warm and moist environment predisposes the area to intertrigo, yeast, and superficial fungal infections.

The mons, labia majora, and perineal body are covered by hair-bearing, keratinized skin that is richly supplied with sebaceous, eccrine, and apocrine sweat glands. At the vulva, cornified skin gradually changes into more delicate mucosa. In a normal adult premenopausal woman, the mons and labia

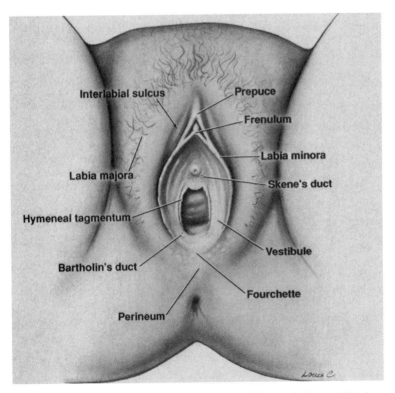

Figure 17-1 Normal topography of the vulva. (From Wilkinson E. Normal histology and nomenclature of the vulva and malignant neoplasms, including VIN. Dermatol Clin. 1992;10;284; with permission.)

majora are somewhat protruberant because of a thick subcutaneous fat pad. Conversely, in postmenopausal and other hypogonadal states, there is a marked decrease in the fat pad and in the number of pubic hairs. Postmenopausal atrophy of the introital epithelium also allows the vascular pattern to become more apparent, a finding also seen after prolonged use of topical steroids. Genital skin has more melanocytes per surface area, so genital skin is normally darker than surrounding skin, and this hyperpigmentation intensifies during pregnancy under the influence of increased levels of estrogen and progesterone.

The labia minora are a pair of thin leaflets of variable size and shape located between the labia majora. The labia minora are covered by lightly keratinized, non-hair-bearing, slightly papillated, squamous epithelium, which lose their keratinized layer at the level of Hart's line (Fig. 17-2). This marks the beginning of the vulvar vestibule, which continues proximally until the hymenal ring, at which level the internal genitalia begin.

The Bartholin's glands are a pair of pea-sized structures that are normally nonpalpable and are located at the 4 o'clock and 8 o'clock positions on the

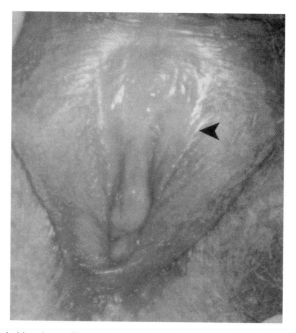

Figure 17-2 Labia minora. The shiny middle portion corresponds to the vulvar vestibule. The arrow points to Hart's line, the lateral border of the vestibule.

posterolateral aspect of the vulvar vestibule. Cysts, abscesses, and, rarely, adenocarcinoma of Bartholin's gland may make this gland apparent, however. The sensory and sympathetic innervation is supplied mainly by the pudendal nerve (S2,3,4), with some contributions from L1 and L2 at the anterior portions of the vulva. The pudendal nerve also supplies the muscles of the pelvic sling, the urethral and anal openings, and their respective sphincters. Thus, damage to the pudendal nerve and herpetic infection of the sacral ganglia can cause symptoms referrable to the urethra, anus, and vulva.

History

Typical complaints pertaining to the vulva include pruritus (itching) with/or without pain (usually experienced as "burning") and the discovery of palpable lesions. Because most patients are not aware of the vulva as an anatomic structure, they will often localize their complaints to the "vagina" when they actually mean the vulva.

A methodical technique for eliciting a gynecologic and sexual history is recommended to preclude missing important information. It should include details about pregnancies, surgeries, contraceptive methods, previous sexually transmitted diseases and their treatments, sexual practices, the number of partners, and whether safe sex is practiced. This is particularly helpful in identifying viral infections that may have recurrent symptoms after periods of latency such as human papilloma virus (HPV) and herpes simplex virus (HSV). Recurrent HSV outbreaks can give rise to a variety of non-specific vulvar symptoms that may pose a diagnostic challenge, but once diagnosed, women can be taught to recognize these for what they are (1). It is helpful to determine whether the vulvar symptoms are constant, intermittent, or only associated with intercourse, and, if dyspareunia is present, to clarify whether it is superficial ("entry" dyspareunia) or deep. Determining the onset of the symptoms (as well as any inciting factors), the duration, and any exacerbating or alleviating factors is helpful. Recall that abnormal vaginal discharge resulting from vaginitis and/or cervicitis is a common cause of vulvar symptoms, usually pruritus at first, but, with time and continued irritation, often vulvar burning. Because the mucosal lining of the urethral orifice can become involved in the inflammatory process of vulvitis, urinary symptoms such as urethral irritation, dysuria, and frequency commonly occur. In addition, severe vulvar burning can result from urine coming in contact with inflamed vulvar mucosa.

It is important to elicit a complete medical history. For example, nongynecologic processes such as Crohn's disease (2), Behcet's syndrome, and infectious mononucleosis (3) may be responsible for vulvar ulcers or erosions (Box

17-1). A dermatologic history that reveals previous diagnoses of diffuse skin processes such as psoriasis, seborrheic dermatitis, and atopic dermatitis may be helpful in identifying the cause of vulvar lesions. A history of concomitant pruritus in a sexual partner or family member might suggest infestation with scabies or pubic lice.

The medication history should include topical and systemic drugs, including over-the-counter and prescription medications. Broad-spectrum antibiotics can predispose to vulvovaginal candidiasis. Certain medications such as nonsteroidal anti-inflammatory agents and antibiotics (e.g., tetracyclines) sometimes cause bullous fixed drug eruptions in the genital area. Irritant or allergic vulvitis may be caused by a wide variety of agents; thus one must carefully identify all of a patient's vaginal or vulvar exposures, from spermicides to sanitary pads to laundry detergents. Intravaginal products and medications can alter the normal bacterial flora of the vagina (often by raising the vaginal pH) and induce vulvar symptoms through the production of abnormal vaginal discharges.

Physical Examination

The physical examination is best performed with the patient in the lithotomy position, with good lighting provided by a floor or overhead lamp that can be directed. The hair-bearing skin should be examined for nits and lice; textural changes; broken-off hairs; scales; crusts; color changes; papules (Figs. 17-3 and 17-4); plaques (Figs. 17-5 to 17-7); nodules, pustules, and ulcers (Fig. 17-8); and erosions. Thickening and accentuation of surface skin markings and broken-off hairs usually result from chronic friction caused by scratching and rubbing (Fig. 17-9). These changes are most often symmetric; asymmetry

---

Box 17-1 Differential Diagnosis of Pustules, Ulcers, and Erosions

- *Pustules*—herpes simplex, candidiasis, pustular psoriasis, Reiter's syndrome, aphthosis associated with inflammatory bowel disease, Behçet's syndrome
- *Ulcers*—herpes simplex, syphilis and other infections (TB, LGV, other STDs), aphthosis, Behçet's syndrome, pyoderma gangrenosum, extraintestinal Crohn's disease, malignancies
- *Erosions*—lichen sclerosus, lichen planus, bullous drug reactions (including Stevens-Johnson syndrome), lupus erythematosus, erosive vulvitis, desquamative inflammatory vaginitis, autoimmune bullous diseases

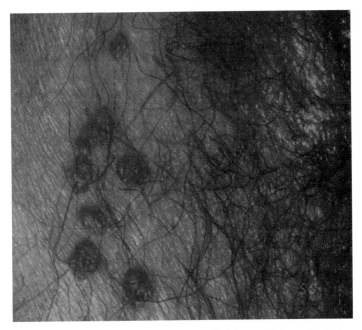

Figure 17-3 Flat warts (HPV). A group of discrete, dark brown, flat papules just medial to the labia majora. Routine histology can differentiate these from seborrheic keratoses and Bowenoid papulosis (VIN III).

suggests the possible presence of an underlying focus of concern such as HPV infection. Side lighting is helpful for the detection of flat warts on the vulva. The presence of a discharge pooling at the introitus is abnormal. When evaluating complaints related to the vulva, speculum exam of the cervix and vagina as well as bimanual examination should always be performed.

It is important to recognize that certain physical findings represent normal variations. For instance, the appearance of the labia minora may vary widely. Some labia are thin and short whereas others are long enough to protrude between the lips of the labia majora. In the latter instance, the free edges of the labia minora may be more pigmented and rugose, and more closely resemble the appearance of the labia majora.

Another important normal variation is the presence of symmetrically disposed papillae along Hart's line, at the fourchette, at the free edge of the hymen, or diffusely over the inner surfaces of the labia minora (4). These benign lesions are frequently misdiagnosed as condylomata acuminata (caused by the human papillomavirus), which can lead to psychological distress and inappropriate destructive therapies. Benign vulvar papillomas are soft, uniform, transluscent, 1 to 5 mm spike-like outpouchings with a capillary at the core

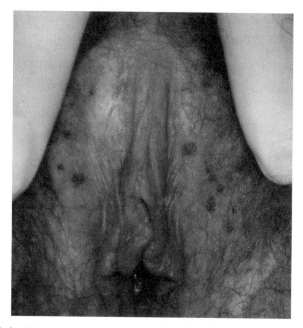

Figure 17-4 Angiokeratomas. Discrete, 1 to 3 mm dark-red papules. These are benign vascular growths. They may arouse concern when solitary and darker in color, because they may be mistaken for a nevus or melanoma. (For color reproduction, see Plate 7 at back of book.)

(Fig. 17-10). Condylomata acuminata, in contrast, are usually firm, opaque, rounded papillae, and often form uneven clumps as a result of multiple papules arising from a single stalk (Box 17-2 and Fig. 17-11). Even routine histology of vulvar papillomas can be misleading because vacuolated cells (which are commonly seen in mucosal biopsies) are often overinterpreted as HPV-infected cells. Experimental studies using DNA hybridization (5) and PCR techniques (6) have been helpful in distinguishing these normal variants from condylomata because such testing typically fails to demonstrate the presence of HPV DNA.

The mucosal surfaces of the vulvar vestibule should be closely examined. The presence of erythema around the ostia of Skene's and Bartholin's ducts or in localized patches within the vestibule should be noted. If severe pain is elicited upon application of light pressure with a cotton-tipped applicator over these inflamed areas, the patient should be queried as to whether she has pain on penile insertion even if this information is not volunteered.

When the physical examination detects suspicious lesions, further evaluation of the vulva may be enhanced by the application of 3% to 5% acetic acid

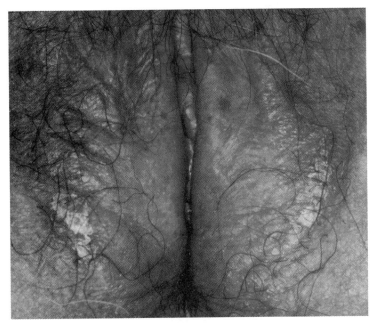

Figure 17-5 Psoriasis. Erythematous papulosquamous plaque with white scales at the outer borders; note scattered nonscaly papules around the major plaque.

(vinegar) combined with the use of a hand-held magnifying glass. Areas of aceto-whitening suggest focal HPV infection or dysplasia but require directed biopsy for definitive diagnosis. It should be noted, however, that aceto-whitening is a normal finding on the inner labia and at the junction of the inferior portion of the vestibule, probably because of the trauma of intercourse or inflammatory conditions such as mild yeast infections (7). Because aceto-whitening lacks both specificity and sensitivity, this technique has not been universally endorsed.

Laboratory Testing and Vulvar Biopsy

When vulvar symptoms or abnormalities are present, it is important to exclude cervicitis and vaginitis as potential sources of the problem by taking specimens from the cervix for chlamydia and gonorrhea and performing wet mount and KOH examinations of the vaginal discharge. Potassium hydroxide solution also facilitates microscopic examination of skin and mucosal scrapings when looking for yeast, fungi, nits, or scabies. Ulcers on the vulva are typically evaluated with culture for herpes simplex virus and appropriately

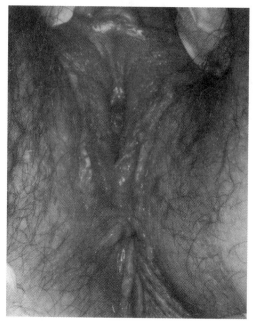

Figure 17-6 Intraepithelial squamous cell carcinoma extending from the vulva to the perianal area in a patient with a 20-year history of condylomata. She complained of pruritus. Paget's disease should be included in the differential diagnosis. (For color reproduction, see Plate 8 at back of book.)

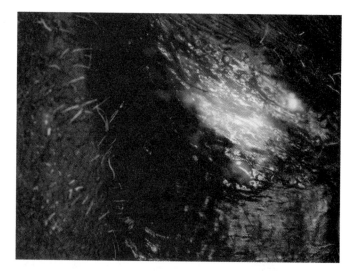

Figure 17-7 Intraepithelial squamous cell carcinoma. A plaque of irregular shiny pink and black papules on the labia majora of an immunosuppressed patient with previous history of condylomata. This lesion is an intraepithelial squamous cell carcinoma. Histology will differentiate this from melanoma. (For color reproduction, see Plate 9 at back of book.)

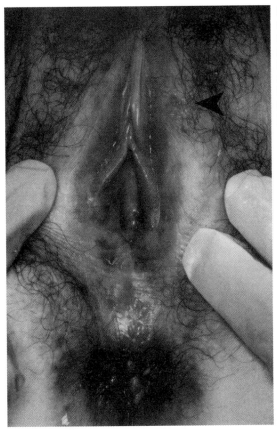

Figure 17-8 Primary herpes simplex with grouped vesicles and multiple superficial erosions in the vulva. There are also perianal condylomata acuminata. It is not unusual to find more than one sexually transmitted disease in a patient.

timed serologic testing for syphilis, but laboratory testing is unavailable for many of the responsible infectious agents (see Chapter 8) and for the noninfectious causes.

The skin biopsy is indispensable in the diagnosis and follow-up of dermatologic conditions of the vulva, and its importance in excluding malignant lesions cannot be overemphasized. Those primary care physicians adept at skin biopsies should feel comfortable performing biopsies of the vulva. After infiltration with 1% lidocaine (usually with epinephrine) a disposable punch biopsy instrument (such as the Keyes punch) can be used on the outer vulva. Mucosal biopsies are performed using the same anesthesia but are better accomplished with iris scissors. For eroded or bullous lesions, the biopsy specimen should be obtained from the edge of a lesion and include adjacent, noneroded mucosa. The specimen should be placed in the formaldehyde solution promptly to prevent dessication of the specimen. Closing the biopsy site with sutures using 6-0 quick-absorbing catgut allows for much faster healing.

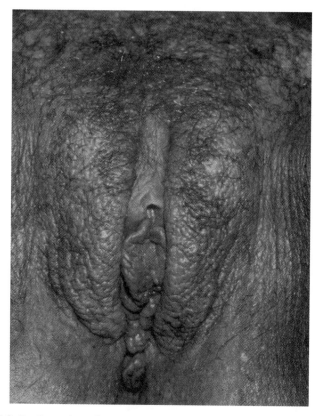

Figure 17-9 Pruritus vulvae. Symmetrical lichenification (skin thickening with increased skin markings) of labia majora with punctate excoriations and absent or broken-off hairs.

When histologic examination suggests of allergic contact dermatitis and the culprit cannot be identified with thorough history taking and/or trials of elimination, skin patch testing can be helpful. Such testing is typically performed by a dermatologist.

General Therapeutic Measures

Clothing worn next to the body should be loose and made of natural, absorbent material. When vulvar dermatitis is acute, one can justify encouraging the patient to stay home from work for at least 48 hr to permit complete freedom from restrictive clothing and to allow enough time for intensive treatment.

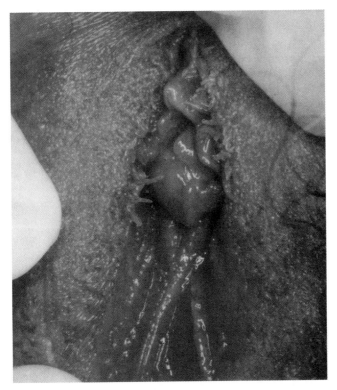

Figure 17-10 Benign vulvar papillomatosis. Uniform, fine, transluscent, individual, long outpouchings of the mucosa. DNA hybridization did not reveal HPV on biopsy.

Baths are useful for cleaning off crusts and macerated scales. During the acute phase, daily baths plus open wet compresses for 20 to 30 min two other times during the day will speed the healing process. Plain tap water, a 1:20 Burow's solution (Domeboro), or colloidal oatmeal (Aveeno) may be used.

In general, ointments are preferred to creams because creams generally contain preservatives, a common cause of contact dermatitis. Midpotency topical steroids such as triamcinolone 0.1% ointment or fluocinolone acetonide 0.025% ointment (Synalar) for 10 to 14 days are generally sufficient to treat an acute problem. Prolonged use leads to the development of striae, folliculitis-type lesions, epidermal atrophy, and telangiectasias. Marked erythema and burning are signs of a rebound phenomenon that may occur upon discontinuation of chronic topical steroid therapy.

Five percent Lidocaine ointment or Emla (lidocaine 2.5% and prilocaine 2.5%) cream is effective for temporary, local pain control in patients with mu-

---

Box 17-2 Differential Diagnosis of Vulvar Papules, Plaques, and Nodules

---

Discrete Papules (<10 mm)

- *Skin-colored to black*—prurigo nodularis (picker's nodules), warts (HPV), vulvar intraepithelia neoplasia (VIN), seborrheic keratoses, acrochordons (skin tags), nevi, basal cell and squamous cell cancers, melanomas
- *Yellowish or grayish-white*—Fordyce spots (apocrine miliaria), molluscum contagiosum, milia, epidermal inclusion cysts
- *Erythematous to purple*—angiokeratomas, cherry angiomas, pyogenic granuloma, varicosities

Confluent Papules and Plaques (>10 mm)

- *Skin-colored to black*—warts, VIN I-III, secondary syphilis, noninfectious granulomas
- *Erythematous (with or without scaling)*—psoriasis, lichen planus, squamous cell carcinoma, extramammary Paget's disease

Nodules

- *Cystic*—epidermal inclusion cyst, Bartholin's cyst, extraintestinal Crohn's disease, hidradenitis suppurativa
- *Doughy*—neurofibroma, lipoma, localized edema
- *Firm*—fibromas, depositions (calcium, amyloid), malignant neoplasms, benign tumors of glandular origin

---

cosal ulcers or erosions and for temporary relief of pain associated with types of vulvodynia.

When pruritus is severe, certain measures may be required in addition to treating the underlying problem. A cold compress or an icebag wrapped in a facecloth applied to the vulva can provide immediate though temporary relief. Because pruritus is most often worse at night, hydroxyzine hydrochloride 25 to 50 mg at bedtime is a useful adjunctive therapy. For patients who do not respond to hydroxyzine and have no contraindications to tricyclic antidepressants, low dose (10 to 25 mg) doxepin or amitriptyline at bedtime is helpful. The patient should be instructed to avoid rubbing the area.

Protective agents such as Desitin, A&D, and zinc oxide ointments serve as excellent barriers and prevent irritating discharges from coming in contact with fragile skin or mucosa. They can be applied over other topical therapies if needed. These agents can be cleaned off with cotton balls saturated with mineral oil.

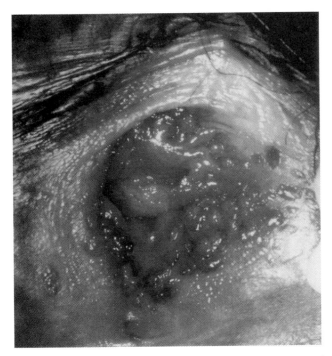

Figure 17-11 Condyloma acuminata (HPV). Asymmetric groups of firm, rounded papillae that are clumped together.

Powders are infrequently required but, when needed, Zeasorb (available over the counter) may be preferred. Its particle size is smaller than standard talc, which allows for greater surface area for absorption and a decreased likelihood of irritating the vulvar tissue.

Dermatologic Abnormalities of the Vulva

As per standard practice for nongenital areas of skin, dermatologic lesions of the vulva are described as macules, papules, patches, plaques, vesicles, or bullae, and secondary changes as crusts, fissures, erosions, ulcers, excoriations, atrophy, and scarring (7). However, the anatomy of the vulva influences the appearance of the lesions. Specifically, the vulva is confined to a tight space characterized by deep folds of skin that are in direct apposition to each other, creating a warm and moist environment with natural occlusion. Because of this, blisters quickly become denuded and are hardly ever seen intact, appearing instead as ulcers or erosions. Likewise, scales quickly become hydrated and manifest as piles of macerated white debris. As a result of increased absorption, wide atrophic striae develop more quickly from the use of topical steroids.

One must be aware that malignant lesions on the vulva can assume a wide variety of appearances: ulcerative, erythematous, proliferative, or hyperkeratotic (8). They may be hypopigmented, hyperpigmented, or erythematous. Indeed, vulvar intraepithelial neoplasia (VIN) can be any of these three colors (Box 17-3). Therefore in order to diagnose cancer in its early stages, vulvar lesions demand both liberal use of biopsy and close patient monitoring during treatment.

Nonmalignant Dermatologic Lesions

The classification of vulvar skin lesions has traditionally been based on distinguishing red, white, and dark lesions. Such organization is helpful in the initial diagnosis of vulvar lesions, but one must remain aware of the wide variability and overlap in the appearances of various lesions. This, together with the highly variable clinical appearance of malignancies on the vulva, necessitates liberal use of biopsy.

Red Lesions

Diffuse erythema of the vulva commonly results from yeast vulvitis or inflammation of the vulva from another infectious vaginitis, and typically resolves with control of the abnormal vaginal discharge. Aside from these causes, irritant and allergic dermatitis, seborrheic dermatitis, psoriasis, and lichen planus are often responsible for erythematous lesions of the vulva. Of course, as previously stated, a red lesion on the vulva may also represent a malignancy.

Seborrhea and Psoriasis
The papulosquamous disorders seborrheic dermatitis and intertriginous psoriasis present as red lesions. Their diagnosis is aided by the presence of skin involvement elsewhere on the body that tend to be confined to the outer, hair-bearing aspect of the vulva.

Irritant and Allergic Vulvitis
Diffuse redness or red lesions on the vulva can be caused by either irritant or allergic vulvitis, both of which result from materials coming in contact with the vagina and/or vulva. Common offending agents include the alcohol and preservatives contained in medicated creams (including those found in anti-yeast preparations), latex condoms, lubricants, sanitary pads, douches, lubricants, formaldehyde in new clothing, detergents, and lubricants. In addition

---

Box 17-3 Differential Diagnosis of Nonpalpable Color Changes on the Vulva

---

Loss of Pigment (May Be Patchy)
Vitiligo
Lichen sclerosus
Post-inflammatory scars
Vulvar intraepithelial neoplasia (VIN)

Hyperpigmentation
Diffuse
    Endocrine causes: Cushing's disease, Addison's disease, pregnancy
    Acanthosis nigricans
    Post-inflammatory
Patchy
    Post-inflammatory
    Lentigines, benign lentiginosis
    Benign vulvar melanosis
    Benign nevi
    Seborrheic keratoses (early)
    Flat condylomata
    VIN
    Melanoma

Red/Purple Discoloration
Diffuse
    Acute vulvitis
    Port-wine stain
    Post-steroid rebound erythema
    Erosive vulvitis
    Erysipelas
Patchy
    Port-wine stain
    Inflammatory dermatoses (e.g., psoriasis, lichen sclerosus)
    Erosive vulvitis
    VIN
    Kaposi's sarcoma, angiosarcoma

---

to identifying and eliminating the culprit agent, the vulvar pruritus can be treated using local measures as previously described, and a brief course (10 to 14 days) of treatment with a mid-potency topical steroid ointment (e.g., triamcinolone 0.1%). A protective barrier such as A& D ointment is often useful in protecting the inflamed area after discontinuing the topical steroids. Allergic or irritant vulvitis most closely resembles yeast vulvitis, but other possible causes of diffuse pruritus (see Fig. 17-9) include dysplasia (VIN) and vulvar condyloma, particularly those warts that are flat and less obvious to the patient.

Lichen Planus

Lichen planus is a rare disease that is typically a purely cutaneous papulosquamous inflammatory condition. However, a severely erosive and scarring variant may involve the vulvovaginal mucosa, sometimes with simultaneous involvement of the mouth. As with the more common lichen sclerosus, lichen planus eventually causes sclerosis and narrowing of the vulvovaginal canal (Fig. 17-12). It is painful, recalcitrant to therapy, and requires long-term follow-up to guard against the development of squamous cell carcinoma.

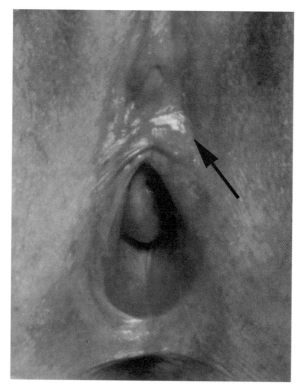

Figure 17-12 Erosive lichen planus of the vulva with narrowing of the opening and complete resorption of the labia minora. Arrow points to white reticulation in interlabial furrow.

Superpotent topical steroids are used as for vulvar lichen sclerosus (see below). Because the erosions of lichen planus also extend into the vagina; however, insertion of 1% hydrocortisone suppositories into the vagina several times a week is a useful adjunct.

The diagnosis of lichen planus and other erosive diseases may be difficult. In general, women with any chronic erosions on the vulva may benefit from referral to a dermatologist when the primary care physician or gynecologist is unable to establish the diagnosis.

White Lesions

Lichen Sclerosus

Lichen sclerosus (previously termed *lichen sclerosus et atrophicus* or *kraurosis vulvae*) is an inflammatory skin disease of unknown etiology that is not uncommon. It can occur in any age group, including children, although postmenopausal women are most often affected. In addition to its association with vulvar cancer, untreated lichen sclerosus can cause marked scarring of the vulvar tissue, severe enough that sometimes patients are left with "keyhole" vaginal openings. Because of its important implications and evolving clinical appearance, the diagnosis should always be confirmed with vulvar biopsy.

Initially, grayish-white, polygonal patches appear but later thin, finely wrinkled skin covers the labia, clitoris, and perianal areas (Fig. 17-13). Associated purpura and erosions attest to the fragile nature of these lesions. Although asymptomatic in a small minority of patients, pruritus is the prominent symptom and may be severe. Lesions can also sometimes be found on nongenital skin and are usually asymtomatic.

In the chronic phase, large atrophic patches develop, and the vulvar skin appears white, soft, and slightly wrinkled but smooth. The perianal area is also often affected; consequently, the area of perineal involvement forms a "figure-eight" or "hourglass" appearance. Because fissures and erosions often complicate this stage, burning pain, dysuria, dyspareunia, and discharge may accompany the pruritus. The chronic stage is also characterized by loss of normal vulvar architecture, such as resorption of the labia minora, which sometimes leads to stenosis of the introitus. The prepuce of the clitoris and the perianal area may also become scarred, which in severe cases may be associated with pencil-thin stools. The risk of squamous cell carcinoma is increased 10-fold to 100-fold, but the overall incidence remains fairly low, affecting 3% to 4% of women with lichen sclerosus (9).

Topical testosterone therapy was previously the treatment for lichen sclerosus, but it has been supplanted by super-potent topical steroids, which are much more effective (10). Clobetasol propionate ointment or cream (Temovate or Cormax) is applied in a very thin layer, twice daily for 2 to 4 months, the du-

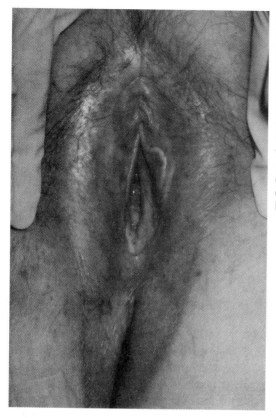

Figure 17-13 Lichen sclerosus. Mucosal atrophy and homogenization of the dermis give rise to a gray, waxy appearance with increased visibility of veins. The right labia minora is completely resorbed, making the vulva asymmetric; the sclerosus extends to the perianal area, causing pencil-thin stools. The condition was reversed by super-potent topical steroids. (For color reproduction, see Plate 10 at back of book.)

ration depending on individual response. Thereafter, maintenance therapy can be accomplished with less frequent use (2 to 3 times a week) of the same preparation or daily use of a less potent one. Because of the albeit low but increased risk of squamous cell cancer of the vulva, women diagnosed with lichen sclerosus should undergo annual pelvic exams. Periodic biopsies of persistently ulcerated or hyperplastic areas should be performed to rule out malignancy.

Vitiligo

Vitiligo may start on the vulva or sometimes be confined to this area. Vitiligo is a purely cosmetic issue. Rarely, lichen sclerosis lacking textural changes may resemble it, but in general the diagnosis of vitiligo can be made without biopsy.

Dark Lesions

Relatively common causes of hyperpigmented lesions on the vulva are seborrheic keratoses, lentigines, nevi, and condylomata. It is important to distinguish these benign causes from malignant melanoma (see Vulvar Melanoma section below).

Vulvar Intraepithelial Neoplasia and Vulvar Malignancies

The following discussion focuses on the more common malignancies of the vulva. Vulvar malignancies are best managed by gynecologic oncologists. However, the importance of the primary physician in detecting these lesions cannot be overstated. Also, the finding of a vulvar squamous cell cancer requires that the physician take steps to carefully exclude malignancy elsewhere in the genital tract, particularly the cervix, as well as the colon and anus.

Overall vulvar malignancies are rare; squamous cell cancer and melanomas are the more common types.

Squamous Cell Carcinoma of the Vulva

VIN is believed to arise from HPV infection, and with time can progress to invasive squamous cell carcinoma of the vulva. VIN I (mild dysplasia), VIN II (moderate dysplasia), and VIN III (marked dysplasia) are analogous to the classification system used to describe pre-invasive lesions of the cervix (CIN). In contrast to CIN, however, VIN most commonly presents as a high-grade lesion (VIN III), yet the risk of malignant transformation from VIN is much lower than that from CIN—about 5% (11). As with premalignant cervical lesions, spontaneous improvement is possible.

VIN is commonly pruritic but may be entirely asymptomatic. Its clinical appearance may vary considerably and include skin-colored, hypopigmented, hyperpigmented, and erythematous lesions. High-grade VIN often presents as a sharply demarcated papule (7). VIN can be a multifocal disease, particularly in younger women (12). Appropriate management includes biopsying multiple lesions, especially the thicker or more hypertrophied ones, to detect possible invasion. Colposcopic examination of the vulva is helpful in directing biopsies by detecting areas of erythema, lichenification, punctation, mosaic patterns, and areas of aceto-whitening.

VIN sometimes causes pruritus and can assume various appearances ranging from a macule that is erythematous, hypopigmented, or dark, to a papule or warty growth.

VIN III can be treated in nonhairy areas with carbon dioxide laser ablation, or medical therapy with 5-flourouracil, which often entails severe, painful desquamation. In hairy areas, surgical excision and closure are advised, because VIN III can extend along hair follicles (11). Fortunately, progression of VIN to squamous cell carcinoma is uncommon, but the likelihood increases with immunosuppression resulting from aging or other causes. The average age at diagnosis of vulvar squamous cell carcinoma is 60 to 65 years, but 10% of all cases occur in younger women in their 20s and 30s (8). Aside from VIN, other risk factors for the development of vulvar carcinoma include other genital carcinomas, chronic vulvar inflammatory disorders (e.g., lichen sclerosus, lichen planus), smoking, and genital warts (13). Interestingly, in older women whose vulvar cancer was attributed to lichen sclerosus, HPV DNA can sometimes but not always be identified, suggesting that sometimes lichen sclerosus acts independently to induce mutations (in a manner analogous to sunlight exposure), but at other times is further influenced by HPV infection. It shall be noted that approximately one third of the time, however, squamous cell cancer of the vulva arises in the absence of any premalignant precursors (13).

Treatment of squamous cell cancer of the vulva depends on the depth of invasion, but it frequently requires radical excision with a 2-cm margin that extends to the deep perineal fascia. Lymph node dissection is usually required. In general, the vulva tolerates radiation therapy poorly, but chemo-sensitizing irradiation with *cis*-platin is sometimes used, typically before surgery in order to shrink the tumor and allow for a less extensive excision.

Vulvar Melanoma

Melanomas of the vulva are uncommon but unfortunately are diagnosed at a later stage than melanomas elsewhere on the body. Although accounting for less than 2% of all dark lesions of the vulva (7), melanoma's aggressive behavior dictates that it be distinguished from the benign causes of hyperpigmentation. Because the clinical appearance of melanoma may differ little from that of benign nevi, lentigo, or foci of chronic irritant dermatitis, biopsy is usually required. Also, because 30% to 50% of melanomas arise from existing nevi (8,13), patient report of a mole having "always been there" should not dissuade the physician from biopsying the lesion when suspicious features are present.

Paget's Disease of the Vulva

Paget's disease of the vulva is an uncommon slow-growing intraepithelial neoplasm. Because the lesion is often pruritic and presents as an erythematous, eczematous-appearing plaque, it is often misdiagnosed. However, the finding of a fiery red background mottled with white hyperkeratotic islands should prompt biopsy. Although it is uncommonly associated with Paget's disease of the breast, a mammary lesion should be excluded as well as lesions in the genital and gastrointestinal tracts. Unlike Paget's disease of the breast, which is associated with an underlying ductal carcinoma, Paget's disease of the vulva rarely signifies an underlying malignancy, but when it does, a palpable mass is generally present (8). Paget's disease of the vulva generally remains intraepithelial, but because of its risk of invasion and recurrence, wide and deep excision followed by careful follow-up are required.

Pruritus Vulvae

Pruritus vulvae describes chronic, idiopathic itching of the vulva. It generally affects the cutaneous, hair-bearing surfaces resulting in hyperpigmentation, scaling, thickening, and accentuation of surface skin markings. The presence of broken-off hairs attests to the chronicity of the friction caused by scratching and rubbing (see Fig. 17-9). These changes are most often symmetrical. The common causes of vulvar pruritus (Box 17-4) should be excluded, namely atopic dermatitis, contact dermatitis, dermatitis secondary to irritating vagi-

---

Box 17-4 Differential Diagnosis of Vulvar Pruritus

Associated with Generalized Pruritus
- *Systemic diseases*—diabetes, chronic renal and hepatic failure, polycythemia vera, Hodgkin's lymphoma, hypo- and hyper-thyroidism
- *Psychogenic*—delusions of parasitosis

Localized to Vulva and Perineum
- *Infestations*—pinworms, pediculosis pubis (lice), scabies
- *Infections*—erythrasma, candidiasis, tinea, HPV
- *Dermatologic conditions*—seborrheic dermatitis, allergic or irritant contact dermatitis, psoriasis, lichen planus, lichen sclerosus, lichen simplex chronicus
- *Neoplasia*—vulvar intraepithelial neoplasia (I-III), squamous cell carcinoma, Paget's disease

With Associated Vaginal Discharge
- *Cervicitis*
- *Vaginitis*—infectious and noninfectious

nal discharges, and vulvar condylomata. Less commonly, VIN presents as an asymmetric, pruritic plaque.

Interrupting the itch-scratch-itch cycle is important. Pruritus vulvae can be treated with potent topical steroids for a trial period of 2 to 3 weeks as well as the other measures described in the General Therapeutic Measures section. The patient should be instructed to avoid rubbing the area. A punch biopsy is often necessary for complete evaluation of these patients.

Bartholin's Gland Cysts and Abscesses

Cysts can develop in a Bartholin's gland, at which time a palpable mass develops, and the patient may suffer pain, sometimes severe enough to interfere with daily activities. If the cyst spontaneously ruptures, the patient only requires hot Sitz baths. However, symptomatic cysts that fail to rupture can be treated by incision just inside the hymenal ring, or just outside of it (but not on the labia), preceded by sterile prep and local anesthesia. Because of the risk of recurrence, many physicians consider simple incision and drainage inadequate, preferring concomitant placement of a Word catheter (14). The catheter is inserted into the stab wound and left in place for approximately 4 weeks to allow formation of a new tract. Sometimes marsupialization or "window" operations become necessary. Recurrent symptomatic Bartholin's gland cysts require surgical excision, which should be performed by a gynecologist in an operating suite because of the risk of bleeding. Surgical excision of Bartholin's gland cysts has also been recommended as initial therapy for the postmenopausal woman because the risk of underlying carcinoma is increased.

Abscesses of the Bartholin gland can also occur. These can be readily distinguished from Bartholin's gland cysts by the pronounced vulvar erythema and edema that accompany the tender visible mass. Abscesses usually develop rapidly over a few days' time and often rupture spontaneously within a week, in which case the patient requires only hot Sitz baths, antibiotics, and analgesics. Early unruptured abscesses may also be treated in this manner until they "point," at which time incision and drainage with placement of a Word catheter can be performed. Historically, Bartholin's gland abscesses have been attributed to infection with gonococcus or chlamydia, but recent data point to other bacterial infections, and antibiotic coverage should be broad (14).

Vulvar Pain Syndromes

Vulvar pain syndromes include pudendal neuralgia and vulvodynia, of which there are different subtypes.

Pudendal Neuralgia

Pudendal neuralgia is characterized by constant burning in the vulvar and perivulvar areas (labia majora, mons, perineum, perianal area, and the upper inner thighs) (15). The vulvar pain of pudendal neuralgia may be accompanied by intermittent sharp, shooting, or lancinating pains that may radiate down one leg in a manner that has been described as "neuralgic" and "sciatica-like". Classic pudendal neuralgia is caused by trauma to the pudendal nerve such as from a pelvic injury, stretching secondary to laxity of the pelvic diaphragm, or an episiotomy scar that develops a neuroma. Recurrent anogenital herpes simplex infection (see Fig. 17-8) may also cause this syndrome). The diagnosis of herpes should be made with a positive HSV culture obtained at the time of an outbreak.

Inspection of the vulva generally does not reveal any lesions, with the possible exception of a surgical scar or HSV lesions. However, neurologic examination reveals an area of sensory loss in addition to shifting areas of allodynia (light touch stimulus that is interpreted as pain). Allodynia is responsible for most patient complaints because even such innocuous stimuli as clothing touching the skin can induce extreme discomfort. Hyperpathia (perception of pain lasting longer than application of the stimulus with a resulting "echo") also can occur, and classically these patients suffer not only introital dyspareunia but pain that can persist long after intercourse, sometimes for days.

Therapy consists of topical anesthetics such as 5% xylocaine ointment applied to the vulva. Tricyclic antidepressants (i.e., amitriptyline or imipramine) often provide substantial relief, and are superior to the selective serotonin reuptake inhibitors (SSRIs). The dose of tricyclics required for pain syndromes is much lower than that necessary for antidepressant action, and a typical starting dose is amitriptyline 10 mg 1 hr before bedtime, doubling the dose every 4 days or so until the desired effect is reached. Usually the dose does not exceed 75 mg; sometimes side effects are limiting. It is important to warn the patient of possible sedation and anticholinergic side effects and clarify that these medications are being prescribed for relief of "nerve pain" and not for depression. Frequently the addition of an anticonvulsant such as diphenylhydantoin (Dilantin), carbamazepine (Tegretol), or gabapentin (Neurontin) is necessary. Patients who fail to respond to such measures may benefit from referral to a specialist. Some of these patients may require a benzodiazepine such as clonazepam (Klonopin). Neither laser vaporization nor surgical excision is indicated for pudendal neuralgia.

Vulvodynia

Vulvodynia (Greek, "vulvar pain") is a general term that by accepted definition denotes unexplained, chronic (greater than 6 month duration) vulvar discomfort, often described as a burning or a sensation of irritation or rawness. The International Society for the Study of Vulvar Diseases (ISSVD) has been helpful in motivating research in this area (15a), but the different causes of vulvodynia remain poorly understood; consequently its management remains frustrating for both patients and physicians. Authors differ in their recognition of subtypes of vulvodynia, but these often include essential vulvodynia and the vulvar vestibulitis syndrome (VVS), the latter being the major cause of chronic vulvar discomfort (16).

The prevalence of vulvodynia is difficult to estimate. It appears to affect Caucasians almost exclusively and, although it can occur at any age, studies reveal a predilection for the reproductive years. Attempts to implicate a history of physical or sexual abuse or previous sexually transmitted diseases have been unsuccessful (17).

When evaluating a patient complaining of vulvar pain, it is important to exclude vulvar dermatoses and chronic vaginal infections because the pain associated with these treatable conditions usually resolves in response to therapy. Microscopic evaluation of the vaginal discharge is important even in the absence of gross findings, because treatment of unusually long lactobacillus with amoxicillin (18) or long curved rods (mobiluncus) with clindamycin vaginal cream has been associated with permanent resolution of vulvodynia in some patients.

When evaluating a patient with chronic vulvodynia it is important to perform microscopic evaluation of the vaginal discharge to exclude curable causes.

Essential Vulvodynia

Essential (or "idiopathic" or "dysesthetic") vulvodynia in many ways clinically resembles pudendal neuralgia but without the stabbing or lancinating neuralgic pains or evidence of preceding trauma or herpes infection. Sensory findings have not been systematically delineated for this condition.

Some believe that essential vulvodynia is a chronic pain syndrome belonging to the family of fibromyalgia, interstitial cystitis, and irritable bowel syndrome. Interestingly, some patients with essential vulvodynia also have one of these pain syndromes. The etiology of this condition is unknown. One theory holds that persistent, local irritation leads to persistent localized pain, which with time alters central processing of stimuli such that light touch becomes interpreted as pain. The area of involvement then gradually expands.

Therapy is essentially the same as for pudendal neuralgia: a topical anesthetic together with a tricyclic antidepressant is usually first-line treatment. In general, patients with essential vulvodynia have had their problem for years and are best managed like any other patient with a chronic pain syndrome. At the risk of sounding defeatist, patients should be counseled that the goal is pain management rather than "cure". Because of the chronicity and other implications of this syndrome, psychological counseling can often help patients cope with this disorder.

Vulvar Vestibulitis

Vulvar vestibulitis is a form of vulvodynia in which pain is confined to the vulvar vestibule during intercourse (16). Superficial dyspareunia is therefore the major complaint and is often severe enough to prevent intercourse. Physical findings are present but subtle and consist of erythema in the vulvar vestibule around the openings of Bartholin's and Skene's glands (the 4 o'clock and 8 o'clock positions). When a cotton-tipped applicator is used to apply light pressure to these erythematous areas, burning pain is elicited.

Milder cases can be treated with topical anesthetics such as Emla or 5% Xylocaine ointment applied 20 to 30 min before intercourse, with petroleum jelly or Astroglide for lubrication. Hydroxyzine hydrochloride 10 to 25 mg at bedtime may be added. The wide range of as yet unproven additional modalities attests to the current lack of understanding of this disorder: a low-oxalate diet in combination with calcium citrate tablets (19), intralesional injections of alpha-interferon at the vulvar vestibule (20), and biofeedback (21). When introital dyspareunia is severe enough to completely prevent intercourse and the patient's quality of life is severely impacted, surgical excision of the vulvar vestibule with mobilization of the vaginal mucosa (vestibulectomy) restores function in approximately 85% of patients (22). Psychological counseling is an important adjunct in the therapy of these patients whether or not they undergo surgery (23). Ablation of tissue with the carbon dioxide laser should not be used, because it appears to exacerbate this condition.

Summary

Many important vulvar diseases may have subtle presentations. Thus, for example, an older woman who reports mild vulvar pruritus should not be assumed to simply be suffering from symptoms of postmenopausal atrophy but should undergo thorough evaluation to carefully exclude such diagnoses as lichen sclerosus, VIN, and squamous cell carcinoma. Other patients may hesitate to even volunteer their vulvar symptoms; this reluctance probably contributes to the difficulty in estimating the prevalence of conditions such as vulvodynia. Clearly these patients could benefit from their physician taking a more active role in eliciting symptoms referrable to the vulva. Also, many important diseases of the vulva may be entirely asymptomatic and go completely unnoticed by the patient.

In summary, careful examination of the vulva is critical and should be a component of every pelvic examination.

REFERENCES

1. **Koelle DM, Benedetto J, Langenberg A, et al.** Asymptomatic reactivation of herpes simplex virus in women after first episode of genital herpes. Ann Int Med. 1992; 116:433-7.

2. **Weber A, Ziegler C, Belinson J, et al.** Gynecologic history of women with inflammatory bowel disease. Obstet Gynecol. 1995;86:843-7.

3. **Taylor S, Drake SM, Dedicoat M, Wood MJ.** Genital ulcers associated with acute Epstein-Barr virus infection. Sex Transm Infect. 1998;74:296-7.

4. **Friedrich EG Jr.** Anatomic Variants in Vulvar Disease, 2nd ed. Philadelphia: WB Saunders; 1983:244.

5. **Moyal-Barracco M, Leibowitch M, Orth G.** Vestibular papillae of the vulva: lack of evidence for human papillomavirus etiology. Arch Dermatol. 1990;126:1594-8.

6. **DeDeus JM, Focchi J, Stavale JN, et al.** Histologic and biomolecular aspects of papillomatosis of the vulvar vestibule in relation to human papillomavirus. Obstet Gynecol. 1995;86:758-63.

7. **Apgar BS, Cox JT.** Differentiating normal and abnormal findings of the vulva. Am Fam Phys. 1996;53;4:1171-80.

8. **Di Saia PJ.** Vulvar and vaginal disease. In: Scott JR, ed. Danforth's Obstetrics and Gynecology, 8th ed. Philadelphia: Lippincott Williams & Wilkins; 1999.

9. **Ridley CM.** Lichen sclerosus. Derm Clin. 1992;10:309-18.

10. **Dalziel KL, Wojnarowska F.** Long-term control of vulvar lichen sclerosus after treatment with a potent topical steroid cream. J Reprod Med. 1992;38:25-7.

11. **Jebakumar S, Woolley PD, Bhattacharyya MN.** Vulvar intraepithelia neoplasia. Int J STD AIDS. 1996;7:10-3.

12. **Jablonska S, Majewski S.** Special aspects of infectious diseases in women: human papillomavirus infection in women. Clin Dermatol. 1997;15:67-79.

13. **Crum CP, McLachlin CM, Tate JE, Mutter GL.** Pathobiology of vulvar squamous neoplasia. Curr Opin Obstet Gynecol. 1997;9:63-9.

14. **Hill DA, Lense JJ.** Office management of bartholin gland cysts and abscesses. Am Fam Phys. 1998;57:1611-6.

15. **Turner ML, Marinoff SC.** Pudendal neuralgia. Am J Obstet Gynecol. 1991;l165:1233-6.

15a. Burning vulva syndrome. Report of the ISSVD Task Force. J Reprod Med. 1984;29:457.

16. **Marinoff SC, Turner, ML.** Vulvar vestibulitis syndrome. Dermatol Clin. 1992;10:435-44.

17. **Masheb RM, Nash JM, Brondolo, Kerns RD.** Volvodynia: an introduction and critical review of a chronic pain condition. Pain. 2000;86:3-10.

18. **Davis GD, Hutchison CV.** Clinical management of vulvodynia. Clin Obstet Gynecol. 1999;42:221-33.

19. **Solomons CC, Melmed MH, Heitler SM.** Calcium citrate for vulvar vestibulitis: a case report. J Reprod Med. 1991;36:879.

20. **Marinoff SC, Turner ML, Hirsch RP, et al.** Intralesional alpha-interferon: cost-effective therapy for vulvar vestibulitis syndrome. J Reprod Med. 1993;38:19-24.[AD2]

21. **Glazer HI, Rodke G, Swencionis C, et al.** Treatment of vulvar vestibulitis syndrome with electromyographic biofeedback of pelvic floor musculature. J Reprod Med. 1995;40:283-90.

22. **Friedrich EG.** Vulvar vestibulitis syndrome. J Reprod Med. 1987;32:110-4.

23. **Schover LR, Youngs DD, Cannata R.** Psychosexual aspects of the evaluation and management of vulvar vestibulitis. Am J Obstet Gynecol. 1992;167:630-6.

CHAPTER 18

Management of Common Breast Problems and Breast Cancer Prevention

BARBARA L. SMITH, MD, PHD

Although most clinical breast care is devoted to the early detection of breast cancer, many physicians see women for symptoms of benign breast disease. In addition, asymptomatic breast abnormalities are often discovered during the course of routine physical examination and mammography. Breast problems commonly seen include discrete palpable masses, vague thickening or nodularity, breast pain, nipple discharge, infections, and, in some practices, abnormalities during pregnancy or lactation. Management of these problems is often challenging, especially because it may be difficult to distinguish benign from malignant breast lesions.

The primary care physician is often responsible for coordinating the follow-up of abnormalities detected by mammography or other imaging modalities. In addition, the primary care physician should evaluate a woman's risk factors for breast cancer, and based on her risk profile, recommend an appropriate screening schedule—or perhaps devise a plan with the goal of cancer prevention. Breast cancer risk must also be assessed when making decisions regarding the use of hormone replacement therapy after menopause. Increasingly, care involves discussion of issues surrounding genetic testing for breast cancer risk genes.

Failure to diagnose breast cancer is one of the most common causes of litigation in medical practice. It is essential to discuss carefully and in detail with the patient any recommendations regarding mammography, ultrasonography, biopsy, referral, or follow-up interval, as well as document the plan in the patient's chart.

Office Evaluation

Evaluation of a breast problem requires a detailed history of the presenting symptoms, a review of previous breast problems, a review of risk factors for breast carcinoma, a thorough physical examination of the breasts, and imaging studies when appropriate.

History

In evaluating a new breast problem, the physician should document the initial symptoms and duration of the abnormality, noting any tenderness of the area of concern, any changes in size or tenderness, and for premenopausal women, any changes that occur with the menstrual cycle. The patient should be asked if she has had any nipple discharge. The history should also note previous breast problems, including breast pain, palpable or mammographic abnormalities, and previous biopsies or cyst aspirations. The date of the last screening mammogram should be noted.

Breast Cancer Risk Factors

Risk factors for breast cancer that should generally be asked about during the history are listed in Box 18-1.

Breast cancer risk may be increased by hormonal and reproductive factors including early menarche (age 11 years or younger), late menopause (age 55

Box 18-1 Established Risk Factors for Breast Cancer

- Older age
- Previous history of breast, ovarian, or endometrial cancer
- History of atypia or CIS on breast biopsy
- Family history of breast cancer
- Hormonal and reproductive factors (e.g., early menarche, late menopause, nulliparity, late first childbirth, elevated endogenous estrogen levels)
- Alcohol use
- Obesity
- Sedentary lifestyle

or older), nulliparity, late age at first live birth (after age 30 years), or use of exogenous hormones (1) (see section on Exogenous Hormones and Breast Cancer Risk later in this chapter).

Breast cancer risk is increased by a positive family history of breast or ovarian cancer. Several breast cancer risk genes have also been identified, including *BRCA1*, *BRCA2*, the Li-Fraumeni syndrome gene p53, and the Cowden disease gene *PTEN*. Familial risk is greatest in the setting of multiple affected relatives, relatives with early onset breast or ovarian cancer, and in families with bilateral breast cancer. Both maternal and paternal sides of the family are now recognized to be relevant in assessing breast cancer risk.

Risk is also increased in women who themselves have had a previous breast, ovarian, or endometrial cancer. Women who have breast biopsies showing histologic findings such as lobular carcinoma in situ (LCIS), atypical ductal hyperplasia, or atypical lobular hyperplasia are also at increased risk. Previous radiation treatments to the breast or chest wall increase the risk of breast cancer, particularly if administered during the teenage years. Hodgkin disease survivors who received mantle irradiation, particularly as teenagers, are now recognized to have significantly increased breast cancer risk (2,3).

Fibroadenomas are benign breast tumors that may also increase subsequent breast cancer risk two- to fourfold, but only when either the histologic findings are complex, adjacent proliferative disease is present, or the patient has a family history of breast cancer (4). It should be emphasized that two thirds of women with benign breast disease do not have these concurrent factors, and their risk is not increased.

Dietary and lifestyle factors are also recognized to have an impact on breast cancer risk. Alcohol intake is associated with an increased risk of breast cancer (5), with a clear increase in breast cancer risk evident beginning with two or more drinks per day. Interestingly, a recent analysis from the Nurses' Health study demonstrated that adequate folate intake can mitigate the effects of large quantities of alcohol on breast cancer risk (6). Although some studies have shown a weak association between higher dietary fat intake and breast cancer risk (7), the majority of studies have failed to detect such a link (8-12). However, obesity, particularly weight gain during middle age (12a), as well as a sedentary lifestyle (13), do appear to be associated with increased breast cancer risk. Although previously there was concern that the use of calcium channel blockers may be associated with an increased risk of breast cancer (14), further review has failed to demonstrate this (15).

Elevated endogenous estrogen levels have been correlated with an increased risk for breast cancer, even when controlling for body mass index (BMI) (16). Related to this finding is the observation that women in the highest quartile of bone mass in the Framingham Study had a threefold increased risk of breast cancer (17).

Lastly, increasing age is an important risk factor for breast cancer. Although breast cancer does occur in young women, nearly half of all new breast cancer cases are diagnosed in women age 65 years and older.

Physical Examination

Physical examination of the breasts includes inspection of the skin, palpation of the breasts, examination of the nipples for discharge, and palpation of the axillary and supraclavicular lymph node areas. The breasts should be inspected with the patient sitting with her hands behind her head and her elbows back to look for asymmetry, dimpling of the skin, and any areas of erythema or edema. The breasts should then be palpated in a systematic fashion with the patient supine and sitting, and tissue should be examined from the clavicle to below the inframammary fold, and from the sternum to the posterior axillary line, taking care to include the subareolar area. If an abnormal area is identified, a careful description of its size, contour, texture, tenderness, and position should be recorded. A diagram of the location of any abnormality noted is extremely useful for future reference.

The nipples and areolae are best examined with the patient in the supine position, first inspecting for any areas of skin breakdown, then squeezing gently to check for discharge.

The axillary nodes lie beneath the hair-bearing skin of the axilla and are examined by the physician pressing his or her fingers inward and upward to check for enlarged nodes. Supraclavicular nodes may be examined with the patient in the supine or sitting position. If any enlarged nodes are discovered, their size, mobility, and number should be recorded. Tenderness of enlarged nodes, which may be more suggestive of a reactive process, should be noted.

Breast Imaging Studies

Many breast problems may require the use of imaging studies for evaluation. Mammography, ultrasonography, and, increasingly, breast magnetic resonance imaging (MRI) are useful in characterizing breast lesions.

Mammography

Mammography is the primary screening imaging modality in the evaluation of breast problems (Figs. 18-1 to 18-6). Masses may be identified and their contour and density, and the presence of microcalcifications determined. It has been suggested that mammography is appropriate in the work-up of a breast problem in women older than 35 years (18), and may be used at an earlier age for breast problems in younger high-risk women.

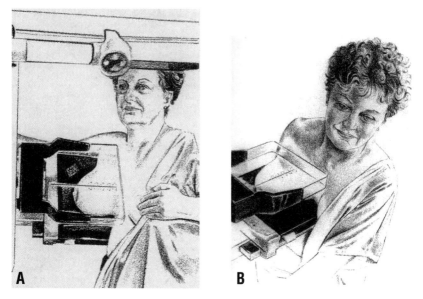

A   B

Figure 18-1 Standard screening mammography includes two views of each breast. *A,* Positioning of the woman for the mediolateral oblique (MLO) view. This view is particularly important because it includes all of the upper outer quadrant and axillary tail. The upper outer quadrant is the most common location for malignancy. *B,* Positioning of the woman for the craniocaudal (CC) view. The CC view is superior to the MLO view in imaging the medial aspect of the breast and overall provides better detail because greater compression of the breast tissue is possible. (From Bassett L. Breast imaging. In: Bland KI, Copeland EM III, eds. The Breast: Comprehensive Management of Benign and Malignant Diseases. Philadelphia: WB Saunders; 1998:648; with permission.)

Despite the overall value of mammography in the evaluation of breast problems, it must be remembered that 10% to 15% of palpable breast cancers are not visualized by mammography. In such cases, the cancer either is not producing calcifications or is a density that is not radiographically different than surrounding normal breast tissue. For this reason, a negative mammogram does not eliminate the need for biopsy of a palpable breast abnormality. Inappropriate reliance on a negative mammogram can result in delays in the diagnosis of a breast malignancy.

Because 10% to 15% of palpable breast cancers are not detected by mammography, a negative mammogram does not eliminate the need for biopsy of a palpable breast abnormality.

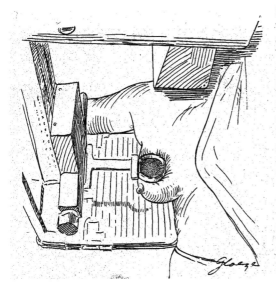

Figure 18-2 Spot compression view. When a mammographic abnormality is detected, additional views may be requested, most commonly the spot compression view. This may be performed in any projection and is often combined with magnification. Focal compression allows for greater detail of the area of concern and may displace overlying tissue that can obscure a lesion. (From Bassett L. Breast imaging. In: Bland KI, Copeland EM III, eds. The Breast: Comprehensive Management of Benign and Malignant Diseases. Philadelphia: WB Saunders; 1998:648; with permission.)

Ultrasonography

Ultrasonography is a confirmatory rather than screening modality useful in determining whether a lesion identified by physical examination or mammography is cystic or solid, and to better define its size, contour, and internal texture. However, ultrasonography cannot detect calcifications, may fail to detect some breast masses, and may misinterpret irregularities in normal breast texture as masses. As is the case for mammography, a negative sonogram result does not eliminate the need for biopsy of a palpable mass.

Magnetic Resonance Imaging and Other Imaging Modalities

Magnetic resonance imaging is a promising addition to breast imaging options. With gadolinium contrast, many malignant lesions enhance relative to normal breast parenchyma. Although some benign lesion such as fibroadenomas also enhance with gadolinium contrast, malignant lesions appear to enhance more rapidly and often to a greater extent.

The sensitivity and specificity of MRI in distinguishing benign from malignant lesions is still being defined. At present its main approved use is to detect leaks in silicone breast implants, where it can identify the ruptured silicone membrane within the silicone gel. Magnetic resonance imaging is also proving useful in identifying occult primary tumors in women presenting with palpable axillary nodes and no palpable or mammographically identified primary breast lesion. In addition, MRI appears to be effective in assessing the

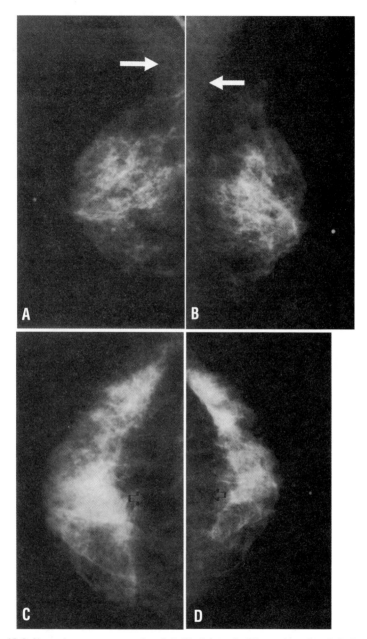

Figure 18-3 Normal mammogram. *A* and *B,* Mediolateral oblique view. *C* and *D,* Craniocaudal view. Left and right views are placed side by side to allow direct comparison and assessment of symmetry. The BB bullet marks the location of the nipple and thereby provides a consistent landmark between images and in certain settings prevents misinterpretation of the nipple as a mass. Note that breast tissue is normally denser in the upper quadrants than in the lower; the area of least density represents retroglandular fat (best seen on the CC view and marked by the open black arrows). A stripe of pectoralis muscle (*white arrows*) should be included in the MLO image to confirm adequate depth of the view.

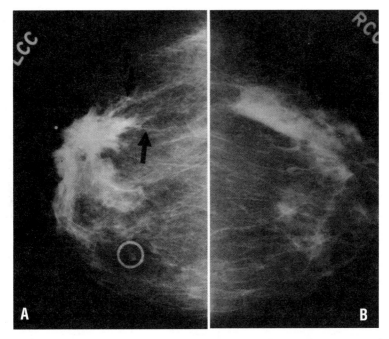

Figure 18-4 Craniocaudal view of a classic spiculated mass. Diagnostic mammography of the left breast was performed for a palpable mass; views of the contralateral breast were performed for comparison purposes and to detect synchronous lesions. The location of the palpable mass was marked with a BB bullet placed on the skin by the technologist. This advanced mass with large radiating spiculations (*arrows*) was ultimately determined to be an infiltrating ductal carcinoma. The circle marker denotes the site of a mole on the skin surface.

extent of vaguely defined tumors, in identifying unsuspected multifocal disease, and in helping to identify patients who are not eligible for breast-conserving surgery. Magnetic resonance imaging can also distinguish locally recurrent tumor from surgical scarring and radiation change after lumpectomy and radiation, although it does not provide reliable readings until 18 months or more after completion of surgery or radiation therapy. The utility of MRI in screening young, high-risk women with mammographically dense breast tissue is being explored.

Nuclear medicine studies such as sestimibi scintimammography and positron-emission tomography (PET) scanning remain primarily investigational tools. Currently neither thermography nor xerography has a role in the evaluation of breast problems.

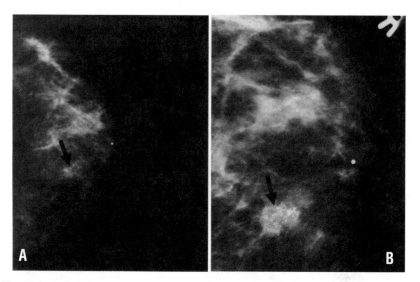

Figure 18-5 Craniocaudal view (*A*) and magnification (*B*) of clustered calcifications (*arrows*) in the right breast: The tight grouping and varying size and shape of the calcifications are features suspicious for malignancy. Magnification view confirms the pleomorphic appearance and highlights the underlying dense mass as well. Pathology ultimately revealed infiltrating ductal carcinoma.

Common Breast Problems

Palpable Abnormalities

Palpable breast lesions include discrete palpable masses, vague thickenings, and generalized nodularity. Discrete masses (i.e., those clearly distinguishable from surrounding normal breast tissue) may be solid or cystic. Clinical examination is not accurate in distinguishing a cyst from a solid mass. Rosner and Baird found that physical examination correctly identified only 58% of 66 palpable cysts (19).

Cysts

If a palpable mass is suspected to be a cyst, aspiration should be used to confirm this, even if the mass was previously shown to be a simple cyst by ultrasonography (Fig. 18-7). Aspiration confirms that the palpable mass corresponds to the lesion seen on ultrasonography and allows a more thorough examination of the surrounding breast tissue.

One should generally attempt to aspirate a breast cyst only when confident that the lump is truly cystic, which is usually ascertained either by ul-

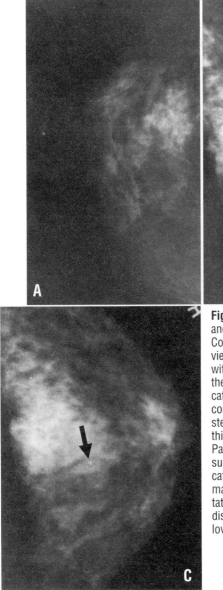
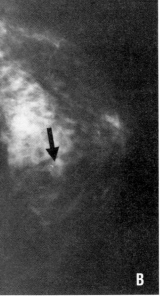

Figure 18-6 Asymmetric tissue and microcalcifications. *A* and *B*, Comparison of left and right CC views helps identify a focal density with associated calcifications in the right breast (*arrow*). Magnification view of right breast (*C*) confirms the findings, and several stereotactic-guided biopsies of this density were performed. Pathology revealed benign tissue—fibrous mastopathy. Calcifications are a common finding on mammograms and, when punctate (small and round) and widely dispersed, they can often be followed with serial mammograms.

trasonography or by patient history of previous aspiration in the same location. The procedure is preceded by a sterile prep. Local anesthesia is avoided because the resulting wheal obscures the location of the cyst. Nonetheless, because a fine-gauge needle is used, most patients tolerate this procedure well.

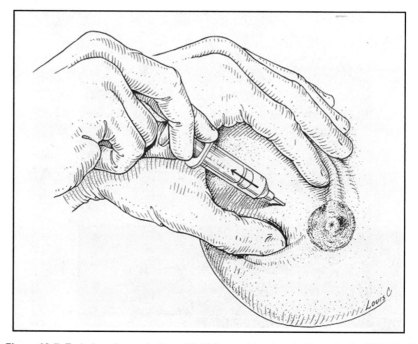

Figure 18-7 Technique for aspiration of fluid from a breast cyst. (From Souba WW, Bland KI. Indications and techniques for biopsy. In: Bland KI, Copeland EM III, eds. The Breast: Comprehensive Management of Benign and Malignant Diseases, vol 2, 2nd ed. Philadelphia: WB Saunders; 1991:809; with permission.)

The cyst is steadied between two fingers. With the other hand braced against the breast or chest wall, a 21-gauge needle is advanced until a change in resistance is felt as the needle traverses the cyst wall and then enters the lumen. The cyst is often deeper than it appears.

If the aspirated fluid is nonbloody and no palpable mass remains after aspiration, the fluid is discarded and cytologic analysis is unnecessary. Ciatto and colleagues found no malignancies among 6747 nonbloody cyst aspirations (20). Blood-stained fluid, on the other hand, suggests the presence of a papillary tumor in the wall of the cyst, which, while more commonly benign, may sometimes be malignant, particularly in older women. Likewise, persistence of a breast lump following aspiration suggests the possible presence of tumor. Both of these situations warrant cytologic analysis of the fluid (21) and biopsy of the mass. Biopsy is generally indicated in this setting even if the cytologic analysis is negative for malignancy.

A third situation for which these measures are undertaken is cyst recurrence. If a cyst is aspirated without previous ultrasound documentation that it was a simple cyst, the patient should be re-examined in 4 to 8 weeks. Fewer than 20% of simple cysts recur after a single aspiration, and fewer than 9% recur after two or three aspirations (22). When the same cyst recurs rapidly after aspiration, it should be reaspirated and the cyst contents sent for cytologic analysis. A biopsy should be performed if the results of the cytologic analysis are suspicious or if the cyst recurs after three successive aspirations. Appearance of a new cyst in a different area of breast tissue, however, does not require this additional work-up, and this cyst should be evaluated and aspirated as a new problem. Additional cysts may be expected in more than half of patients (23).

Solid Masses

Discrete masses within the breast that are solid, either by ultrasonographic criteria or by failing to yield fluid on an appropriately guided aspiration attempt, require a tissue diagnosis to exclude malignancy. Physical examination alone correctly identifies a mass as malignant in only 60% to 85% of cases (24,25), and experienced examiners will often disagree on the need for biopsy of a particular lesion. Boyd and colleagues found that four surgeons uniformly agreed on the need for biopsy of only 73% of 15 palpable masses later shown on biopsy to be malignant (24). Before biopsy, it is appropriate to order a mammogram for a woman older than age 35 to evaluate for synchronous lesions.

Options for biopsy of palpable lesions include fine-needle aspiration biopsy (FNA), core needle biopsy, and open surgical biopsy. Fine-needle aspiration using a 22- to 25-gauge needle may be performed with minimal patient discomfort at the time that a palpable mass is identified on physical examination. In interpreting results, it must be recognized that the false-negative rate of FNA ranges from 1% to 35% (25–27) for palpable lesions. An equivocal diagnosis, nonspecific findings such as normal or fibrocystic breast tissue (which suggests the area of concern may not have been sampled), or any atypical cytologic findings should generally be further evaluated with core needle or open surgical biopsy. The false-positive rate is generally in the 1% to 2% range but may be higher in some institutions (25,26).

Core needle biopsy obtains a 11- to 14-gauge cylinder of tissue from the mass being sampled and is analyzed by conventional pathologic analysis rather than by cytologic analysis (28). As with FNA, the false-positive rate is very low. This technique is more uncomfortable for the patient than FNA as it entails use of a much larger needle and requires that a small nick be made in the skin.

As is the case for FNA, the finding of atypia or any equivocal diagnosis on core biopsy requires open surgical biopsy to rule out malignancy. Core biopsy findings that are discordant with the clinical or mammographic appearance of the lesion should be viewed with suspicion and followed with open surgical biopsy.

For patients who choose or require open surgical biopsy, the standard approach is outpatient biopsy under local anesthesia with or without sedation. In excising the lesion, the surgeon should strive to excise the lesion with a narrow rim of normal-appearing breast tissue.

Vague Thickening or Nodularity

Normal breast texture is often heterogeneous, particularly in premenopausal women. These variations in texture may create areas that feel firmer to palpation than the surrounding tissue, and may or may not be tender. Such areas are of particular concern because it may be difficult to rule out a malignancy such as lobular carcinoma, which produces only a vague mass.

In evaluating an area of concern, the examiner should first compare it with the corresponding area of the opposite breast for symmetry. Symmetric areas of thickening are rarely pathologic. Asymmetric areas, particularly those that are tender, often represent fibrocystic disease and frequently resolve spontaneously. To avoid unnecessary biopsies, such vague areas occurring in premenstrual women should be re-examined after one or two menstrual cycles. If the asymmetry resolves, the finding was most likely due to a benign process, and the patient may return to routine follow-up. Areas of asymmetry that persist, however, must be viewed with some suspicion. Such patients should be referred to a surgeon for evaluation and potential biopsy. It is appropriate to order a mammogram at this point to rule out synchronous lesions in a woman older than 35 years who has not had a mammogram within the past 6 months. Fine-needle aspiration biopsy is generally not appropriate in this setting as tumors that produce only vague masses often have intermingled normal tissue and sampling error can be high. Open surgical biopsy is generally required for adequate sampling to rule out malignancy.

Breast Pain

Breast pain is one of the most common breast symptoms experienced by women, and causes many women to visit their physicians for medical care (29-31). Usually it is concern that the pain is indicative of a serious condition such as breast cancer that motivates the visit. Physiologic breast tenderness varies with the menstrual cycle, with greatest tenderness immediately before the menstrual period, or for some women, mid-cycle. Noncyclic pain may also be observed. The pain may be intermittent or continuous and is often described by the patient as "burning". The pain may be diffuse or primarily in a localized area, and may be asymmetric.

Although breast pain is poorly understood, its cyclic nature and its resolution at menopause suggest a hormonal cause. Several studies have measured circulating estrogen levels in women with breast pain and have found no difference compared with pain-free controls. It has been postulated that progesterone levels may be decreased in women with breast pain, and that the relative balance of estrogen and progesterone influences breast pain. It has also been suggested that thyroid hormones may influence breast pain, based on the observation that the administration of thyrotrophin-releasing factor resulted in a marked increase in prolactin release in a large group of women with breast pain compared with asymptomatic controls (32).

Although breast pain is only rarely caused by breast cancer, evaluation of the patient first requires that malignancy be ruled out. A careful physical examination should be performed and any palpable masses present evaluated as described above. One recent study of 987 patients who presented with breast pain without palpable abnormalities found the incidence of malignancy (0.4%) detected by mammography to be no higher than that seen in the asymptomatic control group referred for routine screening mammography (33). Nonetheless, mammography is generally performed in any woman older than 35 years with persistent, noncyclic breast pain—particularly if the pain is asymmetric—because it is the standard of care and often provides the patient additional reassurance.

It is also important to rule out causes of pain that do not arise from the breast itself, including muscle strain, costochondritis, and pain of pleural or mediastinal origin. Once these less common causes of pain are excluded, efforts should be directed at symptom management.

For the majority of women presenting with breast pain, reassurance that the work-up has shown no evidence of breast cancer or other serious abnormality is the only treatment necessary. The patient may also be reassured that breast pain is usually self-limited, most often resolving within a few months. During the periods of more severe breast tenderness, symptomatic relief may usually be obtained with the use of non-narcotic analgesics, in particular, nonsteroidal anti-inflammatory agents. Lifestyle changes such as elimination of caffeine, chocolate, or salt from the diet, while harmless, are of no proven benefit.

Other remedies may be helpful in women with significant breast pain. Evening primrose oil, one or two capsules taken orally twice per day, has been reported to produce significant or complete pain relief in half of women with cyclic mastalgia (34). This oil, obtained from the evening primrose flower, is high in polyunsaturated oils and may have some prostaglandin-inhibiting effects. Vitamin E at 400 to 800 I/U daily and vitamin B$_6$ at 50 I/U daily also reduces breast pain in some women.

It is advisable to re-examine the patient with new symptoms of breast pain after one or two menstrual cycles to be sure that no palpable abnormality is evolving and to assess her response to conservative treatment. For the rare patient whose breast pain is severe and unresponsive to conservative measures, hormonal pharmacologic therapy may be instituted. Agents that have been used to treat breast pain include danazol (weak androgen analog) (35,35a), bromocriptine (prolactin antagonist), and tamoxifen (estrogen antagonist) (36,37). It should be emphasized that such measures are only very rarely required, and for pain of this severity it would be appropriate to consult a breast specialist.

Nipple Discharge and Other Nipple and Areola Pathology

Discharge may be expressed from the nipples of as many as 60% to 70% of healthy women (38). Physiologic nipple discharge is usually bilateral, appears from multiple ducts, is yellow to green in color, and is produced only with active attempts to express it. This is to be distinguished from galactorrhea, which is a milky discharge that is bilateral and often spontaneous. Galactorrhea, which is almost never caused by a breast malignancy, may be distinguished from physiologic discharge under the microscope by the presence of fat. As many as one third of women with galactorrhea have pituitary tumors, particularly if there is associated amenorrhea. Other causes of galactorrhea include hypothyroidism, chest wall trauma, and

Physiologic nipple discharge is yellow to green in color, is usually bilateral, and is extruded from multiple ducts only with active expression. Galactorrhea, in contrast, is a bilateral milky discharge, often spontaneous, that contains fat droplets when viewed under a microscope. Pathologic nipple discharge is most often unilateral, spontaneous, sometimes bloody, and necessitates that malignancy be excluded.

certain pharmacologic agents. The evaluation of galactorrhea includes measurement of serum prolactin levels and thyroid function tests. If the prolactin level is elevated, an MRI scan of the head should be performed to rule out a pituitary adenoma.

Pathologic nipple discharge is most often unilateral and spontaneous and may be bloody. Although the most common cause of pathologic nipple discharge is a papilloma or other benign process, such discharge may also indicate malignancy and should be evaluated further (39-41). A mammogram should be performed in the evaluation of pathologic nipple discharge for any woman older than 35 years.

Careful physical examination should be performed to identify any palpable masses present. The position of the duct from which discharge is obtained should be documented. Of most concern is spontaneous, single duct discharge, or any discharge that is bloody.

Cytologic analysis of a suspicious nipple discharge is rarely helpful, because surgical evaluation is required even if the cytologic findings are negative. Ductograms are likewise generally not useful, as they rarely provide data that influence the type of surgical procedure performed. Excision of the duct from which the discharge is arising is performed to rule out malignancy (42,43).

Erosion or chronic crusting of the nipple raises the suspicion of Paget's disease of the nipple, a variant of infiltrating or intraductal carcinoma that arises in the terminal ducts to involve the surface of the nipple itself. A biopsy is required to distinguish Paget's disease from benign lesions (e.g., nipple adenomas) or dermatologic conditions (e.g., eczema) that may also involve the nipple and areola.

Breast Infections

Infections of the breast fall into two general categories, lactational infections and chronic subareolar infections associated with duct ectasia.

Infections and abscesses may occur during lactation, particularly during periods of weaning or engorgement. Early-stage infections are treated with oral antibiotics that cover gram-positive cocci, application of warm soaks, and active attempts to keep the breast emptied. Weaning is not necessary during treatment of these early infections, and the infant is not adversely affected by nursing from the breast with the infection (44,45). Once an abscess forms, however, surgical drainage and weaning are usually required. Recurrent infections during lactation are thought to arise from repeated colonization of the nipple by the nursing infant, and in this setting weaning is necessary.

Lactational abscesses rarely form fluctuant masses owing to the network of fibrous septae within the breast (44). Therefore the diagnosis of abscess is established by the presence of fever, leukocytosis, and point tenderness in the breast. Breast abscesses are typically multiloculated, and usually require surgical drainage under general anesthesia. The cavity should be packed open as for any abscess, and weaning is required.

In women who are not lactating, the subareolar ducts of the breast may develop a chronic relapsing form of infection variously known as periductal mastitis or duct ectasia. This condition appears to be associated with smoking and diabetes (43). The infections are most often mixed infections of both aerobic and anaerobic skin flora (46,47). A series of infections result in inflammatory changes and scarring and may lead to retraction or inversion of the nipple, masses in the subareolar area, and occasionally, in a chronic fistula from the subareolar ducts to the periareolar skin (43,48). Palpable masses and mammographic changes mimicking carcinoma may result.

Periductal mastitis initially presents with subareolar pain and mild erythema. If treated at this early stage, warm compresses and oral antibiotics alone may be effective. Antibiotic treatment is often unsuccessful unless anaerobe coverage is included as well as aerobic skin flora. If an abscess has developed, incision and drainage are required in addition to these antibiotics. Repeated infections are treated by excision of the entire subareolar duct complex after the acute infection has completely resolved, with intravenous antibiotic coverage during the perioperative period. Rarely, patients have recurrent infections requiring excision of the nipple and areola (42,49).

Breast Abnormalities in Pregnant or Lactating Women

Physical diagnosis of breast malignancy may be extremely difficult in women who are pregnant or lactating. Although engorgement or diffuse thickening of the breasts may be expected during pregnancy and lactation, distinct masses, asymmetric tissue, or any area of persistent concern to the patient should be evaluated, without waiting for delivery or the elective cessation of lactation. Such patients should be referred promptly to a surgeon for possible biopsy. Biopsy can be performed safely during pregnancy and lactation, and should not be postponed.

The causes of breast masses during pregnancy include all the common breast lesions of premenopausal women, including fibroadenomas, fibrocystic change, fibrosis, and occasionally breast carcinoma. Lactating adenomas are benign lesions that grossly resemble fibroadenomas that may also be seen during pregnancy.

Mammography is generally not performed during pregnancy, as much because of the increased density of breast tissue and resulting decreased mammographic sensitivity as for concern about radiation to the fetus. Mammographic sensitivity is also poor during lactation and for 3 to 4 months after cessation of breastfeeding. Ultrasonography may be useful in distinguishing cystic from solid palpable lesions and for evaluating contour and internal texture.

Abnormalities on Mammography

The use of screening mammography has led to an increase in the number of nonpalpable breast lesions identified. The majority of abnormal mammographic findings, however, represent benign abnormalities. Mammographers have developed a series of criteria by which they grade their degree of suspicion that a given mammographic finding represents a malignancy (20,50-53).

In an effort to minimize the number of biopsies with benign findings, short interval follow-up rather than biopsy is recommended for lesions judged to be "probably benign," with biopsy reserved for lesions that change and become more suspicious during follow-up. Sickles (54) reported prospective follow-up of 3184 consecutive probably benign mammographic abnormalities with a protocol for which repeat mammography was performed at 6 months after the initial finding, 6 to 12 months later, and then annually for two more examinations. Seventeen (0.5%) of these 3184 probably benign lesions subsequently proved malignant on biopsy. Two smaller series found 0.6% (55) and 1.1% (56) rates of malignancy in lesions detected on mammography that were followed as "probably benign". Using this procedure, these authors were able to eliminate several biopsies for which the findings would be benign, and as a result approximately 40% of the lesions that are ultimately recommended for biopsy proved to be malignant (54,56). These results support the balanced use of follow-up with mammography and biopsy to minimize the morbidity and the monetary and psychological costs of unnecessary biopsies that would otherwise be prompted by mammographic screening.

In the past open surgical biopsy with preoperative wire localization was required if biopsy of a nonpalpable lesion detected by mammography or ultrasonography was recommended. Nowadays, especially in settings where high-resolution stereotactic mammography is available, a biopsy of most nonpalpable lesions can be performed by a radiologist using core needle biopsy. This approach uses either stereotactic mammographic or ultrasound guidance and an 11- or 14-gauge core needle, and represents a less invasive and less costly alternative to open surgical biopsy (57-59). Certain lesions still require open surgical biopsy with preoperative wire localization, particularly those located near the skin surface or chest wall or consisting of poorly defined clusters of faint calcifications.

It is important for the ordering clinician to recognize the limitations of core biopsy to be able to correctly interpret its results. Even in skilled hands, core biopsy of a malignant lesion may yield false negative results. If the findings of the core biopsy are discordant with the mammographic findings (e.g., only benign breast tissue is identified after core biopsy of a suspicious, spiculated mass), the biopsy should be repeated or the patient referred for open surgical biopsy.

It must be recognized that pathologic interpretation of certain lesions may be difficult with core biopsy. The small tissue fragment size and potential distortion resulting from core biopsy makes the differentiation of atypia versus carcinoma *in situ* extremely difficult. The finding of atypia on core biopsy requires open surgical biopsy to rule out malignancy, with up to half of such subsequent open biopsies showing carcinoma *in situ*.

In most cases it is recommended that routine mammographic screening be resumed after the results of needle biopsy have proved to be benign. If enough uncertainty remains that 6-month follow-up mammography is recommended, it may be more appropriate to excise the lesion.

For patients who choose or require open surgical biopsy of a nonpalpable lesion, preoperative wire localization of the lesion using mammography or ultrasonographic guidance is required to direct the surgeon to the appropriate area. The surgeon then removes a piece of tissue around the wire in order to include the lesion with a rim of surrounding normal breast tissue, usually with the patient under local anesthesia. A specimen radiograph of the excised tissue is obtained before the patient leaves the operating room to be sure that the lesion is contained within the specimen.

Breast Cancer Screening

Early detection through screening remains the central focus of efforts to reduce breast cancer mortality. At present, three accepted screening modalities are used: mammography, clinical breast examination (i.e., physical examination by a skilled examiner), and breast self-examination (BSE).

Screening Mammography

Mammography can detect many cancers before they form a palpable mass. The long-term prognosis is more favorable for breast cancers detected by mammography alone (60), making mammography a central component of screening programs.

Ages 40 to 49 Years

Although there is general agreement that regular mammographic screening after the age of 50 years results in an approximately 30% reduction in breast cancer mortality (61), there has been considerable controversy about the value of screening mammography in women aged 40 to 49 years.

A 1993 National Cancer Institute meta-analysis of randomized breast cancer screening studies concluded that no benefit from mammographic screening occurred for women aged 40 to 49 at 5 to 7 years follow-up (61). A second NIH Consensus Conference on screening mammography was called in early 1997 to assess new data from ongoing screening studies (62). Ten- to twelve-year follow-up of ongoing Swedish studies was presented, with the Gothenborg and Malmo studies showing significant reductions in mortality in screened women aged 40 to 49. An overview combining these results with the results of other studies showed a 17% to 24% statistically significant reduction in mortality in women aged 40 to 49 who had undergone mammographic screening.

However, another meta-analysis of these and other trials concluded that mammography yielded no reduction in breast cancer mortality for women 40 to 49 years old (63). Careful review of the Swedish trials determined that the apparent mortality benefit often did not occur until 8 to 12 years into the trial, and was actually reflecting the outcome of mammography performed in women in their 50s who enrolled in their late 40s. Only the Canadian National Breast Screening Study 1 trial was designed specifically to test the effectiveness of screening mammography in women aged 40 to 49, and at 7-year follow-up was unable to detect a difference in mortality (64). This study, however, has been criticized for nonrandomization of the study population. It is to be hoped that completion of the Canadian trial, as well as of an ongoing British trial that is enrolling women 40 or 41 years old, may help resolve these conflicting findings and interpretations.

After review of data from the Swedish trials, the National Cancer Institute and the American Cancer Society recommended mammographic screening of women aged 40 to 49, with the American Cancer Society endorsing annual mammography in this age group. In contrast, the American College of Physicians—American Society of Internal Medicine and the Canadian Task Force on the Periodic Health Exam concluded that women younger than 50 should not undergo screening mammography. The NIH Consensus Conference chose an unusual intermediate position, stating that although the data were not compelling enough to recommend screening for women aged 40 to 49, each woman should be provided information to decide for herself whether to undergo screening mammography (65).

Screening mammography in women younger than 50 years is fraught with problems. Because younger women's breasts are more radiographically dense, mammography is less specific. Consequently, a higher proportion of false-positive findings occur, such that it is estimated that nearly one third of women who undergo annual screening beginning at age 40 years will have a mammogram yielding abnormal results and requiring further evaluation over the course of the decade (65). Another problem with screening in this age group is that ductal carcinoma in situ is frequently diagnosed in women undergoing screening mammography in their 40s but little is understood regarding its natural history, clinical significance, or treatment (65). The morbidity and psychosocial consequences stemming from the higher number of false-positive mammographic findings must be taken into consideration when assessing the value of this screening test.

Conversely, because of the higher diversity of breast tissue in younger women, mammography also has a lower sensitivity for detecting carcinoma. In addition to this decreased specificity and sensitivity of mammography in younger women, the relatively low incidence of breast cancer in women aged 40 to 49 years and its more aggressive behavior in this age group make mammography far less cost effective for these patients than for women aged 50 to 69 years (estimated $105,000 per year of life saved in contrast to $21,400) (66).

On the other hand, some authors point out the number of women whose deaths from breast cancer may be prevented through mammographic screening in their 40s and argue that obstacles such as poor cost effectiveness be addressed by taking measures to reduce the charges associated with mammography. Such proponents of mammography for women in their 40s have also recently begun suggesting a fairly frequent screening interval of 1 to $1\frac{1}{2}$ years to help improve efficacy by decreasing the number of "interval cancers" (67).

Other authors point out that the incidence of breast cancer approximately doubles from the age group of 40 to 44 years to the age group of 45 to 49 years (65). Still others note that at the time of menopause, both the sensitivity and specificity of mammography improve, and that perhaps a woman's reproductive stage should influence the timing of initiating mammography rather than an arbitrary age. Some have proposed that the patient be informed of the harms and benefits of screening before age 50 years and take an active role in the decision process (68). Certainly, an individual's risk factors for breast cancer should influence the initiation and frequency of screening mammography (see the section on Management of the Usual High-Risk Patient later in this chapter).

In summary, for women between the ages of 40 and 49 years, there are proponents of various mammography regimens ranging from no screening to annual mammography (Table 18-1). It is hoped that forthcoming data from ongoing trials will help clarify recommendations.

It should be noted that baseline mammography at age 35 years is no longer recommended.

Ages 50 to 70 Years

Mammographic screening is recommended after the age of 50 years, with nearly all analyses demonstrating a 30% reduction in breast cancer mortality in women who receive screening compared with those who do not. Most groups that issue screening guidelines advocate annual mammographic screening after the age of 50 years, although some state that every other year is sufficient and health insurance coverage may only allow for screening every other year.

Ages over 70 Years

An upper age limit for screening has not been defined. Very few women over the age of 70 have been included in screening trials, but the annual incidence of breast cancer increases with increasing age and breast tissue density decreases, reducing the number of false-negative and false-positive readings. Because of comorbidities in this age group, the cost effectiveness of mammography in terms of years of life saved decreases. However, for older women who are in sufficiently good health to tolerate lumpectomy under local anes-

Table 18-1 Recommendations for Screening Clinical Breast Examination and Mammography for Usual-Risk Women

	Recommendations	
Organization	Clinical Breast Examination	Mammography
American Cancer Society American Medical Association American College of Obstetricians and Gynecologists	Annually beginning at age 40	Every 1–2 years beginning at age 40, then annually beginning at age 50
American Academy of Family Physicians	Every 1–3 years at ages 30–39, then annually beginning at age 40	Annually beginning at age 50
American College of Physicians–American Society of Internal Medicine	Annually beginning at age 40	Every 2 years for women aged 50–74
Canadian Task Force on the Periodic Health Exam	Annually at ages 50–69	Annually at ages 50–69
National Cancer Institute	Annually beginning at age 50	Every 1–2 years beginning at age 50; offer patient option of screening in 40s

thesia, it seems reasonable to continue physical examination and mammographic screening.

Clinical Breast Examination

Although mammography can detect many breast cancers at an early stage (Fig. 18-8), as many as 10% to 15% of palpable breast malignancies are not visualized by mammography. These cancers do not produce calcifications or a density radiographically distinguishable from surrounding normal breast tissue. For this reason, clinical breast examination by a skilled examiner, usually a physician or a specially trained nurse, is the second component of most screening programs.

Annual physical examination by a health professional is recommended after age 40 years, although some groups would lower this age to 35 years or younger (see Table 18-1). Many consider it reasonable to include examination of the breasts in any general physical examination of a woman older than age 30 years.

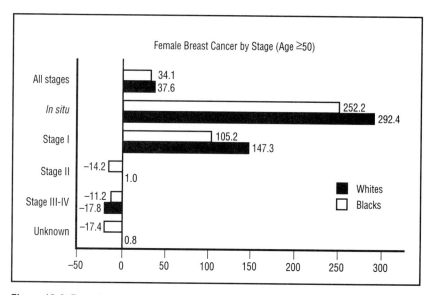

Figure 18-8 From 1983 to 1995 in the United States detection of early-stage breast cancer increased while the incidence of later-stage disease decreased. This reflects the effect
of mammographic screening, which has been endorsed by many health groups since the
mid-1980s. Note that while the increase in the detection of early-stage disease was more
dramatic in blacks than whites, other data demonstrate that survival rates for blacks remain consistently lower than for whites, the reasons for which are not understood. (From
J Natl Cancer Inst. 1998;90:1429; with permission.)

Breast Self-Examination

Breast self-examination (BSE) is the third component of breast cancer
screening programs and is encouraged for all women as a low-risk, low-cost,
and potentially beneficial means to detect breast cancers. The individual
woman is instructed in systematic monthly self-examination to detect palpable abnormalities and is encouraged to report any abnormal findings to her
physician without delay. Although more than 40% of breast cancers are detected by the woman herself (69), there are nonetheless conflicting data about
the efficacy of BSE in reducing breast cancer mortality (70-72).

Self-examination may generate anxiety in some women who perceive
their breasts to be "lumpy" and become alarmed by the irregular texture of
normal breast tissue. Such concern responds well to education and reassurance that some nodularity is normal and that cancers produce hard, distinct
lumps that the woman will, in fact, be able to distinguish from her normal
breast tissue.

Barriers to Screening

Only a fraction of American women adhere to breast cancer screening guidelines. The most common reasons identified for failure to undergo screening are that the woman's physician did not recommend mammography, did not perform a clinical breast examination, or did not instruct the woman in breast self-examination. Physicians and other health care professionals who care for women must continue to address these deficiencies.

Patient factors also contribute to underuse of breast cancer screening programs. Many women incorrectly believe that they do not need to be screened unless they have a symptomatic breast problem. Other women refuse mammography because they fear the discomfort of mammography or are afraid that a lesion may be found. For uninsured and underinsured women, the costs of breast cancer screening may be a significant barrier. These patient-related barriers to screening must be addressed through patient education and reduction of financial obstacles.

Special Screening Situations

Patients Who Have Undergone Cosmetic Breast Surgery

Screening for breast cancer may be more difficult in women who have had cosmetic breast surgery. Reduction mammoplasty and mastopexy generally do not interfere with mammography or physical examination. However, women who have undergone breast augmentation require special mammogram views to minimize the volume of breast tissue obscured by the implant. At a minimum, such women should follow standard screening practices for their age group.

Physical examination is usually not greatly hampered by the presence of implants. Leakage or rupture of an implant can be identified as a change in the size or shape of the augmented or reconstructed breast on physical examination, or with variable success by ultrasonography, mammography, or MRI. Gross rupture is generally treated with replacement of the implant.

Currently no clinical evidence demonstrates that silicone implants increase the incidence of breast carcinoma (73,74). Also, follow-up studies have failed to confirm a link between silicone implants and any autoimmune disorder (75,76). It is generally not recommended that women with intact silicone implants in place have their implants removed.

Women at High Risk for Breast Cancer

IDENTIFICATION OF THE HIGH-RISK PATIENT

A woman's risk of breast cancer may be increased by any of several factors, including personal history of previous breast cancer, personal history of atypia on biopsy, family history of breast cancer, and mutation in a breast cancer susceptibility gene on genetic testing, among others. In practice, the degree of risk for an individual woman is usually estimated by clinical judgment after review of the patient's family history and personal risk factors (see Box 18-1). However, risk can also be calculated by application of mathematical models and rarely, when appropriate, through referral for genetic testing.

Several mathematical models may now be used for assessing breast cancer risk. The Gail model (Table 18-2) is particularly useful for women without a strong family history of breast cancer (77). Risk is calculated based on the patient's age at menarche, age at first pregnancy, first-degree relatives with

Table 18-2 Relative Risk of Breast Cancer According to the Gail Model*

Risk Factor		Relative Risk
Group A. Age of menarche, years		
≥14		1.00
12–13		1.10
<12		1.21
Group B. Woman's current age and number of breast biopsies		
Age <50 years		
0		1.00
1		1.70
≥2		2.88
Age ≥50 years		
0		1.00
1		1.27
≥2		1.62
Group C. Age at first term live birth, years, and number of first-degree relatives with breast cancer		
<20	0	1.00
	1	2.61
	≥2	6.80
20–24	0	1.24
	1	2.68
	≥2	5.78
25–29 or nulliparous	0	1.55
	1	2.76
	≥2	4.91
≥30	0	1.93
	1	2.83
	≥2	4.17

*Recommendations for use: Select one number each from risk factor groups A, B, and C. Multiply the three numbers together to get the summary relative risk.
Data from Gail MG, et al. Projecting individualized probabilities of developing breast cancer for white females who are being examined annually. J Natl Cancer Inst. 1989;1:1879-86.

breast cancer, number of previous breast biopsies, and the presence of atypical hyperplasia on previous biopsies. The Claus model (78) is most useful for women with a strong family history of breast cancer and calculates risk based on current age, first- and second-degree relatives with breast cancer, and age of onset in affected relatives.

Perhaps the most practical way to assess accurately an individual's 5-year and lifetime risk of breast cancer is the Breast Cancer Risk Assessment Tool. Developed by the National Cancer Institute in 1998, this computer program calculates a woman's risk in a few minutes based on her responses to seven risk factor questions. The floppy disk is available to clinicians by ordering online at http://cancertrials.nci.nih.gov or calling 1-800-4-CANCER. Women younger than 60 years with an estimated 5-year risk of breast cancer of 1.7% or higher have been deemed higher risk and may be considered candidates for chemoprevention (see Chemoprevention of Breast Cancer section later in this chapter).

GENETIC TESTING

The tumor-suppressor genes *BRCA1* and *BRCA2* were identified in 1994 and in 1996, respectively. Women who carry mutations of these genes are at high risk for breast cancer and are prone to developing the disease at a younger age. The cumulative risk of breast cancer in women with these mutations is approximately 3% by age 30 years, 50% by age 50 years, and 85% by age 70 years (79). Those carrying the *BRCA1* mutation are also at increased risk for ovarian cancer (see Chapter 13).

Contrary to popular lay opinion, *BRCA1* and *BRCA2* testing are not useful as a widespread screening method. Most cases of breast cancer are sporadic and unrelated. In the United States, only 10% to 15% of breast cancers are believed to be familial, and, of these, only one third are attributable to an inherited mutation in the *BRCA1* or *BRCA2* gene.

To illustrate, the incidence of *BRCA1* mutations in the non-Ashkenazi general population is rare (0.12%), but approximately 1% in Americans of Ashkenazi Jewish descent. In one recent study of 400 American women diagnosed with breast cancer, only 3.3% of white women and 0% of black women were carriers of *BRCA1* mutations. In this study, for those patients whose family histories included both breast and ovarian cancer, or who had at least four relatives affected by breast cancer, the prevalence of the *BRCA1* mutation rose significantly higher, to as high as 33% (79a).

Even most patients with a family history of breast cancer will be found not to have BRCA1 or BRCA2 mutations. Therefore the patient's family history currently remains the primary means by which one assesses increased familial risk.

Recommendations for referral for *BRCA1* and *BRCA2* genetic testing vary widely; however, familial factors to predict mutations were recently published. These include known *BRCA1* or *BRCA2* mutation in a family member, a family history of both breast and ovarian cancer, two or more relatives diagnosed with breast cancer before the age of 50 years, one or more relatives diagnosed with breast cancer before the age of 50 years and Ashkenazi ancestry, male relative with breast cancer, or ovarian cancer plus Ashkenazi ancestry (Box 18-2) (80). A family history of bilateral breast cancer is no longer considered an indication for genetic testing.

The decision to refer a patient for genetic testing must be made carefully and deliberately. Although the testing itself involves only phlebotomy for procurement of DNA from peripheral leukocytes, it is expensive (often exceeding $2600), generally is not covered by insurance, and it may take 6 weeks for results to become available. Pre- and post-test counseling are best provided by a genetics counselor. Informed consent must include understanding the limits of DNA testing (potential for false-positive and false-negative results, but more importantly the incomplete penetrance of these genes), and the potential for experiencing a wide range of emotional reactions. Even those who test negative may suffer survivor guilt. Also, although many states have begun to enact legislation regarding these issues, lack of confidentiality and health insurance and employment discrimination are potential outcomes. Ideally, affected relatives should first be tested for the *BRCA1* and *BRCA2* genes, and the index patient then tested only if their results are positive. Testing centers can be located by contacting http://cancernet.nci.nih.gov/genesrch.shtml or calling 1-800-4-CANCER (1-800-422-6237).

Those women found to be carriers of *BRCA1* and *BRCA2* mutations represent a special subset of high-risk patients; therefore surveillance would be ex-

---

Box 18-2 Family History Risk Factors for Carrying a *BRCA1* or *BRCA2* Mutation

- Known *BRCA1* or *BRCA2* mutation
- Breast and ovarian cancer
- Two or more family members under 50 years of age with breast cancer
- Male breast cancer
- One or more family members under 50 with breast cancer plus Ashkenazi ancestry
- Ovarian cancer plus Ashkenazi ancestry

From Armstrong K, Eisen A, Weber B. Assessing the risk of breast cancer. N Engl J Med. 2000;342:564-71; with permission.

pected to be more aggressive than that for other high-risk patients. A recent task force recommended that beginning between the ages of 18 and 21 years *BRCA1* and *BRCA2* mutations carriers perform monthly breast self-examination, and beginning between the ages 25 and 35 years undergo clinical breast examination annually or semi-annually as well as annual mammography (80a). Those patients with *BRCA1* mutations should also be offered aggressive ovarian cancer screening (see Chapter 13). These recommendations were based on expert opinion only, however, since the efficacy of such surveillance measures is unknown.

The same task force (80a) concluded that research is needed to study the efficacy of various interventions in this specific population. Because of insufficient data, they were unable to recommend for or against prophylactic surgery and could not comment on chemoprevention, but did recommended that such individuals be encouraged to seek care within research protocols. Although the effect of lifestyle modifications has not yet been studied in carriers of *BRCA1* or *BRCA2* mutations, the task force endorsed healthy diet, regular exercise, and avoidance of such carcinogenic agents as cigarettes.

Management of the Usual High-Risk Patient

There are three options for women at high risk for breast cancer: close surveillance, prophylactic mastectomy, or chemoprevention (81).

Close Surveillance

The option of close surveillance is that most often chosen. For women with a previous diagnosis of breast cancer, surveillance protocols are based on the stage of the initial tumor. For women with lobular carcinoma *in situ* (LCIS), atypical hyperplasia, or a family history of breast carcinoma, surveillance should include twice yearly physical examinations by a physician. Mammography should be performed annually after diagnosis of LCIS or atypia. For women with a family history of breast cancer, annual mammography should begin at least 5 years before the age at diagnosis of the youngest affected relative and no later than age 35 years. For women from families with a proven or suspected breast cancer syndrome, annual screening should begin 10 years earlier than the age at the time of diagnosis of the youngest affected relative (82).

> *For women with a family history of breast carcinoma, surveillance should include twice yearly clinical breast examination and annual mammography beginning at least 5 years before the age at diagnosis of the youngest affected relative but no later than age 35.*

Prophylactic Mastectomy

Because prophylactic mastectomy often leaves some residual breast tissue, it does not fully protect against the future development of breast cancer. However, a recent retrospective study of 639 high-risk women who had undergone prophylactic mastectomy found the procedure to be 90% effective in reducing the incidence of breast cancer compared with their sisters (82a). Even with the availability of immediate breast reconstruction this intervention is often unacceptable, however. Now that tamoxifen and other promising agents for reducing breast cancer risk are available, it is expected that even fewer high-risk women will opt for prophylactic mastectomy.

Chemoprevention

For some time, prospective randomized trials have shown that in women diagnosed with breast cancer tamoxifen can reduce the risk of a new contralateral breast cancer by nearly 40% to 47% (83,83a). More recently, the National Surgical adjuvant Breast and Bowel Project (NSABP) Tamoxifen Chemoprevention Trial (P-1 Study) examined the prophylactic effect of tamoxifen taken for 5 years in unaffected women at high risk for breast cancer (84). The study demonstrated a 49% reduction in the risk of invasive breast cancer—results so compelling that the study was stopped early to allow patients assigned to the placebo arm to switch to the active drug. Interestingly, tamoxifen reduced the incidence of estrogen receptor-positive but not receptor-negative breast cancers.

Women in the tamoxifen arm did demonstrate an increased rate of complications, including a 2.5-fold increased rate of endometrial carcinoma and a slight increase in risk of thromboembolic disease (deep venous thrombosis, pulmonary embolism, and possibly stroke). These side effects were seen primarily in women older than 50 years and at the low rates similar to those seen in women taking estrogen replacement therapy. An additional benefit of tamoxifen, however, was a 20% decrease in the incidence of fractures of the hip, radius, and spine. Tamoxifen had no effect on the incidence of coronary artery disease events.

Results of two other smaller trials that tested the efficacy of tamoxifen in the prevention of breast cancer failed to show a significant reduction of breast cancer incidence in women taking tamoxifen compared with those taking a placebo (85,86). However, these two studies had significant methodologic flaws and lacked the statistical power of the P-1 trial (87).

As a consequence of the findings of the P-1 study, tamoxifen has received FDA approval for use as a chemopreventive agent for breast cancer for high-risk women. Eligible women are those older than 35 years who have a risk of developing breast cancer over the next 5 years equivalent to that of a 60-year-old woman (a 1.7% chance). Previous history of lobular carcinoma *in situ* is also an automatic criterion. Risk can be assessed using the Gail model that takes into account patient age, race, age at menarche, age at first live birth, number of first-degree relatives with breast cancer, and previous biopsies, particularly those showing atypical hyperplasia (77). A clinician can determine an individual's risk using the NCI computer program. It should be noted that patients taking tamoxifen must use reliable contraception.

The Multiple Outcomes of a Raloxifene Evaluation (MORE) trial followed more than 7000 women with osteoporosis for a mean of 40 months and determined the effects of this selective estrogen receptor modulator, raloxifene (Evista), on several outcomes (88). One finding was a 76% reduction in the risk of invasive breast cancer during the 3 years of the treatment. As with tamoxifen, raloxifene reduced the risk of estrogen receptor-positive but not receptor-negative tumors.

For postmenopausal women at high risk for breast cancer, HRT is not recommended. However, SERMs may offer such women breast cancer chemoprevention.

Raloxifene also led to a similiar risk of thromboembolic disease (deep venous thrombosis, pulmonary embolism); however, unlike tamoxifen, raloxifene did not increase the risk of endometrial cancer. If longer follow-up confirms these early findings, raloxifene may be preferred over tamoxifen for breast cancer chemoprevention for women who have a uterus.

Another chemoprevention trial underway is the NSABP Study of Tamoxifen and Raloxifene (STAR) Trial. This study will eventually include 22,000 postmenopausal women at high risk for breast cancer and will compare the chemoprevention of tamoxifen and raloxifene (84). Interested patients can sign up for information by mail: NSABP, Box 21, Pittsburgh, PA 15261; by fax: (412) 330-4664; or online: http://www.nsabp.pitt.edu.

Other potential chemoprevention agents include other forthcoming selective estrogen receptor modulators (SERMs), retinoids, protease inhibitors, and new dietary modifications.

Exogenous Hormones and Breast Cancer Risk

Oral Contraceptives

Data suggest that overall there is no significantly increased risk of breast cancer among women who have used oral contraceptives. A meta-analysis of studies examining the possible influence of oral contraceptive use on breast cancer risk (89) found no increase in breast cancer risk among women who had used oral contraceptives when compared with nonusers. However, this analysis found a higher risk of premenopausal breast cancer in woman who had used oral contraceptives for a prolonged period of time before their first pregnancy (89,90). It has been suggested that some of this increased risk observed with prolonged oral contraceptive use before the first pregnancy may actually reflect a delayed first pregnancy or an early menarche, both of which are accepted independent risk factors for breast carcinoma.

Postmenopausal Hormone Replacement Therapy

Hormone replacement therapy (HRT) provides many benefits to postmenopausal women, relieving many of the troubling symptoms of menopause and having a favorable effect on bone density and probably the cardiovascular system as well (see Chapter 16). Recent evidence also suggests possible decreased colon cancer mortality (91) and preservation of cognitive function in older women (92).

In addition, a review of overall mortality among users and nonusers of postmenopausal hormone replacement showed a statistically significant decrease in mortality from all causes (relative risk, 0.80; $p < 0.0001$) among users of HRT. This benefit seemed to be derived mainly from a reduction in mortality from acute myocardial infarction (relative risk, 0.60; $p < 0.001$), but there was also a trend toward decreased mortality from other ischemic heart disease, stroke, and cancer of any type (93). The Nurses' Health Study also found significantly decreased overall mortality among current users of hormone replacement relative to nonusers, with a relative risk 0.63 overall, and a greater reduction for women with cardiac risk factors (94). Given that neither of these studies was a randomized controlled trial, however, all of these results must be considered carefully in light of the possibility that these purported benefits of HRT may actually be merely reflections of the "healthy user effect" or other confounders (see also Chapter 16).

Another important consideration is that HRT does carry attendant risks. It appears to slightly increase the risk of thromboembolic disease and, of more concern, may increase the risk of breast carcinoma.

Many but not all studies have detected a trend toward increased risk of breast cancer among women using HRT for 5 or more years. The Nurses' Health Study found a significant increase in breast cancer risk in current users of HRT, with a relative risk of 1.46 after 5 to 9 years of use (95). Relative risk of death from breast cancer was also similarly increased. A more recent study suggests that the inclusion of progesterone in the HRT regimen further increases the risk of breast cancer (96). Interestingly, increased risk of breast cancer is related to current but not past use of hormone replacement, because the risk returns to that of nonusers within 2 to 3 years of discontinuation of hormone replacement (97).

Meta-analyses have also detected an association between increased breast cancer risk and HRT. One analysis found an approximately 10% overall increase in breast cancer risk among women using HRT relative to nonusers (98). Another meta-analysis that included only studies that met select criteria found a relative risk of 1.3 for breast cancer among women using HRT for more than 15 years when compared with nonusers (99). A Swedish cohort study found that risk increased with duration of use and detected an increased risk of breast cancer after 9 years of HRT (100).

Although it appears that HRT probably increases the risk of breast cancer, some but not all studies have demonstrated that HRT use at the time of diagnosis might be associated with a decrease in breast cancer mortality. One recent study of over 2600 patients with breast cancer found that HRT use afforded protection that appears to wane over time. Among HRT users at the time of diagnosis of node negative disease, the rate ratios for breast cancer mortality compared with those of nonusers were 0.5 until 12 years following diagnosis and 2.2 thereafter (96). Proposed explanations include the possibility that HRT may somehow favorably affect the carcinogenic process, or that it may render the tumor more responsive to treatment. However, the authors acknowledge that several methodologic issues may have led to confounding results.

Recently reported data from the Iowa Women's Health Study of 37,105 women suggest that the use of HRT might be associated only with the less common histologic types of breast cancer, namely medullary, papillary, tubular and mucinous. These tumor types are less likely to metastasize to axillary lymph nodes and overall have a more favorable prognosis. Compared with nonusers, those women who had ever used HRT for 4 years or fewer had a relative risk of developing one of these unusual tumors of 1.81; for those women who had used HRT for more than 4 years, a relative risk of 2.65. No association was found between ever having used HRT and the more common, more aggressive breast cancers, namely ductal carcinoma *in situ* or invasive ductal or lobular carcinoma (101).

Data from the Breast Cancer Detection Demonstration Project, which is following 46,355 postmenopausal women, conflict with these findings, however, because it was found that HRT did increase the risk for lobular and ductal carcinomas (101a). This study also noted that the risk of breast cancer was higher with combined estrogen-progestin replacement than estrogen alone. This adverse effect of progesterone may possibly stem either from the fact that progesterone does not down-regulate estrogen or progesterone receptors in the breast, or from progesterone's effect in the breast of increasing the conversion of estrone to the more potent estradiol (101a).

Another component of this study was that the women were stratified by BMI. Interestingly, only leaner women (BMI $\leq$ 24 kg/m^2 or less) displayed an increased risk of breast cancer upon exposure to either form of HRT. A possible explanation is that heavier women already have higher levels of endogenous estrogen (due to the peripheral conversion of androgens), and the addition of exogenous estrogen had no further effect on breast cell proliferation, because it was already maximally stimulated (101a).

Aside from lean body mass, previous analysis has identified other subsets of patients with significantly increased risk for breast cancer with hormone replacement use. These include women who have a family history of breast cancer (relative risk, 3.4), or who are nulliparous (relative risk, 1.5), have benign breast disease (relative risk, 1.7), or whose first live birth was after age 30 (relative risk, 1.7) (99). It should be noted that other studies have not detected a significantly increased risk of breast cancer among women who take HRT and have a positive family history (102). In regard to this unresolved question, ACP-ASIM has in the past recommended against prescribing HRT in women with a family history of breast cancer (103), but it no longer has an official policy on this issue.

In summary, therefore, evidence is accumulating that postmenopausal HRT probably increases the risk of breast cancer. The increase in risk may be substantially higher for women with other breast cancer risk factors. On the other hand, observational studies suggest that HRT may possibly be associated with a significant reduction in mortality from all causes. In clinical practice, it would seem prudent to weigh the individual woman's cardiovascular and osteoporosis risks against her risks for breast carcinoma when making a decision about the use of postmenopausal estrogens. For postmenopausal women with multiple risk factors for breast carcinoma, or for those who are reluctant to increase their breast cancer risk, it may be prudent to attain cardiovascular and osteoporosis risk reduction through exercise, diet, and other non-hormonal pharmacologic means rather than through HRT. It is hoped that selective estrogen receptor modulators will some day reliably provide both cardiovascular and osteoporosis protection with no increase, and perhaps reduction, in breast cancer risk.

Hormone Replacement Therapy after Breast Cancer

Concerns about possible stimulatory effects of exogenous estrogens on occult breast metastases and about potential increased risk of new primary cancers have left many practitioners reluctant to prescribe HRT for women who have been treated for breast cancer. Only a few studies to date have directly addressed this question (104).

Treatment of Breast Cancer

Ten to twelve percent of American women will develop breast cancer at some time in their lives. Treatment options are increasingly being tailored to the specifics of an individual woman's situation, including her own preferences, and to the specific histopathology and other features of her tumor (105). The majority of women with breast cancer are eligible for breast-conserving surgery, with the option of immediate breast reconstruction open for many women who require or choose mastectomy. Radiation therapy is employed routinely after breast-conserving surgery for invasive breast cancers. New evidence suggests that chest wall radiation after mastectomy may improve survival in women with axillary node metastases (106,107). Adjuvant systemic therapy, chemotherapy, HRT, or a combination of these has been shown to provide significant improvement in survival in women with invasive tumors over 1 cm. or with axillary node metastases.

Summary

The primary care physician must be prepared to address many common breast problems that patients may bring to the office and take measures to exclude the diagnosis of cancer. If the process is determined to be benign, the disease process should be carefully communicated to the patient along with reassurance.

Breast cancer screening represents an important intervention proven to reduce mortality, and its underuse should be corrected. It is incumbent on the primary care physician to educate his or her patients of the benefits of breast self-examination, clinical breast exams, and mammography. Controversies surrounding the timing and frequency of mammographic screening will hopefully be resolved with the completion of ongoing trials.

Those patients at high risk for breast cancer deserve close surveillance and should be offered chemoprophylaxis, involvement in trials, or other interventions. Those at especially high risk for breast cancer due to genetic mutations for tumor suppressor genes should follow unique screening and intervention protocols.

Acknowledgments
The mammograms (Figs. 18-3 to 18-6) in this chapter are reproduced courtesy of David P. Smith, MD, Assistant Professor of Radiology, The Johns Hopkins University School of Medicine.

REFERENCES

1. **Henderson IC.** Risk factors for breast cancer development. Cancer. 1993;71(suppl): 2127-40.
2. **Aisenberg A, Finkelstein D, Doppke K, et al.** High risk of breast carcinoma after irradiation of young women with Hodgkin's disease. Cancer. 1997;79:1203-9.

3. **Bhatia S, Robison L, Oberlin O, et al.** Breast cancer and other second neoplasms after childhood Hodgkin's disease. N Engl J Med. 1996;334:745-50.

4. **Dupont WD, Page DL, Park FF.** Long-term risk for breast cancer in women with fibroadenoma. N Engl J Med. 1994;331:10-15.

5. **Smith-Warner SA, Spiegelman D, Yuan S-S, et al.** Alcohol and breast cancer in women: a pooled analysis of cohort studies. JAMA. 1998; 279:535-40.

6. **Zhang S, Hunter DJ, Hankinson SE, et al.** A prospective study of folate intake and the risk of breast cancer. JAMA. 1999;281:1632-7.

7. **Howe GR, Hirohata T, Hislop TG, et al.** Dietary factors and risk of breast cancer: combined analysis of 12 case-control studies. J Natl Cancer Inst. 1990;82:561-9.

8. **Willett WC, Stampfer MJ, Colditz GA, et al.** Dietary fat and the risk of breast cancer. N Engl J Med. 1987;316:22-8.

9. **Willett WC, Hunter DJ, Stampfer MJ, et al.** Dietary fat and fiber in relation to risk of breast cancer: an 8-year follow-up. JAMA. 1992; 68:2037-44.

10. **Knekt P, Albanes D, Seppanen R, et al.** Dietary fat and risk of breast cancer. Am J Clin Nutr. 1990;52:903-8.

11. **Jones DY, Schatzkin A, Green SB, et al.** Dietary fat and breast cancer in the National Health and Nutrition Examination Survey. I—Epidemiologic follow-up study. J Natl Cancer Inst. 1987;79:465-71.

12. **Mills PK, Beeson WL, Phillips RL, Fraser GE.** Dietary habits and breast cancer incidence among Seventh-Day Adventists. Cancer. 1989;64:582-90.

12a. **Huang Z, Hankinson SE, Colditz GA, et al.** Dual effects of weight and weight gain on breast cancer risk. JAMA.1997;278:1407-11, 1448-9.

13. **Thune I, Brenn T, Lund E, et al.** Physical activity and the risk of breast cancer. N Engl J Med. 1997;336:1269-74.

14. **Pahor M, Guralnick JM, Corti M-C, at al.** Calcium channel blockers and the incidence of cancer in aged populations. Lancet. 1996;348:493-7.

15. **Rosenberg L, Rao S, Palmer J, et al.** Calcium channel blockers and the risk of cancer. JAMA. 1988;279:1000-4.

16. **Thomas HV, Reeves GK, Key TJ.** Endogenous estrogen and postmenopausal breast cancer: a quantitative review. Cancer Causes Control. 1997;8:922-8.

17. **Zhang Y, Kiel DP, Kreger BE, et al.** Bone mass and the risk of breast cancer among postmenopausal women. N Engl J Med. 1997;336:611-7.

18. **Cady B, et al.** Evaluation of common breast problems: guidance for primary care providers. Cancer. 1998:48:49-63.

19. **Rosner D, Baird D.** What ultrasonography can tell in breast masses that mammography and physical examination cannot. J Surg Oncol. 1985;28:308-13.

20. **Ciatto S, Cariaggi P, Bulgaresi P.** The value of routine cytologic examination of breast cyst fluids. Acta Cytol. 1987a;31:301-4.

21. **Hamed H, et al.** Follow-up of patients with aspirated breast cysts is necessary. Arch Surg. 1989;124:253-5.

22. **Leis HP Jr.** Gross breast cysts: significance and management. Contemp Surg. 1991;39:13-20.

23. **Hughes LE, Bundred NJ.** Breast macrocysts. World J Surg. 1989;13:711-4.

24. **Boyd NF, et al.** Prospective evaluation of physical examination of the breast. Am J Surg. 1981;142:331-4.

25. **Layfield LJ, Glasgow BJ, Cramer H.** Fine-needle aspiration in the management of breast masses. Pathol Annu. 1989;24:23-62.

26. **Hammond S, et al.** Statistical analysis of fine-needle aspiration cytology of the breast: a review of 678 cases plus 4265 cases from the literature. Acta Cytol. 1987;31:276-80.

27. **Grant CS, et al.** Fine-needle aspiration of the breast. Mayo Clin Proc. 1986;61:377-81.

28. **Ballo MS, Sneige N.** Can core needle biopsy replace fine-needle aspiration cytology in the diagnosis of palpable breast carcinoma? A comparative study of 124 women. Cancer. 1996;78:773-7.

29. **Preece R, Mansel R, Bolton P.** Clinical syndromes of mastalgia. Lancet. 1976;2:670.

30. **Preece R, Mansel R, Hughes L.** Mastalgia psychoneurosis or organic disease? Br Med, 1978;1:29.

31. **Wisbey J, Mansel R, Pye J.** Natural history of breast pain. Lancet. 1983;2:672.

32. **Watt-Boolsen S, Eskildsen P, Blaehr H.** Release of prolactin, thyrotropin, and growth hormone in women with cyclical mastalgia and fibrocystic disease of the breast. Cancer. 1985;56:500.

33. **Duijm LEM, Fuit GL, Hendriks JHCL, et al.** Value of breast imaging in women with painful breasts: observational follow-up study. BMJ. 1998;317:1492-5.

34. **Pashby NL, et al.** A clinical trial of evening primrose oil in mastalgia, Br J Surg. 1981;68:801-5.

35. **Baker H, Snedecor P.** Clinical trial of danazol for benign breast disease. Am Surg. 1979;45:727.

35a. **Lauerson N, Wilson K.** The effect of danazol in the treatment of chronic cystic mastitis. Obstet Gynecol. 1976;48:93.

36. **Mansel R, Preece P, Hughes L.** A double-blind trial of the prolactin inhibitor bromocriptine in painful benign breast disease. Br J Surg. 1978;65:724.

37. **Fentiman IS, Caleffi M, Brame K, et al.** Double-blind controlled trial of tamoxifen therapy for mastalgia. Lancet. 1986;1:287-8.

38. **Petrakis NL.** Physiologic, biochemical, and cytologic aspects of nipple aspirate fluid. Breast Cancer Res Treat. 1986;8:7-19.

39. **Takeda T, et al.** Cytologic studies of nipple discharge. Acta Cytol. 1982;26:35.

40. **Chaudary M, et al.** Nipple discharge: the diagnostic value of testing for occult blood. Am J Surg. 1982;196:651.

41. **Devitt JE.** Management of nipple discharge by clinical findings. Am J Surg. 1985;149:789-92.

42. **Urban J.** Excision of the major duct system of the breast. Cancer. 1963;16:516-20.

43. **Passaro ME, et al.** Lactiferous fistula. J Am Coll Surg. 1994;178:29-32.

44. **Benson EA.** Management of breast abscesses. World J Surg. 1989; 3:753-6.

45. **Niebyl JR, Spence MR, Parmley TH.** Sporadic (nonepidemic) puerperal mastitis. J Reprod Med. 1978;20:97-100.

46. **Brook I.** Microbiology of nonpuerperal breast abscesses. J Infect Dis. 1988;157:377-9.

47. **Walker AP, et al.** A prospective study of the microflora of nonpuerperal breast abscess. Arch Surg. 1988;123:908-11.

48. **Smith BL.** Duct ectasia, periductal mastitis, and breast infections. In: Harris JR, et al, eds. Breast Diseases. Philadelphia: JB Lippincott; 1991.

49. **Hadfield J.** Excision of the major duct system for benign disease of the breast. Br J Surg. 1960;47:472-7.

50. **Hall FM, et al.** Nonpalpable breast lesions: recommendations for biopsy based on suspicion of carcinoma at mammography. Radiology. 1988;167:353-8.

51. **Moskowitz M.** The predictive value of certain mammographic signs in screening for breast cancer. Cancer. 1983;51:1007-11.

52. **Ciatto S, Cataliotti L, Distante V.** Nonpalpable lesions detected with mammography: review of 512 consecutive cases. Radiology. 1987;165:99-102.

53. **Sickles EA.** Mammographic features of 300 consecutive nonpalpable breast cancers. Am J Radiol. 1986;146:661-3.

54. **Sickles EA.** Periodic mammographic follow-up of probably benign lesions: results in 3184 consecutive cases. Radiology. 1991;179:463-8.

55. **Wolfe JN, et al.** Xeroradiography of the breast: overview of 21,057 consecutive cases. Radiology. 1987;165:305-11.

56. **Helvie MA, et al.** Mammographic follow-up of low-suspicion lesions: compliance rate and diagnostic yield. Radiology. 1991;178:155-8.

57. **Parker SH, et al.** Stereotactic breast biopsy with a biopsy gun. Radiology. 1990;176: 741-7.

58. **Ballo MS, Sneige N.** Can core needle biopsy replace fine-needle aspiration cytology in the diagnosis of palpable breast carcinoma? A comparative study of 124 women. Cancer. 1996;78:773-7.

59. **Meyer JE, Christian RL, Lester SC, et al.** Evaluation of nonpalpable solid breast masses with stereotaxic large-needle core biopsy using a dedicated unit. Am J Roentgenol. 1996;167:179-82.

60. **Bassett L, Liu T, Giuliano A, et al.** The prevalence of carcinoma in palpable versus impalpable mammographically detected lesions. Am J Roentgenol. 1991;157:21.

61. **Fletcher SW, et al.** Report of the International Workshop on Screening for Breast Cancer. J Natl Cancer Inst. 1993;85:1644-56.

62. NIH Consensus Statement. Breast Cancer Screening for Women Ages 40-49. Bethesda, MD: Office of Medical Application of Research. 1997;15:1-35.

63. **Elwood JM, Cox B, Richardson AK.** The effectiveness of breast cancer screening by mammography in younger women. Online J Curr Clin Trials. 25 February 1993; Document 32.

64. **Miller AB, Baines CJ, To T, Wall C.** Canadian National Breast Screening Study. 1— Breast cancer detection and death rates among women aged 40 to 49 years. Can Med Assoc J. 1992;147:1459-76.

65. NIH Consensus Statement. Breast Cancer Screening for Women Ages 40-49. J Natl Cancer Inst Monograph No. 22; 1997:vii-xii.

66. **Salzmann P, Kerlikowske K, Phillips K.** Cost-effectiveness of extending screening mammography guideline to include women 40 to 49 years of age. Ann Intern Med. 1997;127:955-65.

67. **Sickles EA, Kopans DB.** Deficiencies in the analysis of breast cancer screening data [Editorial]. J Natl Cancer Inst. 1993;85:1621-4.

68. **Sox HC.** Screening mammography in women younger than 50 years of age [Editorial]. Ann Intern Med. 1995;122:550-2.

69. **Osteen RT, et al.** 1991 national survey of carcinoma of the breast by the Commission on Cancer. J Am Coll Surg. 1994;178:213-9.

70. **Thomas DB, Gao DL, Self SG, et al.** Randomized trial of breast self-examination in Shanghai: methodology and preliminary results. J Natl Cancer Inst. 1997; 89:355-65.

71. **Foster RS, Worden JK, Costanza MC, et al.** Clinical breast examination and breast self-examination. Cancer. 1992;69:1992-8.

72. **Gastrin G, Miller AB, To T, et al.** Incidence and mortality from breast cancer in the Mama Program for breast cancer screening in Finland, 1973-1986. Cancer. 1994;73: 2168-74.

73. **Deapen DM, Brody GS.** Augmentation mammoplasty and breast cancer: a 5-year update of the Los Angeles study. Plast Reconstr Surg. 1992;89:660-5.

74. **Berkell H, Birdsell DC, Jenkins H.** Breast augmentation: a risk factor for breast cancer? N Engl J Med. 1992;326:1649-53.

75. **Brody GS, et al.** Consensus statement on the relationship of breast implants to connective-tissue disorders. Plast Reconstr Surg. 1992;90:1102-4.

76. Food and Drug Administration General and Plastic Surgery Devices Panel Meeting, 18-20 February 1992, Freedom of Information Services Documents 100714, 107031, and 107032.

77. **Gail MG, et al.** Projecting individualized probabilities of developing breast cancer for white females who are being examined annually. J Natl Cancer Inst. 1989;1:1879-86.

78. **Claus EB, Risch N, Thompson WD.** Autosomal dominant inheritance of early-onset breast cancer: implications for risk prediction. Cancer. 1994;73:643-51.

79. **Easton DF, Ford D, Bishop DT, and the Breast Cancer Linkage Consortium.** Breast and ovarian cancer incidence *BRCA1*-mutation carriers. Am J Hum Genet. 1995;56: 266-71.

79a. **Newman B, MuH, Butler LM, et al.** Frequency of breast cancer attributable to *BRCA1* in a population-based series of American women. JAMA. 1998;279:955-7.

80. **Armstrong K, Eisen A, Weber B.** Assessing the risk of breast cancer. N Engl J Med. 2000;342:564-71.

80a. **Burke W, Daly M, Garber J, et al.** Recommendations for follow-up care of individuals with an inherited predisposition to cancer . II. *BRCA1* and *BRCA2*. Cancer Genetics Studies Consortium. JAMA. 1997;277:977-1008.

81. **Cummings S, Olopade O.** Predisposition testing for inherited breast cancer. Oncology. 1998;12:1227-39.

82. **Lynch HT, Marcus JN, Watson P.** Familial breast cancer, family cancer syndromes, and predisposition to breast neoplasia. In: Bland KI, Copeland EM III, eds. The Breast: Comprehensive Management of Benign and Malignant Diseases. Philadelphia: WB Saunders; 1991.

82a. **Hartmann LC, Schaid DJ, Woods JE, et al.** Efficacy of bilateral prophylactic mastectomy in women with a family history of breast cancer. N Engl J Med. 1999;340:77-84.

83. **Fisher B, et al.** A randomized trial evaluating tamoxifen in the treatment of node-negative breast cancer women who have estrogen-receptor positive tumors. N Engl J Med. 1989;320:479-84.

83a. **Early Breast Cancer Trialists' Collaborative Group.** Tamoxifen for early breast cancer: an overview of the randomised trials. Lancet. 1998;351:1451-67.

84. **Fisher B, et al.** Tamoxifen for prevention of breast cancer: report of the National Surgical Adjuvant Breast and Bowel Project P-1 Study. J Natl Cancer Inst. 1998;90: 1371-88.

85. **Veronesi U, Maisonneuve P, Costs A, et al.** Prevention of breast cancer with tamoxifen: preliminary findings from the Italian randomised trial among hysterectomised women. Lancet. 1998;352:93-7.

86. **Powles T, Eeles R, Ashley S, et al.** Interim analysis of the incidence of breast cancer in the Royal Marsden Hospital Tamoxifen Randomised Chemoprevention Trial. Lancet. 1998;352:98-101.

87. **Pritchard KI.** Is tamoxifen effective in prevention of breast cancer? Lancet. 1998; 352:80-1.

88. **Cummings SR, Eckert S, Krueger KA, et al.** The effect of raloxifene on risk of breast cancer in postmenopausal women: results from the MORE randomized trial. JAMA. 1999;281:2189-97.

89. **Romieu I, Berlin JA, Colditz GA.** Oral contraceptives and breast cancer: review and meta-analysis. Cancer. 1990;66:2253-63.

90. **Wingo PA, et al.** Age-specific differences in the relationship between oral contraceptive use and breast cancer. Obstet Gynecol. 1991;78:161-70.

91. **Calle EE, Miracle-McMahill HL, Thun, MJ, et al.** Estrogen replacement therapy and risk of fatal colon cancer in a prospective cohort of postmenopausal women. J Natl Cancer Inst. 1995;87:517-22.

92. **Yaffe K, Sawaya G, Lieberburg I, Grady D.** Estrogen therapy in postmenopausal women: effect on cognitive function and dementia. JAMA. 1998;279:688-94.

93. **Henderson BE, Paganin-Hill A, Ross RK.** Decreased mortality in users of estrogen replacement therapy. Arch Intern Med. 1991;151:75-8.

94. **Grodstein F, Stampfer MJ, Colditz GA, et al.** Postmenopausal hormone therapy and mortality. N Engl J Med. 1997;336:1769-75.

95. **Colditz GA, Hankinson SE, Hunter DJ, et al.** The use of estrogens and progestins and the risk of breast cancer in postmenopausal women. N Engl J Med. 1995;332:1589-93.

96. **Schairer C, Gail M, Byrne C, et al.** Estrogen replacement therapy and breast cancer survival in a large screening study. J Natl Cancer Inst. 1999;91:264-70.

97. **Colditz GA, Stampfer MJ, Willett WC.** Prospective study of estrogen replacement therapy and risk of breast cancer in postmenopausal women. JAMA. 1990;264:2641-53.

98. **Dupont WD, Page DL.** Menopausal estrogen replacement therapy. Arch Intern Med. 1991;151:67-72.

99. **Steinberg KK, et al.** A meta-analysis of the effect of estrogen replacement therapy. JAMA. 1991;265:1985-90.

100. **Bergvist et al.** The risk of breast cancer after estrogen and estrogen-progestin replacement. N Engl J Med. 1989;321:293-9.

101. **Gapstur SM, Morrow M, Sellers TA.** Hormone replacement therapy and risk of breast cancer with a favorable histology. JAMA. 1999;281:2091-7.

101a.**Schairer C, Lubin J, Troisi R, et al.** Menopausal estrogen and estrogen-prostein replacement therapy and breast cancer risk. JAMA. 2000;283:485-91.

102. **Sellers TA, Mink PJ, Cerhan JR, et al.** The role of hormone replacement therapy in the risk for breast cancer and for mortality in women with a family history of breast cancer. Ann Intern Med. 1997;127:973-80.

103. **American College of Physicians.** Guidelines for counseling postmenopausal women about preventive hormone therapy. Ann Intern Med. 1992;117:1038-41.

104. **Marchant DJ.** Estrogen-replacement therapy after breast cancer. Cancer. 1993;71(suppl): 2169-76.

105. **Hortobagyi GN.** Treatment of breast cancer. N Engl J Med. 1998;339:974-82.

106. **Overgaard M, Jensen MB, Overgaard J.** Postoperative radiotherapy in high-risk post-menopausal breast cancer patients given adjuvant tamoxifen. Danish Breast Cancer Cooperative Group DBCG 82c randomized trial. Lancet. 1999;353:1641-8.

107. **Ragaz J, Jackson SM, Le N, et al.** Adjuvant radiotherapy and chemotherapy in node-positive premenopausal women with breast cancer. N Engl J Med. 1997;337:956-62.

CHAPTER 19

Preconception Care

GERDA ELLEN TAPELBAND, MD

Preconception counseling can be defined as patient education and health care delivered before conception in order to optimize pregnancy outcomes. Recent research has identified specific interventions which, if initiated before pregnancy, decrease congenital anomalies, low birth weight, fetal loss, and maternal complications. The United States ranks 24th in the world in infant mortality, has a major congenital defect rate of 3%, and a low birth weight rate of 7% (1), making this area worthy of public health concern.

Early organogenesis, the crucial stage of fetal development, begins 17 days after conception, a time when most women do not yet realize they are pregnant (Fig. 19-1). The health status of the mother at the time of conception (or even earlier) affects pregnancy outcome, especially in regard to certain exposures such as vitamin A and alcohol, and medical conditions such as diabetes. Moreover, 44.1% of pregnancies in the United States are unintended (2). The benefits of making interventions before conception are therefore obvious.

Preconception counseling can be most reliably provided as a component of health promotion in primary care, especially because many women now receive routine gynecologic care from their internist. Often a patient's first contact with an obstetrician-gynecologist is the first prenatal visit, which is typically at 8 to 10 weeks' gestation (and after the first trimester for 24.5% of women in this country) (3). Therefore the primary care provider should take the initiative. Annual exams, family planning visits, or negative pregnancy tests provide ideal opportunities for preconception counseling.

512

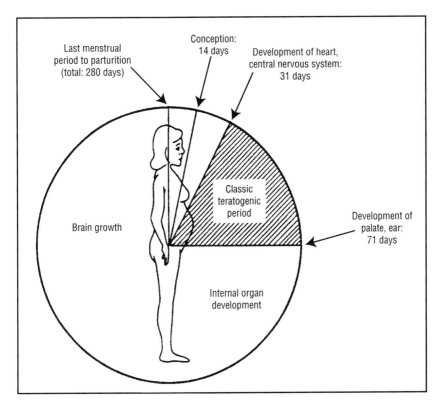

Figure 19-1 Teratogenic period. The importance of preconception care is well illustrated by the pregnancy clock because organogenesis begins 17 days after conception—so early that pregnancy is often yet unrecognized. Shortly thereafter, maternal-fetal transport of substances is established, and until the 10th week of gestation fetal organs are developing rapidly, making them particularly vunerable to substance exposure. Consequently, physicians have traditionally been most concerned about exposures occurring during the first trimester. However, recently it has been postulated that exposures occurring later in gestation may have adverse effects on the offspring's functions and behavior, entities more difficult to assess than anatomic defects. (From Blake DA, Niebyl JR. Requirements and limitations in reproductive and teratogenic risk assessment. In: Niebyl JR, ed. Drug Use in Pregnancy, 2nd ed. Philadelphia: Lea & Febiger; 1988:1-9; with permission.)

Nutrition

Folate and Multivitamins

One of the most important advances in the fight against birth defects has been the discovery of the protective effect of folic acid supplementation against neural tube defects (NTD) such as spina bifida and anencephaly. At present, approximately 4000 affected pregnancies occur yearly in this country.

Folate supplementation before pregnancy and during the first 6 weeks after conception has been shown to significantly decrease NTD in several observational and interventional studies. A Hungarian randomized controlled trial of 4200 women given either a multivitamin with 0.8 mg of folate or a trace element placebo found no NTD in the treatment group, compared with six cases in the placebo group (4). The protective effect is even more significant in women with a previous affected pregnancy. A British randomized controlled trial showed that 4.0 mg daily folate supplementation reduced the risk of subsequent NTD-affected pregnancy by 70% (5). Women with hemoglobinopathies or twin gestations or who take seizure medications also benefit from 4.0 mg daily. This higher dose should be implemented under physician supervision, however, because of the possibility of masking vitamin B_{12} deficiency.

The CDC concluded that folate supplementation could halve NTD rates and therefore recommends

- All women of childbearing age who are capable of becoming pregnant should consume 0.4 mg of folate daily.
- Women with previous NTD-affected offspring should take 4.0 mg of folate daily.
- Supplementation should begin 1 month before conception and continue approximately 3 months after conception.

As a measure to prevent NTDs, all enriched cereal grains sold in the United States as of January 1998 have been supplemented with folate. However, the amount may not be adequate and therefore the CDC's recommendations remain unchanged (6).

There are some data to suggest that the use of multivitamins in the preconception and early pregnancy periods decreases the risk of other congenital anomalies as well. In the Hungarian trial mentioned above, the women given multivitamins with folate had a relative risk (RR) of 0.6 for all congenital malformations (4). Additionally, several case control studies have shown a decreased risk of orofacial clefts and urinary tract anomalies in women taking multivitamins. Therefore one could improve on the CDC instruction by recommending a multivitamin that contains 0.4 mg of folate to all patients at risk for pregnancy.

Despite their public health importance, a 1997 survey showed

All women of child-bearing potential should take a daily multivitamin containing folic acid to decrease the risk of neural tube defects. Supplementation should begin 1 month before conception and should continue for approximately 3 months after conception.

that only 22% of women aged 18 to 45 years old in the United States knew of the CDC recommendations and that only 30% routinely took a daily multivitamin supplement containing folic acid (7).

Vitamin A

The deleterious effects of vitamin A usage were examined in 23,000 women undergoing amniocentesis. Infants of women consuming more than 10,000 IU in supplement form per day had an odds ratio (OR) of 2.4 (confidence interval [CI], 1.3 to 4.4) for all birth defects and 4.8 (CI, 2.2 to 10.5) for defects associated with cranial neural-crest tissue. One infant in 57 had a malformation attributable to vitamin A supplementation. The defects were concentrated among women who had consumed high levels before the seventh week of gestation and, oddly, were greatest in women with high intake only during the 2 weeks before conception (8).

Iron

The net additional requirement for iron in pregnancy is about 1 g, an amount difficult to obtain with the average diet. Supplementation with 325 mg of iron, as found in a multivitamin or prenatal vitamin, is recommended. If the preconception hemoglobin is low, higher doses should be used.

Zinc

Five hundred eighty medically indigent but healthy African-American women with below average zinc levels were randomized to take 25 mg of zinc or no zinc in their prenatal vitamins. Supplementation was associated with greater birth weight (126 g, $p = 0.03$) and head circumference (0.4 cm, $p = 0.02$). The effect size was twice as large in the nonobese women (9). The data in populations with normal zinc levels are mixed.

Weight and Exercise

Almost 10% of American women are obese before conception and thus have increased risk of fetal macrosomia, post-datism, meconium staining, labor abnormalities, and cesarean section. Two large case control studies found obesity doubled the risk of NTD. There was a positive linear relationship, with RR increasing to 4.0 (CI, 1.6 to 9.9) for women weighing over 110 kg. This association was not explained by inadequate folate intake nor did supplementation decrease the risk for obese women (10,11).

In contrast, women who are markedly underweight before pregnancy have increased risk of premature labor and intrauterine growth retardation (IUGR). Those with bulimia and pica are at particular risk. Anorexic women will have difficulty conceiving. The safest time to address obesity and eating disorders is before conception.

Moderate exercise appears safe periconceptionally and in early pregnancy. The American College of Obstetrics and Gynecology no longer recommends limiting maternal heart rate or body temperature but does emphasize the importance of heat dissipation during first trimester exercise and the avoidance of potential abdominal trauma.

Infectious Disease

Infectious diseases are a frequent cause of adverse or complicated pregnancy outcomes. The following are diseases for which preconception counseling can offer protective intervention.

Rubella

Childhood rubella is a mild and frequently subclinical disease characterized by rash, lymphadenopathy, and low-grade fever. However, maternal infection during pregnancy can lead to miscarriage, stillbirth, and a myriad of fetal anomalies. First trimester infection leads to congenital rubella syndrome in 25% of infants, and minor anomalies in up to 85%. Possible sequelae include deafness, cataracts, patent ductus arteriosus, atrial or ventricular septal defects, growth retardation, microcephaly, and mental retardation.

With the widespread immunization of school age children since 1969, a vaccinated birth cohort will eventually replace the 6% to 35% of persons of childbearing age who are currently susceptible. However, there will continue to be loss of protective immunity by adulthood (estimated to be 10%), and immigration without subsequent vaccination (12).

The incidence of congenital rubella dropped dramatically in the mid 1980s, but a resurgence was seen in 1990, when 21 cases were documented in Southern California. Fifty-seven percent of the mothers were United States born. A study demonstrated that over half of the cases had clearly missed opportunities (i.e., office visits with a primary care provider) for adult vaccination before pregnancy (13).

The Immunization Practices Advisory Committee recommends (14)

- Every clinical opportunity for rubella vaccination should be taken: primary care, post-abortion, pre-marital, and post-partum.

- Women without previous vaccination should be vaccinated without screening.
- Women with a probable history of vaccination should have their antibody status confirmed.
- The vaccine should not be given to pregnant women, and women should avoid pregnancy for 3 months after vaccination.

The last recommendation stems from studies demonstrating that rubella vaccine virus can cross the placenta and infect fetal tissue. However, a CDC cohort study of 321 women inadvertently vaccinated within 3 months before to 3 months after conception found no defects compatible with congenital rubella syndrome (14).

Toxoplasmosis

Acute toxoplasmosis during pregnancy conveys an approximately 40% to 50% risk of fetal infection. Infection in the periconception period and first trimester may cause fetal death or the congenital toxoplasmosis syndrome: chorioretinitis, mental retardation, microcephaly, sensorineural hearing loss, and developmental delay.

Because infection with rubella in pregnant women is associated with miscarriage, stillbirth, and fetal anomalies, all women who are not pregnant and who have not received vaccination should be vaccinated without screening. However, pregnant women should not be vaccinated, and pregnancy should be prevented for 3 months after receiving vaccination.

In the United States, 55% to 75% of women of childbearing age are susceptible to toxoplasmosis. Maternal infection affects from 2 to 6 of 1000 pregnancies, causing approximately 3000 cases of congenital toxoplasmosis syndrome each year. Serologic testing is not routine because no vaccine exists; the current strategy for preventing primary infection is universal patient education. All women at risk for pregnancy should be instructed to not eat raw meat, avoid contact with cat feces, wash their hands after handling cats, and wear gloves while gardening.

Varicella

Approximately 10% of adults in the United States are susceptible to varicella. Pregnancy is associated with markedly increased severity of maternal illness; however, congenital varicella syndrome (abnormalities of the skin, limbs, eyes, and central nervous system) fortunately occurs in only 2% of births after first or second trimester infection. Although the overall risk is low, nonpregnant women of childbearing age are a target group for vaccination. Women who report no history of varicella should first undergo serologic testing because many will have had subclinical disease and this series of two vaccinations is relatively expensive. Recurrence of varicella infection, herpes zoster, does not cause fetal infection.

Hepatitis

The United States Preventive Services Task Force (USPSTF) recommends the hepatitis B vaccine for all young adults and older adults in high-risk groups. Women considering pregnancy who have not been vaccinated should be screened because about one third of women who are hepatitis B surface antigen positive will transmit the infection to their infants. Vertical transmision can be reduced by 85% to 95% through prompt administration of HBIG and HBV vaccine to the newborn (15,16). Hepatitis C is vertically transmitted by only 5% to 9% of viremic mothers (17,18).

Sexually Transmitted Diseases

Sexually transmitted diseases (STDs) lead to increased rates of ectopic pregnancy and infertility, and may have specific fetal consequences. Maternal syphilis at any stage of pregnancy can cause spontaneous abortion, premature birth, congenital anomalies, or death. Chlamydia is associated with increased rates of intrauterine death, low birth weight, and post-partum endometritis. Active maternal infection is transmitted to infants in 60% of cases, causing pneumonia or conjunctivitis. Human papilloma virus in the mother's reproductive tract can cause respiratory papillomatosis in the infant.

The USPSTF recommends early pregnancy screening for chlamydia and syphilis in all women, and gonorrhea testing for women at risk of infection (10), although performing the Pap smear and STD screening prior to pregnancy carries certain advantages. Infections or pap smear abnormalities that are detected can be optimally treated without concern for fetal exposure. Primary herpes simplex infection during pregnancy affects the fetus 50% of the time, whereas reactivation disease is transmitted in less than 5% of cases. Pregnant patients with known genital herpes are managed with careful inspection for lesions near the time of delivery (the presence of which might necessitate cesarean section) and, more recently, with suppressive antiviral therapy taken during the last month of pregnancy. One fourth of infected neonates develop disseminated disease, and one third have encephalitis. Prevention of new sexually transmitted infections during pregnancy is critical, and education is warranted in select patients.

Substance Use

Caffeine

Caffeine is consumed by approximately 75% of pregnant women in this country, yet its safety remains controversial. The FDA removed it from the list of compounds considered safe in pregnancy because of animal evidence of teratogenicity, reduced birth weight, fetal death, and developmental abnormalities, as well as human observational data showing high doses associated with IUGR.

The conclusions of two important studies on the effects of caffeine conflict. A prospective cohort study of 431 women with excellent methodology found that moderate consumption of less than 300 mg/day (the approximate caffeine content of a cup of coffee is 107 mg; a cup of tea 34 mg; and a can of cola 47 mg) did not increase the risk of spontaneous abortion (SAB), IUGR, or microcephaly, but there was a nonsignificant trend towards IUGR at doses above 300 mg/day (19). However, a case-control study with 330 cases and 990 controls did find a significant dose-response relationship between caffeine consumption and SAB (20). In the month before conception, high intake (>321 mg/day) was associated with an OR of 1.8 (CI, 1.2 to 2.9). Early pregnancy consumption had a linear association with SAB starting at as little as 163 mg/day (OR, 2.0; CI, 1.3 to 2.9), with high intake associated with an OR of 2.6 (CI, 1.4 to 5.0). This study is weakened by its retrospective ascertainment of caffeine intake and SAB, however. Also, both studies could be confounded by the effect of nausea because women with viable pregnancies are more likely to have taste changes and may consequently decrease their caffeine intake compared with women with nonviable pregnancies.

More recently, a nested case control study measured serum levels of a caffeine metabolite in women who suffered spontaneous abortions before 140 days' gestation and compared them with women who delivered live infants at term. The adjusted odds ratio for spontaneous abortion was higher only for women whose serum levels suggested an intake of at least 6 cups of coffee per day (21).

In summary, high levels of caffeine intake (>300 mg/day) in the month before conception and during early pregnancy must be considered to increase the risk of SAB and probably also IUGR. There is insufficient evidence to conclude that lower levels are unsafe.

Cigarettes

Thirty percent of nonpregnant women aged 18 to 45 smoke, and 21% of women will smoke through their pregnancies (22). There are multiple adverse fetal consequences of smoking, the most significant being a birth weight reduction of approximately 200 g for 10 to 20 cigarettes smoked per day. Smoking is the leading preventable cause of low birth weight. Although the literature is hampered by health-behavior and socioeconomic confounders, multiple observational studies show increased risk of SAB, premature labor and delivery, placenta previa, and placental abruption (23). Children of smokers have a two-fold increase in sudden infant death and higher rates of respiratory infections. Attention deficit hyperactivity disorder (ADHD) may also be associated with smoking because 22% of affected children's mothers smoked during pregnancy compared with 8% of matched controls, significant after controlling for parental ADHD and IQ (24).

Paternal cigarette smoking may also affect the fetus. In addition to increasing the risk of low birth weight, paternal smoking in the 5 years before conception increases the risk of childhood cancer: OR, 1.7; CI, 1.2 to 2.5 for all cancer, OR, 4.5; CI, 1.2 to 16.8 for lymphoma, and OR, 3.8; CI, 1.3 to 12.3 for acute lymphocytic leukemia (25).

Fortunately, smoking cessation by early pregnancy ameliorates many of the deleterious effects. Anti-smoking interventions are more effective in pregnant women, with analysis of seven trials showing a 9.0% higher quit rate (efficacy 10% to 36%) than in nonpregnant smokers. The relapse rate is unfortunately high: 50% at 3 months and 70% at 1 year (26). Nonetheless, cessation counseling and referral to formal programs are primary care interventions that can have a significant impact.

Alcohol

Fetal alcohol syndrome (FAS) can be identified in one per 300 to 1000 live births. It is the leading known cause of mental retardation in the United States The syndrome is characterized by three findings: growth retardation, facial abnormalities (midface hypoplasia, smooth philtrum, short palpebral fissures, and microcephaly), and central nervous system dysfunction (mental retardation and behavioral disorders). The diagnosis requires at least one finding from each category in a child born to a known alcohol-using mother. A milder fetal alcohol effect is estimated to be present in one in 100 births. In addition, alcohol consumption during pregnancy is associated with a two-fold increase in the incidence of SAB and neonatal withdrawal symptoms.

The exact risk incurred by maternal alcohol use is difficult to establish. Studies of children of chronic alcoholics show FAS rates ranging from a low of 6% to a high of 30% to 50% (27,28). Two studies of moderate-heavy drinkers (1 to 2 oz/day absolute alcohol) found approximately 10% of infants had some characteristics of FAS (29,30). However, no difference in pregnancy outcome has been demonstrated with slight-moderate consumption (<1 drink/day). A multivariate analysis of 359 neonates found that the critical period for alcohol-related teratogenicity is around the time of conception (31). The first trimester is the next most vulnerable period. At present there is no established threshold for alcohol effect; therefore the wisest course may be to counsel abstinence.

Because no threshold for fetal alcohol effect has been established, abstinence should be advised.

Recreational Drugs

Substance use is one of the most important risk factors to address before conception. Women considering pregnancy may be particularly receptive to counseling about adverse fetal effects of alcohol and drugs. Conversely, substance-using women who do not want children may become more motivated to use contraception. Failure to screen for chemical dependency in primary care results in missed opportunities. The true prevalence of substance use by pregnant women is difficult to establish. A California population based study (32) of 30,000 women hospitalized for delivery analyzed urine specimens: 5.2% were positive for one or more drugs, 1.9% for cannabinoid, 1.5% for opiates, 1.1% for cocaine (7.8% among African American women), and 6.7% for alcohol. These figures significantly underestimate drug use because urine tests remain positive for only a few hours after alcohol ingestion and for only a few days after drug intake. Overall usage in pregnancy is thought to be much higher, as supported by meconium analysis at a private suburban hospital in Illinois: 6% of privately insured mothers and 12% of Medicaid mothers showed cocaine metabolites (33). Hair analysis of 970 pregnant adolescents and women in inner-city Philadelphia suggested that 28.9% used cocaine (34). This same study found cocaine to be associated with an increased risk of spontaneous abortion (OR, 1.4; CI, 1.0 to 2.1). Despite the difficulties of research in this area, there is little doubt that cocaine is associated with other adverse pregnancy outcomes such as IUGR, preterm delivery, placental abruption, and spontaneous rupture of membranes. Outcomes among pregnant cocaine users in an intensive prenatal program were significantly improved compared with users not in the program, although the outcomes were not as good as in the matched controls (35).

A study of heroin addicts found rates of stillbirth, fetal growth retardation, prematurity, and neonatal mortality three-fold to seven-fold higher than the general population (36). A small percentage of opiate-exposed infants will suffer the full-withdrawal syndrome, characterized by hypertonicity, tremor, irritability, vomiting, diarrhea, and occasionally seizures. When severe, neonatal withdrawal can be fatal. Symptoms usually appear after 1 to 3 days; obstetricians and pediatricians must be advised of patient use and avoid early discharge. Neonatal methadone withdrawal produces similar symptoms, but occurs 3 to 5 days after birth. Perinatal outcomes of patients enrolled in methadone maintenance programs are thought to be comparable with those of nonusers.

Data on the effects of marijuana in pregnancy are scarce. There is a suggestion of increased rates of premature delivery, low birth weight, and small head circumference, but not major malformation.

Despite the difficulties of research in this area, there is little doubt that substance abuse in general is associated with SAB and poor pregnancy outcomes. Helping a woman to abstain from use before conception is clearly the optimal intervention, but initiating multidisciplinary care early in pregnancy also has proven benefit.

Heat Exposure

Milunsky et al conducted a prospective follow-up study of heat exposure and NTD (37). Risk was significantly increased after hot tub exposure in the first 2 months of pregnancy, with a RR of 2.8 (CI, 1.2 to 6.5). Other heat exposures were associated with statistically insignificant increases in NTD: the RR for sauna use was 1.8 (CI, 0.4 to 7.9) and for fever > 100°F was 1.9 (CI, 0.8 to 4.1). Interestingly, there was a dose-response relationship: RR of NTD was 1.9 after exposure to one heat source and 6.2 after exposure to two heat sources. Electric blanket use conveyed no increased risk because it does not increase core body temperature. Because the most vulnerable period is in very early pregnancy, it is important to educate patients in the preconception period. They should be alerted to the risk of hot tubs and saunas and to the need to treat fevers with acetaminophen.

Pregnant patients should be advised to avoid using hot tubs and saunas and to treat fevers with acetaminophen, because heat exposure during pregnancy is associated with neural tube defects.

Occupation

Overall, women who work have better pregnancy outcomes than nonworking women. This reflects the "healthy worker" effect. The data on specific components of work that might be harmful are inconsistent. However, a recent analysis found the key risk factors for preterm labor and low birth weight to be prolonged standing (though not intermittent standing) and long working hours (38).

Specific occupational exposures known to be teratogenic or mutagenic include lead, ethylene oxide, dibromochloropropane, and organic solvents. A prospective controlled study of 125 women who had occupational exposure to organic solvents while pregnant found the risk of major congenital malformations to be 13 times that of matched controls (39).

Ionizing radiation causes SAB, fetal malformation, and low birth weight. The National Council on Radiation Protection recommends total fetal exposure be limited to 0.5 rad. However, no evidence of adverse effects has been found when the fetus is fully shielded while the mother is x-rayed. Video display terminals do not lead to increased rates of SAB (40). Studies from the 1970s and early 1980s found increased rates of SAB in nurses exposed to anesthetic gases and antineoplastics (41,42). Health care workers should exercise caution when handling these agents but be reassured that exposures are significantly lower because of current OSHA standards.

Household products that contain heavy metals or strong solvents, such as oven cleaners, wood-finishing products, and paints, may be harmful to the developing fetus, and pregnant women should minimize such exposure.

Dental Health

A case control study of women who delivered premature, low birth-weight babies found they had significantly worse periodontal disease than mothers whose babies were born at term. Women with the most severe disease had an OR of 7.5 (CI, 2.0 to 28.8) for prematurity and low birth weight (43). A routine preconception dental exam is advisable because x-rays and epinephrine should be avoided after conception.

Genetic Screening

Preconception assessment of genetic risks offers significant advantage. It may influence the desire of some couples to conceive, and it allows for education and decision making outside the emotional context of a pregnancy. There are several recessive genetic disorders that are frequent enough to merit carrier screening in various groups (Table 19-1).

People of Mediterranean, Indian, and Pakistani descent are at risk for beta-thalassemia, whereas Southeast Asians and Africans are at risk for both alpha- and beta-thalassemia. These ethnic groups should be screened with red blood cell indices, and those with low MCVs (50 to 70) tested with hemoglobin electrophoresis to confirm the diagnosis. All African Americans should also be evaluated for sickle cell and other hemoglobinopathies. Approximately one in 12 is a Hgb S carrier, and one in 60 a Hgb C carrier.

People of Eastern European Jewish descent should receive screening for Tay-Sachs disease, a uniformly fatal disease of childhood. Their carrier rate is approximately one in 30. Because the gene is also found in non-Jewish populations (particularly French Canadians), the American College of Obstetricians and Gynecologists (ACOG) also recommends screening for couples with only one member of Eastern European Jewish descent (3).

Cystic fibrosis is the most common lethal autosomal recessive disorder in Caucasians, with a carrier rate of one in 25. Current molecular diagnostic methods detect more than 90% of individuals. Although some controversy remains, a National Institutes of Health consensus panel now suggests offering genetic screening to all couples considering pregnancy.

All patients with a history of recurrent unexplained pregnancy loss or a family history of genetic abnormality such as Down syndrome, fragile X, mental retardation, Huntington's disease, or polycystic kidney disease should be referred for formal genetic counseling.

Advanced Maternal Age

Rates of first births to older women have increased dramatically, such that 20% of American women who have children now begin their families after

Table 19-1 Populations That May Be Considered for Genetic Screening*

Population	Genetic Risk
Mediterranean, Indian, Pakistani descent	Beta-thalassemia
Southeast Asians, Africans	Alpha- and beta-thalassemia
African Americans	Sickle cell; other hemoglobinopathies
Eastern European Jewish descent[†]	Tay-Sachs
Caucasians	Cystic fibrosis

*All patients with a history of recurrent unexplained pregnancy loss or family history of genetic abnormality should be referred for genetic counseling.
[†]ACOG recommends screening for couples with only one member of Eastern European Jewish descent.

age 35. However, many patients are not aware that fecundity declines with age, approximately 18% by age 30 to 35 and 27% after age 35 (44). Preconception counseling may provide an opportunity to discuss this issue as well as the topics of increased maternal and fetal complications.

Maternal mortality increases with age. The rate for women older than 40 is 56 per 100,000 compared with 9.1 per 100,000 in the general gravid population. The data suggest that a healthy woman is at increased risk on the basis of advanced age itself.

Fetal outcomes also worsen with advanced maternal age. A population study of healthy Swedish primagravidas (45) found that those aged 35 to 39 had a significantly higher rate of very low birth weight (OR, 1.9; CI, 1.5 to 2.4), very preterm birth (OR, 1.7; CI, 1.4 to 2.1), and small-for-gestational-age infants (OR, 1.7; CI, 1.5 to 2.0). A Canadian study found an approximate doubling of fetal death for older women even after controlling for co-existing medical conditions (OR, 1.9; CI, 1.3 to 2.7 for ages 35 to 39, and OR, 2.4; CI, 1.3 to 4.5 over age 40). Absolute rates however, remain low, with fetal death at 0.5% to 0.6% and early neonatal death at 0.5% (46).

With increased maternal age, the chance of aneuploid offspring increases. The overall odds of delivering a Down syndrome child are 1 in 600, but at age 35 rise to 1/250, and by age 40 are 1/70. The odds of bearing a child with any chromosomal abnormality are 1/140 at age 35 and 1/40 at age 40. Consequently, patients over age 35 should be offered screening with amniocentesis or chorionic villous sampling once pregnancy occurs.

Medications

The vast majority of drugs have not been, and most likely never will be, adequately studied in pregnancy. Yet 90% of pregnant women in the United States use medications, and 40% of this consumption is during the critical period of organogenesis. Thus the preconception visit is the ideal time to educate patients regarding over-the-counter medications and to review medication regimens in order to maximize maternal therapeutic effect and minimize fetal adverse consequences. It is wise to avoid prescribing FDA fetal risk category D or X drugs at all times to any woman of childbearing potential (Box 19-1). If no alternatives exist, one should advise the patient of the potential risks and of the need for reliable contraception. For a patient planning a pregnancy, the preconception visit allows for adjustment of the medical regimen to one that is considered safe in pregnancy. Often this means switching to older drugs, for which more observational and anecdotal data are available. It is best to educate the patient so that she may participate in the decision-making process because drug exposure in pregnancy can rarely be considered risk-free.

Box 19-1 Fetal Risk Factor Categories*

- **Category A** Controlled studies show no risk to the fetus
- **Category B** No evidence of risk to the human fetus
- **Category C** Risk to the fetus cannot be ruled out
- **Category D** Positive evidence of risk to the fetus

  Despite the known risk, benefits from using the drug in pregnant women may be acceptable in certain clinical settings.

- **Category X** Studies demonstrate fetal abnormalities

  The risk of using the drug during pregnancy clearly outweighs any possible benefit, and the drug is contraindicated in women who are or may become pregnant.

---

*The majority of drugs have been assigned to Category C. Therefore, the use of most drugs during pregnancy requires a careful risk-benefit analysis; ideally the patient should be involved in this decision making. Note that many drugs have not been assigned a fetal risk factor rating. Reference textbooks are therefore important.

Note also that the considerations regarding the safety of medications during lactation differ entirely from those during pregnancy. For example, though diphenhydramine (Benadryl) is considered relatively safe during pregnancy, its use during lactation may sedate the infant and cause inadequate feeding. Consult a pediatric source regarding drug use during lactation.

To generalize, drugs whose benefits usually outweigh risks in pregnancy include digoxin, penicillin, cephalosporins, erythromycin, and clindamycin. Fluoxetine was at one time felt to cause minor anomalies, but a recent prospective controlled study failed to show any detrimental effect (47). Similarly, metronidazole was once thought to have teratogenic effects in humans, but recent meta-analysis of seven studies (48) and a large case control study of more than 30,000 pregnant women (49) found no such risk. Although estrogen and progesterone are contraindicated in pregnancy, no adverse fetal effects have been demonstrated with inadvertant exposure to oral contraceptives or depot medroxyprogesterone. Over-the-counter medications such as acetaminophen, pseudoephedrine, and most cold and cough preparations are generally safe.

Commonly prescribed medications that are known teratogens and should be avoided in pregnancy include ACE inhibitors and receptor blockers (both safe in first trimester), warfarin, ergots, lithium, isotretinoin, and antineoplastics (Box 19-2). Drugs thought to pose mild fetal risk are rifampin, chloramphenicol, trimethoprim, and live vaccines. Tetracyclines cause discoloration of the offspring's deciduous teeth. Fluoroquinolones cause arthropathy in immature animals. Aspirin and NSAIDs in the third trimester may cause premature closure of the ductus arteriosus. Drugs for conditions such as epilepsy, hypertension, and HIV are discussed in the next section.

Box 19-2 Medications To Avoid in the Pregnant Patient*

- ACE inhibitors and receptor blockers[†]
- Amiodarone
- Androgens
- Anticonvulsants (most; see discussion)
- Antifungals (fluconazole, ketoconazole)
- Aspirin
- Baclofen
- Clarithromycin
- Clonidine
- Danazol
- Diuretics
- Fluoroquinolones
- Isotretinoin and other retinoids
- Leukotriene esterase inhibitors

- Lithium
- MAOIs
- Methotrexate and most other anti-neoplastic agents
- Methimazole
- Misoprostol
- NSAIDs (avoid in third trimester)
- Oral hypoglycemics
- Propranolol
- Spironolactone
- Sulfamethoxazole (avoid near term)
- Tamoxifen
- Tetracyclines
- Thalidomide
- Warfarin

*Some of these medications are teratogenic; others may be harmful to the fetus through a variety of mechanisms.
[†]ACE inhibitors and receptor blockers are safe only during the first trimester (i.e., prior to functioning of the fetal kidney).

Disease and Treatment of Disease

This section will address common medical problems whose management requires re-evaluation before conception. Medical complications of pregnancy are beyond the scope of this chapter.

Pregnancy should be discouraged in the following conditions because they are associated with a 30% to 50% historical risk of maternal death: pulmonary hypertension, Marfan's disease with aortic root dilatation, complicated coarctation of the aorta, and diabetes with coronary artery disease (Box 19-3). A smaller but significant risk of mortality (estimated at 5% to 15%) has been seen with mitral stenosis of functional class III or IV, prosthetic heart valves, previous myocardial infarction, atrial fibrillation with aortic stenosis, uncorrected tetralogy of Fallot, and intracranial arteriovenous malformation.

To help ensure normal neurologic development of the fetus, adults with phenylketonuria must return to a low phenylalanine diet before conception. Women with a history of thromboembolic disease or hypercoagulable states are at increased risk for clotting events during pregnancy and should receive

---

Box 19-3 Conditions Associated with Maternal Death

30%–50% Risk
Pulmonary hypertension
Marfan's disease with aortic root dilatation
Complicated coarctation of the aorta
Diabetes with coronary artery disease

5%–15% Risk
Mitral stenosis of functional class III or IV
Prosthetic heart valves
Previous myocardial infarction
Atrial fibrillation with aortic stenosis
Uncorrected tetralogy of Fallot
Intracranial arteriovenous malformation

---

prophylaxis with subcutaneous heparin because warfarin is teratogenic. Systemic lupus erythematosus is associated with SAB, IUGR, and prematurity, but patients without significant complications may attempt conception during periods of disease quiescence.

Chronic Renal Disease

The degree of renal dysfunction is the major determinant of maternal and fetal prognosis. More than 90% of women with mild impairment of renal function without proteinuria or hypertension have a successful pregnancy, compared to only half of patients on dialysis. Women with a baseline creatinine clearance of less than 25 to 30 mL/min are at significant risk of accelerated deterioration of maternal disease as well as fetal loss. Hypertension in the setting of renal insuffiency is the second major predictor. Fetal loss is ten-fold higher if hypertension is present at conception or early pregnancy than if blood pressure is spontaneously normal or well controlled on therapy (50). Thousands of women have now had successful pregnancies after renal transplantation.

Asthma

With proper control of their asthma, most women will have a normal pregnancy and healthy baby. The National Asthma Education Project recommends that asthma be as aggressively treated in pregnant women as in nonpregnant women because the risk of uncontrolled asthma is far greater than the risk of medications (51). Preconception management should focus on avoidance or control of triggers, patient education, baseline spirometry, and institution of home peak flow monitoring.

Medications should be managed in a stepwise manner with inhaled drugs preferred. Animal studies and human experience suggest little potential fetal harm from selective beta-2 agonists, theophylline (with serum levels <12 g/mL), and cromolyn sodium. Daily oral or parenteral corticosteroids are associated with decreased birth weight but not congenital malformations in humans. Inhaled steroids result in very low plasma levels; beclomethasone is the preferred agent because there is the most experience with this drug. There are few data on nedocromil sodium or leukotriene antagonists. Immunotherapy should not be initiated in pregnancy because of the serious fetal consequences in the event of anaphylaxis; however, injections may be continued at the same dose if already ongoing.

Diabetes

Diabetic women are three to four times more likely than health mothers to have offspring with major congenital malformations: 9% have significant cardiac, renal, skeletal, gastrointestinal, or central nervous system anomalies. This rate increases to 20% to 25% if a woman has very poor glycemic control in the first weeks of pregnancy. Diabetes-related malformations occur in the first 5 to 8 weeks after conception, during early organogenesis. Intervention studies clearly demonstrate that malformation rates decrease if tight control is instituted before conception.

In women with diabetes, poor glycemic control during the first weeks of pregnancy is associated with a high rate (20% to 25%) of congenital malformations. Tight control of diabetes should therefore be instituted before conception.

Kitzmiller et al (52) compared birth outcomes for women who underwent intensive management of their diabetes before conception with those referred to the same program after pregnancy was confirmed (average of 12 weeks' gestation). Preconception institution of tight control decreased the fetal anomaly rate to 1.2% compared with 11% in the post-conception group ($P = 0.01$). The Maine Diabetes Project found women who did not receive preconception counseling had an OR of 3.9 (CI, 1.2 to 13.9) for fetal and neonatal death, irrespective of prenatal care (53).

Preconception management of the diabetic begins with assessment of glycemic control and complications with a glycohemoglobin, creatinine clearance, electrocardiogram, and ophthalmologic exam. Oral sulfonylureas should be discontinued before conception because they provide inadequate control. Data are lacking for use of metformin and thiazolidinediones in pregnancy. Most diabetics require insulin during pregnancy, although a minority of patients can remain on diet control alone. Tight control (blood glucose levels of 70 to 100 mg/dL preprandial and 100 to 140 mg/dL 1 hr postprandial) should be instituted, with a goal of near euglycemia at conception. Intensive medical management, home monitoring, and patient education are required to attain these levels. It may be helpful to involve a consultant such as an endocrinologist or obstetrician who specializes in high-risk pregnancy in the preconception period.

Once pregnancy occurs, placental lactogen and cortisol increase insulin resistance, rendering the patient more susceptible to ketoacidosis and sometimes leading to a doubling of insulin requirements. However, insulin requirements often decrease in early gestation because of inadequate intake from nausea or in the third trimester because of placental insufficiency. The fetus is relatively protected against hypoglycemia because neither endogenous nor exogenous insulin crosses the placenta.

Patients with pre-existing complications require special surveillance. Retinopathy accelerates in pregnancy, so patients with eye disease need fundoscopic exams each trimester. Proteinuria increases, but in most cases returns to baseline post-partum. However, 20% to 30% of patients suffer persistent decline in creatinine clearance. Mortality risk increases if macrovascular disease is present.

Many diabetic women are still not getting appropriate care. A 1995 population based study in Michigan found that only one third of gravid women with established diabetes received preconception counseling (54). Given the importance of achieving tight control before conception, primary care providers can dramatically improve outcomes by providing anticipatory guidance to all diabetic women.

Chronic Hypertension

The incidence of chronic hypertension in pregnant women is estimated to be 1% to 5% and is higher among older women, obese women, and black women. Preconception determination of blood pressure provides a valuable baseline. Diastolic blood pressure drops in early pregnancy by 10 to 17 mm Hg to a nadir at 16 to 20 weeks, then rises through the second half of pregnancy to just under pre-pregnancy values.

Most women with mild uncomplicated primary hypertension will have a benign pregnancy course. In the past 30 years, at least seven studies have compared antihypertensive therapy with placebo. Rates of pre-eclampsia, preterm delivery, and perinatal death were no different. In the early trials, there was a higher incidence of fetal loss in untreated women that was not replicated in later trials. However, pregnant women with long-standing, severe hypertension and/or pre-existing cardiovascular or renal disease are at increased risk for superimposed pre-eclampsia, abruptio-placentae, and fetal morbidity. The results of two retrospective trials indicate that, for women with diastolic pressures above 110, antihypertensive therapy decreases the incidence of stroke and cardiovascular complications (55).

The decision to use medications for chronic hypertension around conception and in early pregnancy should take into account the severity of hypertension, target organ risk, and the physiologic decline. A blood pressure of approximately 150/100 is a reasonable treatment threshold. If end organ damage is evident, the threshold should be lowered.

The antihypertensive medication most commonly used in pregnancy is methyldopa. It has been evaluated in numerous studies, and no significant adverse long-term effects have been reported. A small decrease in infant head size was reported in one study, without later effect on growth or intelligence (56). Side effects include transient neonatal hypotension, maternal sedation, and rebound hypertension.

Second-line agents include labetolol (potential side effects: neonatal apnea and bradycardia) and hydralazine (potential side effects: maternal tachycardia and orthostasis and fetal thrombocytopenia) for which there are few clinical trials but extensive experience. Nifedipine has been used frequently and safely in later pregnancy, but periconception and long-term data are needed.

Diuretics should be avoided because they interfere with normal plasma volume expansion. Propranolol has adverse effects on intrauterine growth and hemodynamics, but other beta-blockers are often used. ACE inhibitors and receptor blockers are contraindicated in the second and third trimesters because they are teratogenic, causing such defects as skull abnormalities, limb contractures, craniofacial deformities, and pulmonary hypoplasia. Some of these anomalies are felt to be a consequence of the medication causing hypotension and decreased renal flow in the fetus. Although ACE inhibitors are considered safe in the first trimester, some authors recommend not prescribing them in any woman with childbearing potential, unless for a unique indication.

Seizure Disorders

The fetal anomaly rate in neonates of women with a seizure disorder is two-fold to three-fold higher than in the general population. This is not solely because of anti-epileptic drug teratogenicity because the malformation rate is also slightly increased in children of epileptic women not on medications or in children whose fathers have epilepsy. Nonetheless, women with seizure disorders have a greater than 90% chance of delivering normal infants.

Seizure disorders in the context of desired pregnancy pose a difficult dilemma because most anti-epileptic drugs are FDA category D or worse, yet fetal exposure to the hypoxemia and acidosis associated with a seizure is also potentially harmful, not to mention the maternal risk. Ideally, a woman with a seizure disorder plans her pregnancy well in advance because medication use can often be altogether reconsidered. In select patients and after extensive patient education and counseling (which may be best performed in conjunction with formal neurologic consultation), one can consider a trial of a slow withdrawal taper over 3 months (with close monitoring and appropriate warnings regarding driving, etc.). Those patients that remain seizure-free for a 6-month duration off of their medication can attempt to conceive and maintain their pregnancy without anti-epileptics. A study of patients seizure-free for more than 2 years on a single drug found that 65% remained seizure-free off medications (57). Patients requiring more than one drug or those with complex partial seizures with secondary generalization are less likely to be successful.

If medication is necessary, the goal is to strive for monotherapy at the lowest effective dose before conception. Because there is no agreement on which antiepileptic is least teratogenic, the most recent consensus recommends using the drug that is most effective in preventing seizures in a given patient. Carbamazepine, valproic acid, and phenobarbital are the most commonly used medications. Carbamazepine may increase the risk of NTD to 0.5%, and one small study showed developmental delay. Phenobarbital is associated with cardiac, orofacial, and urogenital malformations. Phenytoin has been linked with a syndrome of mental retardation, prenatal and postnatal growth retardation, and a recognizable pattern of craniofacial and distal phalanx malformations, and is avoided when possible. Valproate-exposed neonates may have a NTD rate of 1% to 2%, and higher rates of cardiac, urogenital, craniofacial, and skeletal malformations. The highest incidence of congenital malformations is in neonates exposed to multiple drugs (58). Data for newer drugs such as gabapentin are lacking. Pregnant patients on any antiepileptic drugs should be encouraged to register in the AED Pregnancy Registry to help define fetal risk (888-233-2334).

Fortunately, only 17.3% of women experience an increase in seizure frequency during pregnancy (59). Decreased protein binding and increased drug clearance in pregnancy mandate frequent level checks and often dose adjustments. Free levels are more specific. To help reduce the risk of adverse fetal effects, patients are often instructed to split their dose and increase the dosing frequency. Patient counseling should also stress the need for good nutrition, health, and sleep patterns before conception. Folate supplementation at 4 mg/day is recommended.

AIDS

Without intervention, more than one fourth of infants of women with HIV become infected perinatally. Transmission risk increases with high maternal viral load, low maternal CD4 count, advanced clinical disease, prolonged rupture of membranes, and premature delivery. It appears to decrease with cesarean section or birth of a second twin vaginally. Breast feeding conveys an additional independent 14% transmission risk and should be discouraged.

The AIDS Clinical Trial Group showed that AZT treatment of infected women antepartum and intravenously intrapartum, and their infants for 6 weeks, reduced the rate of perinatal transmission from 22.6% to 7.6% (60). Treatment was effective regardless of HIV-1 RNA level or CD4 count at entry, and the results persisted at 18-month follow-up (61). Trials studying the use of other antiretrovirals are underway. The International Antiviral Pregnancy Registry is monitoring community-based treatment (800-722-9292, ext 8465). Eighty percent of pregnant women with HIV now use antiretrovirals, and perinatal transmission rates have almost halved. These results justify universal availability of preconception HIV testing.

Women with symptomatic AIDS suffer a slight increase in fetal loss, low birth weight, and preterm delivery. Pregnancy does not appear to accelerate disease progression. Compulsive attention should be given to routine HIV care in seropositive women of childbearing potential. Pneumocystis prophylaxis with TMP-SMX poses a risk of newborn kernicterus or hemolysis and should therefore be dosed two or three times per week. Tuberculosis prophylaxis should be delayed at least until the second trimester. *Mycobacterium avium* and fungal prophylaxis should be deferred. Active disease must of course be treated, but commonly used drugs such as fluoroquinolones, clofazamine, pentamadine, and pyrazinamide should be avoided.

Summary

Preconception counseling is best delivered to all women of childbearing potential, and provides the opportunity to

- Recommend folate (or folate-containing multivitamin) supplementation
- Screen and vaccinate for hepatitis B, rubella, and varicella
- Screen for and treat sexually transmitted diseases
- Review the risk of high-dose caffeine
- Strongly discourage alcohol, cigarettes, and recreational drugs
- Counsel regarding the treatment of fevers and avoiding heat exposure
- Advise patients of their risk for genetic disease

- Assess all medications for teratogenicity, including over-the-counter drugs and vitamins
- Achieve tight control of diabetes before conception
- Re-evaluate the treatment of other medical conditions

REFERENCES

1. **Kalter H.** Congenital malformations: etiologic factors and their role in prevention. N Engl J Med. 1983;308:424-31.

2. **DePersio SR, Chen W, Blose D, et al.** Unintended childbearing. MMWR. 1992;41: 933-6.

3. ACOG Technical Bulletin. Preconception care. Intnl J Gynecol Obstet. 1995;50:201-7

4. **Czeizel AE, Dudas I.** Prevention of the first occurrence of neural tube defects by periconceptional vitamin supplementation. N Engl J Med. 1992;327:1832-35.

5. **MRC Vitamin Study Research Group.** Prevention of neural tube defects: results of the medical research council vitamin study. Lancet. 1991;338:1027-31.

6. **Daly S, Mills JL, Molloy AM, et al.** Minimum effective dose of folic acid for food fortification to prevent neural-tube defects. Lancet. 1997;350:1666-9.

7. Knowledge and use of folic acid by women of childbearing age. MMWR. 1997;46:721.

8. **Rothman KJ, Moore LL, Singer MR, et al.** Teratogenicity of high vitamin A intake. N Engl J Med. 1995;333:1369-73, 1414-5.

9. **Goldenberg RL, Tamura T, Neggers Y, et al.** The effect of zinc supplementation on pregnancy outcome. JAMA. 1995;274:463-8.

10. **Werler MM, Louik C, Shapiro S, Mitchell AA.** Prepregnant weight in relation to risk of neural tube defects. JAMA. 1996;275:1089-92.

11. **Shaw GM, Velie EM, Schaffer D.** Risk of neural tube defect-affected pregnancies among obese women. JAMA. 1996;275:1093-6.

12. **United States Preventive Services Task Force.** Guide to Clinical Preventive Services, 2nd ed. Baltimore: Williams and Wilkins; 1996:269-77, 791-815.

13. **Lee SH, Ewert DP, Frederick PD, Mascola L.** Resurgence of congenital rubella syndrome in the 1990s. JAMA. 1992;267:2616-20.

14. **Immunization Practices Advisory Committee.** Rubella prevention. MMWR. 1990; 39(RR-15).

15. **Beasley RP, Lee GC, Roan C-H, et al.** Prevention of perinatally transmitted hepatitis B virus infections with hepatitis B immune globulin and hepatitis B vaccine. Lancet. 1983;2:1099-1102.

16. **Stevens CE, Toy PT, Tong MJ.** Perinatal hepatitis B virus transmission in the United States: prevention by passive-active immunization. JAMA. 1985;253:1740-5.

17. **Ohto H, Terazawa S, Sasaki N, et al.** Transmission of hepatitis C virus from mothers to infants. N Eng J Med. 1994;330:744-50.

18. **Polywka S.** Low risk of vertical transmission of hepatitis C by breast milk. Clin Infect Dis. 1999;29:1327-9.

19. **Mills JL, Holmes LB, Aarons JH, et al.** Moderate caffeine use and the risk of spontaneous abortion and intrauterine growth retardation. JAMA. 1993;269:593-7.

20. **Infante-Rivard C, Fernandez A, Gauthier R, et al.** Fetal loss associated with caffeine intake before and during pregnancy. JAMA. 1993;270:2940-3, 2973-4.

21. **Klebanoff MA.** Maternal serum paraxanthine, a caffeine metabolite, and the risk of spontaneous abortion. N Engl J Med. 1999;341:1639-44.

22. **Williamson DF, Serdula MK, Kendrick JS, Binkin NJ.** Comparing the prevalence of smoking in pregnant and nonpregnant women 1985 to 1986. JAMA. 1989;261:70-4.

23. Smoking and Reproductive Health. ACOG Technical Bulletin. 1993;180:1-5.

24. **Milberger S, et al.** Is maternal smoking during pregnancy a risk factor for attention deficit hyperactivity disorder in children? Am J Psych. 1996;153:1138-42.

25. **Ji BT, Shu XO, Linet MS, et al.** Paternal cigarette smoking and the risk of childhood cancer among offspring of nonsmoking mothers. J Natl Cancer Inst. 1997;89:238-44.

26. **Mullen PD, Ramirez G, Groff JY.** A meta-analysis of randomized trials of prenatal smoking cessation interventions. Am J Obstet Gynecol. 1994;171:1328-34.

27. **Olegaard R, Sabel KG, Aronsson M, et al.** Effects on the child of alcohol abuse during pregnancy. Acta Paediatr Scand Suppl. 1979; 275:112-21.

28. **Abel EL, Sokol RJ.** Incidence of fetal alcohol syndrome and economic impact of FAS-related anomalies. Drug Alcohol Depend. 1987;19:51-70.

29. **Hansom JW, Streissguth AP, Smith DW.** The effects of moderate alcohol consumption during pregnancy on fetal growth and morphogenesis. J Pediatr. 1978;92:457-60.

30. **Autti-Ramo I, Gaily E, Granstrom ML.** Dysmorphic features in offspring of alcoholic mothers. Arch Dis Child. 1992;67:712-16.

31. **Ernhart CB, Sokol RJ, Martier S, et al.** Alcohol teratogenicity in the human: a detailed assessment of specificity, critical period, and threshold. Am J Obstet Gynecol. 1987;156:33-9.

32. **Vega WA, Kolody B, Hwang J, Noble A.** Prevalence and magnitude of perinatal substance exposures in California. N Engl J Med. 1993;329:859-4.

33. **Shutzman DL.** Incidence of intrauterine cocaine exposure in a suburban setting. Pediatrics. 1991;88:825-7.

34. **Ness FB, Grisso JA, Hirshinger N, et al.** Cocaine and tobacco use and the risk of spontaneous abortion. N Engl J Med 1999;340:333-86.

35. **MacGregor SN, Keith LG, Bachicha JA, Chasnoff IJ.** Cocaine abuse during pregnancy: correlation between prenatal care and perinatal outcome. Obstet Gynecol. 1989;74:882-5.

36. **Fricker HS, Segal S.** Narcotic addiction, pregnancy, and the newborn. Am J Dis Child. 1978;132:360-6.

37. **Milunsky A, Ulcickas M, Rothman KJ, et al.** Maternal heat exposure and neural tube defects. JAMA. 1992;268:882-5.

38. **Gabbe SG, Turner LP.** Reproductive hazards of the American lifestyle: work during pregnancy. Am J Obstet Gynecol. 1997;176:826-32.

39. **Khattak S.** Pregnancy outcome following gestational exposure to organic solvents: a prospective controlled study. JAMA 1999;281:1106-9.

40. **Schnorr TM, Grajewski BA, Hornung RW, et al.** Video display terminals and the risk of spontaneous abortion. N Engl J Med. 1991;324:727-33.

41. **Selevan SG, Lindbohm M-L, Hornung RW, Hemminki K.** A study of occupational exposure to antineoplastic drugs and fetal loss in nurses. N Engl J Med. 1985;313:1173-8.

42. **Cohen E, Brown B, Bruce DL, et al.** Occupational disease among operating room personnel: a national study. Anesthesiol. 1974;41:321-40.

43. **Offenbacher S, Katz V, Fertik G, et al.** Periodontal infection as a possible risk factor for preterm low birth weight. J Periodontol. 1996;67S:1103-13.

44. **Schwartz D, Mayaux MJ.** Female fecundity as a function of age. N Engl J Med. 1982; 306:404-6.

45. **Cnattingius S, Forman MR, Berendes HW, Isotalo L.** Delayed childbearing and risk of adverse perinatal outcome. JAMA. 1992;268:886-90.

46. **Fretts RC, Schmittdiel J, McLean FH, et al.** Increased maternal age and the risk of fetal death. N Engl J Med. 1995;333:953-7.

47. **Kulin NA, Patuszak A, Sage S, et al.** Pregnancy outcome following maternal use of the new selective serotonin reuptake inhibitors: a prospective controlled multicenter study. JAMA 1998;279:609-10.

48. **Burtin P, Taddio A, Ariburnu O, et al.** Safety of metronidazole in pregnancy: a meta-analysis. Am J Obstet Gynecol. 1995;172(2 Pt 1):525-9.

49. **Czeizel AE, Rockenbauer M.** A population based case-control teratologic study of oral metronidazole treatment during pregnancy. Br J Obstet Gynaecol. 1998;105:322-7.

50. **Jungers P, Chauveau D, Choukroun G, et al.** Pregnancy in women with impaired renal function. Clin Nephrol. 1997;47:281-8.

51. **National Asthma Education Project: Working Group on Asthma and Pregnancy.** Management of asthma during pregnancy. NIH Publication 93-3279:17-23, 29-33; September 1993.

52. **Kitzmiller JL, Gavin LA, Gin GD, et al.** Preconception care of diabetes. JAMA. 1991; 265:731-6.

53. **Willhoite MB, Bennert HW, Palomaki GE, et al.** The impact of preconception counseling on pregnancy outcomes. Diabetes Care. 1993;16:450-5.

54. **Janz NK, Herman WH, Becker MP, et al.** Diabetes and pregnancy: factors associated with seeking pre-conception care. Diabetes Care. 1995;18:157-64.

55. **Sibai BM.** Treatment of hypertension in pregnant women. N Eng J Med. 1996;335: 257-65.

56. **Moar VA, Jefferies M, Mutch L, et al.** Neonatal head circumference and the treatment of maternal hypertension. Br J Obstet Gynaecol. 1978;85:933-7.

57. **Callaghan N, Garrett A, Goggin T.** Withdrawal of anticonvulsant drugs in patients free of seizures for two years. N Eng J Med. 1988;318:942-6.

58. **Delgado-Escueta AV, Janz D.** Consensus guidelines: preconception counseling, management, and care of the pregnant woman with epilepsy. Neurology. 1992;42(S5):149-60.

59. **Lopes-Cendes I, Andermann E, Cendes F, et al.** Risk factors for changes in seizure frequency during pregnancy of epileptic women: a cohort study. AES Proceedings. Epilepsia. 1992;33(S3):57.

60. **Connor EM, Sperling RS, Gelber R, et al.** Reduction of maternal-infant transmission of human immunodeficiency virus type 1 with zidovudine treatment. N Eng J Med. 1994;331:1173-80.

61. **Sperling RS.** Maternal viral load, zidovudine treatment, and the risk of transmission of HIV-1 from mother to infant. N Eng J Med. 1996;335:1621-9.

CHAPTER 20

Infertility

MEERA C. KATARIA, MD

JANICE RYDEN, MD

BERT SCOCCIA, MD

Infertility is defined as the inability to conceive after 1 year of regular coitus without contraception (1). This definition of infertility is based on a monthly fecundity rate of 15% to 25%. Approximately 10% to 20% of couples may experience problems conceiving (2). Aside from population growth, other factors that have contributed to the recent increased utilization of fertility assistance include delayed childbearing (for career or other reasons), increased incidence of sexually transmitted diseases, greater societal acceptance of infertility treatment and a decreased number of infants available for adoption.

An important principle in the management of infertility is allowing the couple control of the decision making. Choosing when or whether to initiate infertility investigation should be left to the patient, as should the decision to proceed with any infertility treatment. It is therefore important to provide adequate time at office visits to educate the couple regarding the risks and efficacy of various procedures. Also, because infertility services are expensive and typically incompletely covered by health insurance plans, costs must often be discussed. Before embarking infertility treatment plans, issues of preconception care should be considered (see Chapter 19).

Etiology

Infertility can result from a wide variety of etiologies. A male factor is responsible for 40% of infertile couples (2). Female factors account for 40% of infertility, and a combination of male and female factors account for 10%. In approximately 10% of infertile couples no cause will be found ("unexplained infertility").

Male Factors

Varicocele accounts for 55% of male infertility, followed by testicular failure (15%), vas deferens obstruction or absence (10%), cryptorchidism (10%), semen volume abnormalities (5%), and immunological factors (5%).

Female Factors

Ovulatory dysfunction is present in 40% of women with infertility. Tubal factors account for 30% of women with infertility (3), followed by cervical factors (15%), endometriosis (10%), and immunological factors (5%) (1).

Ovulatory dysfunction may include a wide variety of problems ranging from frank anovulation to intermittent ovulation to subtle dysfunction such as the "luteal phase defect". Common causes of ovulatory disorders include hyperprolactinemia and polycystic ovary syndrome (PCOS). Certain medical conditions (e.g., hypothyroidism, hypercortisolism, late-onset adrenal hyperplasia, androgen-producing tumors of either ovarian or adrenal origin, diabetes) can result in ovulatory dysfunction as well. Anovulation can also stem from congenital hypothalamic dysfunction (e.g., the rare Kallman's syndrome). More commonly, reversible hypothalamic dysfunction can result from such causes as intense exercise training, underweight body habitus, and even caloric restriction without weight loss.

Tubal blockage and peritoneal adhesions are typically due to either previous pelvic inflammatory disease or endometriosis. Even in the absence of mechanical obstruction, mild endometriosis can contribute to infertility. This is postulated to be due to local peritoneal prostaglandin release and immunologic stimulation leading to decreased survival of the sperm, egg, or embryo.

The cervix serves important functions, such as temporary storage and nutritional support of sperm, and produces a meshlike mucus that can filter out debris, bacteria, and sperm lacking favorable motility. Damage to the cervix typically results from cone biopsy or electrosurgical excisions of the cervix or multiple D&C's.

Intrauterine synechiae (Asherman's syndrome) represent scarring of the uterine cavity, a rare sequela of uterine surgery (e.g., D&C for induced abortion or other indications, cesarean section, myomectomy). The patient usually presents with a progressive decrease in the volume of menstrual flow, sometimes with complete secondary amenorrhea. Unexplained infertility may possibly stem from anti-sperm antibodies, the significance of which is unknown, or subtle defects that exceed the sensitivity of available testing. Of the couples who undergo complete infertility assessment, 10% will have no cause identified.

It is important to note that fertility is also affected by the age of the couple, particularly that of the female. A decline in reproductive potential typically begins in women in the early to mid 30s, progresses more rapidly between the ages of 35–40, and accelerates further after age 40 (Fig. 20-1). Although the incidence of endometriosis, fibroids, and exposure to pelvic infections increases as women age, the primary factor is declining ovarian function, which typically precedes menopause by 8 to 10 years. For this reason, the American Society for Reproductive Medicine recommends evaluation after 1 year of infertility for women younger than age 35 but after only 6 months for women age 35 and older.

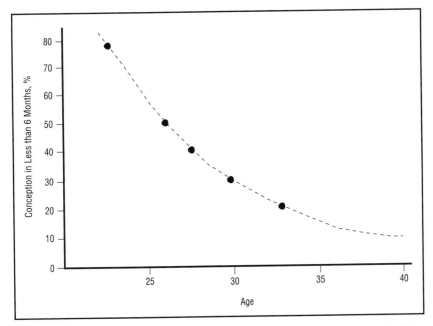

Figure 20-1 Correlation between age and incidence of pregnancy within 6 months. Note that the most significant decline of incidence of pregnancy within 6 months is at 35 years of age. (Modified from Behrman SJ, Kistner RW. Progress in Infertility [1975].)

Initial Evaluation

History

First, a menstrual history should be elicited. Ovulatory cycles are usually regular and range from 21 to 35 days. Further support for ovulation can be garnered by the presence of premenstrual symptoms ("molimina"), experience of *mittelschmerz* (pelvic pain upon ovulation), and the observation of abundant, clear, ovulatory cervical mucous at mid-cycle. Also, by the time of presentation many patients may have already used home ovulation predictor kits that detect the LH surge in the urine. Similarly, a basal body temperature curve demonstrating a 0.5°C (or 1°F) temperature elevation during the luteal phase is supportive of but not definitive for an ovulatory cycle (Fig. 20-2). Absence of these features is suggestive of anovulatory cycles.

If the patient has had longstanding anovulatory cycles (usually amenorrhea or oligomenorrhea), the diagnosis of PCOS should be entertained. Obesity, hirsutism, acne, and multiple ovarian cysts on ultrasound have been classically described; however, it should be pointed out that none of these findings (including polycystic ovaries) is required to make the diagnosis of this endocrinologic disorder of ovarian dysfunction. When laboratory studies fail to confirm the diagnosis of PCOS with an LH:FSH ratio >2, then one must consider other virilizing disorders (e.g., androgen-secreting neoplasm of adrenal or ovarian origin, Cushing's disease, adult-onset adrenal hyperplasia). Typically these causes are distinguishable from PCOS by a more abrupt onset or the presence of more striking physical exam findings (see Chapter 3).

Ovulatory dysfunction may also result from hypothyroidism, hyperprolactinemia, and premature ovarian failure. Because these last three conditions sometimes lack signs and symptoms aside from infertility and mild menstrual disturbances (4), all women undergoing infertility investigation should have these causes excluded (see Hormone Tests).

When the patient's menstrual pattern suggests anovulatory cycles and she has a particularly thin body habitus (especially if less than 85% normal BMI), one should ask about recent weight changes, exercise habits, caloric restriction, and the possibility of eating disorders. Patients should be made aware that sometimes weight gain of only a small amount (for many women, 5 lb) is needed to restore ovulation. Similarly, reducing intensive exercise training to a maintenance regimen is often therapeutic in restoring hypothalamic function (see Chapter 3). Increasing dysmenorrhea and dyspareunia over time may suggest the possibility of endometriosis. Secondary hypomenorrhea (sometimes with progression to amenorrhea) can be due to Asherman's syndrome when the past surgical history also reveals previous pelvic procedures.

One should also take a reproductive history although, excepting such presentations as previous ectopic pregnancy (which may signal possible tubal disease), this information often contributes surprisingly little to the diagnosis of the current infertility problem. However, a history of previous successful conception portends a better prognosis, because pregnancy rates are higher in couples with secondary rather than primary infertility. Spontaneous conception is more likely for couples in whom the period of infertility has been brief (5). Of course, it is also important to take a medical history of the male partner, including whether or not he has previously fathered a child.

Spontaneous conception is more likely for couples in whom the period of infertility has been brief.

A history of pelvic inflammatory disease, previous pelvic surgery, or IUD use can similarly lead one to suspect a possible tubal etiology. It should be noted, however, that chlamydia may cause tubal damage in the absence of overt salpingitis. Previous cone biopsy of the cervix may suggest a cervical cause. It is important to elicit a full medical history as well as a review of systems, because medical problems (e.g., diabetes) may be a source of ovulatory dysfunction. One should investigate the medication use of both partners. Recent discontinuation of medroxyprogesterone acetate (Depo-Provera) may result in a delay in return to fertility that varies widely but may be as long as 22 months. Men treated for hypertension with calcium-channel blockers have a reversible decrease in fertility due to reduced sperm capacitation; therefore another class of medication should be substituted (6).

A substance use history for both partners should also be elicited. Quitting smoking (7-9) and reducing caffeine to no more than 300 mg per day (1 to 2 cups of coffee) has been associated with an increase in fertility (1,10). Alcohol use also appears to affect female fertility in a dose-related manner (11,11a). Marijuana use has been shown to inhibit gonadotropin secretion in both men and women, although its impact on fertility remains to be proven (12). An occupational history should also be elicited from both partners, because exposure to certain solvents, pesticides and dusts has been associated with infertility (13).

When conducting the history one should elicit the couple's pattern of coitus, and take the opportunity to clarify their understanding regarding the fertile period of the woman's cycle. One recent prospective study of healthy women attempting pregnancy found that nearly all pregnancies were attributable to intercourse during a 6-day period that ended on the day of ovulation, with probability of conception increasing as one approached the day of ovulation (Fig. 20-3) (14). This finding implies either a brief life span for ova or a change in the cervical mucus shortly after ovulation that renders it in-

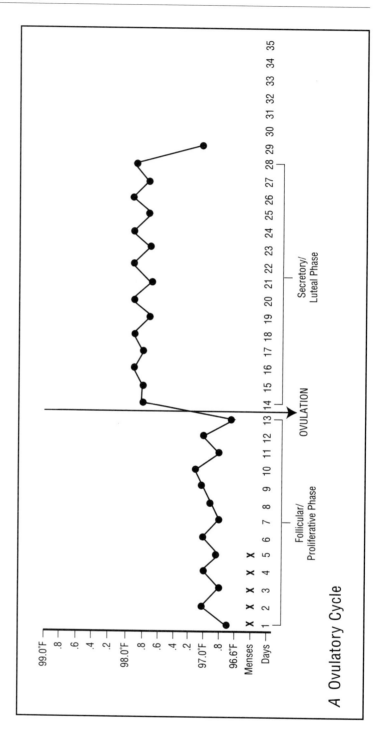

A Ovulatory Cycle

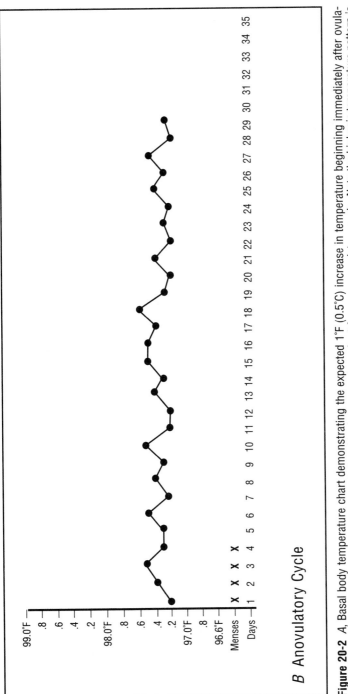

B Anovulatory Cycle

Figure 20-2 *A*, Basal body temperature chart demonstrating the expected 1°F (0.5°C) increase in temperature beginning immediately after ovulation and continuing through the luteal phase. *B*, Basal body temperature chart from an anovulatory cycle. Note the biphasic temperature pattern is lacking.

Patients should be counseled that postponing coitus until evidence of ovulation may result in missed opportunities for conception.

hospitable to sperm passage. On the other hand, these data suggest that sperm may remain viable in the female reproductive tract for up to 5 days. Patients should therefore be made aware that postponing coitus until evidence of ovulation may result in missed opportunities for attempting conception. In addition, this study found no evidence that daily intercourse decreased the likelihood of conception, despite the common belief that spacing intercourse to every other day optimizes fertility.

Physical Examination

The physical examination may uncover signs to suggest the cause of the infertility. The patient's height and weight should be measured and note made of markedly high or low BMI. The thyroid and skin should be carefully examined. Acne or hirsutism (which is sometimes successfully treated and not apparent on exam) may result from a hyperandrogenic state of either ovarian or

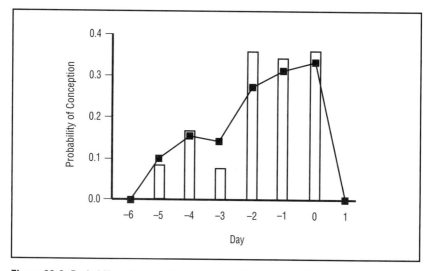

Figure 20-3 Probability of conception on specific days near the day of ovulation. The bars represent probabilities calculated from data on 129 menstrual cycles in which sexual intercourse was recorded to have occurred on only a single day during the 6-day interval ending on the day of ovulation (day 0). The solid line shows daily probabilities based on all 625 cycles, as estimated by the statistical model. (From Wilcox AJ, Weinberg CR, Baird DD. Timing of sexual intercourse in relation to ovulation. N Engl J Med. 1995;333:1517-21; with permission.)

adrenal origin. Expression of nipple discharge on breast exam is often functional but can result from hyperprolactinemia. Obesity and abdominal striae raise concern for possible Cushing's disease or PCOS. The pelvic exam occasionally reveals relevant findings such as clitoromegaly, a pelvic mass, or cul-de-sac nodularity resulting from endometriosis. Testing for chlamydia and gonorrhea is appropriate in the setting of vaginal discharge, evidence of gross cervicitis, or previous history of pelvic infections.

The male partner should also be examined for gynecomastia and undergo genital examination to evaluate the size and consistency of the testicles, and for the presence of a varicocoele. Digital examination of the prostate can help exclude hyperplasia, prostatitis or tumors.

Diagnostic Testing

Basic Tests

When investigating infertility, evaluation of both the male and female partner is warranted, because the likelihood of both partners having impaired fertility is relatively high. By contrast, couples in whom there is only one affected partner frequently compensate for the impairment, conceive spontaneously with only minor delays, and therefore typically never present for infertility evaluation (5). Standard testing for all infertile couples includes semen analysis, hysterosalpingography (HSG) to establish normal anatomy, and laboratory assessment of ovulation (15).

Semen Analysis
Semen analysis should be performed early in the infertility evaluation, because male factors account for 40% of infertility. The man should abstain from intercourse for 2 to 4 days before giving a semen sample collected by masturbation (ideally without the use of lubricants or soap) into a plastic urinalysis cup. Alternatively, silicon (but not latex) condoms can be used to collect a semen specimen. The semen sample must be kept warm (at body temperature) and be delivered to the andrology laboratory within 30 to 60 min after ejaculation.

The normal parameters for a semen analysis have been defined by the 1992 World Health Organization (WHO) manual (Table 20-1). Sperm counts below 20 million/mL (*oligozoospermia*) are associated with decreased male fertility. *Asthenozoospermia* indicates a decrease in motility, where fewer than 50% spermatozoa have forward progression. *Teratozoospermia* is defined as fewer than 30% spermatozoa having normal head morphology. When there is a disturbance of all three variables described above, the term *oligoasthenoterato-*

Table 20-1 Normal Results of Semen Analysis

Volume	≥2 ml
pH	7.2–7.8
Spermatozoa	≥20 million/mL
Motility	≥50%
Morphology	≥30%
White blood cells	<1 million/mL

Data from Rowe PJ, et al. WHO Manual for the Standardized Investigation and Diagnosis of the Infertile Couple. Cambridge Univ Pr; 1993.

zoospermia is used. Ejaculate volume of less than 2 ml is also considered abnormal, as in an increase in white blood cells over 1 million/mL (leukocytospermia), which may indicate a possible prostate infection.

Abnormal findings are usually confirmed with repeat semen analysis; however, it should be noted that the predictive value of abnormalities is often low, because many men with abnormal parameters achieve conception without intervention (5). Nonetheless, men with any of the aforementioned abnormal findings should be referred for urologic evaluation.

Hysterosalpingography

The hysterosalpingogram permits evaluation of fallopian tube patency as well as uterine cavity abnormalities (Table 20-2). HSG can pinpoint abnormalities in the interstitial portion of the tube (salpingitis isthmica nodosa or polyps), the isthmus (obstruction), and the fimbria (hydrosalpinges), or identify peritubular adhesions. In addition, HSG can help uncover uterine abnormalities such as adhesions (Asherman's syndrome), polyps, myomas, bicornuate or subseptate uterus, or anomalies due to DES exposure *in utero*.

HSG is performed under fluoroscopic guidance during the follicular phase of the menstrual cycle, after cessation of menses. The major complication of the HSG is infection, which occurs in 1% to 3% of patients. Some centers prescribe prophylactic doxycycline or azithromycin beginning 1 day before the procedure. Other complications include hypersensitivity reaction to the iodinated contrast, vascular extravasation of the contrast, and pain. To reduce discomfort a nonsteroidal anti-inflammatory agent can be given 1 hr before the procedure (1).

HSG has about a 75% correlation to laparoscopy or hysteroscopy for accuracy, with a false negative rate ranging between 8% and 24% and a false positive rate between 6% and 25%. When the HSG detects hydrosalpinx or evidence of recent infection the patient is prescribed a week-long course of doxycycline. Occasionally laparoscopy is substituted for HSG in the initial infertility evaluation.

Table 20-2 Summary of Diagnostic Tests for Female Infertility

Female Factors	Diagnostic Tests
Cervical	Post-coital test (PCT)
Endometrial	Endometrial biopsy (EB) or progesterone level
Uterine	Hysterosalpingography (HSG) or hysteroscopy or hysterosonography
Tubal	Hysterosalpingography
Peritoneal	Laparoscopy
Ovarian	LH, FSH, estradiol
Hormonal	TSH, prolactin, total testosterone, DHEAS, 17-hydroxyprogesterone
Immunologic	Antisperm antibodies

Hormone Tests

As mentioned previously, measurement of thyroid-stimulating hormone (TSH), prolactin, and follicle-stimulating hormone (FSH) levels should always be obtained, because ovulatory dysfunction resulting from abnormalities in these three areas may not be evident on history or physical exam. Hypothryoidism is diagnosed with a TSH level exceeding 4.5 mU/L. An elevated prolactin level should be confirmed with a second test to rule out physiologic causes such as feeding, sleep, or stress, and the patient's medications should be reviewed to exclude iatrogenic etiologies such as antidopaminergic drugs. Also, it should be noted that hypothyroidism can cause high prolactin values due to lactotrope stimulation by the thyrotropin-releasing hormone (TRH). Those patients with a prolactin level greater than 30 ng/mL should undergo magnetic resonance imaging (MRI) to look for the presence of a pituitary adenoma, which can occur in up to 30% of patients with even minimal prolactin elevations and which should be managed by specialists. Prolactinomas are treated most often with medications (dopamine agonists such as bromocriptine) but sometimes require surgery or radiotherapy.

Lastly, an FSH level is obtained to exclude premature menopause. In any woman age 35 or older both FSH and estradiol levels are measured on the third day of menstruation to evaluate the woman's ovarian reserve. An FSH level greater than 10 mIU/mL with an estradiol level less than 50 pg/mL indicates decreased ovarian reserve and, consequently, a longer time to conception. FSH levels over 25 mIU/mL indicate a likelihood of pregnancy under 5%. An elevated FSH requires confirmatory testing two weeks later to avoid being misled by a pre-ovulatory FSH surge.

The adequacy of ovulatory function can be evaluated by progesterone levels obtained on day 21 of the menstrual cycle, with levels greater than 3 ng/mL providing presumptive evidence of ovulation. Midluteal progesterone levels over 10 ng/mL (in unstimulated cycles) indicate adequate luteal progesterone production. In stimulated menstrual cycles or in the first trimester of pregnancy progesterone levels over 20 ng/mL are considered adequate. It is important to point out that progesterone is produced by the corpus luteum in tonic pulses under the influence of pitutitary LH; therefore a single luteal phase progesterone level may not adequately represent the entire range of peaks and troughs. Thus some consider the endometrial biopsy a superior test (1).

Other Hormone Testing

Notwithstanding the requisite hormone testing (TSH, prolactin, and FSH levels), the commonest cause of anovulation is polycystic ovary syndrome (PCOS). To help confirm this diagnosis one can measure the LH and FSH levels. Patients with PCOS have normal levels but often have an increased LH-to-FSH ratio (usually greater than 2:1). If tested, these patients also have elevated levels of androgens (dehydroepiandrosterone sulfate [DHEA-S] and total testosterone levels). Because estrogen is present due to peripheral aromatization of androgens, a progestin challenge in these patients results in a normal withdrawal bleed.

Congenital hypothalamic dysfunction is most commonly caused by Kallman's syndrome (congenital LHRH deficiency associated with midline anatomic defects and anosmia). Ischemic or traumatic injury to the hypothalamus or pituitary can also disrupt the axis, as can medical problems such as chronic renal failure and cirrhosis (26). In addition, reversible causes such as underweight body habitus, malnutrition, and excessive exercise can cause hypothalamic dysfunction. When gonadotropin levels are measured in these patients, they can be either normal or decreased and therefore such testing is not performed. However, lack of withdrawal bleed in response to a progestin challenge is helpful in confirming the diagnosis. In such patients the ovary is not stimulated to produce estrogen; consequently, these patients require both estrogen and progestin to menstruate. Therefore, once the progestin challenge fails to induce a withdrawal bleed, an estrogen-progestin challenge is next performed by administering conjugated estrogen 0.625 mg orally per day for 25 days with medroxyprogesterone acetate 10 mg orally added for the last 10 days. Patients with hypothalmic dysfunction will experience a withdrawal bleed; failure to respond generally implies an absent or severely damaged endometrium such as that seen with Asherman's syndrome.

Adrenal hyperplasia is a rare but treatable cause of anovulation and virilization. These patients have an enzyme deficiency, usually of 21-hydroxlyase which leads to excess adrenal androgen production. Therefore, for patients in whom significant virilization is detected, one should obtain levels of total testosterone, DHEA-S, and 17-hydroxyprogesterone (17-OHP). Once androgen excess is found, adrenocorticotropic hormone (ACTH) stimulation and measurement of three hormone 17-hydroxy-progesterone levels at times 0 and 1 hr post-injection can confirm the diagnosis (16).

Endometrial Biopsy

The endometrial biopsy (EB) can diagnose luteal phase inadequacy, which is a subtle form of ovulatory dysfunction resulting from altered corpus luteum function. This leads to inadequate progesterone effect on the endometrium and can result in abnormal implantation or early pregnancy wastage, and thus presents clinically either as infertility or recurrent spontaneous abortion (17).

Endometrial biopsy provides histologic evidence of endometrial maturation and is dated according to the criteria established in 1950 by Noyes et al (18). EB is performed 7 to 10 days following ovulation using a flexible plastic catheter. The histologic maturation is compared with the patient's actual cycle day that the biopsy was performed, as determined either from the onset of next menses (day 28) or the day of the preceding LH surge (day 13). A delay of more than 2 days by histologic criteria indicates a luteal phase inadequacy. If the result is abnormal, the biopsy should be repeated. Luteal phase inadequacy may be seen in up to 30% of normal women; however, normally the incidence of recurrent luteal phase defect is only 3% in consecutive cycles.

Endometrial biopsy is an invasive procedure with a complication rate of 3% (excessive pain, vasovagal reaction, uterine perforation, and interruption of pregnancy). However, for the reasons stated above, EB is felt by some to be necessary to diagnose luteal phase inadequacy and to detect polyps or endometritis as well.

Postcoital Test

The postcoital test (PCT) allows evaluation of the interaction between the cervical mucus and the sperm. PCT is performed at the time of ovulation as determined by basal body temperature, ovulation predictor test, or ultrasonography. Following 48 hr of abstinence, intercourse should take place 4 to 12 hr before the scheduled PCT. The patient is advised to refrain from douching.

The mucus can be obtained with an aspirating canula, and it is placed on a slide with an overlying cover slip. The slide can be viewed under the microscope with 100 times magnification. The mucus is observed for clarity, spinnbarkheit ("stretchability"), and quantity. The microscopic exam assesses white blood cells (which when present in a significant number suggest cervicitis and should be treated with doxycycline), sperm number, sperm movement, and sperm forward progression. A count of 5 motile sperm per high power field is considered normal. Absence of sperm in the PCT may indicate a coital problem. Poor sperm motility indicating an immunologic problem occurs in approximately one third of couples with an abnormal PCT (10).

Detection of Ovulation

Three tests permit assessment of the day of ovulation and therefore are helpful in timing either coitus or procedures such as intrauterine insemination: basal body temperature charts, ovulation predictor kits, and ultrasonography.

BASAL BODY TEMPERATURE

Basal body temperature (BBT) is taken every morning immediately upon awakening and recorded (see Fig. 20-2). Body temperature falls to a nadir around the time of the LH surge, then rises shortly thereafter around the time of ovulation. The temperature elevation (approximately 0.5°C or 1°F) is normally maintained for the next 11 to 16 days due to the effect of progesterone on the hypothalamic thermoregulatory center. However, such testing is not always reliable. Elevation of BBT may occur with plasma progesterone elevations as low as 4 ng/mL. Conversely, 10% of ovulating women will have calendars that fail to reflect normal function (19). Lastly, BBT is not very accurate in predicting the timing of ovulation, because it may occur as long as 3 days following the temperature nadir in up to 70% of cycles. In addition to documenting her basal body temperature and menses, it may be helpful for the patient to also record when intercourse takes place; this may assist in diagnosing problems in coital timing or frequency.

OVULATION PREDICTOR KITS

The serum luteinizing hormone (LH) surge occurs between 5 and 9 AM, is detectable in the urine shortly thereafter, and usually induces ovulation 16 to 48 hr later. The sensitivity of the urine LH predictor kits is between 70% and 85%. The kits can be purchased over the counter as a set of 5 tests for approximately $20 to $30.

ULTRASONOGRAPHY

Ultrasonography is the most accurate test for documenting ovulation, with a sensitivity of virtually 100%. However, it is expensive and time consuming. Ovulatory follicles are detected by their size. In unstimulated cycles maximum follicular diameters at ovulation range from 11 to 32 mm, whereas in clomiphene citrate cycles the maximum follicular diameter at ovulation ranges between 18 to 30 mm.

Advanced Tests

As previously discussed, the standard infertility evaluation usually consists of history and physical, semen analysis, hysterosalpingogram, and serum levels of FSH, TSH, prolactin, and luteal phase progesterone levels. For women age 35 and older, measurement of serum FSH and estradiol levels on day 3 of the menstrual cycle is also performed. Often, the post-coital test and endometrial biopsy are employed. The following tests are pursued only when indicated.

Laparoscopy
Laparoscopy is performed when the HSG is abnormal or when the history suggests the presence of pelvic adhesions or endometriosis. Complications include anesthetic adverse events, adhesions, hemorrhage, infection, and bowel or bladder trauma. With the advent of operative laparoscopy, therapeutic intervention can take place at the time of the diagnostic procedure (3,10,19a).

Hysteroscopy
Hysteroscopy further assesses any abnormality that may have been detected in the HSG and can allow for therapeutic intervention. Complications include bleeding, infection, uterine perforation, adhesions, anesthetic adverse events, and fluid absorption (10).

Hysterosonography
Hysterosonography is a vaginal ultrasound-guided test for the evaluation of the uterine cavity. Normal saline injected into the uterus via a small catheter permits visualization of intrauterine pathology such as myomas or polyps. The advantage of this technique over hysteroscopy is that it can determine the extent of intramural involvement of the myoma, thereby suggesting the best surgical approach.

Antisperm Antibodies
Sperm are highly antigenic, and antibodies can sometimes be detected in the female partner. In addition, antibodies can sometimes be detected in the male's own serum (indirect immunobead test) or semen (direct immunobead test) following interruption of the normal barrier via trauma, infection, testicular torsion, or vasectomy reversal. Such testing is therefore done when sperm are immotile in the PCT, after vasectomy reversal, or in the setting of unexplained infertility. Immunoglobulins A and G are considered important, and only head-directed antibodies are felt to interfere with fertilization.

Treatment

Overview

In the case of ovulatory dysfunction, correction of the underlying disorder and/or use of exogenous hormones to induce ovulation can lead to successful ovulation in most cases. However, when premature ovarian failure is diagnosed, infertility must be managed with oocyte or embryo donation when pregnancy is still desired. While surgical repair of obstructed tubes results in low (often less than 30%) subsequent pregnancy rates, laparoscopic resection or ablation of minimal to mild endometriosis can enhance fecundity (20). However, assisted reproductive technology such as *in vitro* fertilization is frequently ultimately necessary. When cervical factors contribute to infertility, the usual treatment is to bypass the cervix with intrauterine insemination (IUI) of washed sperm. Asherman's syndrome is an uncommon cause of infertility but easily corrected with hysteroscopic dissection of the adhesions. Patients with unexplained infertility often conceive successfully with empiric regimens of exogenous hormones that yield superovulation combined with intrauterine insemination. If unsuccessful, these patients are often referred for empiric use of advanced assisted reproductive technology which, because of its relatively high success rate, is used for other causes of infertility as well (21,22).

If premature ovarian failure is the cause of infertility, oocyte or embryo donation is required for pregnancy to be achieved.

Ovulatory Dysfunction

Hyperprolactinemia

For patients with symptomatic hyperprolactinemia (with or without a pituitary adenoma), the treatment of choice is the dopamine agonist bromocriptine. Therapy is started with a dose of 1.25 mg (one-half tablet) each night at bedtime for 1 week. The dose can then be increased to 2.5 mg at night. After 2 weeks the prolactin levels should be repeated and the bromocriptine dose increased by 2.5 mg as needed until prolactin levels are normalized.

Patients who are unable to tolerate oral bromocriptine due to gastrointestinal side effects can use the intravaginal route, often at a reduced dosage. Patients who become pregnant should stop bromocriptine unless they have a pituitary macroadenoma (>1 cm) or note symptoms of tumor enlargement during pregnancy (headache or visual field disturbance).

Patients who fail dopamine agonist therapy may require transphenoidal hypophysectomy or radiotherapy. Also, recall that those presenting with high prolactin levels sometimes merely have hypothyroidism, and this etiology should first be excluded.

Hypothyroidism

Ovulatory dysfunction due to hypothyroidism is easily corrected with thyroid replacement therapy. The starting dose may be estimated based upon body weight but is typically initiated at 75 μg per day. After 4 weeks of therapy the

TSH level can be rechecked and the thyroxine dosage can be increased by 25 µg if necessary. This process is repeated until the TSH is in the range of approximately 1 to 3 mU/L. Note that once the patient taking thyroid replacement becomes pregnant the target TSH is lowered to approximately 1 mU/L.

Polycystic Ovary Syndrome

If the patient with PCOS is overweight, sometimes weight loss alone is adequate to restore ovulation. However, medical intervention is usually required. Recent studies have demonstrated return of ovulatory function by reversing insulin resistance with metformin (23), which can be discontinued once the patient becomes pregnant. Some have also recently begun using the thiazolidinediones for this purpose. In general, however, usually patients with PCOS require ovulation induction with either clomiphene citrate or, if necessary, gonadotropins.

For patients with polycystic ovary syndrome who are overweight, weight loss may be all that is necessary to restore ovulatory function.

Clomiphene citrate is an antiestrogenic compound that increases pituitary gonadotropin (FSH and LH) secretion and folliculogenesis. Therefore use of clomiphene requires an intact hypothalamo-pituitary axis. This can first be confirmed by a withdrawal bleed following progestin challenge of progesterone in oil 100 mg intramuscularly or medroxyprogesterone acetate 10 mg orally per day for 10 days (see Chapter 3). Then, beginning on days 3 to 5 of the progestin-induced menstrual cycle, clomiphene can be started at a dose of 50 mg orally for 5 days. If ovulation does not occur, as determined by basal body temperature or LH surge predictor kit, the dose may be increased by 50 mg per day each month, to a maximum of 150 mg per day. Once the ovulatory dose of clomiphene has been established, an endometrial biopsy to ascertain endometrial adequacy and a post-coital test to rule out cervical mucus problems are often performed. Most patients ovulate at doses less than 100 mg per day, and most conceptions occur within 6 months of initiation of therapy. Because of this, some authorities recommend that clomiphene trials not be continued beyond this time.

Multiple pregnancies occur in 10% of cycles (16) but are usually only twins. Side effects of clomiphene include ovarian enlargement, vasomotor instability, alopecia, urticaria, and visual disturbances (scotomata), but discontinuation of treatment is rare (5).

Recently, concern has been raised about the possible association of fertility drugs and ovarian cancer. Some but not all (24,25) studies have suggested that women using clomiphene or gonadotropins might be at increased risk. It is appropriate to advise patients of this concern but that the data are not yet definitive. It is of note that nulliparity and infertility themselves raise a woman's risk of ovarian cancer, whereas pregnancy, lactation, and oral contraceptives decrease this risk.

Pituitary Dysfunction (and Use of Gonadotropins for Other Causes of Infertility)

For patients with PCOS who fail clomiphene or for patients with conditions that render them without endogenous estrogen production (such as those with hypothalamic dysfunction), intramuscular injections of urinary menotropins (FSH and LH) or subcutaneous injections of recombinent follitropins (pure formulations of FSH alone) are used. Use of these gonadotropins requires availability of ultrasonography and serum estradiol (E2) monitoring seven days a week to minimize the complications of multiple gestations (30%) and severe ovarian hyperstimulation syndrome (1%).

Patients are started on injections of one ampule of gonadotropins (75 IU) daily beginning on day 2 or 3 of the progestin-induced menstrual cycle. The dose may be increased one ampule at a time as necessary until ultrasonography demonstrates follicular development. When there is at least one mature follicle (diameter ≥18 mm) by ultrasonography and the E2 is at least 250 pg/mL, human chorionic gonadotropin (hCG) 10,000 U IM can be given to induce ovulation 36 hr later. To avoid complications, hCG is withheld when the E2 level is greater than 1500 pg/mL or when ultrasonography shows more than four mature follicles and multiple smaller follicles (diameter ≤10 mm). Luteal phase support is given to patients with hypothalamo-pituitary axis dysfunction using either hCG 5000 U one week post-ovulation or progesterone suppositories 25 mg per vagina twice daily for 2 weeks. Complications of gonadotropin use include persistent ovarian cysts and a 30% chance of multiple pregnancy. When patients present with a high-order (≥3) pregnancy, it may be medically indicated to recommend multifetal pregnancy reduction to reduce the risk of prematurity and low birth weight in the remaining fetuses.

Complications of gonadotropin use include persistent ovarian cysts and a 30% chance of multiple pregnancy. Data are inconclusive regarding a possible association with subsequent ovarian cancer.

Ovarian hyperstimulation syndrome is a serious but rare complication (1%). This syndrome is usually associated with exogenous hCG administration and results from increased vascular permeability and extravasation of intravascular fluid. Massive ascites or anasarca, hemoconcentration, and renal and hepatic failure can all ensue, and patients often require monitoring and aggressive management in an intensive care setting (5,26).

Luteal phase inadequacy can be treated with either "superovulation" with clomiphene or gonadotropins, as described above, or with luteal phase supplementation. Luteal phase support must also be given to patients with hypothalamo-pituitary axis dysfunction, using an injection of hCG 5000 U one week post-ovulation, or intravaginal progesterone suppositories for 2 weeks.

Short-acting gonadotropin-releasing hormone (GnRH) agonists, such as intranasal nafarelin acetate and subcutaneous leuprolide acetate, have recently been used in conjuction with gonadotropins (FSH and LH) to prevent premature follicular luteinization. While GnRH agonists have an initial stimulatory effect on gonadotropins lasting 7 to 10 days, they subsequently suppress gonadotropin function, which helps prevent premature luteinization. These drugs are not FDA approved for ovulation and patients should be so informed.

Adrenal Hyperplasia

Adrenal hyperplasia is a rare cause of anovulation that can be successfully treated by partially suppressing adrenal function with corticosteroids. Commonly used regimens include prednisone to 2.5 to 5 mg orally per day and dexamethasone 0.25 to 0.5 mg orally per day. These dosages should be lowered so as to maintain the 8 AM cortisol level above 2.0 µg/dL to avoid total adrenal suppression.

Hypothalamic Amenorrhea

The treatment of choice for the induction of ovulation in hypothalamic amenorrhea is gonadotropin-releasing hormone infusion, with luteal phase support. GnRH may be given in a pulsatile manner with an infusion pump every 60 to 90 min. GnRH may be administered subcutaneously (10 to 20 µg per pulse) or intravenously (5 to 10 µg per pulse), starting on day 2 or 3 of the cycle, and the treatment is monitored every 4 to 5 days with E2 and ultrasonography in a manner similar to menotropin ovulation induction. Ovulation then occurs spontaneously once follicular development produces adequate estrogen feedback to the hypothalamo-pituitary axis to trigger the LH surge. The luteal phase must be supported with either a continued GnRH infusion or as previously described for gonadotropins.

Tubal Disease

Laparoscopic surgery can be used to treat pelvic adhesions, hydrosalpinges, and proximal tubal obstructions. Proximal tubal occlusions can also be recanalized by hysteroscopic approach under laparoscopic control. However, the overall pregnancy rate following these procedures is quite low, about 30%. Because of this, some have recommended *in vitro* fertilization over repair, not only for its superior efficacy but for its lower cost (15). Certainly when extensive tubal disease is present, or following multiple surgical procedures, assisted reproductive technology is recommended, with pregnancy rates of 25% to 30% per cycle (3). In contrast, reversing tubal sterilization with laparotomy and microreanastomosis is relatively effective with an average success rate of 50%. However, following any surgical repair of the fallopian tubes the risk of ectopic pregnancy is increased.

Cervical Factors

Intrauterine insemination (IU) is indicated in cases of poor PCT, low sperm counts, or in cases of unexplained infertility. IUI involves the injection of sperm directly into the uterine cavity, after washing the semen of all prostaglandins. The reported overall pregnancy rate after IUI for cervical factor infertility is 60% to 70%. IUI is also sometimes a helpful adjunct in women taking clomiphene citrate for ovarian stimulation due to the drug's anti-estrogenic effects on the cervical mucous.

Uterine Factors

Uterine myomas large enough to distort the pelvic organs may sometimes result in infertility. Of women with unexplained infertility who are found to have myomas, 50% achieve pregnancy following myomectomy. Uterine adhesions (Asherman's syndrome) can be resected via the operating hysteroscopy or resectoscope. In addition, endometrial polyps, submucosal myomas, and uterine septa can be resected with the same technology (16,19a).

Endometriosis

Laparoscopic diagnosis and treatment of endometriosis has become routine with the advent of operative laparoscopy. Until recently early disease (stages I or II) was left untreated; while it can result in delayed fertility, overall spontaneous pregnancy rates can be as high as 60% to 70%. However, one recent prospective trial demonstrated significant improvement to fertility following laparoscopic ablation of minimal-to-mild endometriosis (20). In cases of advanced disease (stages III or IV), a combined surgical excision and medical suppression with GnRH agonists or danazol has been used successfully, with overall pregnancy rates around 50% to 60%. It should be noted that when used alone without surgery, hormonal treatment improves pain symptoms but not fertility (15,27). When surgical treatment has failed, assisted reproductive technology offers an excellent therapeutic alternative with pregnancy rates of 25% to 30% per cycle.

Immunological Factors

The significance of antisperm antibodies is not well understood, and treatment with corticosteroid suppression has not resulted in increased pregnancy rates. Currently IUI is used initially for three cycles, but assisted reproductive technology (e.g., *in vitro* fertilization) represents the best alternative (see Assisted Reproductive Technology below). Overall pregnancy rates are 30%.

Male Factors

Intrauterine insemination is the treatment of choice in cases of reduced sperm counts. However, when sperm counts are less than 5 million/mL, assisted reproductive technology should be considered, with the option of intracytoplasmic sperm injection (ICSI) in cases of severe male factor. In fact, ICSI technology has almost obviated the need for donor insemination (4). However, when used, therapeutic donor insemination is associated with excellent pregnancy rates, at a fraction of the cost of assisted reproductive technologies (19,28-30).

Unexplained Infertility

Empiric induction of ovulation with clomiphene citrate for 3 to 4 months has been shown to approximately double the pregnancy rate in couples with infertility of more than 3 years' duration (31). If pregnancy fails to occur sometimes adding intrauterine insemination or intraperitoneal insemination improves the fecundability rates (32). Thereafter use of gonadotropins for another 3 to 4 months is often successful. Usually 4 to 6 cycles of ovulation induction may be necessary to achieve pregnancy. The overall pregnancy rate for empiric therapy of unexplained infertility is 30%. When ovulation induction is not successful within 4 to 6 cycles, assisted reproductive technology is undertaken, with pregnancy rates of 25% to 30% per cycle.

Assisted Reproductive Technology

The first test-tube baby conceived via *in vitro* fertilization and embryo transfer (IVF-ET) was born in 1978, and since then assisted reproductive technology (ART) has expanded to include other complex techniques and applications.

ART was originally developed as a treatment for tubal factor infertility; however, it is now also used in the setting of endometriosis and male factor infertility—for which intracytoplasmic sperm injection is also often incorporated. Because of its relatively high success rate, ART is also utilized for unexplained infertility. Although fecundability rates are typically low (often only 15% to 25% per cycle), after six cycles the cumulative probability of pregnancy reaches 60% to 70%. The low rate is attributed in part to a failure of the embryos to successfully implant in the endometrium. In addition, among those embryos that do successfully implant there is a 20% to 30% risk of spontaneous abortion, similar to that seen in the fertile population. Increasing the number of embryos transferred can therefore greatly improve the pregnancy rate. However, this motivation is counter-balanced by a desire to minimize the chance of multiple births, and typically an average of two to three embryos are transferred. Many factors must be considered, and, for example, a greater number of embryos are typically transferred to women older than 40 years, since the rate of spontaneous abortion increases steadily with increasing maternal age.

The various ART procedures are summarized in Table 20-3.

In Vitro Fertilization and Embryo Transfer

Because multiple embryos are desired, controlled ovarian hyperstimulation is used, employing GnRH and gonadotropins as previously described. After close monitoring with ultrasonography and serum estradiol levels, hCG is administered and oocytes are retrieved 34 to 36 hr later (just before egg release). Transvaginal aspiration in a sedated patient is now preferred to avoid exposing the oocytes to the carbon dioxide that is required with laparoscopy. After the oocytes are incubated for 2 to 36 hr in culture media, washed and concentrated sperm are added, and the eggs are examined for fertilization 16 to 18 hr later. Of those that are fertilized, only the normal-appearing eggs are transferred to growth medium. Approximately 48 hr after aspiration of the oocytes, and with the patient in the lithotomy position, embryos in the four- to six-cell stage are transferred into the uterus transcervically via a catheter (33,34). Although a rare complication (<1%), ectopic pregnancy is not completely prevented by in vitro fertilization, and women with previous history of ectopic pregnancy should be advised of such.

Gamete Intrafallopian Transfer

Gamete intrafallopian transfer (GIFT) differs from in vitro fertilization in that fertilization occurs in vivo, in the fallopian tubes. Oocytes and sperm are transferred to one or both fallopian tubes, usually via laparoscopy. This method therefore requires at least one intact fallopian tube and is indicated

Table 20-3 Characteristics of Assisted Reproductive Technology Procedures*

Procedure	Description	Advantages	Disadvantages	Pregnancy Rate	Multiple Pregnancy Rate	Cost per Completed Cycle
In vitro fertilization and embryo transfer (IVF-ET)	Oocytes are fertilized by sperm on *in vitro* culture system; embryo is then transferred to uterus via cervix	Completely bypasses fallopian tubes May be done in unstimulated cycle in women <35 years old Allows micromanipulation of gametes or embryos; incurs lowest cost	Usually requires controlled ovarian hyperstimulation	26%	40%	$8000–$12,000
Gamete intrafallopian transfer (GIFT)	Oocytes and sperm are placed in one or both fallopian tubes, usually via laparoscopic cannulation	May be more acceptable to some patients for religious reasons	Requires normal fallopian tubes; requires laparoscopic gamete transfer; does not allow *in vitro* assessment or micromanipulation of gametes/embryos; higher cost than IVF-ET	29%	34%	$10,000–$14,000
Zygote intrafallopian transfer (ZIFT)	Combines IVF and GIFT; oocytes are fertilized *in vitro*, then zygotes (embryos) are transferred to fallopian tubes	Allows fertilization assessment and micromanipulation of spermatazoa or embryos *in vitro*	Requires normal fallopian tubes; requires laparoscopic transfer of zygotes; requires two separate procedures (one for oocyte retrieval and one for zygote transfer)	30%	36%	$14,000–$16,000
Cryopreserved embryo transfer	Complex multistep procedure to preserve embryos	Allows for transfer of embryos obtained from a previously successful ART cycle Allows for embryo transfer in a "natural" (unstimulated) cycle; low cost	Requires previously successful *in vitro* fertilization	17%	28%	$2000–$3000 per embryo transfer (plus cost of previous oocyte harvesting)
Oocyte donation	Oocyte donated by third party; pregnancy supported by exogenous hormone administration	Allows conception at any time in menopause with medical clearance Alternative to adoption Recipient's fertility becomes that of the age of the oocyte donor Allows for cryopreservation of excess embryos for future embryo transfer	Requires an oocyte donor volunteer; may result in very high risk conceptions in some women over 50 years; high cost	39%	40%	$13,000–$15,000

*Note that these procedures are associated with similar incidences of spontaneous abortion (15% to 20%), ectopic pregnancy (1%), and birth defects (2%).

for conditions such as endometriosis, cervical factor infertility, and unexplained infertility.

Advantages of GIFT over IVF-ET include its superior simulation of natural timing (IVF-ET places the embryos in the endometrium 3 to 4 days early) and less need for specialized equipment and trained personnel. However, disadvantages of GIFT include the need for laparascopy and general anesthesia, and the lack of information regarding the resulting embryos. Moreover, some have pointed out that controlled ovarian stimulation coupled with intrauterine insemination (COS-IUI) differs little from GIFT, yet the former is much less expensive and avoids laparoscopy (33,34).

Zygote Intrafallopian Transfer

Zygote intrafallopian transfer (ZIFT) consists of laparoscopic transfer of embryos into the fallopian tube after oocyte fertilization *in vitro*. Tubal embryo transfer (TET) and pronuclear stage transfer (PROST) are variations of ZIFT that differ only in the developmental stage at which the embryos are transferred. As with GIFT, ZIFT requires at least one intact fallopian tube and is indicated for severe male factor infertility, immunologic infertility, and possibly unexplained infertility (33,34).

Embryo Cryopreservation

Advances in cryobiology have allowed preservation of embryos, thereby decreasing the number of egg retrieval procedures required for serial attempts at IVF or GIFT. Recent improvements in freezing and thawing techniques have led to better outcomes, so that some facilities now report equal pregnancy rates using fresh or frozen/thawed embryos (33,34).

Oocyte Donation

Oocyte donation is required for women with gonadal dysgenesis or postmenopausal women who wish to carry a pregnancy. Also, oocyte donation is sometimes chosen by women with repeated failures at assisted conception or by those with inheritable genetic defects (34).

Adoption

Couples with infertility who are unable to conceive despite the best of efforts need to be counseled about either stopping all fertility treatments and/or considering adoption. Unresolved feelings about infertility may make it very difficult for a couple to accept adoption as an alternative to living childfree, because a couple with impaired infertility must first grieve their loss (22,35). Once the decision has been made to proceed with adoption, the couple must choose between a public adoption agency, with a typical waiting period of 2 years, and private adoption through an experienced attorney. In either case the couple must first wait for the birth mother to give up her child, which can lead to significant distress or disappointment. RESOLVE, a support group for couples with infertility, offers information on various adoption options available to couples at the state and national level (35).

Psychological Considerations

Couples with infertility may experience any of a wide variety of emotional responses. A minority accepts childlessness easily, but many more suffer significant emotional distress because of the diagnosis. Emotional responses can include anger, frustration, grief, depression, resentment, guilt, shock, denial, and anxiety, and it is common for individual partners to have differing responses. Not surprisingly, sexual dysfunction and marital difficulties can ensue. It is important to provide emotional support and counseling for these couples. Allowing patients adequate time at office visits is very important. Local and national support groups are also quite helpful in addressing the emotional roller coaster that couples with infertility may have to endure. Experienced therapists are sometimes needed.

Conclusion

Infertility is an increasingly common problem. Fortunately this condition can often be treated using therapies that range from simple lifestyle changes to applications of complex technology. Familiarity with evaluation and treatment methods can allow the primary care physician to take part in the early investigation and better guide the patient.

REFERENCES

1. **Rowe PJ, et al.** WHO Manual for the Standardized Investigation and Diagnosis of the Infertile Couple. Cambridge Univ Pr; 1993.
2. **Jaffe SB, Jewelewicz R.** The basic infertility evaluation. Fertil Steril. 1991;56:599-613.
3. **Witt BR.** Pelvic factors and fertility. In: Infertility and Reproductive Medicine Clinics of North America. Philadelphia: WB Saunders; 1991;2:371-90.
4. **Hanson MA, Dumesic DA.** Initial evaluation and treatment of infertility in a primary-care setting. Mayo Clin Proc. 1998;73:681-5.

5. Infertility revisited: the state of the art today and tomorrow. The ESHRE Capri Workshop. European Society for Human Reproduction and Embryology. Hum Reprod. 1996;11:1779-807.

6. **Benoff S, Cooper GW, Hurley I, et al.** The effect of calcium ion channel blockers on sperm fertilization potential. Fertil Steril. 1994;62:606-17.

7. **Bolumar F, Olsen J, Boldsen J, and the European Study Group on Infertility and Subfecundity.** Smoking reduces fecundity: a European multicenter study on infertility and subfecundity. Am J Epidemiol. 1996;143:578-87.

8. **Augood C, Duckett K, Templeton AA.** Smoking and female infertility: a systematic review and meta-analysis. Human Reprod. 1998;13:1532-9.

9. **Curtis KM, Savitz DA, Arbuckle TE.** Effects of cigarette smoking, caffeine consumption, and alcohol intake on fecundaility. Am J Epidemiol. 1997;146:32-41.

10. **Russell JB, Ziegler WF.** The overall workup of the female patient. Assisted Reproduction Rev. 1993;3:182-9.

11. **Jensen TK, Hjollund NH, Henriksen TB, et al.** Does moderate alcohol consumption affect fertility? Follow-up study among couples planning first pregnancy. BMJ. 1998; 317:505-10.

11a. **Buck GM, Sever LE, Batt RE, Mendola P.** Life-style factors and female infertility. Epidemiology. 1997;8:435-41.

12. **Smith CG, Besch NF, Smith RG, Besch PK.** Effect of tetrahydrocannabinol on the hypothalamic-pituitary axis in the ovariectomized rhesus monkey. Fertil Steril. 1979; 31:335-9.

13. **Solomon GM.** Reproductive toxins: a growing concern at work and in the community. J Occup Envir Med. 1997;39:105-7.

14. **Wilcox AJ, Weinberg CR, Baird DD.** Timing of sexual intercourse in relation to ovulation. N Engl J Med. 1995;333:1517-21.

15. **Crosignani PG, Rubin BL, and ESHRE Capri Workshop Group.** Optimal use of infertility diagnostic tests and treatments. Human Reprod. 2000;15:723-32.

16. **Scoccia B.** Amenorrhea. In: Conn's Current Therapy—1993. Rakel RE, ed. Philadelphia: WB Saunders; 1993:1052-7.

17. **Ginsburg KA.** Luteal phase defect: etiology, diagnosis and management. Endocrinol and Metab Clin North Am. 1992;21:85-104.

18. **Noyes RW, Hertig A, Rock J.** Dating the endometrial biopsy. Fertil Steril. 1950;1:3.

19. **Blacker C.** Ovulation stimulation and induction. Endocrinol Metab Clin North Am. 1992;21:57-84.

19a. **Chen SH, Wallach EE.** Five decades of progress in management of the infertile couple. Fertil Steril. 1994;62:665-85.

20. **Marcoux S, Maheux R, Berube S, and the Canadian Collaborative Group on Endometriosis.** Laparoscopic surgery in infertile women with minimal or mild endometriosis. N Engl J Med. 1997;337:217-22.

21. **Illions EH, Valley MT, Kaunitz AM.** Infertility: a clinical guide for the internist. Med Clin North Am. 1998;82:271-95.

22. **Hammer Burns L.** An overview of the psychology of infertility. In: Infertility and Reproductive Medicine Clinics of North America. Philadelphia: WB Saunders; 1993; 4:433-54.

23. **Ehrmann DA.** Insulin-lowering therapeutic modalities for polycystic ovary syndrome. Endocrinol Metab Clin N A. 1999;28:423-8.

24. **Modan B, Ron E, Lerner-Geva L, et al.** Cancer incidence in a cohort of infertile women. Am J Epidemiol. 1998;147;11:1038-42.

25. **Shushan A, Paltiel O, Iscovich J, et al.** Human menopausal gonadotropin and the risk of epithelial ovarian cancer. Fertil Steril. 1996;65:13-8.

26. **Rosene-Montella K, Keely E, Laifer SA, Lee RV.** Evaluation and management of infertility in women: the internists' role. Ann Intern Med. 2000;132:973-81.

27. **Wellbery C.** Diagnosis and treatment of endometriosis. Am Fam Physician. 1999; 60:1753-68.

28. **Alikani M, Cohen J.** Advances in clinical micromanipulation of gametes and embryos: assisted fertilization and hatching. Arch Pathol Lab Med. 1992;116:373-8.

29. **Penzias AS, DeCherney AH.** Advances in clinical *in vitro* fertilization. J Clin Endocrinol Metab. 1994;78:503-8.

30. **Van Steirteghem AC, Nagy Z, Liu J, et al.** Intracytoplasmic sperm injection. Assisted Reprod Rev. 1993;3:160-3.

31. **Glazener CM, Coulson C, Lambert PA, et al.** Clomiphene treatment for women with unexplained fertility: placebo-controlled study of hormonal responses and conception rates. Gynecol Endocrinol. 1990;4:75-83.

32. **Crosignani PG, Walters DE, Soliani A.** The ESHRE multicentre trial on the treatment of unexplained infertility: preliminary report. Human Reprod. 1991;6:953-8.

33. **Hummel WP, Kettel LM.** Assisted reproductive technology: the state of the art. Ann Med. 1997;29:207-14.

34. **Forti G, Krausz C.** Clinical review 100: evaluation and treatment of the infertile couple. J Clin Endocrinol Metab. 1998;83:4177-88.

35. **Mednick RA, Mednick E, Ratz O, Barad D.** Adoption: to have a family, not just a pregnancy. In: Infertility and Reproductive Medicine Clinics of North America. Philadelphia: WB Saunders; 1991;2:443-8.

CHAPTER 21

Domestic Violence

JEANNE MCCAULEY, MD, MPH

omestic violence is defined as the use or threat of physical force against a person by a relative or intimate, who may or may not be living in the same household with the abused person. Though this definition does not include verbal abuse, many experts and victims have expressed concern that this form of abuse causes similar harm and also may be a precursor to physical abuse.

Abuse, whether experienced currently, in recent adulthood, or remotely in childhood or adolescence, is associated with both a variety of physical and psychological symptoms and increased health care utilization among women (1-9). Because women rarely volunteer a history of abuse and most physicians do not routinely screen for the problem (10), it often goes unrecognized. However, increased awareness by primary care providers can improve the likelihood of detecting domestic violence, and allow opportunities for intervention.

Crucial to understanding domestic violence is recognition of its complexity. Careful analysis identifies a multitude of reasons why battered women do not simply leave the abusive relationship (11). Financial dependence on the abuser is common, especially since the abuser may take deliberate measures to deny the victim access to liquid assets. Also, abused women often become socially isolated as the partner progressively restricts access to friends, family, and the telephone—and sometimes even to radio and television. The typical pattern of interspersed "honeymoon" periods, wherein the abuser expresses love and tenderness and makes promises to change his behavior, may have a powerful influence in keeping the abused in the relationship, despite the fact that this phase is followed by a recurrence of violence. Commonly experienced emotions such as shame and humiliation contribute to low self-esteem and feelings of helplessness regarding a woman's situation and, ultimately, impede her exit. In addition, abused women recognize that, despite the fact that legislation against abuse is now universal in this country, legal protection and other interventions are nonetheless often inadequate. Most importantly, abused women frequently cannot leave their batterer because they correctly perceive the associated risk of physical harm or even death for themselves or their dependent family members. In fact, the process of leaving the relationship is clearly identified as the most dangerous time for an abused woman (11).

Because leaving the relationship is typically the most dangerous time for an abused woman, careful planning is often important.

Epidemiology

It is estimated that 2 to 4 million women in the United States are physically abused each year and that domestic violence may occur in as many as 1 in every 4 families (12). The prevalence of current domestic violence in adult women presenting to primary care settings has been estimated to range from 5% to 23%; the lifetime adult prevalence ranges from 8% to 44% (9,12-16). Variations in prevalence reflect differing definitions of physical abuse, sociodemographic differences between populations studied, and the use of different types of surveys (e.g., whether or not the survey was anonymous).

Domestic violence tends to be more common among younger women (with the highest prevalence found among those under age 25), women of lower socioeconomic status, and women who are single, separated, or divorced (9,14,17). Prevalence of abuse during pregnancy may be as high as 17% (18). Most studies detect no racial differences in the prevalence of domestic violence (9,19), yet some report higher rates for whites than nonwhites (20,21). It should be emphasized, however, that domestic violence has been documented among women of all ages, races, and socioeconomic backgrounds.

The National Institute of Justice recently estimated the annual medical costs for adult domestic violence at $1.8 billion, with the total annual societal costs (including tangible property loss and impact on the quality of life) to be 67 billion dollars (22).

Health Problems Associated with Domestic Violence

A 24-year-old woman, recently separated, presents with pelvic pain and an abnormal vaginal discharge. She appears depressed. Your differential diagnosis includes such causes as pelvic inflammatory disease, ectopic pregnancy, urinary tract infection, and vaginitis. What other potentially life-threatening diagnosis should be in your differential diagnosis?

Physical Problems

Studies of abused women in both subspecialist and community settings show that these women suffer from a higher incidence of GI disorders, headaches, chronic pain, pelvic pain, and multiple somatic complaints (1-9,23-25). Chronic pelvic pain may be especially common in women sexually abused in childhood (see Chapter 12) (4,5). One study of women presenting to a gynecologic practice found that women reporting childhood abuse had significantly higher reports of severe PMS, frequent "gynecologic problems", and frequent vaginal infections (8).

In the largest study to date of physical symptoms of female, domestic violence victims in a primary care setting, 1952 Baltimore women of diverse socioeconomic background were anonymously surveyed regarding current and past physical and sexual abuse and their physical and emotional health (9). Those women reporting domestic abuse in the previous 12 months reported more physical symptoms in the previous 6 months when compared with those who were not experiencing current abuse (mean 7.3 vs. 4.3). The specific physical symptoms more common in the currently abused than in the not currently abused group are listed in Box 21-1. Interestingly, women abused before age 18 but not as adults had similar high total numbers of physical symptoms, with many of the symptoms resembling those of the women experiencing current domestic violence (25). The specific gynecologic symptoms commonly reported by these two groups of women include vaginal discharge, pain in the pelvis or genital area, and breast pain. Women experiencing current abuse were also found to be slightly more likely to have suffered a miscarriage sometime in their lives than not currently abused women (9).

Box 21-1 Physical Symptoms in Women Experiencing Current Domestic Violence*

- Loss of appetite
- Frequent or serious bruises
- Nightmares
- Vaginal discharge
- Eating binges or self-induced vomiting
- Diarrhea
- Broken bones, sprains, or cuts
- Pain in pelvis or genital area (gynecologic complaints)
- Fainting or passing out
- Abdominal or stomach pain
- Breast pain
- Frequent or serious headaches
- Difficulty urinating
- Chest pain
- Difficulty sleeping
- Shortness of breath
- Constipation

*Symptoms are in order of decreasing frequency; all are significantly more common in the currently abused than in the not currently abused group (9).

These and similar studies suggest that violence, whether experienced in childhood or adulthood, is associated with the appearance of certain physical symptoms. Although no symptom profile is pathognomonic for abuse, a clinician should be particularly alert to the possibility of abuse if a woman presents with multiple physical symptoms. It is unclear whether the physical problems are a direct result of the trauma itself, a heightened sensitivity to pain due to neural damage, or psychological distress associated with the trauma (26).

Psychological Symptoms and Behavior

Studies of patients in primary care and subspecialty settings have shown that a history of violence, either currently or in the past, is significantly associated with depression, anxiety, low self-esteem, somatization, post-traumatic stress syndrome, current and past drug and alcohol abuse, and suicide attempts

(9,18,25-28). It should be noted that in the case of depression, it is not possible to establish a temporal or causal relationship with the violence (19).

There also appears to be a stepwise relationship between the number of episodes of childhood violence and adult health risk behaviors. A questionnaire mailed to 9508 HMO patients revealed that adverse childhood experiences (which include physical, psychological, or sexual abuse, but also violence against the mother and living in a household with members who were mentally ill or suicidal, substance abusers, or ever imprisoned) found that adults who had suffered four or more adverse childhood experiences were three times more likely to have had 50 or greater lifetime sexual partners and 2.5 times more likely to have had an STD (29). In addition, women exposed to such events in childhood were 1.5 times more likely to have had an unintended first pregnancy (30).

Some abused women suffer from post-traumatic stress disorder and consequently may experience difficulty with pelvic exams, resulting either from "flashbacks" or an increased startle reflex. Clinicians should take extra care to explain the exam before touching the patient, have a supportive chaperone in the room, carefully apprise the patient of each step before proceeding, and be especially gentle.

Medical Utilization

While there have been few studies of health care utilization in battered women, the literature suggests that abused women seek health care with disproportionate frequency (22,31,32). One study followed 117 battered women initially identified in an emergency room and compared them with not-abused women. Over the ensuing 5 years, the group of abused women had higher rates of outpatient hospital utilization (77% vs. 50%), medical admissions (420 vs. 119), and psychiatric admissions (69 vs. 1 in the control group) (31).

In another study of the health effects of criminal victimization (consisting partly of domestic violence), outpatient physician visits (excluding psychotherapy) by the women increased 15% to 24% in the year following the crime (32). In this study, which was somewhat limited by a low response rate, victimization was the most powerful predictor of physician visits and outpatient costs (32). Similarly, the large Baltimore study of battered women in a primary care setting found that currently abused women were more likely to have visited an emergency room in the preceding 6 months (9). Rather surprisingly and in contrast to other data, this study did not reveal a higher rate of psychiatric admissions or greater use of antidepressants or anxiolytics among the currently abused. The reason for this discrepancy is unclear; the finding may merely represent under-recognition of patients' psychological distress by practitioners. Study of this same population did find, however, that women abused before the age of 18 were more likely to have had a psychiatric admission (25).

Barriers to Detection

Patient Barriers to Disclosure

The vast majority of abused patients have never discussed the abuse with a physician or other health professional. Most patients do not spontaneously volunteer a history of abuse. One important patient barrier to disclosure is shame. Many abused women feel intense shame about the violence, and they may even deny or conceal the abuse, fearing additional "secondary stigmatization" (additional shame brought on by being ignored, blamed, rejected, or "judged" by a clinician) (33). This secondary stigmatization can contribute significant additional psychological stress to the patient.

Other barriers to patient disclosure include denial that they are "abused women" (even when the physical harm is severe), financial dependence on the abuser, fear of legal custody issues with children, fear of repercussions from other family members, emotional commitment to the abuser, and a sense of helplessness and hopelessness. Fear of retaliation from the abuser represents a particularly important obstacle, because abused women may correctly recognize that interventions resulting from disclosure may ultimately trigger violence by the partner. Abusive partners may also prevent women from seeking routine or emergency health care (34).

Physician Barriers to Detection and Treatment

The majority of physicians do not screen their patients for abuse. Physician barriers to screening include time pressures, fear of opening Pandora's box, uncertainty of how to deal with patient disclosure, and incorrect assumptions about who may be a victim (35,36). Too often, physicians underestimate the prevalence of domestic violence and doubt that victims could be of similar race, financial, or educational background as themselves. Some clinicians still feel that domestic violence is not a medical problem. Others blame the woman, believing that she either precipitated the abuse or is weak by failing to "just leave".

Experts point out that many abused women present to office medical practices rather than emergency rooms, and that these women typically complain of multiple physical problems in addition to psychological distress. Consequently, primary care physicians are in a unique position to identify and address domestic violence. In addition, detection of abuse, either currently or in the past, may alter both the diagnosis and treatment of the medical and psychiatric problems (34).

Screening and Identification of the Abused Patient

The American College of Physicians–American Society of Internal Medicine, the American College of Obstetricians and Gynecologists, and the Academy of Family Physicians all recommend that clinicians "be alert to the possibility of domestic violence as a causal factor in illness and injury" (17).

Certain sociodemographic indicators and psychological or physical symptoms were found to be especially common among currently abused women in the large Baltimore study (Boxes 21-1 and 21-2) (9). The risk of current domestic violence increases dramatically with increasing number of these features. Clinicians might also be alerted to the possibility of abuse based on the medical presentation, pattern of injury, or behavior of a companion (Table 21-1). It is especially important to screen women who have even "mild" trauma or bruises, multiple physical or psychological problems, or a substance-abusing partner.

Some patients may "test" the clinician to "invite disclosure". In this situation, the patient may hint that something is wrong in her personal life or say she is under a lot of "stress" but will not disclose the abuse unless directly "invited to" by a direct question from the clinician. If the patient perceives an indifferent, distant, or uncaring attitude from the clinician, she may "shut down" (33,34). Physician awareness of this practice of subtle hinting and sen-

---

Box 21-2 Risk Factors for Current Domestic Violence

Sociodemographic features
  Age ≤35
  Separated or divorced
  No medical insurance
  Low income
Psychosocial variables
  Depression, anxiety, somatization, or low self-esteem
  Post-traumatic stress syndrome
  Current or previous drug or alcohol abuse
  Suicide attempt
  Physical symptoms (see Box 21-1)

Derived from data from one primary care population (9).

sitivity to the patient's distress may therefore be effective means of uncovering abuse. It should be noted that women may be most likely to disclose abuse when they perceive a situation to be dangerous; thus the clinician should never minimize the seriousness of any reported verbal or physical abuse (34).

Many experts, including the U.S. Preventive Services Task Force (USPSTF) (17) feel that because of the high prevalence of abuse and the reluctance of patients to volunteer this problem, physicians should actively screen all patients for abuse. One study of abuse victims showed the majority favor routine physical abuse screening by health professionals (10).

Domestic violence is grossly under-recognized; consequently, groups such as USPSTF have recommended universal patient screening.

Patients can be screened for abuse either through written questionnaires or orally, though some experts feel that oral interviews are more accurate. If a woman is given a written questionnaire, it should be administered in a private area. Women should not be screened for abuse if accompanied by another person (other than a very young child) because the male or female companion may be the abuser or related to the abuser. Also, it is important to avoid the term *abuse* in screening questions, as many women exercise denial, even when the physical injury is severe. Examples of screening questions are given in Box 21-3.

Management

The therapeutic importance of a clinician affirming that no one "deserves" to be abused, or that a woman is not "stupid" or "weak" for being in an abusive

Table 21-1 Clues to Abuse in the Medical Setting

Patient History	Patient's Companion	Physical Examination
• Story not consistent with injury	• Will not leave patient alone	• Injuries may have central pattern (face, neck, throat, chest)
• Pregnancy, especially presenting late for prenatal care	• Seems overly solicitious	• May hide injuries by long sleeves or tinted glasses
• Time delay between injury and presentation		• May have "defense injuries" on ulnar area of forearm
• History of miscarriage		• May be *no signs* of injury

Box 21-3 Examples of Screening Questions for Abuse

"Violence is so common in today's society that I am screening all my patients for it. Have you ever been kicked, pushed, threatened, or hurt, or has someone forced you to have sexual activities against your will?"
"Everyone fights in relationships. When you fight, what happens?"
"Are you having a lot of relationship stress?"

---

relationship, cannot be underestimated. Additional positive clinician responses include instilling confidence (e.g., "I know that you can get help when you are ready and here are some resources to help you") (34). Many survivors report that this validation, even from one person, helped restore self-esteem.

A clinician is a part of a team and need not "know all and do all" to be effective in treating abuse. Patients recognize the tremendous time pressure encountered by most physicians and do not expect the clinician to solve the abuse problem or spend a lot of time with them. The value of validating the injustice, providing information and available resources, and offering follow-up appointments should not be underestimated because such measures can go a long way toward helping these women.

The mnemonic "RADAR" serves as a practical clinical tool for the clinician (Box 21-4):

R—Remember to ask about the abuse and validate the patient's feelings. Because many abused women are afraid, alone, and "feel stupid" for tolerating the abuse, it is important for clinicians to have an immediate brief empathetic statement of support such as "This must have very hard for you to discuss. I want you to know that I am concerned about you and will do what I can to help." It is of utmost importance to avoid implying that the she did anything to provoke the abuse. One must also avoid minimizing the abuse or telling her that she should "just leave". As previously described, domestic violence is a complex problem and frequently a woman lacks the energy to leave due to depression or low self-esteem, lacks financial or family support, or fears losing custody of her children. Additionally, a woman is felt to be at greatest risk for homicide when leaving an abuser.

A—Ask directly. Because abused women do not commonly present to internal medicine, gynecological, or subspecialist settings with acute injuries, one can argue that in order to identify victims all women should be screened for abuse. Once abused women have been identified, clinicians may wish to screen them for depression, suicidal ideation, and substance abuse.

Box 21-4 Using RADAR to Detect and Treat Abuse

R   **Remember** to ask about the possibility of abuse in a supportive manner

A   **Ask** directly, if possible, "Have you been hit, hurt, threatened?"

D   **Document** findings if the patient agrees

A   **Assess Safety** "If you leave this office, will you be safe tonight?"

R   **Review Options or Refer** to a hotline or counseling center

Adapted from Alpert EJ. Violence in intimate relationships and the practicing internist: new disease or new agenda? Ann Intern Med. 1995;123:774-81.

D—Documentation. Women should be urged to have their abuse documented in the medical chart. Such documentation may help them get protection orders or child custody. Patient complaints should be recorded verbatim. It is important to never write "The patient alleges that she experienced . . ." because the word alleges is pejorative and implies that the clinician doubts the patient's story. If an acute injury is present, a detailed description of the lesions should be documented, with body maps or photographs used if possible (Fig. 21-1).

Patients should be assured that the clinician will not discuss the abuse with the abuser or other family members. Ideally, charts should be kept in a private locked file. Unfortunately, patients can never be completely assured that information in their charts will be known to only the clinician and patient. Patients have been denied life, disability, or health insurance because of medical documentation of abuse, although some states are implementing laws to make this practice illegal.

A—Assess current safety. Women should be assessed for whether they feel they are currently in danger of trauma or death. One way to ask is, "If you leave this office, do you feel that you will be safe today?" If the patient feels that she is in danger, provide a confidential place in the office where she can call a friend, relative, or shelter for a place to stay. Most women will state that they feel that they are safe to leave your office. However, a physician should briefly discuss a safety plan to implement in the event that an argument is escalating. This plan should include an escape route from the residence, storage of extra cash or credit cards in a place outside the home, keeping a spare set of car keys readily available, and having on hand important papers such as birth certificates and insurance cards. Also, a copy of a marriage license may be important if the couple is married and the patient needs an immediate protection order.

R—Referrals. Physicians should be familiar with the nearest shelters and the services that they provide. In addition to shelter care, some shelters offer

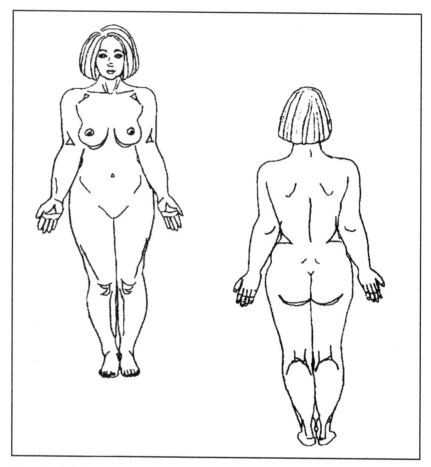

Figure 21-1 Body map used to indicate injury locations.

therapy groups for women, legal advice, or therapy groups for abusers. Social workers and mental health professionals are often knowledgeable about treatment options and local resources. In 1996, a national 24 hour, 7 day a week, toll-free hotline became available (800-799-SAFE).

The role of conjoint therapy (therapy sessions for patient and abuser) remains controversial. Certain couples will benefit if both are motivated and there is no history of antisocial personality disorder in the abuser. The patient should be advised of this option and referred to a mental health specialist if this is her choice.

Follow-Up Care

The physician should remember to always offer the abused patient a follow-up appointment. In addition, the patient and provider may wish to discuss safe times and locations for telephone contact. The physician should be understanding if the patient fails to keep the appointment. Some women are prevented from returning by their abusive partners or simply by their depression. Also, because the pattern of domestic violence often consists of violent episodes alternating with "honeymoon periods", a patient may assume that the abuse has disappeared and she no longer needs help. It is important to acknowledge that decisions surrounding domestic violence are difficult. Assure the patient that the decisions are hers and that you will be available when she needs you.

Summary

Abused women may suffer from many physical and psychological symptoms; thus the primary care physician may represent a critical link for traumatized women to receive care. The first step is for the practitioner to ask about current and past abuse in a nonjudgmental manner. Once an abused woman has been identified, the validation of the difficulties she faces is a simple but important intervention that can aid her mental health. Safety issues should always be assessed, and the patient made aware of appropriate resources. Obtaining a history of abuse may alter diagnostic and treatment strategies. Furthermore, detection and appropriate intervention may save the domestic violence victim's life.

REFERENCES

1. **Drossman DA, Lesserman J, Nachman G, et al.** Sexual and physical abuse in women with functional or organic gastrointestinal disorder. Ann Intern Med. 1990;113: 828-33.
2. **Harber JD, Roos C.** Effects of spouse abuse in the development and maintenance of chronic pain in women. Adv Pain Res. 1985;9:889-95.
3. **Reiter RC, Shakerin LR, Gambone DO, Milborn AK.** Correlation between sexual abuse and somatization in women with somatic and nonsomatic chronic pelvic pain. Am J Obstet Gyecol. 1991;165:104-9.
4. **Walter E, Katon W, Harrop-Griffiths J, et al.** Relationship of chronic pelvic pain to psychiatric diagnoses and childhood sexual abuse. Am J Psych. 1988;145:75-80.
5. **Walker E, Katon WJ, Hansom J, et al.** Medical and psychiatric symptoms in women with childhood sexual abuse. Psychosom Med. 1992;54:658-64.

6. **Briere J, Zaidi LY.** Symptomatology associated with childhood sexual victimization in a nonclinical adult sample. Child Abuse Negl. 1988;12:51-9.

7. **Mullen PE, Romans-Clarkson SE, Walton CA, Herbison GP.** Impact of sexual and physical abuse on women's mental health. Lancet. 1988;12:51-9.

8. **Schei B, Bakketeig LS.** Gynecological impact and sexual and physical abuse by spouse: a study of intrafamily conflict and violence: the conflicts tactics (CT) scale. J Marriage Fam. 1979;41:75-88.

9. **McCauley JM, Kern DE, Kolodner K, et al.** The battering syndrome; prevalence and clinical characteristics of domestic violence in primary medical care internal medicine practices. Ann Intern Med. 1995;123:737-46.

10. **Friedman LS, Samet JH, Roberts MS, et al.** Inquiry about victimization experiences: a survey of patient preferences and physician practices. Arch Intern Med. 1992;152:1186-90.

11. **Alpert EJ.** Violence in intimate relationships and the practicing internist: new disease or new agenda? Ann Intern Med. 1995;123:774-81.

12. **Novello AC.** From the Surgeon General: a medical response to domestic violence. JAMA. 1992;267:31-2.

13. **Rath GD, Jarratt LG, Leonardson G.** Rates of domestic violence against women by male partners. J Am Board Fam Pract. 1989;2:227-33.

14. **Ellicot BA, Johnson MM.** Domestic violence in a primary care setting. Arch Fam Med. 1995;4:113-9.

15. **Hamberger LK, Saunders DG, Hovey M.** Prevalence of domestic violence in community practice and rate of physician inquiry. Fam Med. 1992;24:283-7.

16. **Bullock L, Bullock L, McFarlane J, et al.** The prevalence and characteristics of battered women in a primary care setting. Nurse Pract. 1989;14:47-55.

17. Report of the U.S. Preventative Task Force. Guide to Clinical Preventative Services: Screening for Family Violence. Baltimore: Williams & Wilkins; 1996.

18. **Newberger EH, Barkan JE, Lieberman ES, et al.** Abuse of pregnant women and adverse birth outcomes. JAMA. 1992;267:2370-2.

19. **Bauer HM, Rodriguez MA, Perez-Stable EJ.** Prevalence and determinants of intimate partner abuse among public hospital primary care patients. J Gen Intern Med. 2000;15:811-7.

20. **Gin NE, Rucker L, Frayne S, et al.** Prevalence of domestic violence among patients in three ambulatory care internal medicine clinics. J Gen Intern Med. 1991;6:317-22.

21. **Wagner PF, Mongan P, Hamrick D, Hendrick LK.** Experience of abuse in primary care patients: racial and rural differences. Arch Fam Med. 1995;4:956-62.

22. **Miller TR, Cohen MA.** Victim costs and consequences: a new look. Report to the National Institute of Justice, NCJ 155282; 1996.

23. **Domino JV, Haber JD.** Prior physical and sexual abuse in women with chronic headache: clinical correlates. Headache. 1987;27:310-4.

24. **Moeller TP, Bachmann GA, Moeller J.** The combined effects of physical, sexual, and emotional abuse during childhood: long-term health consequences for women. Child Abuse Negl. 1993;17:623-40.

25. **McCauley J, Kern DE, Kolodner K, et al.** Clinical characteristics of women with a history of child abuse: unhealed wounds. JAMA. 1997;227:1362.

26. **Scarinci K, McDonald-Haile J, Bradley LA, et al.** Altered pain perception and psychosocial feelings among women with GI disorders and a history of abuse. Am J Med. 1994;97:108-18.

27. **Brown GR, Anderson B.** Psychiatric morbidity in adult inpatients with childhood history of sexual or physical abuse. Am J Psychiatry. 1991;148:55-61.

28. **Plichta S.** The effects of women abuse on health care utilization and health care status: a literature review. Womens Health Issues. 1992;2:154-63.

29. **Felitti VJ, Anda RF, Nordenberg D, et al.** Relationship of childhood abuse and household dysfunction to many of the leading causes of death in adults: the adverse childhoold experiences (ACE) study. Am J Prev Med. 1998;14:245-58.

30. **Dietz PM, Spitz AM, Anda RF, et al.** Unintended pregnancy among adult women exposed to abuse or household dysfunction during their childhood. JAMA. 1999;282:1359-64.

31. **Bergman B, Brismar B.** A 5-year follow-up study of 118 battered women. Am J Public Health. 1991;81:1486-9.

32. **Koss MP, Koss PG, Woodruff WJ.** Deleterious effects of criminal victimization on women's health and medical utilization. Arch Intern Med. 1991;151:342-7.

33. **Lim and RI B.** Disclosure of stigmatizing conditions: the disclosure's perspective. Arch Psychiatr Nurs. 1989;2:69-78.

34. **McCauley J, Yurk RA, Jenckes MW, Ford DE.** Inside Pandora's box: abused women's experiences with clinicians and health services. J Gen Intern Med. 1998;13:549-55.

35. **Ferris LE.** Canadian family physicians' and general practioners' perceptions of their effectiveness in identifying and treating wife abuse. Med Care. 1994;32:1163-72.

36. **Sugg NK, Inui T.** Primary care physicians' response to domestic violence: opening Pandora's box. JAMA. 1992;267:3157-60.

CHAPTER 22

Lesbian Health Issues

JOCELYN C. WHITE, MD
AUDREY S. KOH, MD

L esbians are a diverse group of women with unique medical and psychosocial needs. Although 2% to 10% of women are lesbians, they often go unrecognized and may not be cared for adequately by their physicians.
Unfortunately, physicians seldom receive specific training to care for these
patients. This chapter provides physicians with the information necessary to
identify the sexual orientation of patients, take a sensitive social and sexual
history, and address gynecologic issues relevant to lesbians and women sexually active with women (WSW).

Definitions

A woman's sexual orientation is indicative of her potential to respond with
sexual excitement through attraction, fantasy, or behavior to the same sex
(homosexual or lesbian), opposite sex (heterosexual), or both sexes (bisexual).
Sexual orientation can be viewed as having two components, behavior and
identity, which may or may not be congruent in an individual. Of women who
identify themselves as lesbian, most report being currently sexually active
with women or celibate, but 77% of self-identified lesbians report having had
heterosexual coitus at least once in their lives (1). By comparison, WSWs do
not necessarily identify themselves as lesbian or bisexual. They may identify

578

themselves as heterosexual or choose not to identify themselves at all for reasons related to culture, ethnicity, occupation, or peer-support groups.

Practically speaking, women who identify themselves as lesbians have an identity based on emotions, psychological responses, societal expectations, and their own choices. Lesbians comprise a diverse group representing all racial, economic, geographic, religious, cultural, and age populations. Amid this diversity, they have created a culture filled with music, art, literature, history, spiritual beliefs, ethics, and politics. Not all women have access to or feel themselves to be a part of such a community, but it may be an important source of support to many women because it can provide an alternative family or kin group. Community resources may also be useful to physicians looking for lesbian-sensitive referrals for social services, counseling, or peer support.

Communication

Because the two groups of self-identified lesbians and WSWs do not overlap completely, it is challenging to identify, assess, and educate these women in clinical practice. Physicians working with women may find it difficult to take complete social and sexual histories of sexual orientation and sexual activities with women. Consequently, opportunities are lost to assess risk factors for sexually transmitted diseases (STDs), human immunodeficiency virus (HIV), and psychosocial issues. Also lost are opportunities to provide lesbian- and WSW-specific education and disease prevention advice. There are two basic principles for physicians working with lesbians and WSWs: 1) ask questions by using language without heterosexual bias, and 2) take a sexual and social history, even if difficult.

Many lesbians are reluctant to reveal their sexual orientation to physicians for fear of provoking a negative response. Some lesbians do not share this information even when asked directly. At the same time, many physicians are not sure what language to use to respectfully elicit information from lesbian patients. The most commonly used questions often lead to inaccurate or incomplete responses. These questions can also create barriers between the physician and the patient because they assume the latter is heterosexual:

Although many lesbians are reluctant to reveal their sexual orientation to physicians, most appreciate inclusive language that does not assume the patient is heterosexual.

"What form of birth control do you use?" "Are you married or single?" "When was the last time you had intercourse?" are common examples. All of these questions are difficult for lesbians. Because the options given do not necessarily pertain to a lesbian or WSW, the patient must either provide false information or awkwardly stop and explain. The necessity of such an explanation can make the already challenging sexual history even more difficult for both parties. To avoid awkwardness, patients may play along with the assumption of heterosexuality. Physician assumption of patient heterosexuality can have a significant impact on the diagnosis and management of the patient.

Sensitive questions are those that make no assumptions about sexual orientation or behaviors: "Are you single, partnered, married, widowed, or divorced?" "Who is in your immediate family?" "Over your lifetime, have your sexual partners been men, women, or both?" "Is/are you current sexual partner(s) male, female, or both?" "If you become ill, is there someone important whom I should involve in your care?" Because lesbians and WSWs come in all shapes, sizes, ages, colors, and classes, physicians need to use questions without heterosexual bias with all women, not just those they "suspect" of being a lesbian or WSW (Table 22-1).

When taking a sexual history, physicians should use words that patients understand or offer synonyms within the question: "Do you do cunnilingus [or go down] on her?" "Do you do anilingus [or rimming] with her?" "Do you put your fingers in her vagina, anus, or rectum?" Use terms that patients use for activities and body parts. Although it is important to have a professional demeanor, it is more important to convey information accurately and confirm the patient's understanding of the topics discussed. Also remember that in taking a sensitive sexual history it is often helpful for providers to explain that they need information on sexual practices to make an accurate diagnosis or provide appropriate education.

Physicians traditionally learn to ask about sexual orientation during the sexual history. Doing so, however, may heighten provider and patient discomfort. This type of inquiry also limits opportunities to learn about sexual orientation to only those visits in which a sexual history is appropriate. In contrast, the social history is the more comfortable part of the interview in which to first raise these issues. Asking about a relationship, who lives at home with

Table 22-1 Sensitive Questions in History Taking

Social History
Are you single, partnered, widowed, divorced, or married?
Are you in a relationship with a man or a woman?
Who is in your immediate family?
If you become ill, whom should I involve in your care?

Sexual History
Over your lifetime, have your sexual partners been men, women, or both?
Are your current partners men, women, or both?

The social history may be a more comfortable opportunity to elicit the patient's sexual orientation, by asking such questions as "Should you ever become ill is there someone important whom I should involve in your care?"

the patient, or who should become involved in the patient's care if she is seriously ill are useful and comfortable places to begin the discussion of sexual orientation in an open and nonjudgmental manner.

Providers who show a nonjudgmental attitude and use language without heterosexual bias are much more likely to develop trusting relationships with their lesbian and WSW patients. Providers can further improve their relationship in several simple ways: 1) by offering to include a partner in the discussion, 2) by ensuring that a lesbian's partner is treated like any other spouse in the office or hospital setting, including the labor and delivery department and childbirth classes, 3) by including partners in discussions of next-of-kin policies and advance directives, 4) by using hospital and office forms with words that do not assume heterosexual family structures, and 5) by explicitly discussing medical record confidentiality with regard to sexual orientation documentation.

Medical Record Confidentiality

Physicians should thoughtfully consider the implications of placing any documentation of specific sexual behaviors or sexual orientation in the medical record. When possible, it is important to discuss this issue with the patient. Medical records, although ostensibly covered by patient privacy and confidentiality rules, are a legitimate source of concern to lesbians. Medical records have played key roles in legal disputes over child custody or visitation rights, employment issues, and dishonorable discharges from the military. Although it is important for medical reasons to have this information in the chart, an informed consent discussion about these issues with the patient is appropriate. If the patient requests that the information not be entered into the chart, the physician faces a difficult decision. A physician may, in this instance, choose to use a coded entry in the medical record known only to the other clinicians in that setting. The code serves to remind providers of the patient's sexual history or orientation but will prevent inadvertent breaches of confidentiality. Where a coded entry is not possible, and sexual history or sexual orientation information is central to providing care, physicians should inform the patient that this information is being placed in the chart and should discuss with the patient medical record confidentiality and release of information procedures.

"Coming Out" Issues

Society's negative attitude toward or fear of lesbians and gay men is known as *homophobia*. Although lesbian self-esteem is similar overall to that of heterosexual women, some lesbians internalize society's homophobia. These internalized negative thoughts and fears can create a stressful conflict between lesbians' self-perceived sexual orientation and how they reveal this orientation to the outside world.

The process of discovering one's sexual orientation and revealing it to others is known as "coming out" and may begin at any age. Indeed, it may be a life-long process. Coming out involves a shift in core identity that takes place in four stages: 1) awareness of homosexual feelings, 2) testing and exploration, 3) identity acceptance, and 4) identity integration and disclosure to others (2). Social and family attitudes strongly influence the experience of coming out and can cause significant emotional distress in a lesbian. Societal and internalized homophobia may cause the lesbian to perform an often fatiguing "cost-benefit analysis" for every situation in which she considers coming out. When the costs of coming out are perpetually high, a lesbian may become socially isolated or attempt to deny her sexual orientation.

Lesbian adolescents are particularly vulnerable during this process, and any distress incurred from coming out can compound other developmental tasks. Parental, especially maternal, acceptance during the coming out process may be the primary determinant of the development of healthy self-esteem in adolescent lesbians. Sexual-orientation confusion may appear to the physician as depression, diminished school performance, alcohol and substance use, acting out, and suicidal ideation. Indeed, gay and lesbian youth may be at a higher risk for depression and suicide than their peers (3). For these reasons it is extremely important for the physician to identify the sexual orientation of adolescents, to screen for signs of sexual orientation confusion, and to consider distress over sexual orientation in the differential diagnosis of depression and substance abuse.

Psychosocial Issues

Several other psychosocial issues are worth considering in women who identify as lesbian. Depressive distress is higher in lesbians, especially African American lesbians, than in the general population of women. Rates of alcohol abuse in a random population appear to be no greater among lesbians than other women, but heavy use of alcohol and substances may continue later in life among lesbians compared with other women. Domestic violence exists in lesbian couples and is often associated with alcohol or substance abuse by the battering partner. Lesbian-sensitive shelters may be difficult to find but can be a crucial part of management. Finally, hate crimes against lesbians can be a particular source of distress. They may take the form of verbal abuse, property crime, physical or sexual assault, and murder. Recent experience of a hate crime should be considered in the differential diagnosis of all stress-related conditions.

Cancer Risks

There are no population-based studies of gynecologic and breast cancer risk in lesbians. Based on their sexual and reproductive histories, however, the incidence of certain cancers in lesbians as a group may differ from that of the general population of women. Cancer screening decisions in lesbians should therefore be based upon standard screening guidelines for women but influenced by individual risk factors. However, many lesbians fail to get proper screening because of inadequate contact with the health care system. The barriers that affect heterosexuals usually apply, but additional obstacles have been identified. These include a fear of a homophobic medical system (often resulting from past negative experiences), the impact of the common myth of lesbian "immunity" to sexually transmitted diseases and certain cancers, and the lack of health insurance coverage under the partner's policy (4).

Cervical cancer appears less common among lesbians than among bisexual or heterosexual women as suggested by lower rates of dysplasia and abnormal Pap smears (3% vs. 12% and 12% vs. 16%, respectively) (1,5,6). This is most likely because of decreased exposure to such risk factors as early age of first coitus with a male, total number of heterosexual contacts, and infection with human papilloma virus (HPV). In a study of women aged 25–30 years, current cigarette smoking, history of abnormal Pap smear, greater than ten lifetime male partners, and two or fewer years since the last sexual contact with a male partner were associated with a greater likelihood of detecting HPV. However, human papilloma virus can also be transmitted from one woman to another during sexual contact, and cervical cancer has been reported in women who report sexual activity only with women throughout their lifetimes (7). American Cancer Society and American College of Obstetricians and Gynecologists recommendations and other preventive health guidelines give no information for cervical cancer screening in women who are celibate or who are sexually active with women only. In the absence of appropriate data, it is recommended that physicians obtain Pap smears in lesbians and WSWs in accordance with current guidelines for the general population of women.

There is no specific information on breast cancer, endometrial cancer, or ovarian cancer in lesbians or WSWs. Epidemiologic studies suggest an increased risk of breast cancer among nulliparous women, women who are older at first full-term pregnancy, and women who have never breast fed. Many lesbians fall into these categories, and physicians should therefore adhere to current guidelines for breast examination and mammography. Endometrial and ovarian cancer have been reported to occur more frequently in women who have not used oral contraception and those who have not given birth. Based on these risk factors, some lesbians may be at a slightly higher risk for ovarian and endometrial cancers, but the data are not strong enough to support the use of high-risk screening recommendations; therefore physicians should follow standard screening guidelines.

Lesbians older than 40 years may smoke more often, drink alcohol more often, and have a higher body mass index than their heterosexual counterparts (8). No data have been reported on lung, colon, or head and neck cancers in lesbians. Physicians should emphasize the health risks of smoking and alcohol use to lesbians and strongly encourage smoking cessation, low-fat diets, exercise, and responsible use of alcohol.

Sexually Associated and Transmitted Infections

Overall, vaginitis and STDs are less common in lesbians than in bisexual or heterosexual women. There are relatively few data on STDs in lesbian populations, and sampling biases complicate many existing studies. However, ascertainment of sexual behavior rather than identity is the key because the risk for many STDs varies markedly with the type of sexual activity.

Bacterial vaginosis has been found in approximately one third of lesbians seeking gynecologic care (9–11). It has been diagnosed in women who have never had sexual relations and in women with lifetime exclusively female sexual contact. In a study of 101 monogamous lesbians, 73% of index subjects with bacterial vaginosis had a sexual partner with bacterial vaginosis (11). These findings suggest the possibility of female-to-female (FTF) transmission of bacterial vaginosis, probably through mingling of vaginal secretions. This is distinct from bacterial vaginosis in heterosexual couples, in whom sexual transmission has not been clearly demonstrated.

Candida vulvovaginitis among lesbians has been reported at approximately the same or lower rates than heterosexual women (9,12). The vaginal microenvironment plays a far greater role than sexual transmission in the pathophysiology of *Candida* vulvovaginitis. Theoretically, FTF transmission via vaginal secretions, oral or rectal reservoirs, or shared sex toys is possible. Lesbians with frequently recurring *Candida* vulvovaginitis should have their sexual partners evaluated if symptomatic.

Trichomoniasis is uncommon but has been found in 2% to 15% of WSWs (9,12). It has been diagnosed in virginal women and in women who are sexual exclusively with women. Transmission is possible via vaginal secretions or fomites. Thus evaluation and treatment of female sexual partners should be offered, particularly if the partner is symptomatic.

Chlamydia, gonorrhea, and syphilis are very uncommon in lesbians (5,9,12). However, because of the prevalence of chlamydia in the general population and the possibility of asymptomatic infection, physicians should screen for chlamydia in those lesbians who report sexual activity with men since their last negative tests.

Herpes simplex virus (HSV) has been found in 1% to 7% of screened lesbians (5,9,12). Transmission can occur by genital-genital, oral-genital, and oral-oral contact. Information given to lesbians regarding infectivity and treatment should be similar to advice given to heterosexual women but tailored to the sexual practices of lesbians.

HPV is reported at lower rates in lesbians than in heterosexual women (9). As in the general population, genital-genital and fomite transmission are believed to occur in lesbians. Using polymerase chain reaction technology, one researcher found HPV in 35% of lesbians, including 29% of women with lifetime exclusively female sexual contact (7). All HPV DNA types were detected in the cervix, vagina, and vulva, including oncogenic DNA types 16, 18, 31, 33, and 35. This supports the need for lesbians to be regularly screened by Pap smear for lower-tract dysplasia and cancers.

HIV and AIDS

There is little scientific data on lesbians and HIV or AIDS. A Centers for Disease Control (CDC) report on AIDS in lesbians found 164 cases with no cases clearly attributable to FTF transmission. Infection occurred via intravenous drug use or via sex with infected men (13). This compilation is flawed, however, by the CDC's rigid definition of *lesbian* and its narrowly defined risk categories. A study of 18 HIV-serodiscordant lesbian couples found no cases of seroconversion in a 6-month follow-up period (14). There are several case reports of suspected FTF transmission of HIV via menstrual or traumatic bleeding, however.

Lesbians are more likely to be HIV infected than heterosexual women, according to some studies.

The question of sexual behaviors versus sexual orientation or identity is critical with respect to HIV. WSWs may be more likely to take risks generally. Alternatively, women who take risks may be more likely to have sex with other women. Paradoxically, women who identify themselves as lesbians often believe they are not at risk for HIV infection for many reasons, including the fact that they are lesbians. However, a study in New York City found that WSWs are more likely than other women to be HIV infected (15). Similarly, a study of San Francisco Bay area lesbians and bisexual women showed the prevalence of HIV to be higher than that for San Francisco women in general (16). Hepatitis B markers were also detected in 5.4% of the studied women, confirming that many may engage in high-risk behaviors. In this population sample, substance abuse, needle sharing, unprotected sex, and sex with high-risk partners occurred at alarming rates. In general, alcohol and drug use are felt to be important contributors to increased HIV risk by diminishing judgment and vigilance against high-risk behaviors.

HIV virus is present in blood (including menstrual blood), vaginal and cervical secretions, saliva, and breast milk. The virus is present in highest concentrations in the blood. In saliva the concentration is low, and saliva may have additional agents that inactivate HIV (17). Theoretically, FTF infection is riskier with sexual exposure to the infected woman during her menstrual period or with traumatic sexual practices. For the uninfected woman, the risk of becoming infected increases with nonintact skin or mucosa. This may include abrasions from tampon use or anal-receptive sex, STD-associated ulcerations or other lesions, or open skin on the fingers or genitals or in the mouth (e.g., as may result from brushing or flossing) (18). The risk of HIV transmission is also increased when either partner has vaginitis or cervicitis due to the higher concentration of target CD_4 cells in the vagina.

Protective barriers include dental dams, condoms, latex gloves, and household nonmicrowaveable plastic wrap. Water-based lubricant on the side of the barrier that is on the genitals increases touch sensitivity and pleasure. Shared dildos or other sex toys should be boiled, soaked in alcohol, or rinsed in bleach between partners or covered with a new condom before each usage (Table 22-2) (19).

In lesbians without high-risk behaviors, the transmission of HIV is probably low. In such couples, safer sex guidelines should be followed for 6 months until HIV-antibody testing for both partners is negative. However, given the diversity of behaviors among lesbians, and the diversity of women who identify themselves as lesbians or WSW, counseling should be directed to risk-behavior assessment, education, and prevention (18).

Fertility Issues

In surveys of lesbians, 30% to 62% express the desire to parent (8,11,16). The preferred parenting methods reported are: anonymous artificial a donor in-

Table 22-2 Safer Sex for Female-to-Female Sexual Activities

Safe
- Hugging, caressing, dry kissing
- Mutual masturbation

Safer
- Intraoral (wet) kissing with intact oral mucosa
- Tribadism (i.e., rubbing of the genitals on the partner's body) with intact skin
- Using latex barriers with:
  Cunnilingus
  Anilingus
  Digital vaginal or anal penetration
  Dildos or sex toys for vaginal or anal penetration
- Cunnilingus with intact oral/genital mucosa and no menses/genital bleeding
- Anilingus with intact oral/anal mucosa
- Digital vaginal penetration with intact skin and no menses/genital bleeding

Risky
- Anal penetration
- Activities in the presence of menstrual bleeding or other genital bleeding or open
  skin/ulcerative lesions:
  Cunnilingus
  Anilingus
  Digital vaginal or anal penetration
  Sharing sex toys
- Blood-letting sexual activities
  S&M activities that result in bleeding or open wounds (e.g., cutting, piercing, whipping to
  the point of bleeding)

Aids to Safer Sex
- Discussion between sex partners before sexual activity
- Sexual activities while sober, not under the influence of alcohol or other mind-altering drugs
- Latex barriers:
  Gloves, finger cots
  Condoms
  Female condom (Reality)
  Dental dams
- Plastic barriers:
  Nonmicrowaveable plastic food wrap
- Water-based lubricants
- Cleaning sex toys:
  Boil in water for 20 min, *or*
  Soak in isopropanol for 10 min, then rinse in water, *or*
  Rinse three times in diluted bleach (1 part bleach to 10 parts water), then rinse in water

semination (15%–40%), known donor insemination (18%–31%), sex with a man (9%–28%), and adoption (44%–47%). Fertility issues specific to lesbians center on how to obtain and deliver sperm.

Lesbians often require medical assistance to obtain or inseminate sperm. Even though infertility has not been diagnosed, these services fall under the aegis of "infertility treatment". Because infertility services are often excluded from insurance coverage, the expense of becoming pregnant can be prohibitive. Some patients, relatives of patients, and medical personnel may question the effect on children of being raised in a lesbian household or may be inclined to turn lesbians away from these fertility services. Extensive psychological and social science studies have looked at offspring's gender identity, sexual orientation, self-esteem, and social adjustment. There has been no difference detected in children of lesbians, compared with children of heterosexual single- or two-parent households (20). Primary care physicians may support the pregnant or conceiving lesbian by demonstrating a nonjudgmental attitude and by encouraging acceptance of lesbian mothers among members of the fertility and labor and delivery teams. Physicians should encourage partners to participate in all phases of the process as well.

For lesbians who conceive by artificial insemination (AI), the timing of ovulation and insemination is critical. Some patients can accurately detect their own cervical mucous changes or mittelschmerz as signs of ovulation. Many patients, however, do not notice these changes. Basal body temperature charts are retrospective and often unreliable. Serial ultrasonography is highly accurate, but it is costly, time consuming, and retrospective. Urinary luteinizing hormone (LH) measurement with home testing kits is effective and cost efficient.

Optimal cervical mucous occurs during the LH surge, and ovulation occurs approximately 12 to 30 hr after positive urine LH testing. Urine LH should be checked once or twice a day, beginning several days before the expected LH surge. Typically, this would be 16 days before day 1 of the shortest menstrual cycle a patient has had in the previous six cycles. Most home test kits include detailed instructions and guidance.

AI can be performed with fresh or frozen semen. However, because of the risk of STDs, particularly HIV infection, insemination of frozen quarantined semen is recommended. There have been at least 12 reported cases of HIV transmission via AI, including some with the use of frozen specimens. Thus a 6-month quarantine of frozen specimens with ongoing HIV-antibody testing of the donor before release is recommended. Donors should be thoroughly screened with family history for hereditary disease, medical history, lab screening for STDs, semen analysis with freeze-thaw characteristics, and genetic diseases as appropriate.

AI can be vaginal, intracervical, or intrauterine. Using fresh donor semen, monthly fecundities of 15% and cumulative pregnancy rates of 60% to 75%

have occurred with intracervical AI. Frozen donor sperm used intravaginally or intracervically is associated with a reduction in monthly fecundity of 3% to 5% (21). The 6-month pregnancy rate for frozen intracervical AI can be increased from 32% to 78% by performing two consecutive inseminations instead of one AI per cycle (22). These should be done the day of and the day after the urine LH surge.

To further increase monthly fecundity rates (to more than 15% per cycle), intrauterine insemination (IUI) of frozen washed sperm can be performed (23). Sperm must be washed and concentrated to remove seminal plasma components. This reduces the uterine contractions and the risk of anaphylaxis that would otherwise occur with exposure to foreign proteins and leukocytes in the semen. It also isolates the motile sperm, starts the process of capacitation, and concentrates the inseminate to a volume that can be accommodated by the uterine cavity (0.25–0.5 mL).

Legal Issues

Many of the decisions regarding AI revolve around legal issues (24). These are so intrinsic to the process that they will be briefly described. The key question is whether the sperm donor will be recognized as the legal father of the child. Some lesbians choose not to have their donor participate as a father because of court bias toward biological sperm donors over biological lesbian mothers in custody suits. If the intention is that the donor not be recognized as the father, the only fail-safe solution is to use an anonymous donor. For women who use a known donor, some guidance is provided by the Uniform Parentage Act, a 1973 model law that has been adopted in some states. AI "under the supervision of a licensed physician" is one of the criteria required to try to establish that a known donor not have parental rights. Thus women who seek only a donor should be encouraged to inseminate under physician supervision. "Physician supervision" is variably interpreted, but the conservative rendition is insemination performed by a licensed physician. Additionally, if a known donor is used and the donor is not intended to be the legal father, it is important to demonstrate this in as many ways as possible. For example, a donor-recipient agreement, payment for the semen, physician-supervised insemination, keeping the donor's name off the birth certificate, and avoidance of parental-type involvement of the donor with the offspring may be useful ways to keep the intentions legally intact. Allowing interaction that is parental in nature between the donor and the offspring can negate all of the aforementioned safeguards. Such interaction gives support to the legal recognition of the donor as a parent, should the donor contest his rights. An alternative to the known-unknown donor dichotomy is provided by some sperm banks that offer anonymous donor semen with the option for disclosure of donor identity. This is scrupulously defined as disclosure only to the offspring when his/her age of majority is reached.

It should be noted that in some regions, the Uniform Parentage Act has actually been used to bar unmarried women from donor insemination. Thus lesbians planning parenthood should consult a knowledgeable attorney for current, local-jurisdiction advice.

The hostile attitude of some physicians and sperm banks to lesbians or an outright refusal to provide services can be a significant deterrent to becoming pregnant (11,25). Even with more favorable attitudes by physicians, the inconvenience and expense involved in AI force many lesbians to consider using unscreened or inadequately screened private semen donors or having sex with male friends or strangers. These practices make the lesbian patient or her offspring vulnerable to STDs, HIV, custody and paternity challenges, and unexpected hereditary conditions in the offspring. Thus many believe it is ethically justifiable but not obligatory for physicians to provide insemination services to lesbians. A physician who feels unable to provide these services should refer the patient to another provider.

Ovum donation and embryo transfer has been traditionally used by heterosexual couples when the infertile woman is unable to use her own eggs. This technology makes possible the donation of oocytes from one woman to her lesbian partner for gestation. This has obvious social and legal implications for lesbian couples considering motherhood. Some facilities are willing to undertake this procedure with lesbian couples.

Summary

Many physicians are presently caring for lesbians and WSWs without recognizing their sexual orientation or their unique medical and psychosocial needs. Although lesbians appear to have no disease in greater prevalence than other women, they do have transmission, prevention, and screening issues that deserve specific attention. They also have unique fertility issues. Improvement in communication skills and knowledge about lesbian health will allow primary care physicians to provide optimal care for their patients.

REFERENCES

1. **Johnson SR, Smith SM, Guenther SM.** Comparison of gynecologic health care problems between lesbians and bisexual women. J Reprod Med. 1987;32:805-11.
2. **Sophie J.** A critical examination of stage theories of lesbian identity development. J Homosex. 1986;12:39-51.

3. **Remafedi G, Farrow J, Deisher RW.** Risk factors for attempted suicide in gay and bisexual adolescents. Pediatrics. 1991;87:869-75.

4. **Rankow EJ.** Lesbian health issues for the primary care provider. J Fam Practice. 1995;40:486-93.

5. **Robertson P, Schacter J.** Failure to identify venereal disease in a lesbian population. Sex Transm Dis. 1981;8:75-6.

6. **Sadeghi SB, Sadeghi A, Cosby M, et al.** Human papillomavirus infection: frequency and association with cervical neoplasia in a young population. Acta Cytol. 1989;33: 319-23.

7. **Marrazzo JM, Koutsky LA, Stine KL, et al.** Genital human papillomavirus infection in women who have sex with women. J Infect Dis. 1998;178:1604-9.

8. **Bradford J, Ryan C, Rothblum ED.** National Lesbian Health Care Survey: implications for mental health care. J Consult Clin Psychol. 1994;62:228-42.

9. **Skinner CJ, Stokes J, Kirlew Y, et al.** A case-controlled study of the sexual health needs of lesbians. Genitourin Med. 1996;72:277-80.

10. **Berger BJ, Kolton S, Zenilman JM, et al.** Bacterial vaginosis in lesbians: a sexually transmitted disease. Clin Infect Dis. 1995;21:1402-5.

11. **Marrazzo JM, Koutsky LA, Agnew K, et al.** Prevalence and microbiology of bacterial vaginosis in lesbians. International Society for STD Research, Denver, July 1999.

12. **Johnson SR, Guenther SM, Laube DW, Keettel WC.** Factors influencing lesbian gynecologic care: a preliminary study. Am J Obstet Gynecol. 1981;140:20-8.

13. **Chu SY, Hammett TA, Buehler JW.** Update: epidemiology of reported cases of AIDS in women who report sex only with other women, 1980–1991. AIDS. 1992;6:518-9.

14. **Raiteri R, Fora R, Sinicco A.** No HIV-1 transmission through lesbian sex [Letter to the Editor]. Lancet. 1994;334:270.

15. **Bevier PJ, Chaisson MA, Heffernan RE, Castro KG.** Women at a sexually transmitted disease clinic who reported same-sex contact: their HIV seroprevalence and risk behaviors. Am J Public Health. 1995;85:1366-71.

16. **Lemp GF, Jones M, Kellogg TA, et al.** HIV seroprevalence and risk behaviors among lesbians and bisexual women in San Francisco and Berkeley, California. Am J Public Health. 1995;85:1549-52.

17. **Fultz P.** Components of saliva inactivate human immunodeficiency virus. Lancet. 1986;2:1215.

18. **Kennedy MB, Scarlett MI, Duerr AC, Chu SY.** Assessing HIV risk among women who have sex with women: scientific and communication issues. J Am Med Womens Assoc. 1995;50:103-7.

19. Safer Sex Guidelines: Healthy Sexuality and HIV—A Resource Guide for Educators and Counsellors. Canadian AIDS Society; 1994.

20. **Patterson CJ.** Children of lesbian and gay parents. Child Dev. 1992;63:1025-42.

21. **Byrd W, Bradshaw K, Carr B, et al.** A prospective randomized study of pregnancy rates following intrauterine and intracervical insemination using frozen donor semen. Fertil Steril. 1990;53:521-7.

22. **Centola G, Mattox J, Raubertas R.** Pregnancy rates after double versus single insemination with frozen donor semen. Fertil Steril. 1990;54:1089-92.

23. **Silva PD, Meisch J, Schauberger CW.** Intrauterine insemination of cryopreserved donor semen. Fertil Steril. 1989;52:243-5.

24. **Kendell K, (ed).** Lesbians Choosing Motherhood: Legal Implications of Alternative Insemination and Reproductive Technologies, 3rd ed. National Center for Lesbian Rights; 1996:4-9.

25. **Bybee D.** Michigan Lesbian Survey: A Report to the Michigan Organization for Human Rights and the Michigan Department of Public Health. Michigan Department of Public Health and Human Services; 1990.

Index

Color Plates

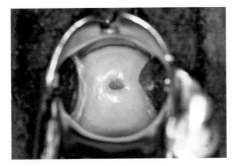

Plate 1. Nulliparous cervix. The nulliparous os is smooth and round. Childbirth or abortion results in a more irregular, "worn" cervix. With close inspection the squamocolumnar junction can be seen just inside the os. For further information, see discussion of Figure 1-5 in Chapter 1 text (where Plate 1 is reproduced in black and white). (From Atlas of Visual Inspection of the Cervix with Acetic Acid. Baltimore: JHPIEGO Corporation; 1999; with permission.)

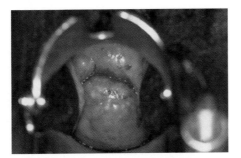

Plate 2. Nabothian cysts are formed when glandular tissue is folded over and covered by squamous epithelium. Nabothian cysts are common, may become quite large, and should not be confused with pathologic lesions. For further information, see discussion of Figure 1-6 in Chapter 1 text (where Plate 2 is reproduced in black and white). (From Atlas of Visual Inspection of the Cervix with Acetic Acid. Baltimore: JHPIEGO Corporation; 1999; with permission.)

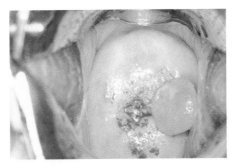

Plate 3. A cervical polyp appears as a finger-like projection in the cervical os and may emanate from cervical or endometrial tissue. Polyps may cause menorrhagia and postcoital bleeding. Although almost always benign, they are usually removed and sent for pathologic evaluation. In postmenopausal women polyps occasionally signal underlying endometrial hyperplasia. For further information, see discussion of Figure 1-7 in Chapter 1 text (where Plate 3 is reproduced in black and white). (From Atlas of Visual Inspection of the Cervix with Acetic Acid. Baltimore: JHPIEGO Corporation; 1999; with permission.)

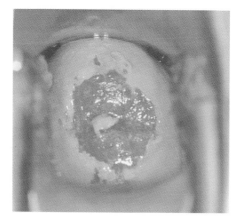

Plate 4. Cervical ectopy (or "ectropion"), defined as the presence of columnar epithelium on the ectocervix, is a normal variant. Here the squamocolumnar junction is obvious at first inspection, at the color change. For further information, see discussion of Figure 1-8 in Chapter 1 text (where Plate 4 is reproduced in black and white). (From Atlas of Visual Inspection of the Cervix with Acetic Acid. Baltimore: JHPIEGO Corporation; 1999; with permission.)

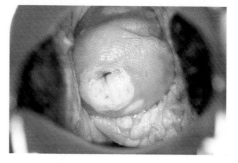

Plate 5. Cervical warts. Warts are more readily seen following the application of dilute acetic acid (vinegar solution). Genital warts are caused by HPV, which is responsible for cervical dysplasia and squamous cell cancers of the cervix. For further information, see discussion of Figure 1-9 in Chapter 1 text (where Plate 5 is reproduced in black and white). (From Atlas of Visual Inspection of the Cervix with Acetic Acid. Baltimore: JHPIEGO Corporation; 1999; with permission.)

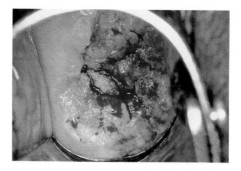

Plate 6. Invasive cancer of the cervix can assume a variety of appearances. Here a dark mass appears on the ectocervix, but at other times a mass may protrude from the cervical os or the cervix may appear densely white. Bimanual examination reveals an enlarged, hard cervix that may or may not be mobile. For further information, see discussion of Figure 1-10 in Chapter 1 text (where Plate 6 is reproduced in black and white). (From Atlas of Visual Inspection of the Cervix with Acetic Acid. Baltimore: JHPIEGO Corporation; 1999; with permission.)

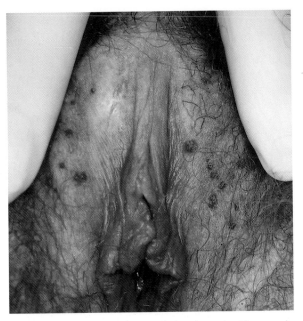

Plate 7. Angiokeratomas. Discrete, 1 to 3 mm dark-red papules. These are benign vascular growths. They may arouse concern when solitary and darker in color, because they may be mistaken for a nevus or melanoma. For further information, see discussion of Figure 17-4 in Chapter 17 text (where Plate 7 is reproduced in black and white). (Courtesy of Maria L. Chanco Turner, MD, Dermatology Branch, National Institutes of Health.)

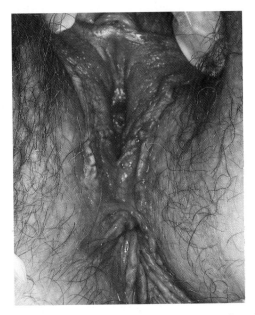

Plate 8. Intraepithelial squamous cell carcinoma extending from the vulva to the perianal area in a patient with a 20-year history of condylomata. She complained of pruritus. Paget's disease should be included in the differential diagnosis. For further information, see discussion of Figure 17-6 in Chapter 17 text (where Plate 8 is reproduced in black and white). (Courtesy of Maria L. Chanco Turner, MD, Dermatology Branch, National Institutes of Health.)

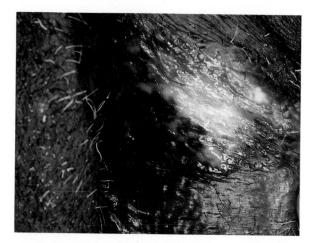

Plate 9. Intraepithelial squamous cell carcinoma. A plaque of irregular shiny pink and black papules on the labia majora of an immunosuppressed patient with previous history of condylomata. This lesion is an intraepithelial squamous cell carcinoma. Histology will differentiate this from melanoma. For further information, see discussion of Figure 17-7 in Chapter 17 text (where Plate 9 is reproduced in black and white). (Courtesy of Maria L. Chanco Turner, MD, Dermatology Branch, National Institutes of Health.)

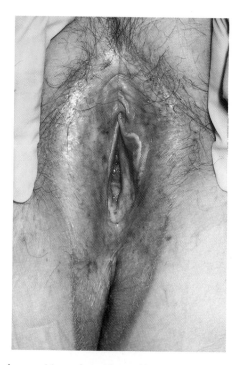

Plate 10. Lichen sclerosus. Mucosal atrophy and homogenization of the dermis give rise to a gray, waxy appearance with increased visibility of veins. The right labia minora is completely resorbed, making the vulva asymmetric; the sclerosus extends to the perianal area, causing pencil-thin stools. The condition was reversed by super-potent topical steroids. For further information, see discussion of Figure 17-13 in Chapter 17 text (where Plate 10 is reproduced in black and white). (Courtesy of Maria L. Chanco Turner, MD, Dermatology Branch, National Institutes of Health.)